51585448

£ 140.00

Medical Law and Ethics

The International Library of Essays in Law and Legal Theory
Second Series
Series Editor: Tom D. Campbell

Titles in the Series:

Medical Law and Ethics

Edited by

Sheila McLean

University of Glasgow, UK

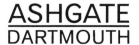

ASHGATE
DARTMOUTH

Published by
Dartmouth Publishing Company
Ashgate Publishing Limited
Gower House
Croft Road
Aldershot
Hants GU11 3HR
England

Ashgate Publishing Company
131 Main Street
Burlington, VT 05401-5600 USA

Ashgate website: http://www.ashgate.com

British Library Cataloguing in Publication Data
Medical law and ethics. – (International library of essays
  in law and legal theory. Second series)
  1. Medical laws and legislation 2. Medical ethics
  I. McLean, Sheila A. M.
  344'.041

Library of Congress Cataloging-in-Publication Data
Medical law and ethics / edited by Sheila McLean.
        p. cm. — (International library of essays in law and legal theory. Second series)
    Includes bibliographical references.
    ISBN 0-7546-2003-4
      1. Medical laws and legislation. 2. Medical ethics. I. McLean, Sheila. II. Series.

  K3601 .M43 2001
  344'.041—dc21   2001022937

ISBN 0 7546 2003 4

Printed in Great Britain by The Cromwell Press, Trowbridge, Wiltshire

Contents

PART III   HUMAN EXPERIMENTATION AND RESEARCH

PART IV   DEATH AND DYING

Acknowledgements

The editor and publishers wish to thank the following for permission to use copyright material.

Ashgate Publishing Limited for the essay: Ann Sommerville (1996), 'Are Advance Directives Really the Answer? And What was the Question?', in Sheila A.M. McLean (ed.), *Death, Dying and the Law*, Aldershot: Dartmouth, pp. 29–47.

Blackwell Publishers for the essays: Sheila A.M. McLean (1990), 'Abortion Law: Is Consensual Reform Possible?', *Journal of Law and Society*, **17**, pp. 106–23; Alastair V. Campbell (1989), 'A Report from New Zealand: An "Unfortunate Experiment"', *Bioethics*, **3**, pp. 59–66; John Griffiths (1995), 'Assisted Suicide in the Netherlands: The *Chabot* Case', *Modern Law Review*, **58**, pp. 232–48, 895–7. Copyright © 1995 The Modern Law Review.

Cambridge University Press for the essay: John Keown (1995), 'Euthanasia in the Netherlands: Sliding Down the Slippery Slope?', in John Keown (ed.), *Euthanasia Examined: Ethical, Clinical and Legal Perspectives*, Cambridge: Cambridge University Press, pp. 261–96.

HarperCollins Publishers for the essay: Ronald Dworkin (1993), 'The Morality of Abortion', in Ronald Dworkin (ed.), *Life's Dominion*, London: HarperCollins, pp. 30–67, 245–7.

Hastings Center for the essays: Susan S. Mattingly (1992), 'The Maternal–Fetal Dyad: Exploring the Two-Patient Obstetric Model', *Hastings Center Report*, **92**, January–February, pp. 13–18; George J. Annas (1988), 'She's Going to Die: The Case of Angela C', *Hastings Center Report*, **88**, February–March, pp. 23–5; John A. Robertson (1991), 'Second Thoughts on Living Wills', *Hastings Center Report*, November–December, pp. 6–9; Joanne Lynn and Joan M. Teno (1993), 'After the Patient Self-Determination Act: The Need for Empirical Research on Formal Advance Directives', *Hastings Center Report*, **23**, January–February, pp. 20–24; Linda L. Emanuel and Ezekiel J. Emanuel (1993), 'Decisions at the End of Life: Guided by Communities of Patients', *Hastings Center Report*, **23**, September–October, pp. 6–14. Copyright © Hastings Center.

Johns Hopkins University Press for the essay: Helga Kuhse (1999), 'Some Reflections on the Problem of Advance Directives, Personhood, and Personal Identity', *Kennedy Institute of Ethics Journal*, **9**, pp. 347–64. Copyright © 1999 The Johns Hopkins University Press.

Massachusetts Medical Society for the essay: Henry K. Beecher (1966), 'Ethics and Clinical Research', *New England Journal of Medicine*, **274**, pp. 1354–60. Copyright © 1966 Massachusetts Medical Society.

David W. Meyers (1970), 'Compulsory Sterilisation and Castration', in David W. Meyers, *The Human Body and the Law*, Edinburgh: Edinburgh University Press, pp. 26–47, 167–73. Copyright © D.W. Meyers.

Oxford University Press for the essays: Margaret Brazier (1999), 'Regulating the Reproduction Business?', *Medical Law Review*, **7**, pp. 166–93. Copyright © 1999 Oxford University Press; Ian Kennedy (1998), 'Research and Experimentation', in Ian Kennedy and Andrew Grubb (eds), *Principles of Medical Law*, Oxford: Oxford University Press, pp. 714–46. Copyright © 1998 Oxford University Press. Reprinted from *Principles of Medical Law*, edited by Ian Kennedy and Andrew Grubb (1998) by permission of Oxford University Press.

Penguin UK for the essay: Jonathan Glover (1977), 'Not Striving to Keep Alive', in Jonathan Glover (ed.), *Causing Death and Saving Lives*, Harmondsworth: Penguin Books, Chapters 7 and 8, pp. 92–116, 304–305. Copyright © 1977 Jonathan Glover.

Princeton University Press for the essay: Allen Buchanan (1978), 'Medical Paternalism', *Philosophy and Public Affairs*, **7**, pp. 370–90. Copyright © 1978 Princeton University Press.

Sweet & Maxwell Ltd for the essay: Gerald Robertson (1981), 'Informed Consent to Medical Treatment', *Law Quarterly Review*, **97**, pp. 102–26.

Taylor & Francis Ltd for the essay: Danuta Mendelson (1996), 'Historical Evolution and Modern Implications of Concepts of Consent to, and Refusal of, Medical Treatment in the Law of Trespass', *The Journal of Legal Medicine*, **17**, pp. 1–71. http://www.tandf.co.uk/journals

T&T Clark Ltd for the essay: J.K. Mason (2000), 'Unwanted Pregnancy: A Case of Retroversion?', *Edinburgh Law Review*, **4**, pp. 191–206.

Yale Law Journal for the essays: Marjorie Maguire Shultz (1985), 'From Informed Consent to Patient Choice: A New Protected Interest', *Yale Law Journal*, **95**, pp. 219–99. Reprinted by permission of The Yale Law Journal Company and William S. Hein Company from *The Yale Law Journal*, **95**, pp. 219–99; Dawn E. Johnsen (1986), 'The Creation of Fetal Rights: Conflicts with Women's Constitutional Rights to Liberty, Privacy, and Equal Protection', *Yale Law Journal*, **95**, pp. 599–625. Reprinted by permission of The Yale Law Journal Company and William S. Hein Company from The Yale Law Journal, **95**, pp. 599–625.

Every effort has been made to trace all the copyright holders, but if any have been inadvertently overlooked the publishers will be pleased to make the necessary arrangement at the first opportunity.

Preface to the Second Series

The first series of the International Library of Essays in Law and Legal Theory has established itself as a major research resource with fifty-eight volumes of the most significant theoretical essays in contemporary legal studies. Each volume contains essays of central theoretical importance in its subject area and the series as a whole makes available an extensive range of valuable material of considerable interest to those involved in research, teaching and the study of law.

The rapid growth of theoretically interesting scholarly work in law has created a demand for a second series which includes more recent publications of note and earlier essays to which renewed attention is being given. It also affords the opportunity to extend the areas of law covered in the first series.

The new series follows the successful pattern of reproducing entire essays with the original page numbers as an aid to comprehensive research and accurate referencing. Editors have selected not only the most influential essays but also those which they consider to be of greatest continuing importance. The objective of the second series is to enlarge the scope of the library, include significant recent work and reflect a variety of editorial perspectives.

Each volume is edited by an expert in the specific area who makes the selection on the basis of the quality, influence and significance of the essays, taking care to include essays which are not readily available. Each volume contains a substantial introduction explaining the context and significance of the essays selected.

I am most grateful for the care which volume editors have taken in carrying out the complex task of selecting and presenting essays which meet the exacting criteria set for the series.

TOM CAMPBELL
Series Editor
Centre for Applied Philosophy and Public Ethics
Charles Sturt University

Introduction

Over the last 20 or 30 years, the discipline of medical law has become an acknowledged area of specialism in most law schools and many medical faculties throughout the world. Although doubt has been expressed about whether or not it qualifies as a discipline separate from other legal areas, medical law has maintained an identity distinct from, albeit related to, more traditional legal disciplines.

In part, this is due to the challenges which dilemmas in health care present, and in large part it results from the almost unique closeness of medical law and ethics in general. The medical lawyer is required to engage with philosophy, medicine, law, nursing and social and political policy. New issues arise constantly, and often only the most sophisticated analysis will suffice to ensure that answers are provided, or at least routes through problems are identified. For this reason, medical law has become one of the most high profile and challenging of legal disciplines.

Apart from its profile, it is not unreasonable to suggest that medical law, and those engaged with it, are at the forefront of analysing and seeking to resolve intensely human, and often distressing, contemporary dilemmas. The developments in the 'new' genetics, for example (to be covered in a separate volume) have posed unforeseen and complex challenges to the way we live our lives, our self-perception and our interrelatedness with others. Long before genetics became a major issue, however, more traditional concerns dominated the field. Superimposed on them was medicine's other great 'revolution' – namely, the capacities of clinicians to circumvent infertility problems in those who would otherwise have had no opportunity to reproduce.

As medicine progresses, so the opportunity – and even need – to use human subjects in research expands. Although a practice with a long history, the treatment of human research subjects has long been controversial, and remains so today. Attempts to balance the interests of the individual with those of the community have sometimes resulted in concerns about the security of the individual research subject, and about the extent to which he or she is truly a volunteer in this process. Equally, the medical maverick finds a central place in this area.

Few subjects can be as emotive as the decisions made by individuals at the end of life. The recognition of the persistent vegetative state forced the law's involvement in matters traditionally thought of as private and required subtle, and controversial, reasoning in the search for a resolution. Equally, the general climate of respect for patients' rights has raised the question of the extent to which people should have rights in choosing their death, in the same way as they have acknowledged rights in choosing how to live.

Although many areas of medical law could have been chosen for this volume, I have confined myself to four broad areas – some new, some traditional. Even within the areas selected, of course, the range of issues which could have been considered is enormous, and selection was difficult. What I have tried to do in this volume is to select those essays which demonstrate most clearly both the legal complexities of the subjects and the human dilemmas contained within them. In a sense, it is invidious to choose some commentaries over others, some authors at the expense of others. What this volume does not claim is that the essays contained in it are undoubtedly the best; rather it asserts an admittedly personal, perhaps idiosyncratic, choice of both topics and commentators, in an effort to display the range and diversity of issues which make up modern medical law. As my intention is partly to demonstrate the nature of the analysis required of medical law, as well as exploring content, it is to be hoped that I will be forgiven for this.

The chapters in this book follow a straightforward plan. Parts I and II consider what might be called the more traditional issues in medical law – negligence, consent to treatment and reproduction. Parts III and IV address more 'modern' problems in medical law – human experimentation and research and issues at the end of life. Although primarily legal in content, the closeness of medical law and ethics is highlighted by the inclusion of some essays which are essentially pure philosophy, but which have direct relevance to the legal issues covered. Indeed, virtually all of the legal essays highlight the jurisprudential nature of the subject. These are not descriptive documents; rather they argue a case, using historical and contemporary explanations to critique and evaluate the law as it currently stands.

Negligence/Consent

In Chapter 1, Marjorie Schultz provides an excellent analysis of the move towards recognizing informed consent as a critical feature of patients' rights, and medical law in the USA. In her lengthy piece, she traces the development of the law in this area, in particular addressing the extent to which patient autonomy has become an interest seen as worthy of protection. Her conclusion, that a new model of authority in the doctor patient relationship is required, carries resonance even many years after this article was written. As she says:

> Medical decisionmaking involves the interwoven, overlapping and often competing claims of personal autonomy and professional competence. The challenge of regulating medical decisionmaking is to allocate the proper weight to each of these values. (p. 82)

Within the existing legal framework, Schultz claims that '[p]rotection of patient autonomy remains derivative rather than direct, episodic rather than systematic' (p. 83).

The creation of legal protection of patient autonomy is taken up by Gerald Robertson in Chapter 2. As informed consent is primarily a feature of US jurisprudence, Robertson explores the extent to which it has implications for UK law. Tracing the history of the development of informed consent in the USA, he re-emphasizes the extent to which it was a device used to enhance respect for patient autonomy. He also, however, concludes that additional, and policy-based, reasoning underlay its creation and absorption into common legal parlance in that country – namely, the desire to expand the liability of physicians. Although UK courts increasingly use the language of informed consent, Robertson points out that it forms no part of UK law. Indeed, that contention holds true even today, although some similarities to the US position may be observed in the approach taken by UK courts. However, Robertson's prediction that English (I would argue each of the UK's jurisdictions) law will probably seek to restrict the applicability of any such doctrine has been borne out in reality. Cases such as *Bolam* v. *Friern Hospital Management Committee*,[1] which have long been criticized for handing over to doctors the power effectively to set their own standards have been absorbed – albeit not in a wholesale manner – into leading cases such as *Sidaway* v. *Board of Governors of the Bethlem*

Royal Hospital and the Maudsley Hospital,[2] leaving the UK in a position whereby the amount of information legally required for a meaningful consent is heavily dependent on what other doctors would tell their patients. Robertson, therefore, was correct to predict that '... the doctrine of informed consent is unlikely to develop in this country and that consequently it will prove to be of limited scope in affording compensation to victims of medical accidents (p. 109).

The law's reluctance to elevate the standard of disclosure required, and thereby to give real meaning to patient autonomy, can partly be explained by the reasons which have traditionally been used to support non-disclosure. These were identified by Allen Buchanan, whose essay is reproduced as Chapter 4 of this volume. He identifies a number of lines of argument, which he subsumes under the general heading of 'Medical Paternalism', and argues that each of them can be defeated. In a powerful exposé of the inherent weakness of arguments for non-disclosure Buchanan indirectly challenges legal subservience to accepted medical practice, although he writes as a philosopher. It is, of course, plausible to argue that, since Buchanan wrote this essay, times have moved on, and certainly we have a generation of doctors and other health care workers growing around us for whom respect for patients is more than merely a mantra without meaning. Nonetheless, the attitude that, for example, patients will be harmed by disclosure about the truth of their condition, still lingers and carries weight. Even in those US states which follow the 'prudent patient' test, developed in the case of *Canterbury* v. *Spence*,[3] the notion of therapeutic privilege forms an integral part of the doctrine. Thus, although the *Canterbury* test seems to focus on the prudent or average patient, rather than on the prudent or average doctor, it remains permissible to withhold information likely to distress the patient. In this way, the withholding of truth, to which Buchanan so strongly objects, is built into even the more radical approach to disclosure of information.

This pattern is repeated on a worldwide basis. In Chapter 3, Danuta Mendelson takes us on a guided tour of the law of consent in much of the English-speaking world. As an Australian, she would doubtless see the case of *Rogers* v. *Whittaker*[4] as a significant development. This was Australia's first major strike against the dominance of the *Bolam* test, and may finally have sounded the death knell of the professional test in Australia. Mendelson's primary concern is to trace the development of the law in respect of consent to treatment and, more significantly, refusal of treatment in a number of countries. She concludes that the supremacy of autonomy in current common law is both unusual and to be regretted:

> Conceptually, the legal right to self-determination is, undoubtedly, a very significant and essential element of modern jurisprudence – people, in general, should be able to exercise control over their bodies in relation to undertaking or cessation of any invasive medical regimen. Nonetheless, there are a number of profound moral and human questions that sit uneasily with the declaratory statements of an ideologically pure notion of personal autonomy. (p. 180)

Whether or not one agrees with the ideology which underpins Mendelson's essay, it has increasing contemporary relevance, given the genetics revolution. The use of individual autonomy as a trumping value certainly has profound consequences when one person's exercise of autonomy may harm that of another person, as may well be the case in genetic conditions. The values of interconnectedness are, arguably, less demanding in the standard medical act, although Mendelson's concentration on the refusal of life-saving medical treatment does shed some light on her concerns about the use of a pure autonomy model, given that such decisions may also impact on others.

Reproduction

Part II of this volume begins with two very different essays on one of the most controversial issues in human reproductive choice – abortion. In Chapter 5 Ronald Dworkin analyses the conservative and liberal approaches to abortion. Of course, his analysis takes account of the fact that it is difficult simplistically to categorize people and their views in this way, but as a tool for analysis it serves the argument well. In his analysis, he focuses on two, potentially extreme, positions, with the Churches representing the 'conservative' perspective and 'feminism' the liberal. His central theme is encapsulated in the following quotation:

> . . . we cannot understand the moral argument now raging around the world – between individuals, within and between religious groups, as conducted by feminist groups, or in the politics of several nations – if we see it as centered on the issue of whether a fetus is a person. Almost everyone shares, explicitly or intuitively, the idea that human life has objective, intrinsic value that is quite independent of its personal value for anyone, and disagreement about the right interpretation of that shared idea is the actual nerve of the great debate about abortion. (p. 244)

In Chapter 6 Sheila McLean also surveys the pro- and anti-choice lobbies' positions on abortion, but from a different perspective. Here, the question is whether or not there is any ground on which agreement could be reached between these positions, and in particular she argues that there is an element of inconsistency in the anti-abortion lobby's arguments. With the exception of those who would always disapprove of abortion, the anti-abortion campaign hinges, she contends, on an inherently disingenuous claim for the moral high ground. Focusing on attempts by anti-choice protagonists to limit the legal availability of abortion to the earliest stages of pregnancy, McLean argues that this position is a complete contradiction of their professed concern with foetal life. Although not proposed as a practical solution, this essay argues that – for the sake of consistency – the anti-choice lobby should argue for minimum time limits rather than maximum ones. In this way, women could be relieved of their unwanted pregnancies and foetuses could also be salvaged.

In Chapter 7 David Meyers provides a clear and shocking account of the policy of non-consensual sterilization carried out in the USA in the twentieth century – a practice apparently endorsed by the public, and certainly by legislators. Most US states had laws in force which permitted, for example, the superintendents of institutions for the 'feeble-minded' to authorize sterilization without reference to the wishes of the individual (usually female). In some cases, women were only released back into the community after surgery to sterilize them, some only finding out many years later just what the operation had been for. Perhaps the most ringing endorsement of this policy can be found in the words of Oliver Wendell Holmes, remembered generally as one of America's most distinguished judges, when he said:

> We have seen more than once that the public welfare may call upon the best citizens for their lives. It would be strange if it could not call upon those who already sap the strength of the state for these lesser sacrifices, often not felt to be such by those concerned, in order to prevent our being swamped with incompetence. It is better for all the world, if instead of waiting to execute degenerate offspring for crime, or to let them starve for their imbecility, society can prevent those who are manifestly unfit from continuing their kind. The principle that sustains compulsory vaccination is broad enough to cover cutting the Fallopian tubes . . . Three generations of imbeciles are enough.[5]

Meyers was one of the first writers to expose this situation, and he concludes:

> There must come a point to which medical advances have perhaps already brought us, where society – represented by a legislative majority – no longer has the right to use its knowledge to manipulate and mutilate the bodies of those it feels somehow do not fit the desired social mould. (Myers, 1971, p. 47)

In Chapter 8 Margaret Brazier addresses the other side of the reproduction coin – not its prevention but its facilitation. The UK is amongst those countries which have chosen to regulate assisted procreation by way of a dedicated statute. While other countries have a much more *laissez-faire* approach to assisted procreation, in 1990 the UK passed the Human Fertilisation and Embryology Act which can trace its genesis to the recommendations of the 1984 *Report of the Committee of Inquiry into Human Fertilisation and Embryology* (the Warnock Report). Although the Act is often held up as an example for other countries, Brazier concludes that:

> Because the British system is built on consensus, regulators, clinicians and scientists work well together. All those strengths benefit patients and promote British reproductive medicine as a success story. The price paid for consensus however is that all too often crucial issues of individual rights, the balance between individual rights and public policy, and issues of conflicting rights are skated over. (p. 298)

There is, she concludes, 'little conceptual depth underpinning British law' (p. 298). This view may well be thought to carry some weight, given the challenges which have arisen already to British law, for example the case of Diane Blood,[6] who sought authority to use semen removed from her dying husband and was effectively precluded from doing so in the UK because of the terms of the legislation (see, further, McLean, 1999). Equally, the cloning of 'Dolly' challenged what legislators had seen as an outright ban on cloning contained in the Act, as the technique used to create Dolly is not specifically covered by it. In light of this attempted ban, the recent parliamentary agreement to permit stem cell research, including cloning, seems to go against the spirit of the Act, yet the amendment will once again place British scientists in a position envied by many of their European colleagues whose countries prohibit research of this nature.

Yet, despite her critique of the law, Brazier also sees its benefits, and concludes that, both in the UK and elsewhere in Europe, countries have 'sought to fashion a scheme of regulation acceptable to its own culture and community . . .' (p. 324). Nonetheless, she suggests, those with the wealth and the technical know-how will be all too able to bypass the regulations in force by use, for example, of the Internet. Arguably this is an insurmountable problem, even were there to be a genuine drive for harmonization of laws. Already, people travel within Europe to obtain services – Mrs Blood was able to receive treatment at a clinic in Belgium, thanks to the Court of Appeal's insistence that she, like all citizens of the European Union, was entitled to move freely throughout Europe for services, including medical services. It seems unlikely that a global – even a European – consensus on the principles underpinning the availability of assisted reproductive techniques is attainable.

In Chapter 9 Susan Mattingly explores one possible model of pregnancy – namely, viewing the woman and the foetus as two distinct patient entities. Although the impetus for viewing pregnancy in this way might have been to generate foetal 'rights', Mattingly convincingly points out that this essentially backfires. If woman and foetus are viewed as separate patients, then there are potentially more obstacles to treating foetuses (since this involves invading the woman's body) rather than fewer. Duties are owed to both patients in this description of pregnancy, but '. . . the injunction against harming one patient involuntarily to help another is virtually absolute' (p. 328). In addition, of course, viewing the foetus and the pregnant woman as separate and distinct entities, generates the 'conflict' between them and poses problems which are difficult to resolve. As Draper has said:

> . . . in the maternal versus foetal conflict model, whoever wins, pregnant women lose. Resolving the conflict in favour of the mother gives her the liberty and the sole burden for deciding whether or not the foetus will live; she alone must sacrifice or live with the consequences. If the conflict model is resolved in favour of the foetus, women lose out again, since the sacrifice for saving life is extracted from them and them alone . . . (Draper, 1992, p. 1).

The implications of generating foetal 'rights' are further considered in Chapter 10 where Dawn Johnsen describes what she calls 'a dangerous conceptual move' (p. 335). Conceding that foetal rights had, at that time (1986), seldom been used to trump women's decisions, she nonetheless – and rightly – indicates the very real potential that such incidents may become more common. The range of ways in which women may harm embryos and foetuses by engaging in activities which are perfectly lawful is substantial, yet concentration on the foetus may lead to a situation where women's basic rights to live as they choose are damaged, if not rendered nugatory, at least for the duration of a pregnancy. Tracing the history of legislative and other activity with direct relevance to protecting the foetus, Johnsen argues that there is a resonance between the tradition of keeping women in the sphere of private (that is, family) life and out of the workplace, and the current trend in developing foetal rights.

Chapter 11 is a short, but immensely poignant, analysis by George Annas of one case in which the true consequences of prioritizing foetuses over women became distressingly clear. In his brief account of the tragic case of Angela Carder, Annas exposes the extent to which the law may collude with medicine to limit women's rights in the interests of salvaging their foetuses. In a hard-hitting critique of the judgment in this case (subsequently overturned after Angela Carder's death) Annas says that the judges:

> . . . treated a live woman as though she were already dead, forced her to undergo an abortion, and then justified their brutal and unprincipled opinion on the basis that she was almost dead and her fetus's interests in life outweighed any interest she might have in her own life or health. (p. 361)

Since Ms Carder's case, courts both in the USA and the UK have, on occasion, continued to place the interests of the foetus on a par with, or occasionally above, the rights which live and competent women are generally conceded to hold. From the advances in medical technology have come a plethora of ethical and legal dilemmas. If nothing else, this situation shows the extent to which progress is seldom value-neutral and has the potential to challenge the analytical skills, and sheer humanity, of the law.

In the final chapter of Part II, J.K. Mason moves us on to a different, but related, topic. Chapter 12 provides a thoughtful and intelligent analysis of *McFarlane* v. *Tayside Health Board*,[7] a Scottish case which was ultimately decided in the House of Lords. As the supreme civil court in the UK, the House of Lords in this judgment has effectively bucked the trend of permitting recovery of damages for the additional costs of bringing up a child born after the parents had attempted to ensure, in this case by contraceptive surgery, that they would have no further children. Mason expertly exposes the inconsistencies in approach by tracing the history of what are often called wrongful birth cases (although he believes that *McFarlane* is in fact a case of what he calls wrongful pregnancy) in the UK. However labelled, *McFarlane* has apparently reversed a trend, which was observable both in the UK and in other countries, of moving away from the 'child as a blessing' policy towards the recognition of the reality of the additional costs associated even with a wanted and much loved child. Arguably, the House of Lords, for reasons which do not stand up well to scrutiny, have simply replaced one policy-based approach with another, but not necessarily better, one. This essay invites us to examine what happens when policy is presented draped in the cloak of reason. As Mason concludes, 'it is difficult to see the House of Lords' judgements in *McFarlane* as other than a scholarly and thoughtful elaboration of a single word – distaste – and it could be argued that we are entitled to disclosure of better grounds on which to reverse an established line of decisions' (p. 377).

Human Experimentation and Research

Part III of this volume returns to consent issues, but now in the context of the use of human beings in research and experimentation. Arguably, the most important essay ever written on this subject makes up Chapter 13. Henry Beecher's shocking exposé of research practices in the USA heralded ever closer scrutiny of the aims and methods of human research. In this short, but passionate, essay Beecher generated serious doubts about the adequacy of international and national control over the use of human subjects in research. In this area above all it might have been anticipated that monitoring would be close and demanding. Following the Nazi atrocities of the Second World War, the Nuremberg Code, developed out of the war crimes trials, was expected to ensure that humans were never again subject to such cruelty. The first Principle of the Code demands that free and voluntary consent is given before research can be ethical or legal, yet Beecher concludes, somewhat unhappily, that some subjects of experiments '. . . would not have been available if they had been truly aware of the uses that would be made of them' (p. 381).

Beecher gives 22 examples of unethical research, although he was also able to claim that many more could be identified. This essay, first published in 1966, is, of course, somewhat elderly, and it might be thought that its age militates against its inclusion. However, to imagine that unethical research or experimentation does not continue to occur would be naïve, and Beecher's contribution reminds us how easy it may be, even in a sophisticated community, for dubious research to occur. This is so despite the increasing scrutiny of research protocols by ethics committees.

Alastair Campbell in Chapter 14 brings us more up-to-date with his brief analysis of the experiment conducted on women cancer patients in a New Zealand Hospital which came to light in 1987. Despite increased surveillance of the use of human subjects and the existence of an international code dedicated to human experimentation and research – the Declaration of Helsinki – one doctor was able to use women, without their knowledge and over a period of 15 to 20 years, to test his own hypothesis that cervical carcinoma *in situ* would virtually never progress to invasive cancer. Women were, therefore, not offered the standard available treatment. An Inquiry was set up, which discovered – amongst other things – that the fact of this experiment had been known to the hospital authorities, yet no one tried to stop it and no extra care was provided for the women concerned. Although condemning the experiment, Campbell nonetheless takes some comfort from the thoroughness of the Committee of Inquiry's work, and concludes that its report is '. . . a powerful endorsement of the centrality of ethical issues both in professional education and in the public debate about the quality of health care' (p. 396).

In Chapter 15 Ian Kennedy undertakes a thorough analysis of the law in this area, viewed from the UK perspective and incorporating European Directives. Although he does not attempt a full-blown critique of existing regulation of human subject research, the model which he demonstrates is potentially of value in the assessment of the pitfalls into which researchers may fall. In addition, the UK model can usefully be contrasted with regimes in force in other jurisdictions.

Death and Dying

The final section of the book concerns issues at the end of life. Many of the essays here are relatively brief, but they are designed to provide the reader with a taste of the range and complexity of issues which arise when decisions are made at the end of life.

In Chapter 16 Helga Kuhse discusses a contentious aspect of end-of-life decisions – the living will debate, holding, against Robertson's argument in Chapter 17, that the fact that people can in fact be apparently happy in, for example, a demented condition does not mean that this should take precedence over previously expressed wishes. She also explores the notion of psychological continuity, and notes that '[g]iven that the continuity between mental states admits of degrees, the issue of when one person has been replaced by another remains somewhat vague' (p. 441). Indeed, she notes the argument that:

> As long as strong psychological connections continue to exist, there is little reason to doubt that the executor of the advance directive and the patient are the same person. Similarly, there is little reason to doubt that a patient who has slipped into a persistent vegetative state and has irreversibly lost the capacity to experience states of consciousness is not the same person as the executor of the advance directive. The reason is not that the patient is a *different* person, but rather that with the permanent loss of the ability to experience *any* psychological states, the patient is . . . no longer a person. (p. 441)

Persons, for Kuhse, are 'conscious beings, who have the capacity for rationality, self-consciousness, and purposive agency; they have the ability to see themselves as existing over time, that is, they are not only living in the present, but have the mental capacity to span time' (p. 442).

Kuhse's refutation of Robertson's approach, therefore, hinges critically on the distinction between persons and non-persons. As she says:

> . . . those who argue that advance directives rest on a confused understanding of personal identity may well be correct, but acceptance of that position does not by itself provide sound reasons for overriding refusals of life-sustaining treatment. Rather, an examination of plausible understandings of the concepts of 'person,' 'human individual,' and 'interests' may well lead one to conclude that the implementation of advance directives will, other things being equal, be justified, even when the now incompetent patient is not experiencing suffering and distress, and seemingly is capable of experiencing some simple but psychologically disjointed pleasures. (p. 447)

In Chapter 17, we move to John Robertson's essay, critiqued by Kuhse in the previous chapter. In this essay Robertson has 'second thoughts' about living wills and, in a brief, but influential, analysis of the rationale for living wills, he seeks to expose their inherent confusion. In seeking to control life (or more accurately, death) after loss of competence, the presumption of proponents of the living will is that it permits individuals to retain control over the manner of their dying when they are no longer able to express their values or decisions. Robertson, however, makes one very telling point. As he says:

> The problem, however, is that the patient's interests when incompetent – viewed from her current perspective – are no longer informed by the interests and values she had when competent. The values and interests of the competent person no longer are relevant to someone who has lost the rational structure on which those values and interests rested. Unless we are to view competently held values and interests as extending to situations in which, because of incompetency, they can no longer have meaning, it matters not that as a competent person the individual would not wish to be maintained in a debilitated or disabled state. (p. 452)

Thus, Robertson concedes the values apparently embodied in respecting the living will, but would suggest that there is an inherent fallacy or confusion surrounding their enforcement. A classic example of this tension might well be the competent person who, having witnessed what has happened to an elderly relative, makes out a living will indicating that, should they become demented, they would not wish to have any life-sustaining treatment, even antibiotics, made available. That same person, however, once demented, might in fact be, for all intents and purposes, perfectly happy. This is a powerful image, and one which doubtless has influenced the views of organizations such as the British Medical Association which counsels that advance statements should be followed only when they are well-informed and specific as to the conditions included and the treatments which are unacceptable.

The value of advance directives is also taken up by Joanne Lynn and Joan Teno in Chapter 18. Writing in the aftermath of the passing of the Patient Self-Determination Act (PSDA), in the USA, they avoid the theoretical for the practical. In their view, '[f]ormal advance directives are not worth much unless they can be shown to improve decisionmaking' (p. 457). Their plea, therefore, is for sound empirical research into the actual, as opposed to the theoretical, impact of the PSDA which was 'intended to encourage patients to claim their rights in regard to decisionmaking' (p. 455). In sum, they argue that 'advance directives have been proposed as the answer to the problem of how to empower patients so that they maintain control of their care even when incompetent. We have not yet shown that directives will answer that need' (p. 458).

Chapter 19 comes from two commentators who have written extensively on proxy decision-making, and whose voices in this field are highly influential. Staying with the subject of advance directives, Linda and Ezekiel Emanuel take the debate one important step forward, recognizing the doubts that have been expressed about the extent to which advance directives actually can, or do, enhance patient choice. The limitations on advance directives can be categorized as personal – the inability of the individual to understand all relevant issues, and their potential to change their mind – and procedural. The latter relates to the fact that in few countries, with the possible exception of Denmark, do people actually make an advance declaration in any event. Evidence abounds that people may not understand medical information, and decisions made on flawed understanding may not, therefore, actually serve the purpose claimed for advance directives. Equally, the option of appointing proxy decision-makers to carry out the wishes of the now incompetent person has been shown to be flawed. Not only do the Emanuels find evidence that people do not talk things through thoroughly with a designated proxy (assuming that they appoint one) but that '[t]he patient's prior wishes and proxy predictions of the patient's prior wishes in circumstances other than the patient's current health overlap only from 33 to 68 percent of the time' (p. 462).

However, there are also others for whom end-of-life decisions must be taken, and where no prior wishes are recorded. In an effort to ensure that these patients may also benefit from the control that the advance directive seems to permit, they propose that 'default guidelines based on a "local patient community medical directive"' should be considered for 'incompetent patients with no advance directives' (pp. 463–64). These, they suggest, could be drawn up by surveying a randomly selected group of other patients in the health care facility, using robust survey methodology. Second, guidelines could then be developed by an institutional committee with broad representation from both medicine and beyond. Third, the preliminary conclusions of these committees should be put to the test by involving the wider public, and the guidelines should be widely publicized. As to implementation, they conclude that:

> When an incompetent patient lacks an advance directive, the health care team would interpret the default directive to apply to the patient's situation in the same way that it currently interprets personal instructional directives. (p. 465)

Although they concede that the use of the default directive would be likely to be infrequent, their proposals are designed to 'help realize the ideal of patient autonomy in life-sustaining treatment decisions for the underrepresented group of patients who have no advance directive' (p. 468).

These proposals are manifestly contentious because, for some, they may simply represent a move towards formalizing, under the cloak of respectability and democracy, the premature ending of some lives. From the other perspective, of course, they represent a genuine attempt to balance the rights of those who have made prior choices with those who have not. In light of people's continued apparent apathy about making such choices, and the increasing numbers of people who will die after a period of incompetence, the Emanuels have at least provided a further twist to the debate about advance directives.

Finally, in Chapter 20, Ann Sommerville gives a clear and thoughtful account of the approach to advance directives in the UK, and explores the approach of the British Medical Association. In concluding that 'advance directives – at least in their present form – may not be the best or only answer for people with deteriorating mental facilities . . .' (p. 488), she nonetheless argues that their real value may in fact lie in the opportunity they can, or should, provide for dialogue between doctor and patient.

In Chapter 21, John Keown provides a compelling critique of the Dutch approach to euthanasia and assisted suicide. Until last year, these remained outlawed in the Netherlands, although tolerated providing that certain criteria are met. A well-known opponent of legalizing euthanasia, John Keown highlights what he sees as the reality of the Dutch situation by analysing the available figures in such a way as to demonstrate that the actual incidence of euthanasia in the Netherlands is considerably higher than officialdom will admit. Although the Dutch experience is often held up as an example which the rest of the world could follow, it is not without its critics, even on grounds different from those Keown identifies. For example, the regulations which currently govern euthanasia require that doctors report cases before they know whether or not they will be prosecuted (arguably, likely to lead to significant underreporting), and the system is essentially based on medical paternalism rather than on the rights of patients to act autonomously in choosing when to die. Keown's opposition is more fundamental than that, and there is no doubt that his analysis of the rate of doctor-assisted dying in the Netherlands is disturbing. If his analysis can be criticized, however, this would be on the basis that no comparison is made with the rates of doctor-assisted deaths in jurisdictions which continue to outlaw both euthanasia and assisted suicide. Doubtless, these figures are unlikely to be readily available, but it does mean that Keown is unable to compare like with like.

In Chapter 22 John Griffiths discusses one of the more controversial cases in the history of euthanasia in the Netherlands – the *Chabot* case. Arguably, it is decisions such as this which add fuel to the concerns expressed by Keown and other commentators. Although public acceptance of euthanasia in the Netherlands seems to exist, before this case the general presumption had been that it would be available primarily to those suffering from physical problems, and certainly not to those whose mental condition was in doubt (not least because of the requirement for a free and voluntary consent). The facts of this case, however, moved the debate forward and expanded the groups who might be able to take advantage of the Dutch approach. Here, a doctor assisted a woman suffering from an 'adjustment disorder consisting of a depressed mood, without psychotic signs, in the context of a complicated bereavement process' (p. 530) to die (without, interestingly, arranging for her to be examined by other colleagues, although he had sought their advice). In carrying out this action Dr Chabot technically could be said to have operated beyond the strict confines of the regulations laid down, but the Court of Appeals accepted that assistance with dying could be extended to those who were not suffering from a somatic or terminal condition.

This ground-breaking decision has been the subject of much ethical and legal debate, as – for some commentators at least – it shows that the slippery slope argument does work: tolerance of assisted dying in extreme cases becomes tolerance in less extreme circumstances, or in cases where there may be concerns about the requesting individual's capacity. Griffiths concedes that there is evidence of 'medical practices which shorten life, in the cases of non-competent or of competent but not-consulted patients' (p. 542) and agrees that the data are 'a matter of concern' (p. 542). Nonetheless, as he points out:

> There is really not a shred of evidence that the frequency of this sort of behaviour is higher in the Netherlands than, for example, in the United States; the only thing that is clear is that more is known about it in the Netherlands. In short, there is no reason to assume . . . a causal relationship between limited legalisation of euthanasia and 'lack of control' over other sorts of medical behaviour. (p. 542)

Griffiths also notes that Dutch euthanasia law, with the *Chabot* case, seems 'to have taken a decisive step away from the doctor-centred approach which has dominated legal development up to now . . . toward patient self-determination' (p. 541). The consequences of this, of course, might be that the qualifying characteristics which must presently be satisfied could be limited or removed altogether, making a request for assisted death from anyone, irrespective of their medical condition, acceptable. This would, of course, not be uncontroversial. Many of those who have, however reluctantly, reduced or lost their opposition to assisted death, have done so on the basis that for some people, in the final stages of a terminal illness, the suffering involved may be so great that they should have the right to receive help in dying 'with dignity'. However, the possibility that such groups could also include those who are simply tired of life, or those who are of arguable competence, will probably cause concern. Logically, of course, it could be argued that if people are allowed to act in a self-determining manner, then it should be irrelevant what is the basis for their decision, in much the same way as the competent adult (and in one UK case, the paranoid schizophrenic[9]) has the right to refuse life-sustaining treatment on any and all grounds.[10] This, however, is a long way from the attitudes of most people, and is not reflected in the only jurisdiction in the world – Oregon – that has legalized assisted suicide, subject to conditions such as that the person must be terminally ill and within months of death. It remains to be seen whether the decision about who can rightfully receive assistance in dying will ultimately be awarded to the individual him- or herself or left in the hands of doctors and medical diagnoses.

In the final chapter of the volume the reader is directed towards the seminal and influential work of Jonathan Glover, represented here in his book, *Causing Death and Saving Lives*. Although almost any part of this book could have been selected, I have chosen to highlight two chapters which tackle head-on the issue of whether or not killing is always wrong. This is an important question, as it underpins much of the debate about voluntary euthanasia, non-voluntary euthanasia, assisted suicide and many other end-of-life decisions.

Significantly, Glover seeks to persuade the reader of the fallacy of the acts/omissions doctrine, at least in some circumstances. If persuaded by his argument, this could have wide-ranging consequences for doctors and the law, as this distinction is routinely used to maintain the right of doctors not to keep someone alive while at the same time maintaining the current prohibition on actively assisting death. Glover says that it is 'hard to believe that the medical policy of refraining from killing in cases where "not striving to keep alive" is thought morally right is a justifiable rule of thumb when the importance of what is at stake is fully appreciated' (pp. 561–62). This sentiment was addressed in the judgment of Lord Mustill in the case of *Airedale NHS Trust* v. *Bland*, where he said:

> The conclusion that the declarations can be upheld depends crucially on a distinction drawn by the criminal law between acts and omissions, and carries with it inescapably a distinction between, on the one hand what is often called 'mercy killing', where active steps are taken in a medical context to terminate the life of a suffering patient, and a situation such as the present, where the proposed conduct has the aim for equally humane reasons of terminating the life of Anthony Bland by withholding from him the basic necessities of life. The acute unease which I feel about adopting this way through the legal and ethical maze is I believe due in an important part to the sensation that however much the terminologies may differ, the ethical status of the two courses of action is for all relevant purposes indistinguishable.[8]

Glover concludes that '. . . except for differences of side-effects, the arguments against killing are really good arguments in favour of saving lives' (p. 571). This surely offers an effective, and important, challenge to current medical practice and to the attitudes of courts in the UK and elsewhere. Indeed, current legal approaches to end-of-life decisions may be categorized as a similar attempt at obfuscation of the real reasoning to that which Mason identified in Chapter 12.

Conclusion

As I said at the beginning of this Introduction, this somewhat eclectic mix of essays is designed in part to demonstrate to the reader the breadth of issues covered by medical law, as well as to stimulate further reading in this area. The congruence or dissonance of accepted ethical standards with the legal approach should also have become clear, as should the fact that seldom is there an easy or a 'right' answer to the problems thrown up by modern medicine. Given the impossible task of selection, I have chosen to focus on readable and thoughtful contributions which clearly expose the issues of fundamental rights, values and interests characterizing modern medical practice and law. Of course, many equally thoughtful and readable contributions have not found their way into this volume, just as many areas are not covered. Space precludes a general overview of every issue in medical law and ethics. However, what follows provides a taste of the complexities of this subject, and will hopefully stimulate further reading in this dynamic area of law.

Notes

 1 [1957] 2 All ER 118.
 2 [1985] 1 All ER 643 (House of Lords).
 3 464 F 2d 772 (DC, 1972); on appeal 409 US 1064.
 4 [1993] 4 Med. LR 79.
 5 *Buck* v. *Bell* 274 US 200, at p. 207.
 6 *R* v. *Human Fertilisation and Embryology Authority, ex parte Blood* [1997] 2 All ER 687.
 7 2000 SLT 154: [1999] 4 All ER 96.
 8 12 BMLR 64 at p. 132.
 9 *Re C* [1994] 1 All ER 819.
10 *Re T* [1992] 4 All ER 649.

References

Draper, H. (1992), *Women, Forced Caesareans and Antenatal Responsibilities*, Working Paper No. 1, Feminist Legal Research Unit, Liverpool: University of Liverpool.

McCullough, L.B. and Chervanak, F.A. (1994), *Ethics in Obstetrics and Gynaecology*, Oxford: Oxford University Press.

McLean, S.A.M. (1999), 'Creating Postmortem Pregnancies: A UK Perspective', *Juridical Review*, p. 323.

Meyers, D. (1971), *The Human Body and the Law*, Edinburgh: Edinburgh University Press.

Warnock, M. (Chair) (1984), *Report of the Committee of Inquiry into Human Fertilisation and Embryology*, Cmnd 9314, London: HMSO.

Part I
Negligence/Consent

[1]

The Yale Law Journal

Volume 95, Number 2, December 1985

From Informed Consent to Patient Choice: A New Protected Interest

Marjorie Maguire Shultz†

INTRODUCTION

Judges and legal scholars have long asserted the importance of patient autonomy in medical decisionmaking. Yet autonomy has never been recognized as a legally protectable interest. It has been vindicated only as a by-product of protection for two other interests—bodily security as protected by rules against unconsented contact, and bodily well-being as protected by rules governing professional competence. Neither bodily security nor bodily well-being, however, is an adequate surrogate; they do not coincide with autonomy. Nor is autonomy merely a formal issue. Decisionmaking by competent professionals does not provide an adequate substitute for patient choice. Injuries that arise from invasion of patients' interest in medical choice are both substantial and distinct.

Part I of this Article explains the importance of patient autonomy and describes how existing doctrines protect that value. Part II examines gaps and flaws in that current scheme of protection. Part III analyzes clusters of cases in which greater vindication of patient autonomy has begun to

† Lecturer, Boalt Hall School of Law, University of California, Berkeley. B.A. 1962, College of Wooster; M.A.T. 1964, University of Chicago; J.D. 1976, University of California, Berkeley. I am deeply grateful to William Fletcher, Robert Cole, Meir Dan-Cohen and Jane Staw; each gave invaluable assistance during the development of this Article. I am also much indebted to my research assistants and seminar students: Susan Raffanti, Dena Belinkoff, Catherine Fisk, Tina Stevens, Jon Polland and Allyn Taylor.

The Yale Law Journal   Vol. 95: 219, 1985

emerge, and urges that these developments should be generalized. Part IV recommends the creation of a distinct and independently protected interest in patient autonomy.

I. Starting Points

A. *The Importance of Patient Autonomy*

Individuality and autonomy have long been central values in Anglo-American society and law. In general, the more intense and personal the consequences of a choice and the less direct or significant the impact of that choice upon others, the more compelling the claim to autonomy in the making of a given decision.[1] Under this criterion, the case for respecting patient autonomy in decisions about health and bodily fate is very strong.[2]

The very fact that health care choices are extremely important, however, generates fear that individuals will make mistakes. The complex and esoteric nature of modern medicine necessitates advice from experts. Needed perspective and emotional support can be provided by family and friends. Given that medical choices affect the quality and even the length of life itself, individuals making such choices may well be urged to seek all the help, in terms of both love and knowledge, that they can find. Ultimately, however, the stake of both experts and loved ones is less intense than that of the patient whose well-being is directly affected.[3] Patients' preferences, therefore, ought generally to be controlling.

---

1. Perhaps the most articulate advocate of this view was John Stuart Mill:

    [T]he sole end for which mankind are warranted . . . in interfering with the liberty of action of any of their number, is self-protection. . . . The only part of the conduct of any one, for which he is amenable to society, is that which concerns others. In the part which merely concerns himself, his independence is, of right, absolute. Over himself, over his own body and mind, the individual is sovereign.

    J. MILL, ON LIBERTY 6 (1873).
2. The classic statement of this value in the medical context is that of Judge Cardozo in Schloendorff v. Society of N.Y. Hosp.: "Every human being of adult years and sound mind has a right to determine what shall be done with his own body; and a surgeon who performs an operation without his patient's consent, commits an assault . . . ." 211 N.Y. 125, 129–30, 105 N.E. 92, 93 (1914). A more recent statement of the importance of patient autonomy is found in 1 PRESIDENT'S COMM'N FOR THE STUDY OF ETHICAL PROBLEMS IN MEDICINE AND BIOMEDICAL AND BEHAVIORAL RESEARCH, MAKING HEALTH CARE DECISIONS 2–4 (1982) [hereinafter cited as MAKING DECISIONS]. *See generally* Goldstein, *For Harold Lasswell: Some Reflections on Human Dignity, Entrapment, Informed Consent, and the Plea Bargain*, 84 YALE L.J. 683 (1975) (critiquing inadequate protection of self-determination in three disparate processes, including informed consent to medical intervention).
3. In Western medicine, deference to the patient's interest is rooted in the Hippocratic tradition. *See* R. VEATCH, A THEORY OF MEDICAL ETHICS 21–25 (1981). In legal terms, the deference to the patient's interest is rooted in the doctor's status as a fiduciary. *See* Canterbury v. Spence, 464 F.2d 772, 782 (D.C. Cir.), *cert. denied*, 409 U.S. 1064 (1972). Under these principles, the doctor's interests in income, prestige and convenience, as well as in her own professional opinions and preferences, constitute a less immediate and compelling claim to authority than that which derives from the patient's status as the bearer of consequences. On occasion, however, doctors may have ethical, religious or professional convictions that lead them to wish to refuse some services. *See infra* note 349.

Protecting Patient Choice

B. *Implications for the Doctor-Patient Relationship*

Although the principle of individual autonomy is widely endorsed in theory, its practical implications for the doctor-patient relationship are controversial. Individuals exercise their autonomy in medical decisionmaking by arranging for needed professional services. Presumably, these individuals remain the source of authority and can choose to delegate all or only some of their control to professionals.[4] Yet, ironically, the most significant threat to patient autonomy comes from the very doctors whom patients hire. Because of their knowledge and traditional role, doctors often preempt patient authority.

Although scholars have proposed various models to describe or prescribe the distribution of power within the doctor-patient relationship,[5] for a number of years one view dominated professional ideology and customary practice. Under that view, the patient was seen as making only one key decision, to place herself in a given doctor's care, thereby delegating all subsequent authority to the doctor.[6] Such a model assumed that the patient lacked the technical ability to make medical decisions, and that expertise justified the doctor's making decisions on the patient's behalf.

In the past several decades, however, new developments have strengthened the argument that patient autonomy should receive more than pro forma respect. Advancing medical technology has greatly expanded the options available to the patient. Increased knowledge has heightened

---

4. Such a right flows from the contractual nature of the doctor-patient relationship. A patient's decision to forego information and consent procedures is typically called a waiver under informed consent doctrine. *See* Meisel, *The "Exceptions" to the Informed Consent Doctrine: Striking a Balance Between Competing Values in Medical Decisionmaking*, 1979 WIS. L. REV. 413, 453-60 (discussing waiver exception) [hereinafter cited as Meisel, *Exceptions*]. The difficult issue is determining when such a waiver has been made by the patient.

5. *See, e.g.*, R. BURT, TAKING CARE OF STRANGERS: THE RULE OF LAW IN DOCTOR-PATIENT RELATIONS (1979) (proposing extensive dialogue rather than black and white rules of thumb); Branson, *The Secularization of American Medicine*, HASTINGS CENTER STUD., Nov. 1973, at 17 (advocating that science no longer be regarded as "religion," and that doctors assume more modest, less "priestly" role); Childress, *Metaphors and Models of Medical Relationships*, 8 SOC. RESP.: JOURNALISM, L. MED. 47 (1982) (analyzing various models of medical relationships); May, *Code, Covenant, Contract, or Philanthropy*, HASTINGS CENTER REP., Dec. 1975, at 29 (espousing "covenant" as most inclusive and satisfying model of obligation); Szasz & Hollender, *A Contribution to the Philosophy of Medicine: The Basic Models of the Doctor-Patient Relationship*, in 97 A.M.A. ARCHIVES OF INTERNAL MED. 585 (1956); Veatch, *Models for Ethical Medicine in a Revolutionary Age*, HASTINGS CENTER REP., June 1972, at 5 (pointing out significance of choice of relationship model).

6. *See* 1 MAKING DECISIONS, *supra* note 2, at 19; Meisel, *The Expansion of Liability for Medical Accidents: From Negligence to Strict Liability By Way of Informed Consent*, 56 NEB. L. REV. 51, 77-80 (1977) (tracing legal requirements imposed upon doctors from early days of minimalism to more demanding contemporary times) [hereinafter cited as Meisel, *Expansion*]. Under earlier models, detailed disclosure to and consent by the patient played a role only insofar as they were thought to be essential to the therapeutic outcome. Pernick, *The Patient's Role in Medical Decisionmaking: A Social History of Informed Consent in Medical Therapy*, in 3 MAKING DECISIONS, *supra* note 2, at 1, 14.

The Yale Law Journal   Vol. 95: 219, 1985

awareness of how much remains unknown.[7] Debate and conflict within the medical community are widespread and public.[8] Differences in experts' advice can often be resolved only on the basis of risk and value preferences. This medical uncertainty accentuates the need for professional advice, but it also strengthens the case for ultimate decision by the person whose life is directly involved.

Medical choice increasingly depends on factors that transcend professional training and knowledge. As medicine has become able to extend life, delay and redefine death, harvest and transplant organs, correct abnormality within the womb, enable artificial reproduction, and trace genetic defect, questions about values have come to the fore in medical decisionmaking. Health care choices involve profound questions that are not finally referable to professional expertise.[9]

In the face of value pluralism, factual indeterminacy, and increasing options, patient autonomy has become a central principle of both popular[10] and philosophical[11] analysis of medical decisionmaking. Self-care and consumer movements have applied that principle, seeking to shift the balance away from professional dominance and toward individual knowledge and control.[12] Although medical traditions historically have downgraded

---

7. *See* J. KATZ, THE SILENT WORLD OF DOCTOR AND PATIENT 183–84 *passim* (1984) (discussing pervasiveness of medical uncertainty).

8. Newspaper articles describing medical differences of opinion are common. *See, e.g.,* Brooks, *New Hope is Offered to Victims of Stroke and Potential Victims,* Wall St. J., July 16, 1984, at 1, col. 1; *Top Surgeon Sees No Future for Artificial Heart,* N.Y. Times, Feb. 14, 1984, at D2, col. 3.

9. *See* Veatch, *Generalization of Expertise,* HASTINGS CENTER STUD., Nov. 1973, at 29.

10. *See, e.g.,* Enright, *What Does Society Really Want from Doctors?: More Disclosure,* MED. ECON., May 29, 1978, at 77 (reporting public preferences for greater information); Peck, *What Does Society Really Want from Doctors?: Greater Accountability,* MED. ECON., May 29, 1978, at 93, 105–11 (discussing growing accountability of doctors to consumers); *Going to Hospital? Stick up for Your Rights,* U.S. NEWS & WORLD REP., Oct. 1, 1984, at 61 (interview with Norma Calhoun, Pres., National Soc'y of Patient Representatives) (advising patients how to gain greater role in decisionmaking); *The Patient Has a Right to Know,* N.Y. Times, June 15, 1984, at A26, col. 1 (editorial discussing need for disclosure about health care provider costs and results). The Presidential Commission found that the vast majority of respondents to its survey wanted information and participation in medical decisions. 1 MAKING DECISIONS, *supra* note 2, at 17.

11. *See, e.g.,* J. CHILDRESS, WHO SHOULD DECIDE? PATERNALISM IN HEALTH CARE (1982) (classifying types of paternalism and analyzing their justification in medical contexts); Dworkin, *Autonomy and Informed Consent,* 3 BIOETHICS REP.: LITERATURE 309 (1983) (clarifying special role of autonomy in justifying medical consent norms); Gordon, *The Doctor-Patient Relationship,* 8 J. MED. & PHIL. 243 (1983) (from perspective of religious humanist, emphasizing need for physician to respect autonomy of patient).

12. *See* P. STARR, THE SOCIAL TRANSFORMATION OF AMERICAN MEDICINE 391–92 (1983) (describing movements exhibiting distrust of professional dominance). A leading theorist of self-care in medicine is Ivan Illich. *See* I. ILLICH, MEDICAL NEMESIS: THE EXPROPRIATION OF HEALTH (1976). Both alternative care and self-care have become major influences. *See, e.g.,* BOSTON WOMEN'S HEALTH BOOK COLLECTIVE, THE NEW OUR BODIES, OURSELVES: A BOOK BY AND FOR WOMEN xiii (1984) (one stated goal of book is "to reach as many women as possible with the tools which will enable them to take greater charge of their own health care").

Protecting Patient Choice

patient autonomy,[13] doctors, too, have begun to recognize and accept patient demands for more information and control.[14]

The law's response to pressures for greater recognition of patient autonomy has been ambivalent.[15] Existing rules repudiate the view that the mere hiring of a doctor transfers all authority from patient to doctor. Yet full vindication of patient autonomy interests would necessitate placing final authority regarding important decisions in the hands of any patient having the capacity and the desire to exercise it.[16] I shall argue that precisely such a model for the allocation of authority is appropriate, but, as Part II will demonstrate, no such guarantee of patient autonomy is currently mandated by the law.

C. *Existing Legal Protection of Patient Autonomy*

Although the doctor-patient relationship ordinarily arises through contract,[17] courts have deemed patients incapable of bargaining with doctors over the quality of medical services. Doctors' performance has therefore been monitored under standardized tort rules that govern professional

---

13. Jay Katz traces the history of nondisclosure and failure to share decisions with patients throughout the history of Western medicine. J. KATZ, *supra* note 7, at 1–29. He points out the direct conflict between the medical norm of "custody" and the legal norm of personal liberty. *Id.* at 2.

14. *See, e.g.,* Novack, Plumer, Smith, Ochitill, Morrow & Bennett, *Changes in Physicians' Attitudes Toward Telling the Cancer Patient,* 241 J. A.M.A. 897, 897 (1979) (reporting dramatic reversal in attitude among doctors from 1961 to 1979 over whether to tell patients they have cancer); *see also* Harris & Associates, *Views of Informed Consent and Decisionmaking: Parallel Surveys of Physicians and the Public,* in 2 MAKING DECISIONS, *supra* note 2, at 17, 18, *passim* (physicians reported positive attitudes toward disclosure).

15. This point is developed particularly by Jay Katz. *See* J. KATZ, *supra* note 7; Katz, *Informed Consent—A Fairy Tale? Law's Vision,* 39 U. PITT. L. REV. 137, 138 & nn.1–39 (1977) [hereinafter cited as Katz, *Informed Consent*]. The point is also explored in White, *Informed Consent: Ambiguity in Theory and Practice,* 8 J. HEALTH POL., POL'Y & L. 99 (1983).

16. The province of this discussion is decisionmaking by the autonomous patient who is able to and wants to make her own choices. Traditional exceptions to informed consent doctrine—situations where an emergency exists, where the patient waives the authority to make choices, or where the patient lacks decisionmaking capacity—are not affected by this analysis. Waiver is technically not an exception to respect for autonomy, because it is itself an expression of choice. The other exceptions track the most commonly recognized circumstances under which beneficence, even in the form of paternalism, may justifiably displace autonomy. *See* Dworkin, *Paternalism,* 56 MONIST 64, 76–84 (1972). The most extensive treatment of exceptions is in Meisel, *Exceptions, supra* note 4. Determining patients' decisionmaking capacity can be very problematic. *See* Roth, Meisel & Lidz, *Tests of Competency to Consent to Treatment,* 134 AM. J. PSYCHIATRY 279 (1977) (describing five possible standards for determining competency). Moreover, issues may arise regarding temporary or situation-specific incapacity. *See, e.g., In re* Yetter, 62 Pa. D. & C.2d 619 (Northampton County Ct. 1973) (patient's confinement in mental hospital did not mean she lacked capacity to refuse medical treatment); Nishi v. Hartwell, 52 Hawaii 188, 473 P.2d 116 (1970) (disclosure of side effect of treatment might have had adverse effect on patient).

17. *See, e.g.,* Gray v. Grunnagle, 423 Pa. 144, 166, 223 A.2d 663, 674 (1966) ("[T]he agreement between the physician and his patient is contractual in nature . . ."). The consensual origins of the relationship are especially emphasized in Epstein, *Medical Malpractice: The Case for Contract,* 1976 AM. BAR. FOUND. RESEARCH J. 87, 119. Entry into a contract for services is typically, though not always, the basis for imposition of physician duties of care.

The Yale Law Journal   Vol. 95: 219, 1985

malpractice rather than under contractual criteria of individual expectation.[18] Mainly as a derivative matter, the patient's interest in self-determination has also been analyzed under tort theories.[19]

1. *Battery*

Patient autonomy was initially identified with and subsumed under an interest in physical security, protected by rules proscribing unconsented touch.[20] Medical care often involves touching, and may be considered battery if the touching is unconsented.[21] By mandating patient consent to specific procedures, battery doctrine counters the implication that doctors acquire authority to make decisions simply by virtue of the contract for professional services. Moreover, professional competence is no defense to a medical battery action.[22] Under battery analysis, the patient's wishes take priority over even the fully competent recommendation of a doctor, unless an exception applies.[23] Apart from traditional defenses, the right to be secure against unconsented touching is close to absolute.[24] Application of battery doctrine to medical care thus establishes an uncompromising baseline of protection for patients' self-determination.

Despite the capacity of battery doctrine to protect a degree of physical

---

18. *See* Epstein, *supra* note 17, at 91–96 (discussing interplay of tort and contract principles in doctor-patient relationship). Under tort law, the same fear about inadequacy of lay judgment—here the judgment of jurors rather than patients—leads courts to concede most regulation of professional competence to the profession itself. W. KEETON, D. DOBBS, R. KEETON & D. OWEN, PROSSER & KEETON ON THE LAW OF TORTS § 32, at 188–89 (5th ed. 1984) [hereinafter cited as PROSSER & KEETON]. Epstein conceives of this as supplying an omitted contract term by incorporating custom of the trade. Epstein, *supra* note 17, at 110.

19. The question of self-determination might be analyzed as a problem of the scope of an agency, to be determined by contract between principal and agent. Some commentators have urged a more contractually oriented analysis of medical relations. *See, e.g.,* Epstein, *supra* note 17.

20. *See* Pernick, *supra* note 6, at 29–30; *see also* C. FRIED, MEDICAL EXPERIMENTATION: PERSONAL INTEGRITY AND SOCIAL POLICY 14–18 (1974) (discussing evolution of these doctrines).

21. PROSSER & KEETON, *supra* note 18, § 9, at 39.

22. W. PROSSER, HANDBOOK OF THE LAW OF TORTS § 18, at 104 (4th ed. 1971).

23. Under battery doctrine, the competent patient's choices are largely unfettered. Legal restrictions may arise from the protectable rights of other individuals. The state, for example, may compel vaccination. Jacobson v. Massachusetts, 197 U.S. 11 (1905). Public policy restrictions on individual choice are, however, hotly debated. *See, e.g.,* Bouvia v. County of Riverside, No. 159780 (Cal. Super. Ct. Dec. 16, 1983) (order denying preliminary injunction against forced feeding). Moreover, constitutional privacy decisions have contracted the scope of permissible intervention in medical choice. *See, e.g.,* Roe v. Wade, 410 U.S. 113 (1973) (privacy right to choice concerning abortion); Andrews v. Ballard, 498 F. Supp. 1038 (S.D. Tex. 1980) (privacy right of patients to choose form of treatment violated by state restrictions on performance of acupuncture); Satz v. Perlmutter, 362 So. 2d 160 (Fla. Dist. Ct. App. 1978), *aff'd,* 379 So. 2d 359 (1980) (state interest in preserving life does not override competent but mortally sick patient's right to refuse treatment).

24. C. FRIED, *supra* note 20, at 16. Damages range from symbolic recompense for purely dignitary injury, to compensation of physical or economic injury resulting from unconsented touching (no matter how well intentioned or expertly conducted), to punitive awards for particularly culpable touchings. RESTATEMENT (SECOND) OF TORTS §§ 901, 903, 905, 907, 908 (1979); *see also* PROSSER & KEETON, *supra* note 18, § 9, at 40–41 ("Since battery is a matter of the worst kind of intentions, it is a tort which frequently justifies punitive damages.").

Protecting Patient Choice

autonomy in patients' relations with doctors, many aspects of the medical care relationship do not fit comfortably within the battery model. Doctors lack the antisocial motivation usually associated with intentional torts such as battery.[25] Further, unlike in the typical battery case, the patient usually has given a degree of consent to the doctor's treatment, if only in the broad sense that the patient has sought medical care from the doctor.

Once courts began more thoroughly to examine the subtleties of the doctor-patient relationship, the difficulties inherent in applying battery analysis to problems of medical consent became impossible to ignore. On the one hand, a general consent to treatment given without awareness of risks, prognoses, and options was seen as an insufficient basis upon which to authorize treatment, even medically defensible treatment.[26] Yet to hold that such uninformed consent was invalid, thereby subjecting doctors to actions for battery, threatened to yield unacceptably harsh results. Given the absolute nature of battery, the narrowness of its defenses, and the breadth of its remedies, doctors could end up paying significant damages after providing faultless medical treatment, simply because some minor informational aspect of the consent process was questioned.[27]

---

25. This point is stressed in many cases, *e.g.*, Trogun v. Fruchtman, 58 Wis. 2d 596, 599, 207 N.W.2d 297, 313 (1973).

26. *See* Canterbury v. Spence, 464 F.2d 772, 782 (D.C. Cir.), *cert. denied*, 409 U.S. 1064 (1972).

27. *See, e.g.*, Berkey v. Anderson, 1 Cal. App. 3d 790, 804, 82 Cal. Rptr. 67, 77 (1969) (issue of technical battery raised by failure to disclose risks of myelogram); Fogal v. Genesee Hospital, 41 A.D.2d 468, 344 N.Y.S.2d 552, 559 (1973) (failure to disclose risks of using hypothermia blanket cognizable under theory of assault and battery rather than negligence); Congrove v. Holmes, 37 Ohio Misc. 95, 308 N.E.2d 765 (C.P. Ross County 1973) (summary judgment for plaintiff for damages for paralysis of vocal cords resulting from thyroidectomy, where physician did not warn of risks); Cooper v. Roberts, 220 Pa. Super. 260, 286 A.2d 647 (1971) (assault and battery theory applies where doctor failed to inform patient of collateral risks of perforation of stomach during gastroscopic examination).

These results are possible because battery doctrine employs a very simple analysis of causation. *See* Plant, *An Analysis of "Informed Consent,"* 36 FORDHAM L. REV. 639, 666 (1968) [hereinafter cited as Plant, *Analysis*]. Presumably this is because ordinarily a battery defendant's conduct is assumed to be antisocial and not deserving of the protection of more thorough causal analysis. PROSSER & KEE-TON, *supra* note 18, § 9, at 35, § 43, at 263; Riskin, *Informed Consent: Looking for the Action*, 1975 U. ILL. L.F. 580, 583-84. Thus, battery analysis does not inquire whether the patient would have consented if the doctor had acted properly. Battery doctrine treats the consent, if flawed, as *completely* invalid. *See* W. PROSSER, HANDBOOK OF THE LAW OF TORTS, § 32, at 165 (4th ed. 1971). The likely result would be recovery of all damages, even if the injury was likely to have occurred in any case because the patient would have consented. *See* Riskin, *supra*, at 583-84, 601; *cf.* King, *Causation, Valuation and Chance in Personal Injury Torts Involving Preexisting Conditions and Future Consequences*, 90 YALE L.J. 1353 (1981) (critiquing tendency in present tort law to confuse issues of causation and valuation).

If battery doctrine had continued to be applied to medical consent, some more sophisticated (and more fair) fashion of handling causation and damages might have developed. Such a development might parallel earlier decisions in cases of medical battery that allowed a set-off for benefits derived from unauthorized treatment to reduce damages for injury to a dignitary interest. *See, e.g.*, Mohr v. Williams, 95 Minn. 261, 104 N.W. 12 (1905) (taking into account benefits from unauthorized operation on plaintiff's ear); McCandless v. State, 3 A.D.2d 600, 162 N.Y.S.2d 570 (1957) (award for unauthorized abortion reduced by offset for improvement in condition), *aff'd*, 4 N.Y.S.2d 797, 149 N.E.2d 530, 173 N.Y.S.2d 30, (1958). *But see* D. DOBBS, LAW OF REMEDIES 182 (1973) (question-ing wisdom of offsetting for benefits received in context of intentional tort). However, the transfer of

The Yale Law Journal   Vol. 95: 219, 1985

Discomfort with treating doctors under a doctrine aimed at antisocial conduct has prompted most jurisdictions to limit the battery action to those relatively unusual situations where a medical procedure has been carried out without *any* consent, rather than where the consent has merely been insufficiently informed.[28] The modern allegation of battery typically arises when consent to a particular procedure is given and a different or additional procedure is carried out.[29] The relative infrequency with which battery claims arise today should not, however, obscure the fact that battery doctrine retains a critical philosophical and practical function in protecting patient self-determination.

2. *Informed Consent*[30]

Most litigation about patient autonomy now occurs over doctors' nondisclosure of information, analyzed as an issue of professional negligence.[31] Doctors' responsibility for professional care of patients' physical

---

most disclosure issues to analysis under negligence doctrine removed the necessity for such a development.

28. *See, e.g.*, Cobbs v. Grant, 8 Cal. 3d 229, 240, 502 P.2d 1, 8, 104 Cal. Rptr. 505, 512 (1972) ("We agree with the majority trend. The battery theory should be reserved for those circumstances when a doctor performs an operation to which the patient has not consented."); Trogun v. Fruchtman, 58 Wis. 2d 596, 598–600, 207 N.W.2d 297, 312–13 (1973) (explaining why battery action is appropriate where operation is unauthorized but not where only issue is nondisclosure). At least one state has abolished any action for medical battery. *See* ARIZ. REV. STAT. ANN. § 12-562(B) (1982).

29. *See, e.g.*, Reddington v. Clayman, 334 Mass. 244, 134 N.E.2d 920 (1956) (question of battery presented where surgeon allegedly removed child's uvula during operation for removal of tonsils and adenoids); Hively v. Higgs, 120 Or. 588, 253 P. 363 (1927) (where consent given to operate on septum of nose, removal of tonsils constitutes battery).

The most difficult decisions concern the scope of a consent. *See, e.g.*, Kinikin v. Heupel, 305 N.W.2d 589 (Minn. 1981) (upheld jury verdict on battery theory regarding removal of more of breast than patient intended); Gray v. Grunnagle, 423 Pa. 144, 223 A.2d 663 (1966) (patient's claim that he consented only to exploratory surgery, not to laminectomy, should have gone to jury on battery claim); *see also* A. ROSOFF, INFORMED CONSENT: A GUIDE FOR HEALTH CARE PROVIDERS 8–13 (1981) (discussing factors leading courts to accept or refuse battery theory in disputes over scope of consent).

30. The literature on informed consent is voluminous. Some of the articles that emphasize the importance of patient autonomy include: J. KATZ, *supra* note 7, at 104–64; J. KATZ & A. CAPRON, CATASTROPHIC DISEASES: WHO DECIDES WHAT? 82–85 (1975); Epstein, *supra* note 17, at 87, 119; Goldstein, *supra* note 2, at 695 nn.27–29; Katz, *Informed Consent, supra* note 15; Meisel, *Exceptions, supra* note 4, at 413–22; Riskin, *supra* note 27; White, *supra* note 15. For additional sources on the doctrine, see Capron, *Informed Consent in Catastrophic Disease Research and Treatment*, 123 U. PA. L. REV. 340 (1974); Hagman, *The Medical Patient's Right to Know: Report on a Medical-Legal-Ethical, Empirical Study*, 17 UCLA L. REV. 758 (1970); Meisel, *Expansion, supra* note 6; Meisel & Kabnick, *Informed Consent to Medical Treatment: An Analysis of Recent Legislation*, 41 U. PITT. L. REV. 407 (1980); Plant, *Analysis, supra* note 27; Plant, *The Decline of "Informed Consent,"* 35 WASH. & LEE L. REV. 91 (1978); Waltz & Scheuneman, *Informed Consent to Therapy*, 64 Nw. U.L. REV. 628 (1969); Note, *Informed Consent and the Dying Patient*, 83 YALE L.J. 1632 (1974); Note, *Informed Consent in Medical Malpractice*, 55 CAL. L. REV. 1396 (1967); Note, *Restructuring Informed Consent: Legal Therapy for the Doctor-Patient Relationship*, 79 YALE L. J. 1533 (1970) [hereinafter cited as Note, *Restructuring*]. For a review and synopsis of the vast array of empirical studies in the area, see Meisel & Roth, *Toward an Informed Discussion of Informed Consent: A Review and Critique of the Empirical Studies*, 25 ARIZ L. REV. 265 (1983).

31. PROSSER & KEETON, *supra* note 18, §§ 15, 30, at 106, 165.

Protecting Patient Choice

well-being gives rise to various specific duties, one of which is the provision of sufficient information to allow a patient's decision to be intelligently informed. To recover for nondisclosure under the rules of professional malpractice, the patient must first show a violation of the duty to inform, defined in many states by the standard of expert professionals.[32] Second, the nondisclosure must be shown to have caused a harm cognizable under negligence doctrine. Most states have adopted an objective standard of causation in medical informed consent cases.[33] This standard requires the patient to show that the undisclosed information would have induced not just this patient, but a reasonable patient, to withhold consent to the treatment in question.[34]

3. *The Justifying Prototype*

The shift to negligence analysis made apparent analytic and practical sense.[35] Although some critics decried losses to patient autonomy that would result from emerging negligence rules,[36] current legal protection of patient autonomy has generally been deemed adequate. That judgment, however, rests upon assumptions that are insufficiently examined and ultimately erroneous.

Assumptions that have implicitly governed the debate over patient autonomy are exposed in a prototypical example of informed consent that is frequently used in discussion and reflected in litigation.[37] The doctor pro-

---

32. For a state by state summary, see 3 MAKING DECISIONS, *supra* note 2, at 206–45. *See also* J. AREEN, P. KING, S. GOLDBERG & A. CAPRON, LAW, SCIENCE AND MEDICINE 384 n.4 (1984) (interpreting evidence gathered in MAKING DECISIONS as follows: "[A]s of 1982, 26 states that had declared law on informed consent had adopted a professional standard of disclosure, 19 a patient-oriented standard, and 6 had no law on the subject.").

33. *See* 3 MAKING DECISIONS, *supra* note 2, at 197, 206–45. Although commentators have urged the subjective standard, *e.g.*, Katz, *Informed Consent, supra* note 15, at 163–64, only one state at present seems to have explicitly embraced it, *see* Scott v. Bradford, 606 P.2d 554, 559 (Okla. 1980).

34. *See, e.g.*, Canterbury v. Spence, 464 F.2d 772, 791 (D.C. Cir.), *cert. denied*, 409 U.S. 1064 (1972).

35. Protection of patient choice was thought to contribute to the "malpractice crisis" and health care cost escalation. *See* Bly v. Rhoads, 216 Va. 645, 222 S.E.2d 783 (1976); J. LUDLUM, INFORMED CONSENT 41–42 (1978); Adams & Zuckerman, *Variation in the Growth and Incidence of Medical Malpractice Claims*, 9 J. HEALTH POL., POL'Y & L. 475, 485 (1984) (principle of informed consent is significantly associated with higher annual rate of claims after 1972); Miller, *Informed Consent: I*, 244 J. A.M.A. 2100, 2102 (1980).

36. *See, e.g.*, Goldstein, *supra* note 2, at 691; Katz, *Informed Consent, supra* note 15, at 139; Meisel, *Expansion, supra* note 6, at 112.

37. Not all elements of the prototype are evident in every case or every discussion, but they recur often enough to be a legitimate composite. For instance, surgical cases overwhelmingly dominate the exhaustive list of cases summarized by Rosoff. *See* A. ROSOFF, *supra* note 29, at 471–520 (case index). A number of the leading and most frequently discussed cases involve such a prototype. *See, e.g.*, Canterbury v. Spence, 464 F.2d 772 (D.C. Cir. 1972) (undisclosed risks of surgery), *cert. denied*, 409 U.S. 1064 (1972); Cobbs v. Grant, 8 Cal. 3d 229, 502 P.2d 1, 104 Cal. Rptr. 505 (1972) (same); Salgo v. Leland Stanford Jr. Univ. Bd. of Trustees, 154 Cal. App. 2d 560, 317 P.2d 170 (1957) (same).

poses crucial surgery to a seriously ill patient. The surgery offers the patient's best hope for recovery; no viable alternatives exist. The surgical intervention is competently recommended and competently carried out. The doctor's only failing is nondisclosure of a low-probability risk of complication, such as the possibility of allergic reaction to the anesthetic. The allergic reaction occurs, the patient suffers injury, and the doctor is sued for failure to secure informed consent.

The surgery in the prototype is an invasive touching that requires consent; if there is a conflict between doctor and patient over the advisability of doing the surgery, the competent patient's choice will prevail, as required by battery doctrine. Under modern analysis, the consent, if given, remains valid,[38] and issues of nondisclosure will be analyzed under negligence doctrines governing duties to inform. There will be recovery only if the disclosure is one that would have been made by competent doctors, if a reasonable person in the patient's position would have refused the surgery had the disclosure been made, and if the injury is cognizable under standard negligence principles.

In the context of this example, those limitations seem reasonable; the potential for injury appears to be rather slight. As a reasonable person, the patient would presumably have agreed to the surgery even had the omitted disclosure been made. After all, the information that is undisclosed concerns a remote risk, the patient is seriously ill, and the surgery is the only viable treatment. Thus, although individualists will stress that in not disclosing all the facts the doctor has injured the patient's dignity and integrity,[39] many—perhaps most—will on these facts construe such an injury to be largely symbolic. Moreover, a patient who would not have consented to the surgery on these facts is aberrational. The idiosyncratic and the symbolic do receive some protection under the rules of battery: Basic, if not fully and exhaustively informed, consent is required in surgical cases. Where other important interests such as fairness to doctor-defendants or medical cost escalation are involved, it may plausibly be argued that such absolute protection need not be extended to the relatively less crucial disclosure of information about remote risks.

On the other hand, the argument continues, in a situation where the doctor's recommendation of surgery was one that a reasonable person would not have accepted had disclosure been made (as might be the case if the illness were minor and the undisclosed risk severe or likely to occur), in all likelihood the recommendation itself was probably "wrong." If the

---

38. Under earlier analyses, evidence of the nondisclosure regarding a possible allergic reaction would have invalidated the consent, potentially yielding recovery under a battery theory for all consequences of the surgery no matter how faultlessly performed. *See supra* note 27.

39. *See, e.g.,* Goldstein, *supra* note 2.

Protecting Patient Choice

recommendation was wrong, it would presumably be sanctioned under the mainstream rules governing professional competence. Thus, if the informed consent action involved nondisclosures that led to reasonably avoided and significant harms, it would seem to be largely duplicative of an action in professional negligence.

Consequently, although autonomy remains an important value in theory, the prototypical example makes strong protection of patient choice seem largely unnecessary in fact. The patient's interest in autonomy is conceded basic protection under battery rules. Beyond that, under the prototype, the autonomy interest tends to be seen as either mainly symbolic or highly aberrational on the one hand, or as largely redundant to protections under competence-regulating negligence rules on the other. Thus, in the prototypical case, present doctrines may be argued to provide adequate protection for patient autonomy.

But the prototypical case is not representative of the full range of cases in which the autonomy interest is implicated. The conclusion regarding the adequacy of current protection of patient autonomy derives from the prototype's unwarranted assumptions, first, about the respective roles of physical contact and information in medical choice, and second, about the relationship between injuries to autonomy and injuries to physical well-being. As a result, the prototype both underestimates the degree to which professional preemption of patient autonomy can occur and overestimates the degree to which regulation of medical expertise provides an adequate backup for doctrines safeguarding patient choice. Part II challenges these assumptions and demonstrates how they have led to unacceptable flaws in present legal protection for patient autonomy.

II. FLAWS IN EXISTING PROTECTION OF PATIENT AUTONOMY

A. *Choices That Involve No Physical Touching Receive No Protection Under Battery Doctrine*

The doctrinal prototype described above assumes that important medical decisions are implemented through actual physical touching. Defining the scope of an autonomy interest in terms of physical contact with the body has intuitive appeal and offers a certain simplicity of administration. But ultimately, physical contact is too literal a demarcation for what is a much broader, non-tangible interest in patient choice.[40]

---

40. Just as electronic sophistication made earlier notions of search and seizure insufficient and required the expansion of privacy protection beyond limits on purely physical invasions, *see* Katz v. United States, 389 U.S. 347 (1967), modern medical care requires a more flexible, less literal definition of the interest in patient autonomy than can be achieved through analysis based on physical contact.

Health care choices of vast consequence can be made and implemented without such bodily contact as predictably triggers battery analysis. Most notably, this occurs when a doctor makes a decision not to act. For instance, a doctor's judgment that a given level of diagnostic clarity is sufficient, that an acceptable outcome of treatment has been achieved, or that no medical treatment can be administered, each has potentially grave ramifications for the patient. As much as any that involve literal touching, such judgments implicate important autonomy interests; yet under touch-oriented rules they need not receive the patient's consent.

For example, in initial testing to determine the cause of eye problems, the patient in *Gates v. Jensen*[41] showed results consistent with borderline glaucoma. The doctor undertook further diagnostic testing, and ultimately concluded that the patient's problems derived not from glaucoma but from contact lens irritation. He chose not to perform further tests that could with greater certainty have determined the presence or absence of glaucoma. Instead, the doctor prescribed treatment for what he thought to be the problem. After Ms. Gates became legally blind, it was determined that she did have glaucoma, and that it could have been treated and controlled had it been identified earlier.[42] The doctor's decision not to undertake further diagnostic testing for glaucoma was not expressed as a recommendation to the patient. Rather, the doctor exercised his own judgment unilaterally, on the patient's behalf. Yet, because the doctor's judgment involved no touching of Ms. Gates' body, there was no potential battery: No consent to this "non-action" was required under that doctrine.

The choice of which Ms. Gates was deprived—whether to undergo further testing for glaucoma—was certainly as important as the one she was given—whether to undergo treatment for the contact lens problem. Analyzed in terms of her interest in autonomy rather than her literal physical security, this patient's opportunity to adopt, reject or modify the doctor's unvocalized "recommendation" of inaction should have received as much protection as the choice about the contact lens treatment.

Because the prototypical touching over which the vast bulk of doctor-patient litigation has taken place is surgery,[43] not even all *actions* by doctors will trigger battery analysis of patient consent. Where medical proposals involve less discrete or less invasive conduct than surgery, protection for the patient's interest in choice becomes correspondingly attenuated.[44] For instance, only one court seems to have applied battery

---

41. 92 Wash. 2d 246, 595 P.2d 919 (1979) (en banc).
42. *Id.* at 250, 595 P.2d at 924.
43. *See* A. ROSOFF, *supra* note 29, at 471–520 (index of cases litigated, by category).
44. Thus in the survey conducted for the President's Commission by Harris Associates, 53% of doctors indicated that they sought neither written nor oral consent for prescriptions, and 43% sought neither type of consent for blood tests. 2 MAKING DECISIONS, *supra* note 2, at 168. Outside the realm

Protecting Patient Choice

rules to the prescription of medication, and that case involved atypical factors.[45] Writing a "No-Code" order in a patient's chart, like a choice not to write such an order, will not require patient choice under touch-triggered rules.[46] Consent requirements also may not be triggered when there is a continuing course of action, even when new information makes new choices available. Thus, when a patient enters a hospital, a consent form for hospitalization, including routine physical touching, is normally signed. If, however, after some period of treatment it becomes clear that a given patient's condition is medically hopeless, the patient may not get a renewed opportunity to consent to the doctor's recommended course of treatment. Where the doctor in effect recommends continued hospitalization by failing to recommend possibilities such as going home to die or going to a hospice, her recommendations may well be imposed by default.

Thus, although courts have explained their concern over patient consent in terms of autonomy values,[47] by confounding autonomy with control

---

of surgery or major and invasive diagnostic tests, there is little clarity about when specific consent is required, as has been demonstrated by the empirical research of Meisel and Lidz. *Id.* at 328–35.

45.   The aberrant case is Mink v. University of Chicago, 460 F. Supp. 713 (N.D. Ill. 1978) (for discussion of case, see *infra* Part III(A)(1)). Most prescriptions are not analyzed as potential battery. *See* 2 MAKING DECISIONS, *supra* note 2, at 333–34; 3 MAKING DECISIONS, *supra* note 2, at 16–17. Two possible reasons not to apply battery analysis to prescriptions can be suggested. First, although physical consequences may be significant, the doctor does not touch the patient at all. The doctor's behavior in prescribing drugs is essentially judgmental and intellectual. Second, battery analysis may be rejected because patients are deemed to have consented through their voluntary use of the drugs. Such implied consents are often suspect, however. *See* A. ROSOFF, *supra* note 29, at 5–6. Because courts do not in these instances analyze whether the implied consent is valid, it seems likely that no potential battery is perceived.

Compare the partly analogous problem of patient control over forced feeding. *See, e.g.,* Bouvia v. County of Riverside, No. 159780 (Cal. Super. Ct. Dec. 16, 1983) (refusing to restrain hospital from force-feeding a patient who wished to die); *see also* Dresser, *Feeding the Hunger Artists: Legal Issues in Treating Anorexia Nervosa,* 1984 WIS. L. REV. 297 (analyzing legal grounds for force-feeding anorexics).

46.   If mentally competent and sufficiently aware, patients could initiate such decisions. However, it is hard for patients to focus on available options unless someone isolates these options from business as usual and makes them visible. The tendency toward passivity and inertia among the ill is widely acknowledged. *See* Parsons, *Epilogue* to THE DOCTOR-PATIENT RELATIONSHIP IN THE CHANGING HEALTH SCENE 445–46 (E. Gallagher ed. 1978).

Although some doctors may voluntarily consult with patients, little in their professional training will encourage them to do so. Professor Katz analyzes doctors' disinclination to initiate consultation as "a systematic and intentional omission based upon deeply held professional beliefs that silence is in the patient's best interest." J. KATZ, *supra* note 7, at 58.

The President's Commission for the Study of Ethical Problems in Medicine and Behavioral Research found that only 52% of physicians say they would initiate discussion of resuscitation with a patient in the last stages of a degenerative disease; 38% said they would not do so. 2 MAKING DECISIONS, *supra* note 2, at 226. By contrast, 79% of the public feels that a decision between aggressive and supportive therapy should be made by the patient. Only 12% feel the physician should make the decision unilaterally and 8% think it should be made jointly; 24% believe the patient should control. J. KATZ, *supra* note 7, at 224–25. Professor Katz notes the special difficulties faced in communicating honestly about death. *Id.* at 215–25. *See also* Comment, *A Structural Analysis of the Physician-Patient Relationship in No-Code Decisionmaking,* 93 YALE L.J. 362 (1983) (patient should control decisions whether or not to resuscitate through system of informed consent).

47.   *E.g.,* Natanson v. Kline, 186 Kan. 393, 406, 350 P.2d 1093, 1104 (1960) ("Anglo-American

over physical contact they have left significant medical choices insulated from patient control. Although safeguarding the body's physical perimeter is important, medical care is affirmatively sought, and contact with the body is a relatively unexceptional aspect of that care. The maintenance of personal autonomy in a situation of dependence on expert knowledge and skill is both more subtle and more significant. If the key issue is knowledge and choice regarding the fate of one's body, there is no meaningful difference between a decision that will be implemented by touching the body and one that will be implemented without doing so. Physical invasions have symbolic importance, and they constitute one important class of situations in which autonomy interests are involved. To treat that subcategory as co-extensive with the autonomy interest as a whole, however, creates grave deficiencies in the protection of the broader interest.

B. *Negligence Doctrine Embeds Protection of Patient Choice Within the Interest in Physical Well-Being*

Informed consent is a subcategory of professional negligence doctrine.[48] Standard negligence analysis protects an interest in physical well-being. The doctrine of informed consent injects into the established framework of negligence a concern with patient choice that would otherwise be absent. It recognizes that one way that actionable physical injury may occur is through the failure to disclose information that would have resulted in non-consent to treatment. The concern with choice does not, however, rise to the level of a fully protected interest under negligence doctrine. Rather, choice remains encapsulated within the dominant interest in physical well-being.

The subordination of choice that results from its submergence within the negligence analysis of physical injury reflects a pervasive fear that plaintiffs making such claims will recover when they have not "really" been injured, or that doctors will be held liable when they have not "really" done anything wrong. Moreover, the tendency to assume that reasonable people choose as their doctors tell them to leads to a conclusion that patients' choices will in any event mimic professionals' competent choices. Any "real" and deserving injuries would then be remedied under standard (i.e. non-choice oriented) professional negligence analyses. The importance of separately protecting patient autonomy would greatly diminish.

The following sections trace the distortion of the interest in choice that

---

law starts with the premise of thorough-going self-determination."); Pratt v. Davis, 118 Ill. App. 161, 166 (1905), *aff'd*, 224 Ill. 300, 79 N.E. 562 (1906) (consent prior to surgery is essential to maintenance of right to inviolability of individual).

48. PROSSER & KEETON, *supra* note 18, § 32, at 189–93.

Protecting Patient Choice

takes place at each stage of the standard negligence analysis and demonstrate that although the chain of assumptions that informs that analysis
may be accurate with reference to the prototype, these assumptions are
false as applied to nonprototypical cases.

1. *Duty to Disclose: Physical Contact Revisited*

Because informed consent is the doctrinal category that introduces a
concern about patient autonomy into the standard negligence analysis,
whether or not a case is classified as one of informed consent often determines whether patient autonomy will receive *any* protection. Although
many aspects of informed consent have been exhaustively discussed, little
attention has been paid to when the doctrine is applied. The physical parameters of battery analysis are definitional and unsurprising. More unexpected is the fact that, as this section will demonstrate, negligence analysis also uses physical contact to determine when to impose a duty to
disclose for purposes of securing informed consent. Negligence analysis
may employ physical contact as a limiting device on professional duty because habits of thought have been carried over from battery. Or, as discussed above, the limitation may reflect suspicion about the legitimacy of
the informed consent action.[49] Whatever the reason, adoption of physical
contact as the triggering concept for negligence duties creates additional
gaps in the protection afforded to patient choice.

a. *The Duty to Disclose Will Be Abandoned*

A New York decision, *Karlsons v. Guerinot*,[50] illustrates how a duty of
disclosure may be abandoned where facts do not fit the standard prototype
of a proposal to touch. The plaintiff, a thirty-seven-year-old woman, alleged negligent care based on her doctor's failure to perform amniocentesis, a procedure that would have identified Down's Syndrome in her
fetus early enough to perform an abortion. She also alleged denial of informed consent based on her doctor's failure to inform her of the existence
of the amniocentesis procedure. Allegedly as a result of these failings, she
bore a defective child whom she would rather have aborted. She and her
husband sought damages for pain and suffering, mental anguish, and for
medical and other expenses of rearing the child.[51]

In *Karlsons* the court held that, in the absence of any proposed touch-

---

49. Such an approach would be comparable to special limiting requirements on actions for emotional distress. *See* RESTATEMENT (SECOND) OF TORTS § 46(2)(b) (1965).

50. 57 A.D.2d 73, 394 N.Y.S.2d 933 (1977).

51. Although several other causes of action are alleged in the case, *id.* at 75, 394 N.Y.S.2d at 934,
these are the ones crucial to the analysis here.

ing or invasion of the body, no issue of informed consent could properly be raised:[52]

> Although [our earlier] pronouncement of the scope of the [informed consent] doctrine seems broad on its face, its application has consistently been limited to those situations where the harm suffered arose from some affirmative violation of the patient's physical integrity such as surgical procedures, injections or invasive diagnostic tests.[53]

Resting its conclusion on both common law and statutory grounds,[54] the court affirmed the lower court's dismissal of the informed consent cause of action.[55]

How serious a problem was the dismissal of the informed consent count?[56] In instances of invasive touching, battery doctrine dictates that patients are to make decisions about their own care. A doctor's responsibilities for professionally competent care must then be to know, to advise and recommend, and to implement, but *not* to decide.[57] I have argued that autonomy interests are as compelling where non-invasive decisions are involved as they are where touching is proposed. However, where no touching is proposed, patient decisionmaking may be ignored not only under

---

52. Wrongful birth actions have surfaced in the wake of new genetic technology and altered public policy. Although they were originally treated as presenting standard medical malpractice and consent issues, special rules have now emerged in these cases. *See generally* Capron, *Tort Liability in Genetic Counseling*, 79 COLUM. L. REV. 618 (1979) (examining liability for birth of child with condition that if diagnosed early enough would have led parents to avoid such birth); Collins, *An Overview and Analysis: Prenatal Torts, Preconception Torts, Wrongful Life, Wrongful Death and Wrongful Birth: Time for a New Framework*, 22 J. FAM. L. 677, 695 (1983–84) (courts agree parents may state some cause of action based on wrong information, but disagree on proper measure of recovery); Robertson, *Civil Liability Arising from "Wrongful Birth" Following an Unsuccessful Sterilization Operation*, 4 AM. J.L. & MED. 131 (1978) (analyzing actions in both tort and contract for wrongful birth). In Part III, *infra*, I will argue that the need for different rules is not as situation-specific as analysis in these cases has suggested.

53. 57 A.D.2d at 87, 394 N.Y.S.2d at 939 (citations omitted); *accord* Malloy v. Shanahan, 280 Pa. Super. 440, 443, 421 A.2d 803, 804 (1980) ("The doctrine of informed consent has been applied only to suits involving surgical operations or procedure, wherein 'an operation without the patient's consent is a technical assault.' ") (quoting trial court, in turn quoting Gray v. Grunnagle, 423 Pa. 144, 155, 223 A.2d 663, 669 (1966)).

54. The court acknowledged that the statute it cited was not in effect at the time these facts took place. *Karlsons*, 57 A.D.2d at 82 n.4, 394 N.Y.S.2d at 939 n.4. Nevertheless, the court viewed the statute as providing an indication of legislative inclinations.

55. The *Karlsons* court also rejected the plaintiff's theory that disclosure of the procedure was required under the branch of informed consent dealing with disclosure of alternatives. *See infra* Part II(C).

56. Some patients may know about amniocentesis, unlike other medical information, independently of medical sources. The possibility of independent knowledge, however, should not reduce the scope of the doctor's duty. Rather, it should constitute an affirmative defense, with the doctor bearing the burden of proving the plaintiff's actual knowledge or the applicability of a common knowledge exception.

57. For a discussion of battery rules, see *supra* Part I(C).

Protecting Patient Choice

battery analysis, but also under negligence doctrine. Where choice is not identified as an interest, courts will impose no duty to disclose in order to inform the patient's consent. Yet, in these instances, receiving information from the doctor is the only way a patient can become aware of a pending choice. Nondisclosure here is tantamount to loss of the choice interest itself; only issues of professionally competent care remain.

Karlsons illustrates precisely that outcome. Having denied the existence of any issue of informed consent because of the absence of a proposal to touch, the court observed:

> [T]he alleged undisclosed risks did not relate to any affirmative treatment but rather to the condition of pregnancy itself. *Allegations such as these have traditionally formed the basis of actions in medical malpractice and not informed consent.*[58]

Using the framework of malpractice, the court only inquired into whether the treatment that the doctor recommended and actually implemented constituted professionally competent care of physical well-being. Thus, the sole issue regarding amniocentesis that the court allowed to be considered was: Did defendant doctors breach their duty of professional care "by not properly diagnosing the condition of the child"?[59]

The doctor's failure to recommend amniocentesis (and to implement it, thereby discovering those facts that the test would have revealed) might have been argued to be a failure of competent care. However, it is quite likely that what the court formulated as "not properly diagnosing the condition of the child"[60] would not have constituted professionally incompetent care, particularly in 1973.[61] Amniocentesis involves risks to the fetus. The test was not uniformly used in 1973, and the doctors could competently have held differing opinions about whether such a test should have been recommended.[62] Moreover, non-medical values about the ultimate issue, abortion, are so disproportionately important in the chain of decisions that the medical risks of amniocentesis pale by comparison. Thus, unless such recommendations are made purely on the basis of such medical matters as risk to the fetus, there is significant danger that a doctor's advice regarding amniocentesis might improperly be influenced by his personal values with regard to the issue of abortion. An expression of such

---

58. 57 A.D.2d at 82, 394 N.Y.S.2d at 939 (citations omitted and emphasis added).
59. *Id.* at 78, 394 N.Y.S.2d at 936.
60. *Id.*
61. *See* Capron, *supra* note 52, at 670–71. Professor Capron discusses the difficulty of establishing a standard of practice regarding new fields or procedures like genetic counseling. *Id.* at 620–25. Precisely the same facts that make difference of professional judgment acceptable make the case for disclosure and patient decision more compelling. *See infra* Part III.
62. *See* discussion of the limits of competence regulation *infra* Part III.

an opinion might be appropriate if the patient requested it, but absent such a request, the doctor might well claim that he properly made no recommendation regarding amniocentesis as a prelude to possible abortion.

For these reasons, it might have been both easy and legitimate for the doctor in *Karlsons* to defeat any allegation that failure to diagnose the fetal abnormality constituted professionally incompetent care.[63] Yet there should have been an additional issue derived from the concern with patient choice: Did the defendant doctors breach their duty to protect the patient's autonomy interest by not informing her of the existence of a test, amniocentesis, which could have been used, if the patient so chose, to detect fetal abnormalities? Protection of that interest was lost when the absence of a proposal to touch prompted the court to eliminate issues of disclosure from the case.[64]

Injuries arising from invasion of the interest in choice may be factually similar to injuries arising from failures of competent care. In *Karlsons*, if the doctor's failure to recommend amniocentesis had been judged to constitute professionally incompetent care, the resulting harm would have been the same as if injuries resulted from an invasion of the interest in choice: The parents would have had a child they would not otherwise have had. The possibility of such overlap may easily be construed as meaning that informed consent is nothing but a second, easier bite at the same apple of malpractice recovery.[65] Yet, although the injuries overlap, the analysis differs, because the interests at stake are different. Liability may legitimately be found under one analytic theory, although there is none under the other. If both concerns are to be vindicated, it is crucial to keep the two issues analytically distinct.

Where *Karlsons* illustrates loss of the choice interest in a pre-care diagnostic setting, *Kelton v. District of Columbia*[66] reflects an analogous gap in analysis of post-care nondisclosure. Six years after the delivery of her

---

63. The result would likely be tougher on the doctor if the issue were failure to know of amniocentesis. Such a failure to know of the procedure probably would be found professionally incompetent. Presently, issues of knowledge are often left unexamined because rules do not require inquiry beyond what the doctor recommended or did. The result may be that both incompetence (of knowledge) and inappropriate substitution of judgment go unremedied. For a discussion of the limits of competence regulation, see *infra* Part III. In any case, no such issue of the doctor's knowledge was formulated in *Karlsons*.

64. Professor Capron alludes to this problem but does not pursue it except to suggest that the goals of informed consent are applicable even though there is a lack of touching. Capron, *supra* note 52, at 629–30 n.36.

65. There is a suggestion of such attitudes in Meisel's description of how informed consent functions, Meisel, *Expansion*, *supra* note 6, at 74–77, and in Epstein's critique of the doctrine in which he states that there are "simply no principled limits to a doctrine of informed consent," Epstein, *supra* note 17, at 124.

66. 413 A.2d 919 (D.C. 1980).

Protecting Patient Choice

second child by Caesarian section, the plaintiff underwent exploratory surgery to determine why she had been unable to become pregnant a third time. Her surgeon discovered that there were scars on her fallopian tubes that were consistent with the performance of a tubal ligation or some surgical trauma. The plaintiff sued the doctor who delivered her second child. She alleged that she had not consented to any tubal ligation, nor had she been told of any intentional or accidental surgical intervention affecting her fallopian tubes. Her complaint alleging an unconsented sterilization (battery) was barred by the statute of limitations. However, the plaintiff also claimed that the doctor had breached a separate duty to *tell* her of the damage to her fallopian tubes, and that that claim regarding nondisclosure was timely under negligence limits.

If the plaintiff's allegations were true, she had been injured in several ways. She had been deprived of fertility without her knowledge or consent. The actions that produced this physical harm may have constituted either battery (if intentional) or negligence (if accidental). But the failure to disclose both the physical facts and the doctor's knowledge regarding how the damage came about constituted a different and additional harm. Even after the surgical trauma took place, Ms. Kelton still had a prospective interest in choice. Had she known about the scarring of her tubes, she might have sought surgical repair. At the very least, she would not have had to undergo additional surgery to determine why she was unable to conceive. Disclosure of the scarring would also have allowed her to exercise choice regarding non-medical consequences of the medical facts. Properly informed, Ms. Kelton might have sought to adopt further children, or she might have elected to file suit for the initial injury (the unconsented ligation).[67]

The *Kelton* court, like the *Karlsons* court, allowed a touch-based definition of disclosure requirements to eliminate the patient's interest in these choices. Distinguishing a leading informed consent case, *Canterbury v. Spence*,[68] as involving a failure to disclose risks of prospective surgery, the *Kelton* court upheld a dismissal under timeliness provisions on the ground that there was no cause of action other than battery.[69] The court

---

67. Loss of opportunity to file the battery action may not have been attributable to the doctor's failure to disclose the injury that had occurred. The plaintiff did not file a timely battery action when she did later discover the injury. It is not necessarily the case, however, that a similar delay would have occurred had she been informed earlier. In any event, the other injuries to her interest in choice could not be so easily dismissed.

68. 464 F.2d 772 (D.C. Cir.), *cert. denied*, 409 U.S. 1064 (1972).

69. The court may have seen the disclosure cause of action as a subterfuge to get around the statute of limitations in the "real" battery action. If the court was hostile to the disclosure action for this reason, it underscores the tendency to "see" choice-based disclosure issues within a narrow, precut pattern. For discussion of the duty to disclose malpractice, see Vogel & Delgado, *To Tell the Truth: Physicians' Duty to Disclose Medical Mistakes*, 28 UCLA L. Rev. 52 (1980) and *infra* Part

stated: "Thus a breach of duty to disclose [lack of consent] is not actionable in negligence unless it induces a patient's uninformed consent to a risky operation from which damages actually result."[70] The court's statement implies the following: Consent and consent-oriented disclosure duties arise only in surgery cases and only in advance of a proposed intervention, and such duties extend only to disclosure of the risks posed by the proposed intervention itself. This formulation of the rule ignores various types of disclosure essential to protection of patient autonomy.[71] Thus, while the court recognized that the patient's choice interest may have been violated if a tubal ligation was intentionally performed without the patient's consent, it failed to understand that a choice interest was also implicated in the nondisclosure of the facts after the intervention had occurred. As in *Karlsons*, analysis of disclosures essential to the protection of autonomy was foreclosed because the issue arose outside the touch-based parameters of the informed consent prototype.

b. *The Duty to Disclose Will Be Transposed*

Where a case does not involve physical touching, the issue of disclosure may not wholly disappear, as it did in *Karlsons* and *Kelton*. Instead, a duty to disclose may be considered, but analysis of that duty will shift when a case is not identified as one of informed consent. Where nothing signals the involvement of patient autonomy, duties to disclose will be transposed into issues about professional care of physical well-being. *Roark v. Allen*,[72] a 1982 case decided by the Texas Supreme Court, illustrates this pattern.

The plaintiffs were the parents of a baby allegedly injured during a breech birth. After the delivery, the defendant doctors noticed forceps indentations on the infant's head. They considered the possibility that the indentations might indicate a fractured skull, but after further examination decided that there was no fracture. No one informed the parents of the possibility of a skull fracture, nor were x-rays, which would have revealed the fracture, ordered. Weeks later, bilateral fractures of the infant's skull were detected and the problem was then corrected. The parents sued the obstetrician for negligent use of forceps and their family doctor for

---

III.
70. 413 A.2d at 922.
71. The court's statement also ignores the fact that failure to disclose information may in some situations actually be a failure to provide competent care. *See, e.g.*, Crosby v. Grandview Nursing Home, 290 A.2d 375 (Me. 1972) (failure of physician to advise regarding care of injured foot). The court probably makes this error because it assumes a usage whereby verbal communication necessary to competent care of physical well-being is called "instruction" or "advice."
72. 633 S.W.2d 804 (Tex. 1982), *aff'g in part, rev'g in part*, 625 S.W.2d 411 (Tex. Ct. App. 1981).

Protecting Patient Choice

failure to inform them of the possibility of skull fracture. The jury found for the plaintiffs against both doctors.[73]

The failure of the family doctor to inform the parents of the possibility of skull fracture is the primary concern here. The Texas Supreme Court objected to the lower court's use of informed consent theories to analyze this issue. According to the court, informed consent applies "only to medical procedures which have yet to be performed and . . . it is inapplicable . . . where the patient has already undergone the proposed treatment and been injured."[74] Characterizing this type of nondisclosure as "a totally different cause of action" from informed consent,[75] the court analyzed it as a problem of ordinary negligence and reversed the trial court's judgment for the plaintiff. The *Roark* court's method of arriving at that decision betrays the transposition of interests that occurs when informed consent analysis is deemed inapplicable.

The plaintiffs and the lower courts had posed this nondisclosure as a breach of a duty to protect the parents' interest in choice; they called it an action for lack of informed consent. Once the supreme court decided that informed consent doctrine did not apply, it abandoned the interest in choice and analyzed disclosure in light of the traditional negligence interest in professionally competent care of physical well-being. The court observed that expert testimony was essential to evaluate the duty because "diagnosis of skull fractures is not within the experience of the ordinary layman."[76] This characterization shifted the issue from one of informing about possible courses of action to one of diagnosing skull fractures. The

---

73. *Id.* at 807–08. The Texas Supreme Court affirmed the court of appeals' reversal of the verdict against the obstetrician, albeit on a different ground (that although he was negligent in his use of the forceps, the causal connection between this negligence and the baby's injuries was not sufficiently established). *Id.* at 811. *Roark* illustrates that, even where there is a finding of incompetent care that produces a harm factually similar to the harm resulting from invasion of autonomy, analysis of the autonomy interest would not be redundant.

74. *Id.* at 808. The court seems unwilling to acknowledge that the distinction between pre-care and post-care is largely semantic. This case could be described as one involving a need for further diagnosis and care as a result of birth injuries. Indeed the trial court used just such a phrasing. *Id.*

75. *Id.*

76. *Id.* at 809. At the time the facts occurred, Texas also required expert testimony to establish the standard of care in informed consent actions. *See* Wilson v. Scott, 412 S.W.2d 299, 302 (Tex. 1967). The way the issues are posed in these two actions, however, differs. In an informed consent action, the law itself establishes that there is a choice to be made by the patient; only then does it require medical evidence regarding what a competent doctor would have disclosed to the patient making that choice. Thus *Wilson*, the leading Texas informed consent case, states: "Physicians . . . have a duty to make a reasonable disclosure to a patient . . . based upon the patient's right . . . to exercise an informed consent . . . . [That duty is measured by what a reasonable doctor] would have disclosed to his patient about the risks incident to a proposed diagnosis or treatment . . . ." *Id.* at 301–02. If the law had required the patient's consent (here to a recommendation that the indentations need not be x-rayed), some disclosure, at least of the existence of a choice to be made, would have been necessary. By contrast, where no issue of informed consent is recognized, unless expert testimony is offered regarding the need to disclose, there may be no information given about the very existence of a choice to be made.

The Yale Law Journal   Vol. 95: 219, 1985

defendant's own testimony had been used to establish the standard of care. Asked whether the correct medical procedure would be to advise of the possibility that such a fracture existed, he replied, "Yes, if the fracture was assumed to be there."[77] The supreme court reversed a jury verdict for the plaintiffs, saying there was *no evidence* to support it because "the evidence is uncontroverted that Dr. Allen assumed a fracture did not exist."[78] What began as a question of informing patient choice ended as an issue of the doctor's diagnostic accuracy.[79]

Similarly, in *Sinkey v. Surgical Associates*,[80] the court began with an alleged duty to inform the parents of a child patient (regarding the opinions of a consulting radiologist) and transposed it into a different issue: Was the reading of the x-ray professionally competent? Again, the information was unconnected to any prototypical proposal to touch; the case was not identified as one of informed consent. Yet an interest in choice was probably the basis on which the plaintiff parents alleged that the information should have been communicated to them.[81] The Iowa Supreme Court affirmed a directed verdict for the defendant, saying:

> The second allegation of negligence is based on an asserted duty to advise the patient that the x-ray finding was consistent with appendicitis and that the radiologist's impression was appendicitis. . . .
> . . . .
> *We find no evidence to support the allegation of an incorrect interpretation of the x-ray* [by the attending doctor who diagnosed tonsilitis] *and hold that under these circumstances the doctor had no duty to advise the patient* of the fact that the condition shown in the x-ray was also consistent with appendicitis.[82]

If the allegation were that the doctor should have diagnosed the appendicitis, the competence of the x-ray reading would be critical. Where patient knowledge and choice are the concern, however, the competence of the reading is not the issue.

---

77.   Allen v. Roark, 625 S.W.2d 411, 415 (Tex. Ct. App. 1981), *aff'd in part, rev'd in part*, 633 S.W.2d 804 (Tex. 1982).

78.   Allen v. Roark, 633 S.W.2d at 809.

79.   This decision may have been technically acceptable. The court, however, could easily have taken the "yes" part of the defendant's answer as sufficient, particularly where it reversed the decision under a "no evidence" standard. Even if failure to make such a recommendation was not shown to be incompetent, as the court concluded here, the issue of disclosure for choice should still have remained live. As between the doctor and the parents, it ought to have been the parents' choice whether to incur risks and costs in order to determine with greater accuracy whether or not fractures were present.

80.   186 N.W.2d 658 (Iowa 1971).

81.   Where professionally competent care is the interest which requires verbal communication, that communication tends to be denominated "diagnosis," "advice," or "recommendation." Where the term "disclosure" is used, it ordinarily conveys a concern about patient autonomy.

82.   186 N.W.2d at 661 (emphasis added).

Protecting Patient Choice

Policies for evaluating the competence of doctors' diagnoses differ significantly from those involved in patient choice. The uncertainty of medical judgment legitimately excuses a failure to diagnose correctly, if the judgment was carefully and reasonably made. Such uncertainty should not, however, excuse a failure to disclose information that would have permitted a patient to exercise a different choice. Indeed, the more uncertain the medical judgment involved, the more reason there is to excuse a wrong diagnosis. But, the more uncertain the medical judgment, the less acceptable is the doctor's substitution of her judgment for the patient's. The courts in *Roark* and *Sinkey* applied notions of uncertainty appropriate to analysis of competent care rather than to analysis of disclosure to protect choice. Had the absence of a prototypical proposal to touch not prevented these issues from being recognized as questions of informed consent, the courts would, I think, have been less likely to make this mistake.[83]

2. *Duty To Disclose—Physical Contact Transcended?*

A requirement to disclose alternatives is sometimes mentioned in informed consent cases.[84] If broadly applied and interpreted, such a requirement could close some of the identified gaps in protection of choice, but the requirement to disclose alternatives is itself constricted by concepts centered on touching. Many jurisdictions impose no such disclosure requirements.[85] When they do, the mandate is typically to disclose only al-

---

83. The central tenet of classical informed consent doctrine is disclosure of risks, i.e., possible but uncertain occurrences. *Roark* is a relatively pure type under which the interest in choice is wholly abandoned. Sometimes when a case not falling within the prototypical boundaries of informed consent is treated as an instance of ordinary negligence, it is unclear whether the court analyzes disclosure as a duty derived from an interest in choice or from one in professionally competent care. Stills v. Gratton, 55 Cal. App. 3d 698, 127 Cal. Rptr. 652 (1976), provides an interesting example. The court's selection and discussion of facts, duty, standard of care, and damages reflect alternating and somewhat inconsistent concerns first with choice and then with competent care. Although, as a case treating disclosure under ordinary negligence doctrine, *Stills* provided a greater than average degree of protection for patient choice, that result was shaped by several atypical factors. The case involved the completeness of an abortion, a subject about which sensitivity to choice has been heightened. *See infra* Part III. Further, because two different doctors were involved, disclosure was factually separated from professional care. The same result might not be forthcoming in other circumstances.

84. *E.g.*, Scott v. Bradford, 606 P.2d 554, 557 (Okla. 1979); Siegel v. Mount Sinai Hosp., 62 Ohio App. 2d 12, 21, 403 N.E.2d 202, 209 (1978); Natanson v. Kline, 186 Kan. 393, 410, 350 P.2d 1093, 1106 (1960).

85. According to Andrews, only 10 of 23 statutes governing informed consent specifically require that the doctor disclose alternatives to treatment. Andrews, *Informed Consent Statutes and the Decisionmaking Process*, 5 J. LEGAL MED. 163, 197 (1984). Only a few cases squarely hold a doctor liable for failure to disclose alternatives. One such case is Archer v. Galbraith, 18 Wash. App. 369, 379, 567 P.2d 1155, 1161 (1977). *But cf.* Dunham v. Wright, 423 F.2d 940, 946 (3d Cir. 1970) (disclosure of alternatives not actionable when doctor determines patient has "no alternative"). Even when the issue is raised, courts often leave it to the jury, making no requirement as a matter of law. *See, e.g.*, Masquat v. Maguire, 638 P.2d 1105 (Okla. 1981) (for discussion of case, see *infra* note 133).

The Yale Law Journal   Vol. 95: 219, 1985

ternative treatments, not alternative diagnostic data, theories of the case, or courses for case management.[86] Disclosure requirements are rarely applied to situations of aftermath disclosure,[87] to situations in which no change in continuing treatment is proposed, or to situations where either no treatment is possible or none is proposed. Thus, the alternatives rule does not extend far enough to encompass many situations identified here as gaps in autonomy protection.

Developments in two states suggest potentially broader changes in the limitations that derive from negligence requirements for physical contact. In *Gates v. Jensen*,[88] the Washington Supreme Court selected the doctor's possession of knowledge, rather than his proposal to touch, as the occasion for a duty to inform the patient's choice. The court held that an ophthalmologist had an obligation to inform the patient of test results showing possible glaucoma even though he did not propose either to test further for that condition, or to treat it.

The jury found for the doctor on the plaintiff's claim that the ophthalmologist's failure to diagnose her glaucoma was professionally incompetent. Yet the doctor's failure to tell the patient that her tests showed borderline symptoms of the disease, and that further testing for it was

---

Andrews notes that only 14 percent of physicians surveyed by the President's Commission considered information about alternatives to be integral to informed consent. Andrews, *supra*, at 197. The enactment of statutes specifying exactly what alternatives are to be disclosed in particularly controversial circumstances provides further evidence of the inadequacy of general statutory or common law requirements. *E.g.*, CAL. HEALTH & SAFETY CODE § 1704.5 (West Supp. 1985) (failure to disclose alternative treatments of breast cancer constitutes unprofessional conduct). For a further discussion of the inadequacy of the present alternatives rules, see *infra* Part II(C).

86. For example, in one Washington case, Thornton v. Annest, 19 Wash. App. 174, 574 P.2d 1199 (1978), the defendant doctor performed a hysterectomy during exploratory surgery on the plaintiff, who had severe pelvic inflammatory disease. The plaintiff appealed a jury verdict for the defendant on the ground that the doctor's total failure to disclose alternatives should have entitled her to a partial directed verdict on the issue of informed consent. Concluding that the plaintiff's alleged alternatives were alternative methods of diagnosing rather than alternative treatments, the court upheld denial of the directed verdict. It stated that "[o]nly feasible and available treatment must be disclosed." *Id.* at 179, 574 P.2d at 1203. Under the court's analysis, no disclosure of alternative approaches to diagnosis is required, at least as a matter of law. As in *Karlsons*, when disclosure disappeared from the analysis, only the interest in professionally competent care remained. The court held that the jury might legitimately have concluded that the defendant had complied with the proper standard of care "in *performing* the exploratory surgery as a method of diagnosing plaintiff's symptoms." *Id.* at 180, 574 P.2d at 1203 (emphasis added).

Many cases discussed in this article (*Karlsons, Roark, Sinkey, Keogan*) involve disclosure about alternative diagnostic theories; others could be so characterized if artificial pre/post-care distinctions were abandoned (*Kelton*). In these cases the notion of disclosing alternatives did not convince the courts to accept an informed consent theory of the case. In *Karlsons*, disclosure under an alternatives theory was expressly rejected.

87. Judgments made by a doctor in the aftermath of medical intervention could be described as being the diagnostic process for a potential next stage of decision. Thus diagnosis could, at its most expansive, mean "alternative knowings." As this Article shows, however, courts have tended to freeze concepts like "diagnosis" and "consent" into narrow and literal meanings. Some more flexible and generic concept would be necessary to trigger adequate disclosure.

88. 92 Wash. 2d 246, 595 P.2d 919 (1979), *rev'g* 20 Wash. App. 81, 579 P.2d 374 (1979).

Protecting Patient Choice

possible, deprived her of the choice whether to consent to his recommendation that no further investigation of glaucoma be undertaken. Under the traditional approaches discussed above, the interest in that choice might well have been ignored.

No battery action would lie in *Gates* because there was no unconsented touch. Nor, under the interpretation employed by cases like *Karlsons*,[89] *Kelton*[90] or *Roark*,[91] would there be an obligation to disclose under informed consent doctrine. In accord with such interpretations, the defendant in *Gates* claimed that because he was still engaged in diagnostic assessment and had not yet recommended treatment, no duty to disclose had arisen.[92] But unlike courts in the cases discussed above, the Washington court did not allow the absence of a proposal to touch to eliminate the patient's interest in disclosure and choice.[93]

Although it purported only to apply existing informed consent law, the Washington court articulated what might have become a significant new standard: It ordered that a doctor should disclose whenever he has knowledge of a potentially dangerous abnormality in the patient's body.[94] Under this test, the occasion for disclosure would not be a proposed act of touching, but the doctor's possession of significant knowledge about the medical condition of the patient. The *Gates* standard, if allowed to develop, could have superceded touch-based boundaries that limit protection of patient choice interests to particular stages of treatment or to types of proposed intervention.

---

89. 57 A.D.2d 73, 394 N.Y.S.2d 933 (1977). *See supra* text accompanying notes 50–65 (discussing *Karlsons*).

90. 413 A.2d 919 (D.C. 1980). *See supra* text accompanying notes 66–71 (discussing *Kelton*).

91. 633 S.W.2d 804 (Tex. 1982). *See supra* text accompanying notes 72–79 (discussing *Roark*).

92. The intermediate court explicitly adopted this view in affirming the trial court's refusal to give informed consent instructions. 20 Wash. App. at 87, 579 P.2d at 377. Timeline factors *per se* continue to be suggested by some authors as appropriate considerations in creating duties of disclosure. *See* Comment, *Informed Consent in Washington: Expanded Scope of Material Facts that the Physician Must Disclose to His Patient*, 55 WASH. L. REV. 655, 667–70 (1980).

93. Unlike the court in *Thornton*, 19 Wash. App. 174, 574 P.2d 1199 (1978) (for discussion of case, see *supra* note 86), the court in *Gates* also refused to distinguish between diagnostic theories and proposals to treat for purposes of triggering a patient's interest in disclosure. *Gates*, 92 Wash. 2d at 250, 595 P.2d at 922.

94. In its summary of the facts, the court mentions that Ms. Gates asked about the result of the doctor's tests and was told that everything was all right, but the court does not characterize the problem as misrepresentation. The court phrased its broadened concept of an affirmative duty as follows: "The existence of an abnormal condition in one's body, the presence of a high risk of disease, and the existence of alternative diagnostic procedures to conclusively determine the presence or absence of that disease are all facts which a patient must know in order to make an informed decision on the *course which future medical care will take*." 92 Wash. 2d at 251, 595 P.2d at 923 (emphasis added). Although an improvement on a touch-based trigger, this formulation is still not optimal. It might not, for instance, encompass disclosure of the availability of amniocentesis.

Although the *Gates* court purported only to apply the rule of Miller v. Kennedy, 11 Wash. App. 272, 522 P.2d 852 (1974), *aff'd*, 85 Wash. 2d 151, 530 P.2d 334 (1975), *aff'd en banc*, 91 Wash. 2d 155, 588 P.2d 734 (1978), it is *Gates* which created a new standard not dependent on touching.

Gates was decided in a context of intense conflict over the adequacy of standards of professional negligence.[95] As a by-product of its dissatisfaction with the limitations of traditional competence regulation, the court seems to have become particularly sensitive to the unfairness entailed in relying on the judgment of professionals instead of patients.[96] However, faced with new medical facts, the same court, in *Keogan v. Holy Family Hospital*,[97] sharply limited the potential of *Gates*. In circumstances analytically similar to *Gates*,[98] five justices refused in *Keogan* to impose a duty of disclosure based on possession of knowledge.[99] Instead, like the court in *Karlsons*, they reverted to the assumption that, apart from instances involving touching, regulation of the doctor's competence was the only important issue.[100]

Gates has been criticized as interfering with proper professional judgment, indulging in the fantasy that a patient can "correct the reasonable errors of his physician."[101] Yet *Gates* glimpsed what *Keogan* lost sight of: Although the patient is not more competent in making judgments assessing the likelihood of a particular disease, she is more competent in deciding whether she wishes to undergo more tests and spend more money in order to be more certain about the diagnosis in her case.

---

95. In Helling v. Carey, 83 Wash. 2d 514, 519 P.2d 981 (1974), the court had held that reasonable prudence may require a standard of care higher than the prevailing professional standard. The state legislature responded by enacting WASH. REV. CODE ANN. § 4.24.290 (West Supp. 1986), requiring a plaintiff to demonstrate that the practitioner "failed to exercise that degree of skill, care, and learning possessed at that time by other persons in the same profession . . . ." The *Gates* court, however, interpreted the statute in a fashion that allowed it to continue to apply the doctrine of *Helling. See* 92 Wash. 2d at 253–54, 595 P.2d at 924.

96. Because doctors are incompetent only when they fail to act as other doctors would, there is no external referent by which to judge what are, essentially, questions of utility, e.g., how much certainty about the presence of glaucoma is adequate. The patient could provide a determinate referent by deciding the personal value of additional tests or procedures. Another source for such evaluations would be social decisions allocating collective resources through collective cost-benefit analyses. In *Gates* the court used both tools. It expanded a doctor's obligation to respect patient choice, and it permitted a societal cost-benefit analysis of the adequacy of care by allowing a jury to decide that reliance on the prevailing professional standard was insufficient.

97. 95 Wash. 2d 306, 622 P.2d 1246 (1980).

98. A doctor had obtained results suggesting but not confirming that heart disease was a possible cause of plaintiff's chest pains. As in *Gates*, the doctor concluded that problems other than heart disease lay at the root of the patient's symptoms, and made no disclosure of the possibility of heart disease or of the test results. The patient later died from a heart attack. *Id.* at 307–08, 622 P.2d at 1249.

99. *Id.* at 330–31, 622 P.2d at 1261. The precedential effect of the opinion is uncertain. Justice Horowitz's opinion, purporting to be the opinion of the court, was joined by two other justices on the matter of disclosure under *Gates*. The dissent, refusing to apply *Gates*, however, was signed by five justices. A rehearing was granted, but the case was settled before the rehearing was held. Thus *Keogan* did not directly reverse *Gates*, but it did undermine the holding.

100. Five justices signed an opinion stating that, "[i]f Dr. Snyder was negligent because he should have discovered Keogan's diseased heart and failed to do so, that is what should be alleged and proved . . . . This court with its benefit of hindsight should not now enter the fray . . . with rulings as a matter of law as to what the doctor should have told the patient." *Id.*

101. Comment, *supra* note 92, at 673.

Protecting Patient Choice

Several recent California cases have also taken steps away from physical contact as the definitive occasion for choice-oriented disclosure. In *Truman v. Thomas*,[102] a thirty-year-old woman several times declined to have a Pap Smear that her gynecologist recommended, sometimes saying she could not afford it, sometimes saying simply that she did not feel like it. She eventually died of cervical cancer, and a wrongful death suit was filed alleging the doctor's negligent failure to inform her of the risks of refusing the test. The majority concluded that the case was controlled by *Cobbs v. Grant*,[103] the leading California case on informed consent. It held that instructions should have been given allowing the jury to consider whether the doctor had breached a duty by failing to inform the patient of the risks of refusing the recommended test.[104]

Although the majority appropriately rested its holding on *Cobbs*, the facts in *Truman* differed from the traditional informed consent facts to which *Cobbs* is typically applied. The fact that the patient decided not to have the test meant that the doctor would not touch her. Both the court of appeal majority and the supreme court dissenters stressed that requiring disclosure in such a situation would be a serious and undesirable expansion of the basic doctrine.[105] In their view, apart from traditional requirements for consent to physical contact, people should do as their competent doctors tell them,[106] and protection against incompetent care is therefore

---

102. 27 Cal. 3d 285, 611 P.2d 902, 165 Cal. Rptr. 308 (1980), *rev'g* 155 Cal. Rptr. 752 (Ct. App. 1979).

103. 8 Cal. 3d 229, 502 P.2d 1, 104 Cal. Rptr. 505 (1972).

104. *Truman*, 27 Cal. 3d at 294–95, 611 P.2d at 307–08, 165 Cal. Rptr. at 313–14. A Pap Smear involves physical touching and would therefore require both consent and information about risks. However, no disclosure of remote or minor risks is required. A Pap Smear is virtually risk-free. The risks attach primarily to *refusal* to undergo the recommended test. It is therefore, technically, the alternatives branch of informed consent doctrine that actually requires disclosure. Refusal is a self-evident alternative, but the risks of not having a Pap Smear might not be common knowledge and, therefore, ought to be disclosed.

105. 155 Cal. Rptr. at 757–59; 27 Cal. 3d at 297–301, 611 P.2d at 909–11, 165 Cal. Rptr. at 315–17.

106. According to the court of appeal majority, "[i]t does not follow that the doctor should be required to protect his patient from the patient's lack of judgment." 155 Cal. Rptr. at 757. Furthermore, "[i]t is nonsensical to claim that [a patient] goes to the doctor for advice he will not thereafter follow . . . ." *Id.* at 759. Similarly, according to Judge Clark, writing for the supreme court dissenters, "[w]hen a patient chooses a physician, he or she obviously has confidence in the doctor and intends to accept proffered medical advice [, and it is] reasonable to assume that a patient who refuses advice is aware of potential risk." 27 Cal. 3d at 299, 611 P.2d at 910, 165 Cal. Rptr. at 316.

The supreme court dissenters raise one legitimate issue. There seems a danger here that doctors will be held liable if they fail to get patients' consent, or if a "bad" outcome results from honoring the patient's choice. The *Truman* majority forestalled that problem by holding that if the plaintiff would have refused the test even if fully informed, no liability should result. 27 Cal. 3d at 294, 611 P.2d at 907, 165 Cal. Rptr. at 313. Thus, although it ordinarily uses a reasonable person standard of causation in informed consent cases, the court adopted a subjective person standard here. That decision handled the immediate problem but failed to address the analogous unfairness created by the use of the reasonable person causation standard in the more usual informed consent case. *See also infra* text accompanying notes 127–31, 212–13, 294–309.

all that should be required. The closeness of the outcome in *Truman*,[107] decided in a jurisdiction where concern for patient autonomy has traditionally been vigorous, suggests that the perception of an essential nexus between physical contact and choice is still very strong.

On its facts, *Truman* created a rather modest extension of duty. However, a subsequent California case, *Jamison v. Lindsay*,[108] described a potentially broader obligation to disclose. The plaintiff sued a pathologist for failing to inform either the surgeon or herself of the presence of immature tissue in a tumor removed from her body or of a controversy among pathologists over whether or not such tissue increases the odds of later malignancy. Again, because there was no proposed physical contact, the court of appeal upheld the trial court's refusal to give informed consent instructions, and affirmed a jury verdict for the defendant doctors.[109] Unlike other courts,[110] however, the *Jamison* court did not allow its conclusion that informed consent did not apply to eliminate disclosure as a duty imposed to protect patient autonomy. It observed that, pursuant to the broadened duties of disclosure suggested by *Truman*, an instruction regarding a duty to disclose information necessary for informed decision-making regarding *whether to seek additional treatment* following surgery would have been appropriate.[111] Such a duty would necessarily make possession of information rather than proposed physical contact the occasion for disclosure.[112] Despite the breadth of its theories, *Jamison's* rather stringent procedural rulings[113] barred any actual implementation of those

---

107. The intermediate court's 2-1 decision that no duty was appropriate, 155 Cal. Rptr. 752, was reversed by a bare 4-3 majority of the supreme court, 27 Cal. 3d 285, 611 P.2d 902, 165 Cal. Rptr. 308.

108. 108 Cal. App. 3d 223, 166 Cal. Rptr. 443 (1980).

109. "[N]o treatment or tests had been proposed by respondents. The informed consent theory and appellant's proposed instructions on the duty of a physician to disclose . . . 'regarding the proposed . . . postoperative treatment' were inapposite [because] . . . [a]fter the surgery, respondents did not propose any therapy as to which appellant would have been entitled to make an informed decision." *Id.* at 230, 166 Cal. Rptr. at 446.

110. *See supra* Section B(1).

111. 108 Cal. App. 3d at 231, 166 Cal. Rptr. at 447. Despite this observation, the court held that because the trial court had no responsibility to edit proposed instructions, no reversible error resulted. *Id.*

112. Using that new standard, *Jamison* would require post-intervention disclosure in much the same way that *Gates* extended pre-intervention disclosure.

113. For example, the plaintiff argued on appeal that the nondisclosure should have been analyzed under the reasonable person rather than the expert standard of care. Although agreeing that the broadened duty of disclosure as judged by the lay standard could legitimately have been alleged under ordinary negligence law rather than informed consent doctrine, the appellate court nevertheless held that the plaintiff herself invited the error by requesting an instruction incorporating the expert standard of care. 108 Cal. App. 3d at 232, 166 Cal. Rptr. at 448. Yet, presumably, the plaintiff's lawyer, having characterized the issue as one of informed consent, would have assumed that the lay standard regarding disclosure would have been invoked under that theory, and therefore would have seen no need to request such instructions with reference to the ordinary negligence aspect of the case. The assumption that informed consent doctrine would apply does not seem unwarranted. The appellate court itself cited *Truman* and *Cobbs* (both labeled as informed consent cases), and indicated its recog-

Protecting Patient Choice

theories in the case.[114] It thus remains uncertain whether future plaintiffs can use *Jamison* to achieve broader protection for patient autonomy.

These cases strain to transcend the traditional, touch-based limits on disclosure duties protecting patient autonomy. The standards they suggest would require more disclosure of a different genre of information. A *Gates* or *Truman* standard would require that doctors disclose the process and reasons by which they arrive at their recommendations, rather than simply provide boilerplate warnings about recommendations that are to be accepted as foregone conclusions. It would also require that, even if a doctor deems care satisfactorily completed, and thus recommends no further treatment, she would have to disclose what she *knows* about the patient's condition and prospects as a result of earlier interventions.

Such information could produce a different kind of patient participation than has resulted from disclosure requirements under traditional informed consent.[115] Rather than being a yes/no gatekeeper regarding a single preselected option,[116] the patient could act on broader information that would provide the basis for meaningful participation in medical decision-making. These cases envision a patient actually making choices, including choices that differ from what the doctor deems "reasonable."[117]

nition that the disclosure issue was essentially one involving patient choice. Yet the court refused either to flex its interpretation of the scope of informed consent doctrine or to allow the plaintiff instructions appropriate to a choice theory of the case, however labeled. When the court transferred the disclosure analysis from informed consent to ordinary negligence, the parallel request for an appropriate standard of care instruction should have been deemed similarly transferred.

The plaintiff also challenged the trial judge's instruction, which stated that the pathologist had a right to make a professionally competent judgment between alternative medical procedures. The pathologist, the plaintiff argued, was choosing between beliefs or conclusions that should have been disclosed. The court agreed that the alternative methods instruction was inappropriate. But because the plaintiff did not properly raise this argument at trial, the court refused to consider it on appeal. *Id.* at 233, 166 Cal. Rptr. at 448.

114. In another substantive ruling that prevented broadened disclosure, the court refused to apply the principles of express warranty to the doctor's assertions about the plaintiff's condition, even though he did not disclose known controversy regarding those assertions. *Id.* at 234, 166 Cal. Rptr. at 449. Although the court's conclusion probably reflected traditional resistance to the use of contract principles in medical cases, it was explained on premises linked to a touch-oriented model. The court said the statement came *after* the surgery, and no consent to treatment was based on it. However, from the vantage point of choice, the inaction that was based on the statement was just as significant.

115. Some commentators seem to have given up on the law's ability to create more than a pro forma role for patients. The President's Commission, describing informed consent as having created only a "duty to warn," 1 MAKING DECISIONS, *supra* note 2, at 20, seems to have adopted a rather pessimistic view of the law's role, and has turned its attention to medical education and public opinion to create the "shared decisionmaking" it envisions.

116. *See id.* at 24, 29 (litigation process forces examination of disclosure of risks concerning particular procedure rather than evaluation of entire doctor-patient relationship).

117. Thus in *Truman* the patient made her "unreasonable" choice at least partly for economic reasons. The Pap Smear seemed of less value to her than it seemed to the doctor and she rejected his advice. 27 Cal. 3d at 290, 611 P.2d at 904, 165 Cal. Rptr. at 310. In some sense the case is like that of a Jehovah's Witness whose refusal of a blood transfusion is honored. *See, e.g., In re* Melideo, 88 Misc. 2d 974, 390 N.Y.S.2d 523 (Sup. Ct. 1976). But our willingness to give public recognition to the conflicts of value in the two cases may differ. Although religious conviction is a palatable as well as a constitutionally protected reason for being "unreasonable," we are less sure about lack of funds, a

The Yale Law Journal   Vol. 95: 219, 1985

Although the expansions of duty undertaken in *Gates, Truman* and *Jamison* could be significant, the potential impact of these three cases is questionable. Although not directly overruled, *Gates* was emasculated by *Keogan. Truman* requires disclosure about a course of inaction, but its informed refusal stance is unusual and renders it vulnerable to a narrow, touch-oriented interpretation. The relevant parts of *Jamison* are dicta, expounded by an intermediate court, and the case has not been followed or much discussed. There is little indication of these approaches being adopted in other jurisdictions. If the duty suggested in these cases were actually to take root and develop, it would increase protection for patient autonomy. Whether even such an expanded protection would be adequate to ensure patient choice, however, is the subject of the next section.

3. *Other Elements of the Analysis Which Distort Patient Choice*

Although the *Gates-Truman* approach could bring some instances of patient choice not involving physical contact within the ambit of negligence duties, adoption of this approach would not affect the distortion of choice that occurs at other stages of the informed consent analysis. Informed consent doctrines remain embedded within the different, and often inconsistent, interest in physical well-being. Although various of the specific doctrinal rules of informed consent have been extensively criticized,[118] the role played by interest definition in diluting the vindication of autonomy has not been adequately challenged.

a. *Standard of Care*

Advocates of autonomy have argued that the standard for disclosure in informed consent cases should be what a reasonable patient would want to know rather than what the average competent doctor would actually disclose.[119] Because doctors are trained to take active responsibility and are

---

vastly more frequent factor influencing patient choice. Increased protection of individual choice will highlight potentially unpleasant realities about the correlation of wealth and access to health care under our system. But the difficulty of those issues is no excuse for abandoning analytic clarity concerning the relevant interests. *See infra* Part IV(C).

118. Autonomy-oriented critics have objected to two principal aspects of the doctrine of informed consent: the standards of care and of causation. *See, e.g.*, J. KATZ, *supra* note 7, at 48-84 (criticizing professional standard of care and noting that causation requirements conflict with dignity of individual and right to self-determination); Katz, *Informed Consent, supra* note 15, at 169 (standard of care with respect to disclosure confuses need for medical knowledge to establish risks of proposed procedures with need for medical judgment to establish limits of disclosure); Note, *Restructuring, supra* note 30, at 1555-59 (criticizing professional standard of disclosure). These rules have survived partly because they are logical outgrowths of the way interests are defined under current doctrine.

119. *See, e.g.*, J. KATZ, *supra* note 7 (advocating disclosure based on patient self-determination rather than medical expertise); J. KATZ & A. CAPRON, *supra* note 30, at 114 (goal of full and frank partnership between physician and patient); Comment, *Informed Consent in Medical Malpractice*, 55 CALIF. L. REV. 1396, 1407 (1967) (proposing full disclosure of all known risks); Note, *Restructur-*

Protecting Patient Choice

concerned first and foremost with *outcomes*, historically they have been reluctant to disclose risks and share decisionmaking.[120] If doctors evaluate the adequacy of disclosure, even when it is designed to protect choice, they will naturally respond in terms of these traditions.[121]

Professional expertise, therefore, is not the appropriate determinant of how much disclosure is desirable or adequate for purposes of patient choice. Where the ultimate issue is defined as protection from physical injury, however, absent a painstaking parsing of the sub-issues, professional expertise will seem both central and sufficient to measure duties of care. A substantial minority of states, responding to the identification of the subsidiary choice interest, have adopted a reasonable patient standard to measure the content and adequacy of disclosure.[122] But most states, responding to physical well-being as the protected interest, have chosen professionalized standards of care as both natural and justified.[123] The difference of rules reflects the internal conflict within the hybrid doctrine; the dominance of the professional standard reflects the dominance of physical well-being as the ultimately protected interest. If choice were an independently protected interest, the role of medical expertise could more appropriately be delimited.

b. *Causation*

Medical cases potentially impose enormous liability. Fearing that patients' testimony would be self-serving and biased by hindsight,[124] courts have felt it necessary to subject hypothetical reconstructions of individual choice to standardized criteria.[125] In informed consent cases, plaintiffs

ing, supra note 30, at 1559–66 (urging adoption of "reasonable patient standard"). Perhaps the best known objection to the professional standard was expressed by Judge Robinson in Canterbury v. Spence: "Nor can we ignore the fact that to bind the disclosure obligation to medical usage is to arrogate the decision on revelation to the physician alone." 464 F.2d 772, 784 (D.C. Cir.), *cert. denied*, 409 U.S. 1064 (1972).

To some degree, the conflict over the standard for disclosure reflects the difference between contractual and tort norms. Causes of action in contract look to the reasonable expectations of the promisee; professional negligence actions in tort look to the specialized competencies and practices of the professional group.

120. This fact is thoroughly documented by J. KATZ, *supra* note 7, at 1–29.

121. For example, in Dunham v. Wright, 423 F.2d 940 (3d Cir. 1970), a case involving death as a result of thyroid surgery, the court affirmed the trial court's refusal to grant a judgment n.o.v. on the issue of informed consent after a jury verdict for the doctor. The plaintiff claimed that the doctor's failure to disclose alternative methods of treatment rendered the patient's consent defective. The court, however, quoted with apparent approval the doctor's assertion that the patient had had no alternatives. *Id.* at 946. It seemed completely unaware that the doctor may have simply characterized his expert recommendation in a fashion that justified the foreclosure of the patient's interest in choice.

122. J. AREEN, P. KING, S. GOLDBERG & A. CAPRON, *supra* note 32, at 384 n.4.

123. *Id.* (twenty-six states use professional standard of care).

124. *See, e.g.*, Canterbury v. Spence, 464 F.2d at 790–91 (subjective standard "places the physician in jeopardy of the patient's hindsight and bitterness").

125. *Id.* at 791. *But see* Scott v. Bradford, 606 P.2d 554, 559 (Okla. 1980) (refusing to jeopardize

must show that, had the contested disclosure been made, a reasonable person would not have consented to the treatment.[126]

Such a standard invites both juries and doctors to make the too easy and superficial assumption that reasonable people do what their competent doctors tell them to do.[127] Moreover, as commentators have argued, the choices made by reasonable others are not an appropriate screening criterion where the value at issue is personal autonomy.[128] Yet where physical well-being is the protected interest, choice is placed in the role of factual cause, linking breaches of duty to the occurrence of harm. Analyzed in this way, what began as a concern for individual autonomy almost necessarily comes to be subjected to standardizing and oversimplifying criteria that are alien to individuality.

"right to know" by imposition of "reasonable man" standard). In some unusual instances an objective standard of causation will work to disadvantage doctors. In such instances even jurisdictions that ordinarily employ an objective standard may switch to a subjective one. Of course, the problem of self-serving testimony is removed in these instances, but the substantive illegitimacy of the objective standard in the ordinary case is also indirectly acknowledged by these decisions. *See, e.g.*, Truman v. Thomas, 27 Cal. 3d 285, 294, 611 P.2d 902, 907, 165 Cal. Rptr. 308, 313, (1980) (satisfying "prudent person test" necessary but not sufficient for recovery by plaintiff); *see also* Guebard v. Jabaay, 117 Ill. App. 3d 1, 10, 452 N.E.2d 751, 757-58 (1983) (upholding jury verdict for defendant/physician because, given plaintiff's active sports life, she would have been *less* likely than reasonable person to choose undisclosed alternative to doctor's suggested treatment).

126. Almost all jurisdictions have adopted the objective standard. 3 MAKING DECISIONS, *supra* note 2, at 197. In tort law generally, decisions about how to handle causal questions regarding what would have happened had greater information been provided have not always paralleled the treatment of the issue in medical informed consent cases. Thus, for example, in products liability cases involving failure to warn, courts have not asked whether a warning, if one had been given, would have been heeded. These cases consequently never reach the question of whether that judgment should be assessed in individual or in reasonable person terms. *See, e.g.*, McCormack v. Hankscraft Co., 278 Minn. 322, 154 N.W.2d 488 (1967) (in reversing judgment n.o.v. for defendant, court found evidence sufficient to uphold jury verdict in favor of child injured by boiling water in vaporizer where manufacturer failed to warn despite lack of evidence regarding effectiveness of hypothetical warning). *But see* Cunningham v. Charles Pfizer & Co., 532 P.2d 1377 (Okla. 1975) (failure to warn of statistically small risk of paralysis rendered consent defective; case remanded for new trial with plaintiff entitled to rebuttable presumption that warning would have been heeded with ultimate test being objective one). For a discussion of failure to warn in products liability cases, see Keeton, *Products Liability—Inadequacy of Information*, 48 TEX. L. REV. 398 (1970). Manufacturers and doctors may differ in their ability to absorb the costs of accidents, but doctors can probably prevent invasions of patients' choice more easily than manufacturers can prevent injuries from products. The comparatively personalized setting of the doctor-patient relationship should make discussion and evaluation of warning information more useful than written product warnings. The different treatment of the issue in products liability cases at least suggests that it is not essential to employ the causation analysis currently used by the courts in informed consent. *See also infra* text accompanying notes 212-13, 294-308.

127. *See, e.g., supra* note 106.

128. *See* Meisel, *Expansion, supra* note 6, at 112. Judge Burger made the point forcefully when discussing an opinion by Justice Brandeis. He observed that:

> Nothing in this utterance [by Brandeis] suggests that Justice Brandeis thought an individual possessed these rights only as to *sensible* beliefs, *valid* thoughts, reasonable emotions, or *well-founded* sensations. I suggest he intended to include a great many foolish, unreasonable and even absurd ideas which do not conform, such as refusing medical treatment even at great risks.

Application of the President & Directors of Georgetown College, 331 F.2d 1010, 1017 (D.C. Cir. 1964) (Burger, J., dissenting) (emphasis in original).

Protecting Patient Choice

In many tort actions, factual cause is relatively clear. Even in those actions where actual causation is less certain, an all-or-nothing resolution may yet be justified on grounds that, under a balance of probabilities test, the injury either was or was not causally connected to the negligent act.[129] Invasions of autonomy, however, involve an especially complex and probabilistic analysis. There are multiple issues: Did the doctor's nondisclosure materially invade the patient's interest in choice? What would the patient have chosen had her choice been protected? What would have happened, medically, had the alternate choice been made? Such complexities are unmanageable within the yes/no framework of factual cause; compressed into a single question, they become oversimplified.

Under such a simplified analysis, if individual criteria were used, the very existence of any injury would seem to turn solely on the rather shaky reed of the plaintiff's hindsight testimony. It is not surprising that courts faced with such a compacted ultimate issue moved to adopt objective standards of reasonableness to address the question.[130] If, on the other hand, choice were an independently protected interest, the factual cause issue would be narrower and simpler—whether the patient's right to choose had been encroached upon as a result of a doctor's failure to disclose.[131]

To be sure, difficult problems of uncertainty, prediction and credibility would remain regarding what would have happened had the patient been given the choice. However, with choice as the protected interest, these problems would be assessed as questions of the valuation of an injury that was acknowledged to have taken place. The framework of valuation is better adapted to the resolution of such probabilistic issues than is the traditional analysis of factual cause. Moreover, questions regarding what redress should be available to remedy the invasion of choice would then be analyzed, appropriately, as issues of sanctioning policy rather than of the factual existence of harm.

c. *Categories of Compensable Harm*

Where battery was preoccupied with physical touch, negligence vindicates physical well-being.[132] Many invasions of patient autonomy do re-

---

129. For example, even if the defendants were negligent, if their negligence was, more probably than not, *not* a substantial factor in plaintiff's injury, no liability is warranted. *See* J. FLEMING, AN INTRODUCTION TO THE LAW OF TORTS 109-11 (1967). And where the question of factual cause is complicated by the presence of two tortious factors, if either could, more probably than not, have produced the injurious result, liability is warranted. *Id.*

130. *See* King, *supra* note 27 (criticizing courts' frequent conflation of issues of causation and valuation).

131. Some standard of materiality would be needed. *See infra* text accompanying note 285.

132. While physical injury is the central theme of negligence doctrine, other types of injury may be cognizable. For example, damages for emotional distress may be recovered in conjunction with infringement of other interests, *see* RESTATEMENT (SECOND) OF TORTS § 905(b) (1977), or in their

The Yale Law Journal   Vol. 95: 219, 1985

sult in physical injury as it is traditionally defined. Although such injuries would seem to fit standard negligence definitions of harm, they often go unredressed because, as demonstrated above, the analysis of duty, breach, or cause differs where the protected interest is physical well-being rather than choice. In addition, preemption of patients' authority by doctors may also give rise to injuries that are real but intangible, or to physical outcomes that are arguably not "injurious" except from the individual's vantage point. These outcomes may be excluded from negligence doctrine's definitions of harm. Thus, a patient not told about a method of sterilization that is more reversible than the one performed may have difficulty convincing a court that nonreversibility is a cognizable physical injury.[133] A patient who alleges that, properly informed, she would have chosen a lumpectomy rather than a radical mastectomy might find it hard, under existing negligence rules, to characterize the successful operation that removed her breast and eradicated her cancer as having "injured" her.[134] Similarly, the patient with a desire to go home or to a hospice to die, who is instead maintained alive by hospital machinery, might have difficulty establishing "injury" under definitions of an interest in physical well-being rather than choice.[135] And, at least when such cases were first liti-

---

own right, under rules governing the interest in freedom from emotional distress, *see id.* at § 46.

133. *See, e.g.*, Masquat v. Maguire, 638 P.2d 1105 (Okla. 1981). The doctor admitted he did not inform Ms. Masquat of alternative procedures or of their differing degrees of reversibility. The court held that the doctor's nondisclosure would not support either a battery or an informed consent action because of the absence of "causal linkage between some unrevealed risk and the injuries complained of." *Id.* at 1107.

Intangibility of injury might also play a role in barring redress in cases where doctors' nondisclosure arguably deprived patients of a *chance* to obtain a preferable outcome. If more sophisticated concepts of measurement were devised to value a chance, these "ordinary" physical injuries might arguably be analyzed as injuries attributable to a lapse of professionally competent care. If the chance is lost because the doctor's conduct fell below professional standards, that would be appropriate. Many deprivation of a chance cases, however, are better characterized as injuries to choice. The uncertainty of medicine dictates that doctors should not be accountable for perfect outcomes. Precise measurement of lost chances might suggest such accountability. Competence standards can and should require a substantial threshold of knowledge, judgment, and action. Yet beyond demanding conformity to professional standards, the law should leave the weighing of which chances are worth taking to the judgment of the individual affected. *See infra* text accompanying notes 217–31.

134. Despite the controversial nature of the surgery, no case has been discovered dealing with deprivation of choice regarding lumpectomy as opposed to mastectomy, which suggests that such a cause of action would not presently be cognizable. *Cf.* Hanks v. Doctors Ranson, Swan & Burch, Ltd., 359 So. 2d 1089, 1093 (La. Ct. App.) (for discussion of case, see *infra* text accompanying notes 147–49), *cert. denied*, 360 So. 2d 1178 (La. 1978).

135. The "right to die" examples, although anecdotally familiar, do not seem to have reached the courts—at least as disputes between individuals. *But see Court Hears Dead Man's Arguments in Right-to-Die Case*, San Francisco Chron., Nov. 9, 1984, at 10, col.1 (family filed $10 million civil damage suit against hospital for not respecting family member's wish to be disconnected from respirator). The paucity of such litigation in the literature suggests lacunae in the cause of action as presently conceived. In addition, the societal interest in such decisions is still being litigated. *See generally* J. AREEN, P. KING, S. GOLDBERG & A. CAPRON, *supra* note 32, at 1077–1147 (presenting interdisciplinary viewpoints on legal, social, and ethical issues in regulation of death decisions); PRESIDENT'S COMM'N FOR THE STUDY OF ETHICAL PROBLEMS IN MEDICINE AND BEHAVIORAL RESEARCH, DECIDING TO FOREGO LIFE-SUSTAINING TREATMENT (1983) (re-examining way decisions are and

Protecting Patient Choice

gated, the patient who gives birth to an unwanted child because of a doctor's failure to provide choice-protecting information may have difficulty showing harm.[136]

Conclusions about the reality of injury and about whether conduct is deserving of sanction ultimately depend both on how the underlying interest is defined and on how accurately the consequences of its invasion have been traced. In both respects, existing analysis that vindicates patient autonomy only in an indirect fashion has produced a pattern of protection for that interest that is flawed in critical ways.

C. *The Insufficiency of Negligence Protection*

The preceding sections document how choice is subordinated and distorted at every stage of the negligence analysis. Under the prototype identified at the outset, this weak form of protection offered by informed consent doctrine governs only comparatively peripheral questions. Thus, where the doctor proposes surgical intervention, the occurrence of that intervention will necessarily be within the patient's awareness, and, hence, to some degree, control. Furthermore, medical custom has accepted a need for at least some basic consent in such circumstances.[137] Finally, most states retain some legal requirement under battery doctrine that the patient's consent be sought.[138] Under modern views, that requirement does not demand that the patient's consent be highly informed. However, because courts often treat blanket consents as being of questionable validity,[139] the basic consent requirement for battery in fact necessitates *some* disclosure regarding the specific proposal. Under the prototype, what is

---

ought to be made about whether to forego life-sustaining treatment). Once the parameters of patient autonomy in regard to death decisions are more clearly established, litigation over infringement of those rights by private parties such as doctors and hospitals will likely begin in earnest, as was the case when resolution of constitutional disputes over abortion gave rise to large numbers of private law actions concerning wrongful birth, life, conception, etc.

136. Wrongful birth cases will be discussed in Part III as examples of the emergence of an interest in choice similar to the one suggested here.

137. 2 MAKING DECISIONS, *supra* note 2, at 81. Virtually all doctors report obtaining consent for inpatient surgery.

138. 1 MAKING DECISIONS, *supra* note 2, at 22; *see also supra* text accompanying notes 28–29.

139. *See, e.g.*, Rogers v. Lumbermens Mutual Casualty Co., 119 So. 2d. 649 (La. Ct. App. 1960) (operation for removal of reproductive organs tortious when plaintiff only consented to removal of appendix); Gray v. Grunnagle, 423 Pa. 144, 167, 223 A.2d 663, 674 (1966) (general consent signed upon admission to hospital may be found inadequate). *But see* Kennedy v. Parrott, 243 N.C. 355, 362, 90 S.E.2d 754, 759 (1956) (absent proof to contrary, consent to major operation will be construed as general in nature and surgeon may extend operation to remedy any condition in area of original incision). *See generally* 23 OHIO REV. CODE. ANN. § 2317.54 (Page 1981) (example of statute requiring consent forms to be particular and specific); 1 MAKING DECISIONS, *supra* note 2, at 106 (Joint Commission on Accreditation of Hospitals requiring separate consent forms be signed for any procedure or treatment "for which it is appropriate"); A. ROSOFF, *supra* note 29, at 283 (warning doctors that blanket consent forms are often legally defective).

left to be litigated under a negligence/informed consent theory is mainly nondisclosure concerning collateral risks.[140]

Disclosure of collateral risks tends to be additive and elaborative, comparatively unimportant,[141] particularly if only one course of action is under discussion.[142] As between doing nothing and accepting the recommendation, a patient's decision is driven by the pains and problems of the disease or illness that brought her to the doctor in the first place. Subjecting the patient's interest in receiving such information to professional standards of care and reasonable patient standards of causation seems relatively unobjectionable.

In nonprototypical situations, the contrast is stark. Where the doctor in effect recommends inaction (or continuing action or non-touching action), that recommendation can be implemented without the patient's awareness. Such decisions cannot be physically "sensed" by the patient. As a matter of medical custom, they are viewed as issues of professional competence rather than patient choice.[143] Existing touch-oriented legal doctrines inappropriately reinforce that conclusion.

Yet in these instances, information does not merely elaborate collateral risks but is itself the *sine qua non* of choice, the sole means by which the patient can become aware of highly consequential courses of medical management. Information in these cases is far more important than is most collateral risk information; without disclosure, self-executing judgments will be made by the doctor. The problem is illustrated by *Hanks v. Ranson*.[144] In *Hanks*, the plaintiff's healthy breast was amputated after a competently administered but mistaken diagnostic test. The plaintiff complained that the doctor had not told her of a more diagnostically accurate two-step procedure that would have separated surgery from the diagnostic biopsy. No protection regarding such an alternate choice will be forthcoming under battery doctrine. Consent was given to the very procedure per-

---

140. Under negligence analysis the predominant issue is disclosure of risks of the proposed procedure. *See* 3 MAKING DECISIONS, *supra* note 2, at 195; Andrews, *supra* note 85, at 195.

141. Current doctrines are preoccupied most with that information which is least important. This may explain why the doctrine itself is commonly perceived to be rather insignificant. Thus Katz calls it a "Fairy Tale." Katz, *Informed Consent*, *supra* note 15; *see also* Meisel, *Expansion*, *supra* note 6, at 90 (calling informed consent in 1960's a "paper tiger"). Doctors frequently perceive the legal doctrine to be an albatross. *See, e.g.*, Katz, *Informed Consent: Is It Bad Medicine?* 126 WESTERN J. MED. 426 (1977) (anesthesiologist argues that "informed consent" is useless legal doctrine and that patients complain of being told "too much"). Seventy-nine percent of the public feels that the primary purpose of consent forms is to protect doctors from lawsuits. *See* 2 MAKING DECISIONS, *supra* note 2, at 160.

142. Given the weakness of present rules regarding disclosure of alternatives, this will typically be the situation. *See supra* text accompanying notes 84–87.

143. As the intervention becomes less like the prototypical surgery, there is a rapid fall-off in perceived need to seek consent. *See* 2 MAKING DECISIONS, *supra* note 2, at 168, 335. This is true even though medication decisions, for example, may involve greater risks than surgery. *See id.* at 335.

144. 359 So. 2d 1089 (La. Ct. App.), *cert. denied*, 360 So. 2d 1178 (La. 1978).

Protecting Patient Choice

formed; no consent is presently required for the doctor's decision *not* to use the two-step alternative because that decision involved no physical contact. Moreover, despite acknowledged non-disclosure of the alternative,[145] the court upheld a verdict for the defendant even though jury instructions on informed consent made no reference to disclosure of alternatives. Recharacterizing the issue as one of risk, the court held that the risk of a wrong diagnostic outcome was "remote," and thus need not be disclosed.[146]

Information about alternative courses of action is different than information about collateral risks. Though remote side effect risks of a single option may be comparatively unimportant, even a slightly greater risk, for example, of unnecessary amputation may be sufficient to cause the patient to choose an alternative. Under current informed consent doctrine, however, protection of the opportunity to choose an alternative may either wholly disappear, as in *Hanks*, or be eroded by the distortions that flow from the negligence interest definition.[147] Thus, even had the court in *Hanks* required disclosure of alternatives, vindication of a breast cancer patient's interest in making the choice between one- and two-step procedures should not depend upon whether doctors typically disclose that information, upon whether reasonable patients would make the same choice as the patient, or upon standardized definitions of physical injury. Yet with regard to nonprototypical choices, that will be the result if only current negligence analysis is employed.

Current doctrine perceives nearly all informational issues to be problems of professional knowledge and duty; negligence has become the ordinary category for analysis of nondisclosure.[148] Thus, when informa-

---

145.   *Id.* at 1091. Even if disclosure is required, some fact patterns involving alternatives may not be characterized as "injury" where the protected interest is physical well-being. *See* Masquat v. Maguire, 638 P.2d 1105, 1106–07 (Okla. 1981).

146.   359 So. 2d at 1093.

147.   *Cf. Masquat*, 638 P.2d 1105 (for discussion of case, see *supra* note 133); Thornton v. Annest, 19 Wash. App. 174, 574 P.2d 1199 (1978) (for discussion of case, see *supra* note 86). In part, these cases reflect appellate deference to jury verdicts on the basis of norms regarding the judge-jury function. But they also make clear the inadequacy of current legal protection of patient autonomy under existing doctrines.

148.   One authority did not succumb to this perception. Professor Plant suggested that nondisclosure of information about the "nature and character" of proposed treatment should trigger a claim for battery, while information about collateral risks could be adequately treated under negligence. Plant, *Analysis, supra* note 27, at 648–50 (correlating different types of nondisclosure with different legal actions). The suggestion, however, has not been widely followed. Professor Plant himself later observed that "[u]ltimately almost all informed consent cases came to be treated as falling in the negligence area." Plant, *Decline, supra* note 30, at 92. An occasional court picked up the distinction, *see*, *e.g.*, Hales v. Pittman, 118 Ariz. 305, 309, 576 P.2d 493, 497 (1978); Gaston v. Hunter, 121 Ariz. 33, 57, 588 P.2d 326, 350 (Ct. App. 1978), but their efforts have had little effect. Indeed, it is not likely coincidental that the jurisdiction whose courts incorporated this approach became the first to adopt a statute abolishing actions for medical battery. *See* Ariz. Rev. Stat. Ann. § 12-562 (Supp. 1979).

Moreover, Plant's approach still assumes that important choices will involve physical touching. The

The Yale Law Journal   Vol. 95: 219, 1985

tional gaps in the protection accorded to choice have been perceived at all, they have been "corrected" by expanding the scope of the duty to secure informed consent.[149] The narrow disclosure-of-alternative-treatments approach or the broader *Gates*-type extension of informed consent[150] would bring more information concerning such decisions to the attention of the patient than do other formulations of the duty to secure informed consent. But the solution is less than adequate. The protection offered to patient autonomy under the informed consent doctrine is weak, distorted by an analysis rooted in the standard negligence interest definition. Although such analysis arguably provides adequate vindication for choice interests regarding collateral risk information, it is difficult to justify when it constitutes the sole protection accorded to patient choices regarding entire courses of action (or inaction). Yet that will be the result where battery/consent requirements are not triggered because no touching is proposed.

Only a few states have even extended the doctrine of informed consent to impose any duty of disclosure in circumstances that involve no physical contact.[151] Others have actually moved in the opposite direction: They have abolished all actions for medical-care battery, leaving only a negligence action to protect all aspects of patient choice.[152] Such a policy does nothing to correct existing weaknesses of negligence doctrine; at the same time, it deprives even those instances of choice that do involve physical contact of any vindication other than that available under negligence doctrines. The move to abolish battery seems to be an outgrowth of legitimate frustration with certain aspects of the intentional tort analysis. Yet it may also derive from an uncritical assumption that if negligence/informed consent analysis seems to be doing an adequate job with some aspects of patient choice protection, it may legitimately be applied to all aspects. Such a conclusion is seriously mistaken. If that mistake is not corrected, and some better approach to the problem put forth, the move to abolish medical battery actions might expand, further undermining the limited protection the law currently accords to patient autonomy.

---

types of information under discussion here are not easily characterized as being about the "nature and character" of a proposed intervention.

149. This is the result, for example, of an expansion to cover prescription of drugs, to require disclosure of alternative treatments, or more broadly, to require disclosure of important information, as the Washington court did in *Gates*.

150. *See* Gates v. Jensen, 92 Wash. 2d 246, 595 P.2d 919 (1979) (en banc). For further discussion of this case, see *supra* text accompanying notes 88–101.

151. *See supra* Part II(B)(1)(b).

152. *See, e.g.*, Ariz. Rev. Stat. Ann. § 12-562 (Supp. 1979).

Protecting Patient Choice

III. TOWARD GREATER PROTECTION OF PATIENT CHOICE

A. *Factors Strengthening Patient Choice*

In the case law, two factors seem to strengthen patient claims to information and choice. When there is a relatively crystallized conflict of interest, or when there is a recognizably heightened electiveness, the protection accorded to patient autonomy is likely to be stronger than it would otherwise be. Although neither factor has been clearly articulated or consistently applied, each can be discerned as an emerging influence.

1. *Conflict of Interest: Disqualifying the Doctor*

The principal conflict of interest within the doctor-patient relationship derives from the fact that doctors' incomes rise when patients consume health care services that those same doctors recommend and provide.[153] While that issue is frequently implicit in conflicts about care, it is rarely raised in litigation, presumably because most patients have only an indirect economic stake in the health care they receive.[154] In a few areas, however, litigation raising clear problems of conflict of interest does arise.

a. *Expansion of Battery Doctrine*

Only one court has accepted a battery theory as applicable to the prescription of drugs.[155] Although the holding in *Mink v. University of Chi-*

---

153. Although the incentive to over-service is somewhat reduced because many doctors are paid according to time expended rather than procedures performed, this is not true of some specialists. For example, surgeons are paid mainly when patients accept their recommendations. This relatively direct conflict of interest may partly explain why patient choice is most aggressively protected under battery's consent requirements in surgical cases. Moreover, the potential pharmaceutical, hospital, or laboratory profits that are available to doctors greatly undermine the effectiveness of the payment-for-time concept in offsetting the conflict of interest. *See* Relman, *Dealing With Conflicts of Interest*, 313 NEW ENG. J. MED. 749 (1985) (expressing concern that doctors' entrepreneurial profit-making desires weaken both professional ethics and public trust). The concept also does not remove doctors' economic incentives to recommend time-use itself.

154. Despite their indirect stake in, for example, insurance premiums, patients are not the most obvious financial losers when excess care is provided. Few patients file suit alleging only that they were given more care than they needed, i.e. that they paid for unnecessary care. *See* Salis v. United States, 522 F. Supp. 989, 994–96 (M.D. Pa. 1981). The main objectors to such care would be third-party payors. These organizations tend to pursue political and market methods of cost control. *See* Blumstein & Sloan, *Redefining Government's Role in Health Care: Is a Dose of Competition What the Doctor Should Order?*, 34 VAND. L. REV. 849, 856–59, 863–64 (1981); Havighurst, *Competition in Health Services: Overview, Issues and Answers*, 34 VAND. L. REV. 1117, 1123 (1981). Moreover, since the main conceptual structure of physician accountability is professional competence rather than patient (or indirectly, payor) choice, over-care will rarely be negligent, though it may constitute a violation of patient choice.

155. Several courts have applied negligence theories of informed consent to drug prescription. *See, e.g.*, Hamilton v. Hardy, 37 Colo. App. 375, 549 P.2d 1099, 1104–05 (1976); Trogun v. Fruchtman, 58 Wis. 2d 596, 592–604, 207 N.W.2d 297, 307–15 (1973). At least one case holds drug prescription to be strictly a therapeutic decision, requiring no disclosure to or consent by the patient. *See* Malloy v. Shanahan, 280 Pa. Super. 440, 421 A.2d 803 (1980).

cago[156] was unusual, the federal district court apparently decided that only battery, from among existing doctrinal tools, provided sufficient protection to these patients' autonomy in the face of their doctors' conflict of interest.

During their prenatal care, the *Mink* plaintiffs were administered DES pursuant to a research experiment evaluating the effectiveness of the drug. Suing under both battery and negligence theories, plaintiffs claimed injuries from the increased risk of cancer to their daughters and from personal emotional distress arising from this threat to their children.

As noted in Part II, the application of battery analysis to these facts would ordinarily have been questionable on several grounds.[157] Although pills may have serious physical consequences, prescribing them does not involve the kind of touching traditionally associated with battery. Moreover, the plaintiffs had consented to prenatal care. Under prevailing standards,[158] miscarriage prevention would seem to fall within the ordinary scope of prenatal care; the fact that patients voluntarily ingested the pills would also typically have constituted consent.[159] Yet when the plaintiffs' claim was characterized as one alleging professional negligence, it failed. Even if nondisclosure were found to violate medical community standards, a questionable matter at best, the plaintiffs alleged no injury cognizable under negligence doctrine.[160]

Thus under existing medical consent law, the plaintiffs in *Mink* were trapped between the absence of unconsented touch on the one hand and the lack of injury to physical well-being on the other. Yet the court sensed an injury to patient choice that it was unwilling to ignore; it accepted a

---

156. 460 F. Supp. 713 (N.D. Ill. 1978).

157. *See supra* note 45.

158. The court itself stated the Illinois standard for battery to be a "total lack of consent by the patient." 460 F. Supp. at 717 (footnote omitted).

159. Exactly what the patients were told is a matter of some uncertainty. According to Mark Debofsky, of the office of the plaintiffs' attorney, various plaintiffs testified that doctors told them, "I want you to take these pills to help you through your pregnancy," "I want you to take these vitamins." Mr. Debofsky did not feel that the court's acceptance of the battery claim was premised on affirmative misrepresentation. Telephone interview with Mark Debofsky (Oct. 1984).

160. 460 F. Supp. at 720. *Cf.* Rogers v. Okin, 478 F. Supp. 1342, 1388 (D. Mass.) (no injury under negligence/informed consent because patients have not yet developed tardive dyskinesia, the primary risk/side-effect of medications they were forced to take), *aff'd in part, rev'd in part on other grounds*, 634 F.2d 650 (1st Cir. 1979). The inability to recover under negligence concepts of harm is a common thread in *Mink* and *Rogers*. The *Rogers* court's award of injunctive relief against forced medication based on constitutional grounds is analogous to the acceptance of a battery characterization in *Mink*: Each provided vindication for the patients' interests in choice independent of the definitions and standards of professional negligence. Given the *Rogers* court's constitutional holding, in which it explicitly stated that the competence of the professional recommendation was not sufficient to overcome or satisfy the patients' privacy right to refuse forced medication, it is theoretically though not pragmatically surprising that the court rejected a battery action and held that, although an informed consent action might be appropriate, it would be judged by standards of professional practice. *Id.* at 1387.

Protecting Patient Choice

battery characterization of the nondisclosure in *Mink* rather than allow that injury to go unredressed. The court set aside the absence of physical contact, stating that "[t]he gravamen of a battery action is the plaintiff's lack of consent, not the form of touching."[161] It also determined that the issue regarding consent was sufficient to go to the jury under a battery theory.

In explaining its decision, the court referred to performance of "substantially different *acts.*"[162] The description seems inapposite, however, for it is not the *acts* that were different. Rather, the essential complaint in *Mink* was that the patients were not given crucial information before consenting. Although nondisclosure about medication is typically analyzed, if at all, as an issue of professional negligence,[163] the particular nature of this undisclosed information caused the *Mink* court to deviate from that pattern. What the doctors did not disclose was their research purposes.[164] Although the court does not use the term "conflict of interest," that seems the essential framework from which its decision derives.

A doctor's specialized knowledge and powerful role make her a fiduciary to those who depend on her. Consequently, the doctor owes undivided loyalty to her patients.[165] This duty of loyalty constrains and legitimates whatever power the doctor has to advise or act on behalf of the patient. In *Mink*, however, the doctors' judgments were potentially influenced by research motivations. This violation of the doctor's fiduciary obligation of loyalty increased the court's concern that the dependent patient have the opportunity to control decisions.[166] Typically, where conflict of interest is

---

161. 460 F. Supp. at 717 n.4. The court observed that if the medicine had been administered by injection, touching would have been present. *Id.* at 718.

162. *Id.* (emphasis added).

163. *See supra* note 155. Certainly omitting to tell patients the content of a drug is common, *see* 2 MAKING DECISIONS, *supra* note 2, at 334, and such omission is not perceived as subjecting a doctor to liability. Failure to disclose side effect risks is treated as an issue of professional negligence.

164. Thus it is not the nature of the doctors' medical intervention that is at issue but their *motivation* for intervening.

165. RESTATEMENT (SECOND) OF AGENCY § 387 (1957).

166. *See* RESTATEMENT (SECOND) OF AGENCY § 390 comment a (1957). *But see* Burton v. Brooklyn Doctors Hosp., 88 A.D.2d 217, 452 N.Y.S.2d 875 (1982), which held that researching doctors were negligent in subjecting a premature baby to an experiment involving usage of high quantities of oxygen that eventually blinded the baby. Incompetent care, together with occurrence of injury cognizable under negligence analysis, rescued *Burton* from the problem faced by the court in *Mink*; there was no discussion of battery here. The court's analysis of disclosure, however, was seriously flawed. The court reversed a jury verdict of negligence against the treating doctor for not disclosing the experimentation by his colleagues, about which he knew, to the baby's parents. In so doing, it stated that the doctor did nothing wrong. It concluded that because "no evidence was offered of any continuing obligation on his part to obtain informed consent once his order was countermanded by a superior, the verdict against him based on failure to obtain informed consent cannot stand." *Id.* at 227, 452 N.Y.S.2d at 881–82. Although it is correct to say there was no incompetent *care* by this doctor, dismissal of the disclosure issue seems wrong. The court's "no evidence" characterization is puzzling, because it stated that the hospital imposed on the treating doctor the duty of informing parents, and that he testified that he could not remember informing them. *Id.* Although here the loss

The Yale Law Journal   Vol. 95: 219, 1985

involved, even a showing of competence is insufficient to immunize a fiduciary from liability.[167] A fiduciary must not only justify the substantive adequacy (the competence) of the transaction, but must also disclose it and seek the agreement of the client.[168] The *Mink* court's acceptance of a battery characterization is what prevented either the presence of professional competence or the absence of an injury to physical well-being from immunizing the conduct of the doctors.

The *Mink* decision demonstrates circumstances that call for stronger vindication of patient choice. It suggests the needed transition from physical parameters of consent toward a more intangible notion of medical choice. Furthermore, it transcends the dichotomy that places basic consent under battery doctrine while assigning issues of disclosure to negligence theory. Finally, it reveals that guaranteeing professionally competent care of physical well-being does not sufficiently safeguard patient autonomy.

b. *Application of General Fiduciary Principles*

When medical intervention leads to harm, the doctor who may be guilty of malpractice and does not wish to disclose pertinent facts has interests that directly conflict with those of the patient.[169] Such situations do not lend themselves to a *Mink*-type battery analysis. Some courts, sensing the underlying conflict, have achieved a similar result by analyzing these issues of disclosure under general principles of fiduciary duty. The duty to disclose for purposes of informed consent is a specific instance of such a fiduciary duty,[170] yet, for several reasons, a generic fiduciary duty to dis-

---

could be laid on other more culpable defendants, the court's analysis of nondisclosure leaves much to be desired. Again, the inadequacy stems in part from a refusal to examine disclosure in non-prototypical situations.

167. *See* RESTATEMENT (SECOND) OF AGENCY § 381 comment d (1957). A conflict of interest might, of course, cause the doctors to provide a level of care that falls below the professional standard of competence. If so, they would be liable for the results of that incompetence. There was no contention in *Mink* that the doctors had provided incompetent care at the time the drugs were administered. At the time, DES (a man-made estrogen) was widely prescribed as a miscarriage preventive. Note, *DES and a Proposed Theory of Enterprise Liability*, 46 FORDHAM L. REV. 963, 964 & n.4 (1978). The FDA did not withdraw DES from the market until 1971. Sindell v. Abbott Laboratories, 26 Cal. 3d 588, 594, 607 P.2d 924, 925, 163 Cal. Rptr. 132, 133, *cert. denied*, 449 U.S. 912 (1980).

168. Where an agent, even with the knowledge of the principal, acts on the agent's own account in a transaction, that agent "has a duty to deal fairly . . . *and* to disclose . . . all facts which the agent knows or should know would reasonably affect the principal's judgment, unless the principal has manifested that . . . he does not care to know them." RESTATEMENT (SECOND) OF AGENCY § 390 (1957). The limitation implied here by the qualifier "reasonably" is not nearly so restrictive as the reasonable person causation standard employed in informed consent cases: The actual individual client remains the decisionmaker, and the "unless" clause clearly tilts the requirement in favor of disclosure. Another analogy may be drawn from lawyer-client relations. *See* MODEL RULES OF PROFESSIONAL CONDUCT Rule 1.7(b) (1982) (requires both adequate representation and disclosure/consent).

169. *See* Delgado & Vogel, *supra* note 69, at 52 (proposing duty on all members of medical team to disclose any malpractice they have witnessed).

170. Canterbury v. Spence, 464 F.2d 772, 782 (D.C. Cir.), *cert. denied*, 409 U.S. 1064 (1972),

Protecting Patient Choice

close sometimes more effectively vindicates patient interests in autonomy than do the narrower duties that have crystallized under ordinary rules of medical consent.

Fiduciary responsibilities are imposed in order to regulate relationships marked by dependency and disparity of power.[171] Although technical expertise is the main reason a power inequity exists, such expertise is not the sole measure of the fiduciary's responsibility. Where the possibility of conflict of interest exists, the fiduciary's accountability for disclosure and accountability for competence are separate and cumulative, not alternative. Thus, analysis under general fiduciary principles is less likely than analysis under informed consent doctrines to narrow the obligation of disclosure or to confuse the issues of patient choice with those of professional competence.[172]

For example, where there is failure to disclose in the aftermath of a medical intervention, no proposal to touch or treat is made, and thus battery doctrine will not protect patient autonomy. The absence of proposed physical contact could also mean that no disclosure would be required under rules of informed consent.[173] Yet conflict of interest may trigger analysis under general fiduciary principles, requiring disclosure of all information that might be material to the patient.[174] Unlike the duties specified under battery or informed consent doctrines, such a duty has no limitation based on time or stage of treatment. It is triggered not by physical contact, but by the more flexible and general criterion of possession of relevant information.[175] Thus, under fiduciary principles, where malpractice has likely occurred, nondisclosure of the relevant facts may be remediable in an independent cause of action,[176] or may provide plaintiff a reason to toll the statute of limitations in a malpractice action that would otherwise be barred.[177]

---

draws on this earlier and broader concept of fiduciary duty to impose the specific informed consent duty.

171. *See* Frankel, *Fiduciary Law*, 71 CALIF. L. REV. 795 (1983) (emphasizing control of discretionary and unequal power as common theme in fiduciary law).

172. *But see* Delgado & Vogel, *supra* note 69, at 67 (noting that, although doctors are frequently characterized as fiduciaries, duties of disclosure imposed on them have been less extensive than those imposed on other fiduciaries). Outside of conflict of interest, fiduciary law, too, exhibits some ambivalence about the role of professional standards. *See infra* note 187.

173. *See, e.g.,* cases cited *supra* Part II(B)(1); *see also* Delgado & Vogel, *supra* note 69, at 69–71 (noting limited scope of informed consent duties).

174. *See* Nixdorf v. Hicken, 612 P.2d 348, 354 (Utah 1980) (duty to disclose applies to material information).

175. Such a standard is like the one developed in Gates v. Jensen, 92 Wash. 2d 246, 595 P.2d 919 (1979) (for discussion of case, see *supra* Part II(B)(2).

176. *See, e.g., Nixdorf,* 612 P.2d at 352 n.7.

177. Some courts impose an affirmative duty under which mere silence is tantamount to concealment. *See, e.g.,* Stafford v. Shultz, 42 Cal. 2d 767, 270 P.2d 1 (1954). Other courts require active misrepresentation or silence regarding a known certainty before tolling the statute. *See, e.g.,* Nardone v. Reynolds, 333 So. 2d 25, 34–40 (Fla. 1976).

Moreover, once a duty of disclosure is imposed under general fiduciary principles, there may be less tendency at other stages of the analysis to confuse the patient's interest in the information with issues of competent physical care.[178] Thus, expert testimony may be less likely to be required to establish the standard of care,[179] and defenses might be more narrowly drawn.[180] As in battery analysis, factual cause will tend to be presumed; no inquiry will likely be made regarding what a reasonable person would have done had the disclosure been made.[181] Remedy for a breach of fiduciary duty in circumstances involving conflict of interest may also be broader than if the action were one in ordinary negligence.[182]

Despite their tendency to broaden liability and remedy, however, several factors limit the capacity of general fiduciary duties to resolve problems identified here. First, a relatively crystallized conflict of interest may be necessary before courts decide that such principles should apply. If even the conflict of interest inherent in situations of alleged malpractice

---

178. *But see Nardone*, 333 So. 2d 25. The plaintiffs urged that doctors' nondisclosure of a possible cause of their son's deteriorated condition after brain surgery should toll the statute of limitations in their action for malpractice. The plaintiffs knew of the boy's condition but not why he had suddenly become worse. They were informed only that "these things happen." *Id.* at 29. The court held that the doctors had no affirmative duty to disclose their speculations as distinct from their certainties regarding causes. *Id.* at 39. Given the prevalence of uncertainty in medical knowledge, this distinction places severe constraints on the affirmative duty to disclose. *See also infra* text accompanying notes 215-31. *Nardone* illustrates that even the taint of fiduciary conflict of interest will not always be sufficient to cause a court to strengthen the protection it gives to patient autonomy.

179. Where disclosure of possible malpractice is at issue, the physical injury arises because of allegedly incompetent care, but the legal problem regarding *disclosure* of the harm has nothing to do with professional expertise. This may be more easily recognized in these cases because, intuitively, outcome disclosure is less likely than pretreatment disclosure to be characterized as a question of professional competence. *But see* Lopez v. Swyer, 115 N.J. Super. 237, 251, 279 A.2d 116, 124 (1971) (employing medical community standard of disclosure despite issue of possible malpractice).

The issues of standard of care here may simply parallel the debate over the standard of care in informed consent cases. States that use a reasonable person standard to decide issues of informed consent are likely to use the same criterion under general fiduciary analysis. Yet the influence probably flows the other way. Awareness of the breadth of fiduciary responsibilities may make a court more likely to choose the lay standard of disclosure even where the context is proposed treatment.

180. For instance, the defense of therapeutic privilege may not apply. Utah's informed consent statute, for example, has such a privilege, UTAH CODE ANN. § 78-14-5(2) (1977), which would presumably not apply where a court invoked the broad duty derived from fiduciary principles in *Nixdorf*, 612 P.2d 348.

181. *See, e.g., Nixdorf*, 612 P.2d 348; *Stafford*, 42 Cal. 2d 767, 270 P.2d 1; *Lopez*, 115 N.J. Super. 237, 279 A.2d 116.

182. *E.g.*, had the court imposed a duty to disclose facts to the plaintiff in *Kelton*, 413 A.2d 919, she might have recovered damages flowing from deprivation of her interest in making decisions not only about possible medical intervention, but also about litigation, possible adoption, etc. *See supra* text accompanying notes 66-71.

Delgado and Vogel discuss injuries that may result from nondisclosure of malpractice that are different from those arising from the malpractice itself. Economic harm in particular may be more easily recognized where the conceptual framework is one of general fiduciary responsibility rather than disclosure in the context of treatment per se. Delgado & Vogel, *supra* note 69, at 89; *see also* Hart v. Browne, 103 Cal. App. 3d 947, 163 Cal. Rptr. 356 (1980) (lost opportunity to file malpractice action because of negligence of doctor advising about whether another physician was guilty of malpractice).

Protecting Patient Choice

does not always trigger a duty to disclose,[183] general fiduciary principles would probably be ineffective to generate more aftermath disclosure where malpractice is unlikely.[184] Yet even where no malpractice judgment would be likely, doctors possess information that could be vital to their patients.

Second, decisions involving broad fiduciary principles of disclosure have most frequently arisen in the context of requests to toll the statute of limitations. In such cases, the duty to disclose is imposed for the limited purpose of removing a technical defense to malpractice. The underlying protected interest is still in some sense the same as that in professionally competent physical care.[185] It is less clear whether such a fiduciary duty of disclosure would be recognized as an independent action—i.e., as protecting an interest in patient knowledge and choice rather than as a reason to remove barriers to redress of injuries resulting from a violation of professional care.[186]

Thus, general fiduciary principles can ameliorate limitations on protection of patient choice under existing medical consent doctrines, but such principles are, at present, likely to be invoked only in limited circumstances for limited purposes. A more general fiduciary principle might yet emerge with sufficient coherence and force to solve the problems identified in this Article.[187] In the meantime, principles governing fiduciary conflict of interest have important implications for the protection of patient choice.

---

183. *See* Kelton v. District of Columbia, 413 A.2d 919 (D.C. 1980) (no duty to disclose scarring of fallopian tubes that occurred during caesarian birth); *Nardone*, 333 So. 2d at 39 (no duty to disclose conjecture about cause of relapse).

184. *See, e.g.*, Roark v. Allen, 633 S.W.2d 804 (Tex. 1982) (no duty to disclose factual condition about which doctors made competent but mistaken judgment). *But see* Tresemer v. Barke, 86 Cal. App. 3d 656, 150 Cal. Rptr. 384 (1978) (duty to warn former patient when later learned of dangers of IUD).

185. Damages in the delayed malpractice action may not be identical to what they would have been had the problem been disclosed at the outset. *See* Delgado and Vogel, *supra* note 69, at 89.

186. One court has recognized an independent action. *Nixdorf*, 612 P.2d 348. Another, without clearly addressing the relevant issues, declined to recognize any independent duty of aftermath disclosure. *Kelton*, 413 A.2d at 922.

187. LeBlang & King, *Tort Liability for Nondisclosure: The Physician's Legal Obligations to Disclose Patient Illness and Injury*, 89 DICK. L. REV. 1, 24–26 (1984), suggest that a broad fiduciary duty of disclosure is already emerging. However, many of the cases they annotate could be grounded on other analyses, such as the duty to provide competent care. Thus, the extent to which such cases really rest on and protect patients' autonomy interests, as the authors claim, is questionable.

Moreover, although a broad fiduciary duty surmounts some problems identified here, it is not immune to others. An agent's duty to "act on behalf of the principal," *see* RESTATEMENT (SECOND) OF AGENCY § 13 comment a (1957), may conflict with his accountability to the control of the principal. *Id.* at §§ 13, 14. In most agency relationships, this tension is resolved by contractual allocation of authority. *See id.* at § 376. But in professional relationships, contract is a weak and rarely used tool. In its absence, achieving adequate control by the principal (in professional settings, the client) is further complicated by incorporation of professional standards of conduct into agency rules. *Id.* at § 379 comment c (discussing obligations of professional agent in traditional agency terms). To the extent that professional standards provide a basis for measuring competent performance, they constitute no problem. To the extent that they become a substitute for control by the client, they present the same difficulties that are inherent in the rules now governing medical consent.

2. *Heightened Electiveness: Empowering the Patient*

Just as conflict of interest sometimes prompts courts to require special choice-protecting disclosure, so a factor that might be called "heightened electiveness" seems to produce more aggressive and independent protection of patient choice. I use the term "heightened electiveness" to denote cases where the special role of personal values or preferences causes a court to have greater than ordinary concern about patient choice. Two types of fact patterns seem presently to be perceived as possessing this characteristic: (1) those involving elective, especially cosmetic surgery; and (2) those involving procreation, including sterilization, pregnancy, and birth. Both cosmetic surgery and birth/procreational procedures are, to a significant degree, optional. No progressive and threatening disease drives the patient to undergo medical treatment. The patient seeks some affirmative outcome instead of warding off an encroaching evil. Furthermore, both types of decisions are recognized as highly personal, involving either the uniqueness of personal appearance or the deep personal values and consequences inherent in procreation and parenting.[188] Where heightened electiveness is present, courts sometimes analyze a case in terms of doctrines other than professional negligence, or alternatively, they may use the framework of professional negligence but adapt it in some fashion that increases the protection afforded to choice.

a. *Analysis Under Contract Principles*

A court may strengthen protection of patient choice by classifying the problem as one of contractual obligation, but few medical cases are analyzed under contractual theories. Those that are so analyzed emphasize the definiteness of the doctor's promise.[189] Although that factor may play a role, it is probably not generally dispositive. The certainty of the doctor's promises in such cases is not markedly greater than that in disputes where contractual analysis is denied.[190]

---

188. *See, e.g.*, Roe v. Wade, 410 U.S. 113 (1973) (right to abortion based on constitutional right to privacy); Griswold v. Connecticut, 381 U.S. 479 (1965) (access to birth control information protected by constitutional right of privacy). Procreation cases have to a considerable degree been analyzed as situation-specific, and they are indeed unique. However, these cases also illustrate unresolved issues that are generally present in current doctrines protecting choice.

189. *See* Depenbrok v. Kaiser Found. Health Plan, 79 Cal. App. 3d 167, 144 Cal. Rptr. 724 (1978) (patient may recover for breach of contract if doctor clearly promised a particular result); Guilmet v. Campbell, 385 Mich. 57, 188 N.W.2d 601 (1971) (allegation of specific, clear, and express promise sufficient to go to jury on contract theory). The critical problem is to distinguish between therapeutic reassurance and binding commitment in a setting of inherent uncertainty. As one annotator has aptly commented, "Despite the statement of some courts that [therapeutic reassurance and contractual promise] are quite distinct, there appears to be a 'gray area' . . . ." Annot., 43 A.L.R.3d 1221, 1226 (1972).

190. Thus promises such as "to cure him of bladder trouble," Marty v. Somers, 35 Cal. App.

Protecting Patient Choice

The more important factor leading courts to apply contractual doctrines is the electiveness of the medical intervention. A striking number of the cases employing contractual analysis involve cosmetic surgery or procreative choice.[191] The choice in these cases is often whether to have medical treatment at all, rather than simply what kind of treatment to choose for a condition that requires some treatment. Although courts ordinarily interpret doctors' positive descriptions of potential outcomes as harmless therapeutic reassurance, they are more willing in cases of elective treatment to believe that the doctor induced the treatment,[192] and accordingly more willing to hold the doctor accountable for her promised results rather than solely for the competence of her efforts.

Under tort law, the patient's interest in choice is analyzed under the rules of battery and informed consent; vindication of choice is often diluted. By contrast, contract vindicates patient choice directly. Injury to expectation is judged from the perspective of the actual patient and encompasses, but is not confined to, physical injury; physical contact is irrelevant; professional competence is not dispositive of duty.

b. *Analysis Under Battery Principles*

Battery doctrine, too, provides greater protection for choice than does negligence analysis. Battery applies where there has been no consent at all.[193] Decisions about whether a battery theory may be invoked are most difficult where the finding of no consent rests on whether a treatment is deemed to exceed a consent given to some different or lesser procedure. Although fact patterns vary considerably, cosmetic surgery or procreation

---

182, 182, 169 P. 411, 412 (1917), and that a doctor "could and would cure" an osteopathic problem, Kershaw v. Tilbury, 214 Cal. 679, 689, 8 P.2d 109, 113 (1932), have been held not to state a cause of action in contract. A promise to make the patient's hand "100% good," Wilson v. Blair, 65 Mont. 155, 177-78, 211 P. 289, 297 (1922) (Farr, J., dissenting), *overruled on other grounds*, Klemens & Son v. Reber Plumbing & Heating Co., 139 Mont. 115, 360 P.2d 1005 (1961), was unenforceable because it was not given for separate consideration, an approach that is merely a different way to defeat a contract characterization. *See also* Herrera v. Roessing, 533 P.2d 60 (Colo. Ct. App. 1975) (doctor's statement that patient would not get pregnant after tubal ligation mere opinion, not contractual guarantee). According to Lane and Hirsh, "Courts will look for 'buzz' words such as 'I guarantee' or 'I promise you,'" before upholding a cause of action in contract. Lane & Hirsh, *The Broken Promise: Physician's Breach of Warranty*, 89 CASE & COM., Sept.-Oct. 1984, at 3, 8.

191. *See, e.g.*, Depenbrok v. Kaiser Found. Health Plan, 79 Cal. App. 3d 167, 144 Cal. Rptr. 724 (1978) (promise that tubal ligation would prevent pregnancy); Sullivan v. O'Connor, 363 Mass. 579, 296 N.E.2d 183 (1973) (plastic surgery on nose); Stewart v. Rudner, 349 Mich. 459, 84 N.W.2d 816 (1957) (promise to perform Caesarian section); Hawkins v. McGee, 84 N.H. 114, 146 A. 641 (1929) (plastic surgery on hand). *But see* Herrera v. Roessing, 533 P.2d 60 (Colo. Ct. App. 1975) (statements about tubal ligation did not create contract).

192. *See, e.g.*, *Hawkins*, 84 N.H. 114, 146 A. 641 (relying on repeated solicitations of doctor to uphold contract claim).

193. *See* Cobbs v. Grant, 8 Cal. 3d 229, 240, 502 P.2d 1, 8, 104 Cal. Rptr. 505, 512 (1972).

The Yale Law Journal   Vol. 95: 219, 1985

cases also stand out among those that allow the battery characterization in such circumstances.[194]

c. *Negligence Analysis Under Altered Interest Definition*

Heightened electiveness sometimes causes courts to adapt standard negligence doctrines in ways that strengthen protection of patient choice. Such adaptations are particularly likely to occur in cases involving procreation.

Actions for wrongful birth have encountered multiple analytic difficulties under standard negligence doctrines. When these cases first emerged, courts were extremely reluctant to define the birth of a child,[195] particularly a healthy child,[196] as an injury. When constitutional protection of procreation deflected public policy objections to birth-as-injury,[197] analytic problems came to the fore. The birth of a child, especially a normal child, was difficult to encompass within a definition of protected interest as avoidance of physical injury.[198] If the unwanted child was physically defective, the absence of physical harm might seemingly be finessed, but new

---

194. In his exhaustive analysis of informed consent cases, Professor Rosoff discusses the circumstances under which a limited consent may be used to validate a more extensive operation. *See* A. ROSOFF, *supra* note 29, at 8–13. As cited by Rosoff, the cases refusing to extend consent include a sterilization, Wells v. Van Nort, 100 Ohio St. 101, 125 N.E. 910 (1919), a cosmetic addition to surgery, Lloyd v. Kull, 329 F.2d 168 (7th Cir. 1964), and a hip prosthesis, Cathemer v. Hunter, 27 Ariz. App. 780, 558 P.2d 975 (1976). By contrast, the cases accepting an extension of consent as valid involved the reduction of a fracture, McGuire v. Rix, 118 Neb. 434, 225 N.W. 120 (1929), and an appendectomy and rupture of cysts, Kennedy v. Parrott, 243 N.C. 355, 90 S.E.2d 54 (1956). Rosoff specifically mentions that where medical intervention affects reproductive capacity, ordinary rules about extension of consent may not apply. A. ROSOFF, *supra* note 29, at 8–12. For other decisions upholding battery claims for surgery, see Meretsky v. Ellenby, 370 So. 2d 1222, 1224 (Fla. Dist. Ct. App. 1979) (tip of nose alteration presents battery claim despite statute deeming written consent sufficient to relieve doctor of liability); Kinikin v. Heupel, 305 N.W.2d 589 (Minn. 1981) (breast reduction beyond patient consent constitutes battery); Bang v. Charles T. Miller Hosp., 251 Minn. 427, 88 N.W.2d 186 (1958) (consent to prostate resection does not bar claim of battery where possible severance of sperm cords not disclosed).

195. Gleitman v. Cosgrove, 49 N.J. 22, 31, 227 A.2d 689, 693 (1967).

196. *See, e.g.*, Shaheen v. Knight, 6 Lyc. Rptr. 19, 11 Pa. D. & C.2d 41 (Lycoming County Ct. 1957); Comment, *Wrongful Pregnancy: Recovery for Raising a Healthy Child*, 10 N. KY. L. REV. 341 (1983).

197. *See* Boone v. Mullendore, 416 So. 2d 718 (Ala. 1982); Cockrum v. Baumgartner, 95 Ill. 2d 193, 447 N.E.2d 385, *cert. denied*, 464 U.S. 846 (1983); Christensen v. Thornby, 192 Minn. 123, 255 N.W. 620 (1934); Gleitman v. Cosgrove, 49 N.J. 22, 227 A.2d 689 (1967); Collins, *supra* note 52, at 691–93.

198. *See, e.g.*, Howard v. Lecher, 42 N.Y.2d 109, 112, 366 N.E.2d 64, 66, 397 N.Y.S.2d 363, 365 (1977) (parents "were made to bear no physical or mental injury, other than the anguish of observing their child suffer"); Hickman v. Myers, 632 S.W.2d 869, 870 (Tex. Ct. App. 1982) ("A parent cannot be said to have been damaged by the birth and rearing of a normal, healthy child."). In significant part this concern is discussed as a problem of damages—their intangibility, their uncertainty, and the difficulty of balancing benefits and burdens. *See, e.g.*, Public Health Trust v. Brown, 388 So. 2d 1084, 1085–86 (Fla. Dist. Ct. App. 1980) ("[T]he intangible but all-important, incalculable but invaluable 'benefits' of parenthood far outweigh any of the mere monetary burdens involved."); Rieck v. Medical Protective Co., 64 Wis. 2d 514, 518, 219 N.W.2d 242, 244 (1974) ("Every child's smile, every bond of love and affection, every reason for parental pride . . . . [T]hese are intangible benefits, but they are nonetheless real.").

Protecting Patient Choice

analytic problems arose. It was hard to view the child's physical defect as a harm *to the parent*,[199] yet parents often brought suit on their own behalf, alleging breach of duties owed to them.[200]

Delineations of duty also derive from definition of interest. It was easier to tolerate the unusual nature of the injury involved in these cases if the breach was of a duty that was familiar to negligence doctrine. Such a duty might be an ordinary one of competent care, breached, for instance, by a botched procedure or misdiagnosis.[201] Or it might be a duty of disclosure stemming from the subsidiary choice interest under informed consent, breached for instance, by a failure to disclose risks.[202] Where, however, not only the injury but the duty as well was unusual, it was doubly difficult for a court to recognize this cause of action.[203]

One court solved these analytic problems in a procreation case by redefining the protected interest from physical well-being to an intangible concept of choice. *Berman v. Allen*[204] spoke of the plaintiff's injury as one of being "deprived of the option of making a meaningful decision as to whether to abort the fetus."[205] There is little difficulty in recognizing the birth of either a healthy or a defective child as an injurious consequence if the protected interest is choice. Further, such a formulation easily recognizes parents as plaintiffs in their own right. The redefinition of protected interest also allowed *Berman* to impose a rather unusual duty. In circumstances similar to those in which the court in *Karlsons* found no such duty,[206] the *Berman* court recognized an obligation to preserve the parents' choice by informing them about the availability of amniocentesis

---

199. *See* Howard v. Lecher, 42 N.Y.2d 109, 112, 366 N.E.2d 64, 66, 397 N.Y.S.2d 363, 365 (1977). Capron, *supra* note 52, at 642, effectively critiqued the treatment of parents as bystanders.

200. For a list of cases, see Collins, *supra* note 52, at 693-95 nn.81-84.

201. One of the first cases to allow recovery for the birth of a healthy child was Custodio v. Bauer, 251 Cal. App. 2d 303, 59 Cal. Rptr. 463 (1967), in which a negligent surgical sterilization failed to prevent pregnancy. *See* Troppi v. Scarf, 31 Mich. App. 240, 187 N.W.2d 511 (1971) (negligent filling of birth control pill prescription resulted in unwanted pregnancy); Dumer v. St. Michael's Hosp., 69 Wis. 2d 766, 233 N.W.2d 372 (1975) (wrongful birth derived from negligent failure to diagnose rubella).

202. *See* Harbeson v. Parke-Davis, Inc., 98 Wash. 2d 460, 472, 656 P.2d 483, 491 (1983) (health care providers have duty "to impart to their patients material information as to the likelihood of future children's [sic] being born defective").

203. Although in Karlsons v. Guerinot, 57 A.D.2d 73, 394 N.Y.S.2d 933 (1977), the court did recognize the parents as appropriate plaintiffs, the only duty the court recognized was that of providing competent physical care. *See supra* text accompanying notes 50-65.

204. 80 N.J. 421, 404 A.2d 8 (1979).

205. *Id.* at 430-31, 404 A.2d at 13. *Harbeson*, 98 Wash. 2d at 478, 656 P.2d at 494, involving a more typical breach of duty—the failure to inform a woman plaintiff of risks involved in becoming pregnant while taking epilepsy medication—uses similar language: "Mrs. Harbeson ought to have been informed in order to intelligently exercise her judgment whether to have further children."

206. Like the plaintiff in *Karlsons*, 57 A.D.2d 73, 394 N.Y.S.2d 933, the plaintiff in *Berman* was in her late thirties at the time of the pregnancy. Both women claimed their doctors had a duty to inform them about amniocentesis in order to determine possible fetal abnormality. In both cases the babies were born with Down's Syndrome.

The Yale Law Journal   Vol. 95: 219, 1985

even though no analysis of informed consent would ordinarily be triggered.[207] With choice as the directly protected interest, such a duty of disclosure was both more obvious and more legitimate. The touch-based boundaries of disclosure under informed consent doctrine could be discarded.

Despite its imposition of an unusual duty, *Berman* did not follow its redefinition of interest with an altered standard of care.[208] Other courts, however, have altered the standard of care in cases of heightened electiveness. The Iowa Supreme Court, for instance, although acknowledging that it usually employed a medical community standard in cases of informed consent, adopted a reasonable person standard in a case involving a vasectomy.[209] It explicitly rested that decision on the elective and personal nature of the medical treatment involved.[210]

Berman's redefinition of protected interest did alter its analysis in another crucial way. Although choice is routinely assessed by an objective standard in informed consent actions where it provides the causal link to physical injury,[211] the *Berman* court used a subjective, individualized standard, asking only what these particular parents would have done.[212] This individualized approach emerges naturally where choice itself becomes the protected interest.[213]

Finally, with reference to analysis of damages, *Berman* asserted that because the doctors neither caused nor could have ameliorated the baby's defects, a comprehensive award of tort damages would be out of proportion to defendants' culpability. The court held that the parents could recover damages for emotional distress, but could not recover for the costs of

---

207. *See supra* Part II(B)(1).

208. It adopted the medical community standard. The court accepted without discussion the plaintiffs' characterization of the issue as one to be measured by "accepted medical standards." 80 N.J. at 424, 404 A.2d at 10.

209. Cowman v. Hornaday, 329 N.W.2d 422 (Iowa 1983); *cf.* Cross v. Trapp, 294 S.E.2d 446 (W. Va. 1982) (adopting reasonable person standard in case involving male impotence as result of prostate resection). West Virginia previously had no case law or statute governing informed consent.

210. *Cowman*, 329 N.W.2d at 427. In jurisdictions that routinely employ the lay standard in informed consent cases any special impact of the procreation fact pattern is obscured. *See, e.g., Harbeson*, 98 Wash. 2d 460, 656 P.2d 483.

211. *See* 3 MAKING DECISIONS, *supra* note 2, at 197 (virtually all states employ objective standard of causation).

212. *Berman*, 80 N.J. at 431–32, 404 A.2d at 14. New Jersey apparently has no case or statutory law on causation apart from *Berman*. *Cf. Harbeson*, 98 Wash. 2d 460, 656 P.2d 483, which also adopts without comment a subjective analysis of causation in a procreation case. *Id.* at 482–83, 656 P.2d at 494. Washington clearly employs an objective standard of causation in other informed consent cases, making this decision unique to the procreation context. *Cf.* Steele v. St. Paul Fire & Marine Ins. Co., 371 So. 2d 843, 851 (La. Ct. App.), *cert. denied*, 374 So. 2d 658 (La. 1979) (in hysterectomy case involving young woman, court applied objective person standard but used "in the circumstances" provision of the standard to particularize it to an unusual degree to individual plaintiff).

213. The court did not comment on its divergence from the norm of objective causation. It may simply have responded intuitively to the shift it had made in the structure of the action.

Protecting Patient Choice

rearing the child. As a matter of sanctioning policy, the court's decision might be wise, but the assertion that the doctors did not cause the baby's defects is argumentative at best. It is true that the doctors did not cause the baby's defects in the way that professional malpractice might have caused such injuries. By the court's own logic, however, the protected interest here was choice. The doctors *did cause* a deprivation of choice. The culpable conduct was a failure to inform that prevented the parents from being able to choose to terminate the pregnancy. Thus, a more apt phrasing of the court's concern would be that invasion of the parents' interest in competent care was more culpable than invasion of their interest in choice, thereby justifying a difference in damages.[214] Regardless of whether one agrees with *Berman*'s resolution of the damages problem, the issue is appropriately one of policy about sanctioning, rather than one of causal connection. Defining choice as the protected interest helped to clarify the difference; *Berman*'s explicit focus on comparative culpability rather than on the existence of injury was a step in the right direction.

B. *The Limits of Professional Competence: Generalization of the Patterns*

Conflict of interest undermines the doctor's claim to authority, and special values or preferences intensify the patient's right to control. If either factor is present, courts may alter the overall classification of the action or shift sub-elements within standard analyses in order more clearly to identify and protect patient choice. These exceptions ought not to be narrowly delimited. The issues are pervasive and the rationale is more inclusive than courts have yet recognized. Individuals and their preferences are inherently unique. Professional competence can provide only limited resolu-

---

214. *Berman* might be characterized as specifying an additional set of circumstances in which there may be recovery for infliction of emotional distress. It is probably more accurate, however, to describe the court as limiting, for reasons of sanctioning policy, the recovery it is willing to allow for invasion of its newly defined interest in choice. Other courts might prefer different solutions to the problem of determining what extent and type of recovery is appropriate in these cases. A decision to protect choice does not settle difficult issues of sanctioning policy; it merely clarifies the questions. *See* Collins, *supra* note 52, at 695–700; *infra* Part IV.

The court's decision in *Berman* that emotional distress damages are the only appropriate remedy for this deprivation of choice finds a precursor in Vara v. Drago, 24 A.D.2d 888, 264 N.Y.S.2d 660 (1965). In *Vara*, the defendant failed to tell the plaintiff of his discovery, two months before her due date, that her fetus had died. On appeal, the court affirmed an award of damages for mental anguish *only*. Unless these damages are conceived as the result of outrageous intentional conduct, they were unusual, especially in 1965. RESTATEMENT (SECOND) OF TORTS §§ 46-48, 905 comment c (1977). Freestanding emotional distress damages have only recently been accepted in negligence actions. *See*, *e.g.*, Molien v. Kaiser Found. Hosp., 27 Cal. 3d 916, 616 P.2d 813, 167 Cal. Rptr. 831 (1980). *Vara* can possibly be explained as a variant on the cases having to do with handling of dead bodies, PROSSER & KEETON, *supra* note 18, at 328-30, but the court makes no reference to those cases. More likely, there was some inchoate sense of an injury akin to what I have labeled here as an interest in patient knowledge and choice.

tion of limited questions. The proposition that regulation of professional competence cannot substitute for vigorous protection of patient choice is, then, a matter of general rather than exceptional applicability.

1. *Medical Uncertainty: The Basis of Electiveness*

Implicit in any assumption that competence can adequately substitute for choice is a medical world in which expertise either points in a single direction or, at least, can best choose such a direction from among competing alternatives. Though the idea is comforting, no such world exists.[215] A moment's reflection will suggest long lists of things medicine does not fully know or understand, from the cause of the common cold to the cure for cancer. Although doctors are trained to present a face of decisiveness to patients, they are often only sure about their uncertainty.[216]

Medical uncertainty destroys the possibility of a single right answer, leaving many answers to compete. Specializations and schools of thought in medicine have strenuous and unresolved differences. In terms of quality of care, traditional malpractice law can assure that a doctor's behavior is proper as judged by the norms of at least one recognized school of thought.[217] Strictly as a matter of competence regulation, it is fair that a doctor should not be penalized for a careful, good faith recommendation of a given reputable approach to care. Yet conformity to a particular school of thought does not assure that that viewpoint best fits the circumstances and preferences of the patient. Because there is no certainty about who is right, the patient should receive information about divergent views and be allowed to arrive at her own decision.

Moreover, competence regulation does not guarantee the best possible or the most care; doctors are penalized only if they fall below a minimum threshold of reasonable professional behavior, evidenced legally by what the average doctor in good standing in her profession actually does.[218] Although doctors' knowledge or advice can be appropriately evaluated by reference to what other competent doctors do, questions of how sure one should be about the fact that no skull fracture is present,[219] that an abor-

---

215. J. KATZ, *supra* note 7, at 165-206. Professor Katz, himself a doctor, comprehensively documents both the prevalence of uncertainty and doctors' discomfort in admitting it to their patients.

216. *"There is no certainty about the available knowledge, but its uncertainty can be specified."* J. KATZ, *supra* note 7, at 183-84 (emphasis in original). Medical training forces doctors to present at least an impression of certainty, even in the face of uncertainty. *Id.* at 184.

217. PROSSER & KEETON, *supra* note 18, § 32, at 186-87.

218. *Id.* Prosser notes that while the "averageness" concept refers to professionals in good standing, even "of these it is not the middle but the minimum common skill which is to be looked to." *Id.* at 187. Furthermore, some states still adhere to the locality rule, a further limitation on the standard of care. *Id.* at 164.

219. Roark v. Allen, 633 S.W.2d 804 (Tex. 1982).

Protecting Patient Choice

tion is complete,[220] that immature cells in excised tissue do not signal cancer,[221] that glaucoma,[222] heart disease,[223] or cervical cancer[224] is not developing, that a fetus does not have detectable genetic defect,[225] or that a breast is not unnecessarily amputated[226] are not ultimately questions that can be settled by medical expertise. At bottom, they are questions of allocating scarce resources, personal or societal.[227] Expertise per se provides data and experiential wisdom to inform decisions, but it cannot strike the ultimate balance. Like other questions of utility and value, such issues should be referred to the individual who will enjoy the benefits and suffer the consequences of the choice.[228]

Both courts and doctors have been quick to accept uncertainty as a justification for flexing and softening the standards of professional competence, and appropriately so. They have been less quick to recognize uncertainty's implications for patient self-determination.[229] Although medical

---

220. Stills v. Gratton, 55 Cal. App. 3d 698, 127 Cal. Rptr. 652 (1976).

221. Jamison v. Lindsay, 108 Cal. App. 3d 223, 166 Cal. Rptr. 443 (1980).

222. Gates v. Jensen, 92 Wash. 2d 246, 595 P.2d 919 (1979) (en banc).

223. Keogan v. Holy Family Hosp., 95 Wash. 2d 306, 622 P.2d 1246 (1980) (en banc).

224. Truman v. Thomas, 27 Cal. 3d 285, 611 P.2d 902, 165 Cal. Rptr. 308 (1980) (en banc).

225. Karlsons v. Guerinot, 57 A.D.2d 73, 394 N.Y.S.2d 933 (App. Div. 1977).

226. Hanks v. Doctors Ranson, Swan & Burch, Ltd., 359 So. 2d 1089 (La. Ct. App.), *cert. denied*, 360 So. 2d 1178 (La. 1978).

227. Societal judgment might, of course, override individual choice, as in the case of scarce resources (*e.g.*, organ transplants), or because of public financing of health care. Helling v. Carey, 83 Wash. 2d 514, 519 P.2d 981 (1974) (en banc) (failure to test for glaucoma in patients under 40 is negligent despite conformity to professional standard of care), offers one example of a judicially administered societal intervention into the question of how much care/certainty is enough. The practical effect of *Helling* is to demand a standard response by all doctors to all similarly situated patients, and to brand as culpable any professional who fails to make that response. This issue might be better addressed, however, at the level of individual choice, as suggested here. For further discussion of societal considerations, see *infra* text accompanying notes 326–33.

228. There is a reluctance to think of professions in market terms. For a classic description, see, *e.g.*, Hughes, *Professions*, 92 DAEDALUS 655, 657 (1963) (identifying distinctive traits of a profession, including principle of credat emptor rather than caveat emptor); Newmark v. Gimbel's, Inc., 54 N.J. 585, 258 A.2d 697 (1969) (distinguishing professionals from commercial actors in terms of which legal rules are appropriate for regulation of conduct). This view has hindered awareness of medical care as a service traded for money, or as necessitating active consumer evaluation in order to maximize utility. Recently a great deal more attention has been given to the need for active consumer decision-making and tighter market controls in health care, mainly as a result of concern about rising medical costs. *See, e.g.*, 42 C.F.R. § 476.2–3 (1984) (Department of Health and Human Services regulations requiring disclosure by professional standards review organizations of costs and performance records of medical care providers); *A Special Symposium: Market-Oriented Approaches to Achieving Health Policy Goals*, 34 VAND. L. REV. 849 (1981).

Several major developments in law reflect and support this trend. *See, e.g.*, Arizona v. Maricopa County Medical Soc'y, 457 U.S. 332 (1982) (applying antitrust laws to professions); Bates v. State Bar of Arizona, 433 U.S. 350 (1977) (analogous case, Arizona Supreme Court rule prohibiting professional advertising held unconstitutional); Virginia State Bd. of Pharmacy v. Virginia Citizens Consumer Council, Inc., 425 U.S. 748 (1976) (state statute prohibiting professional advertising by pharmacists held unconstitutional).

229. The Washington Supreme Court's unusually intense awareness of how uncertainty limits the effectiveness of competence regulation (in *Helling* and *Gates*) probably motivated its expansion of protection for choice in *Gates*. *See supra* note 96.

The Yale Law Journal   Vol. 95: 219, 1985

uncertainty heightens the need for professional *advice*, it also strengthens the case for lay *choice*.

Choosing among alternative courses of action implicates individual characteristics of the patient, such as career, age, and gender, as well as personal attitudes and values, from religious belief to risk aversion. A preference for surgical treatment of a back problem or, alternatively, for long-term rest and traction, may depend on the patient's job or lifestyle. A woman's preference for a radical mastectomy as opposed to conservative surgery or chemotherapy may depend more on her body image, age and career than on medically expert knowledge.[230]

The elective quality of plastic surgery and the personal character of procreation are easily perceived. Less recognizable is the fact that the uncertainty and diversity of medical opinion necessarily turn much of medical decision-making into an exercise in electiveness. If cost-benefit comparisons (financial and otherwise) are not made by the patient, there is a significant danger that decisions will reflect the doctor's attitudes and values rather than the patient's.[231]

2. *Conflict of Values: Close Analogue of Conflict of Interest*

The conflict of loyalties in *Mink v. University of Chicago* was crystallized in a way that made recognition of the affront to patient autonomy relatively easy. Conflicts of interest differ from what might be labeled conflicts of judgment or value mainly in terms of the degree to which such

---

230. For an illustration, see J. KATZ, *supra* note 7, at 90–93, 182–84. Similarly, a woman's preference for separating the diagnostic biopsy from the final surgery may be controlled by her attitudes toward bodily disfigurement and risk aversion. *Cf. Hanks*, 359 So. 2d 1089 (no liability for nondisclosure of possibility of separating biopsy from amputation; breast removed after erroneous diagnosis).

There are countless other examples suggesting the need for a different allocation of authority between doctors and patients. Is it better to exercise or not to? Experts disagree. *See A Warning About the Exercise Experts*, San Francisco Chron., Sept. 14, 1984, at 24, col. 1. The choice may depend more on how vital exercise is to the patient's mental and emotional well-being or to a family's pattern of activities than on purely medical recommendation. What form of birth control is best? The answer may depend on sexual habits more than on medical conclusions about safety or effectiveness. Are coronary artery bypass operations desirable? That could depend on what changes a person is willing and able to make in exercise and stress patterns. Yaeger, *Bettering the Odds: Cardiologists Focus Efforts on Prevention of Heart Attacks*, Wall St. J., July 2, 1984, at 1, col. 1; *see also* M. MILLMAN, THE UNKINDEST CUT: LIFE IN THE BACKROOMS OF MEDICINE 90–151, 217–49 (1978) (discussing medical management of mistakes and the overselling of coronary bypass in the face of its uncertain value). Is it better to take time to do a fluid culture to determine whether antibiotics will be effective against an infant's constant ear infections or to turn immediately to standard drugs? The choice may depend on the weight one places on unknown risks associated with powerful chemicals. Etcetera.

231. J. KATZ, *supra* note 7, at 173–74, describes a doctor whose recommendations in favor of radical surgery rather than more conservative approaches were influenced more by his attitudes toward his father and his mentor than by scientific evidence. For other examples, see *id.* at 131–41, 175–84; Hilfiker, *Making Medical Mistakes*, HARPERS, May 1984, at 59. Hilfiker argues that doctors need to accept and have others accept their errors. This is clearly true. It also, however, underscores the need for sharing difficult decisions with the people whose lives depend on them.

Protecting Patient Choice

crystallization is present. Even the best doctor is influenced by various motives, concerns and goals—many of which may not be as benign from the vantage point of patient interests as the medical research in *Mink*. Concerns about income, prestige, and professional independence affect a doctor's recommendations in indirect ways. Even relatively nonselfish factors such as commitments to particular scientific assumptions or medical techniques, as well as personal or professional values, affect the judgments made by doctors regarding the care of patients.

Moreover, doctors as a group are, like other groups, subject to error, to intellectual or professional fashion, to blindspots and myopia. Group-typical behavior is not necessarily either wrongful or incompetent, but neither will it be carefully evaluated by standards of competence that are set by the actual practice of the group itself. Blindspots associated with group characteristics can bend doctors' preferences in ways that differentiate those preferences from those of their patients. For example, doctors as a group are professionally committed to lifesaving. In the past they have tended to interpret "lifesaving" as meaning the maximum extension of biological life. Recently, with demands for "death with dignity," it has become apparent that large numbers of lay persons have different preferences than those that doctors have chosen to implement.[232] Similarly, for years most doctors have been male. As a result, doctors as a group may well have had different preferences about gender-related medical issues such as birth control, procreation, and breast cancer than the population they treated.[233]

---

232. Public policy concerning the right to die is being reconsidered in light of changing medical facts and social values. As that process advances, disputes about the relative authority of doctors and patients can be expected to increase. In Bartling v. Superior Ct., 163 Cal. App. 3d 186, 209 Cal. Rptr. 220 (1984), a patient suffering from five serious diseases asked the hospital to remove his life-sustaining apparatus. The hospital refused and the superior court upheld the hospital. Although the decision was reversed on appeal, reversal came after the patient died. More courts are accepting right to die pleas. *See, e.g.*, Satz v. Perlmutter, 362 So. 2d 160 (Fla. Dist. Ct. App. 1978), *aff'd*, 379 So. 2d 359 (Fla. 1980); *In re* Conroy, 98 N.J. 321, 486 A.2d 1209 (1985). *But see* Bouvia v. County of Riverside, No. 159780 (Cal. Super. Ct. Dec. 16, 1983) (order denying preliminary injunction against forced feeding). Despite this trend, many people still find themselves in conflict with individual doctors, hospitals and courts over their rights to control decisions about their treatment where death is likely. An estimated five million Americans have made living wills stating their wish not to be artificially kept alive where there is no hope of recovery. Nelson, *Doctors Debate Right To Stop 'Heroic' Effort To Keep Elderly Alive*, Wall St. J., Sept. 7, 1982, at 1, col. 1, 20, col. 2.

233. *See generally* G. COREA, THE HIDDEN MALPRACTICE: HOW AMERICAN MEDICINE TREATS WOMEN AS PATIENTS AND PROFESSIONALS (1977) (tracing effects of male domination of medical profession on health care received by women); B. EHRENREICH AND D. ENGLISH, COMPLAINTS AND DISORDERS: THE SEXUAL POLITICS OF SICKNESS (1973) (tracing history of institutional sexism in health care); Morrow, *Women's Health Care and Informed Consent: Who Should Decide What Is Best For Women—Patients or Doctors*, 9 GOLDEN GATE U.L. REV. 553 (1978–79) (discussing factors that have contributed to current problems in women's health care and capacity for change through use of informed consent); Note, *Coerced Sterilization Under Federally Funded Family Planning Programs*, 11 NEW ENG. L. REV. 589 (1976) (discussing effectiveness of regulations guarding against coercive sterilization); Watchorn, *Midwifery: A History of Statutory Suppres-*

The Yale Law Journal   Vol. 95: 219, 1985

Decisions made in a climate of conflicting values or judgments are every bit as consequential to patients as those made when there are conflicts of interest. And it is, after all, the fact that she will have to live with the consequences of the medical choice upon which the patient's claim to authority preeminently rests. As the above examples suggest, there is good reason to be alert to professional advisors' inchoate divisions of loyalty. Indeed, such divisions should be presumed as a given of human nature; the only meaningful safeguard is assurance of the opportunity for patient rather than professional choice.

Not only have some types of conflict been more readily identifiable, some have also been thought more culpable. Conflict of interest has been traditionally viewed as a more serious problem than conflict of value and judgment. The lesson of *Mink*, however, is that there need be no implication of doctor wrongdoing in the narrow sense of that word to justify aggressive protection of patient choice.

In comparison to the crass self-interest of acting to suppress a lawsuit, the conflict of interest in *Mink*[234] was relatively benign, involving research presumably undertaken for the good of society. The comparatively good intentions of these doctors might once have shielded them from criticism.[235] However, sensitivity concerning patient self-determination has increased. The concept of wrong itself has evolved: Wrongfulness here is the illegitimate usurpation of authority. No matter how benign their goals, or how competent their recommendations, the University doctors' research had the potential to distort their decisionmaking.[236] *Mink* allowed the jury to consider, without reference to the constraints of negligence analysis, whether the doctors' substitution of their judgment for that of their patients was permissible.[237]

The problem of unjustified paternalism in medicine transcends the

---

sion, 9 GOLDEN GATE U.L. REV. 631 (1978-79) (tracing legislation affecting the midwife's opportunities).

234. Mink v. University of Chicago, 460 F. Supp. 713 (N.D. Ill. 1978).

235. For extraordinary documentation of relatively casual attitudes toward patient consent where the advancement of science is involved, see J. KATZ, EXPERIMENTATION WITH HUMAN BEINGS (1972); Boffey, *Medical Experimentation: Everybody's a Critic*, San Francisco Chron., Dec. 2, 1984, at 19, col. 1.

236. Biased decisionmaking is the reason universities and other research organizations funded by the government are now required to conduct extensive institutional review of all research conducted on human beings. *E.g.*, Dept. of Health and Human Services, Regulations on Protection of Human Subjects, 45 C.F.R. §§ 46.101-46.117 (1984). *See* Robertson, *The Law of Institutional Review Boards*, 26 UCLA L. REV. 484 (1979). In addition, many private hospitals and treatment centers are establishing their own ethics and decisionmaking review procedures. *See* Kleiman, *Hospital Philosopher Confronts Life's Basic Issues*, N.Y. Times, Jan. 23, 1984, at B1, col. 5.

237. 460 F. Supp. at 717. In the context of bodily contact, differences of judgment and value are presumed and autonomy protected; it is not necessary to demonstrate a conflict of interest in order to justify the patient's right of control. As I have demonstrated, however, current legal doctrines do not adequately protect against unjustified paternalism where only information is involved. *See supra* Part II.

Protecting Patient Choice

boundaries of traditional conflict of interest.[238] The medical profession holds relatively strong ethical and disciplinary ideals proscribing conflicts of interest,[239] but its norms about deference to patient autonomy in instances of conflict of judgment or value are seriously underdeveloped. Moreover, legal analysis of fiduciary and professional responsibility is only gradually becoming attentive to these subtler problems of allocating authority.[240] Because contractual arrangements that govern divisions of authority in most commercial agency relationships are all but absent in professional-client settings,[241] the need for legal rules that establish the limits of professional authority is especially great.

---

238. *See generally* J. CHILDRESS, WHO SHOULD DECIDE? PATERNALISM IN HEALTH CARE (1982) (classifying types of paternalism and analyzing when it is unjustifiable in medical decisionmaking).

239. One of the seven Principles of Medical Ethics adopted by the A.M.A. in 1980 states that "a physician shall . . . strive to expose those physicians deficient in character or competence, or who engage in fraud or deception." JUDICIAL COUNCIL, AM. MEDICAL ASS'N, CURRENT OPINIONS at ix (1984) (Principle II); *see also id.* § 4.04 at 14 (requiring physician to disclose ownership in health care facilities); *id.* § 6.03 at 24 (prohibiting fee-splitting). "The symbol of the profession . . . portrays a group whose members have altruistic motivations and whose professional activities are governed by a code of ethics which . . . condemns misuse of professional skills for selfish purposes." Becker, *The Nature of a Profession,* in 2 THE SIXTY-FIRST YEARBOOK OF THE NATIONAL SOCIETY FOR THE STUDY OF EDUCATION 27, 36 (1962).

Although the A.M.A. Code includes general requirements that the physician shall "respect the rights of patients", *id.* at ix (Principle IV), and shall "deal honestly with patients," *id.* (Principle II), Katz traces the long history of nondisclosure and failure to share decisions with patients. J. KATZ, *supra* note 7, at 1–29. Professor Katz notes the direct conflict between the medical norm of "custody" and the legal norm of personal liberty. *Id.* at 2.

240. The doctrine of informed consent in medicine is part of that effort. J. KATZ, *supra* note 7, at 28, points out that the "recent interest in disclosure and consent," following a "history of silence," could not be expected, as yet, to have altered centuries of contrary medical tradition.

Struggles over professional authority and client control have also emerged within the legal profession. *See* Bell, *Serving Two Masters: Integration Ideals and Client Interests in School Desegregation Litigation,* 85 YALE L.J. 470 (1976); Burt, *Conflict and Trust Between Attorney and Client,* 69 GEO. L.J. 1015 (1981); Spiegel, *Lawyering and Client Decisionmaking: Informed Consent and the Legal Profession,* 128 U. PA. L. REV. 41 (1979); *cf.* Jones v. Barnes, 463 U.S. 745 (1983) (failure of attorney to honor client directive regarding nature of arguments made on appeal did not deprive client of effective counsel). The new ABA Model Rules of Professional Conduct make a greater effort to deal with the issue of client choice and professional disclosure than either the comparable medical rules or the earlier legal rules. MODEL RULES OF PROFESSIONAL CONDUCT Rule 1.4 (1982). Explanations of the legal background for the model rules refer to the RESTATEMENT (SECOND) OF AGENCY § 381 (1958) as a basis for broad disclosure obligations. *See* T. MORGAN & R. ROTUNDA, PROBLEMS AND MATERIALS ON PROFESSIONAL RESPONSIBILITY 175, 177 (2d ed. Supp. 1983).

241. RESTATEMENT (SECOND) OF AGENCY § 376 (1958) anticipates that the extent of an agent's authority will be determined by the terms of the agreement between agent and principal. Although the doctor-patient relationship typically originates from a contract, the terms of the relationship are not usually explicitly bargained for. Instead, the professional model has presumed unquestioning client trust, *see* Hughes, *supra* note 228, at 657, and what courts are fond of calling "abject dependence." *See, e.g.,* Cobbs v. Grant, 8 Cal. 3d 229, 242, 502 P.2d 1, 9, 104 Cal. Rptr. 505, 513 (1972). These presumptions are obviously in conflict with respect for patient consent and control.

The Yale Law Journal   Vol. 95: 219, 1985

c. *Conclusion of Part III*

Where conflict of interest disqualifies the doctor or heightened electiveness intensifies the patient's claim to autonomy, courts have acted to overcome distortions and omissions that have plagued existing legal protection
of patient autonomy. The rationale for such exceptions needs to be generalized. Professional competence does not satisfy the goals of patient autonomy. Medical uncertainty forces a high degree of election in decisionmaking, and extra-medical values necessarily shape resulting choices. The
conflicts of value and judgment that are inherent in all human decision
are both consequential and problematic. Thus, preemption of authority in
circumstances where competent adults may be consulted regarding their
own fate is unjustifiable. Patient choice ought to be a fully and independently protected legal interest.

IV. A NEW INTEREST IN MEDICAL CHOICE

A. *The Interest is Desirable and Congruent with Other Doctrines*

Serious deficiencies exist in the protection presently accorded to patient
autonomy. Both as a matter of omission and as a matter of exception, the
present doctrinal schema is inadequate and inconsistent. A new model for
the allocation of authority between doctors and patients is needed. A patient should be able to avail herself of a doctor's services without depriving
herself of the opportunity to control significant care choices.[242] Patients
should, of course, be free to delegate authority, but such delegation should
not be required or presumed. Giving patients control over medical choices
would delimit doctors' authority and their responsibility. At the same
time, such control implies that new obligations would be placed on doctors
to facilitate and defer to patients' choices. To effectuate such a relationship, the direct creation of an independent interest in medical choice
would be preferable to the indirect vindication now derived through protection of other, related interests.

Creating direct legal protection for patient autonomy would be consis-

---

242. The principle of patient control involves a degree of conflict with professional ideology. Doctors are not supposed to be accountable, insofar as professional decisions are involved, to laypersons.
Freidson observes that "the most strategic distinction [between professions and non-professions] lies in
legitimate, organized autonomy . . . the right to control its own work . . . . [P]rofessions are deliberately granted autonomy, including the exclusive right to determine . . . how the work should be
done." E. FREIDSON, PROFESSION OF MEDICINE: A STUDY OF THE SOCIOLOGY OF APPLIED
KNOWLEDGE 71–72 (1972). Although the conflict might in theory be resolved by differentiating between the "how" and the "whether" of work, doctors have not traditionally been attentive to such
distinctions. *See* J. KATZ, *supra* note 7, at 30–47. The concern about professional independence is
partly directed against organizational control by laypersons rather than against control by individual
patients. Even medicine's organizational independence, however, is threatened by increasingly bureaucratic forms of health care delivery and lay-initiated financial controls on medical decisionmaking.

Protecting Patient Choice

tent with other recent legal developments. The legal duty to facilitate patient choice by disclosing information is likely to be construed as an affirmative duty, and perhaps, therefore, to be resisted under common law
traditions. Yet the line dividing an affirmative duty from a prohibitive one
is largely semantic. The duty to protect patient choice may also be described as prohibitive: It instructs the doctor-agent not to substitute her
judgment for that of the patient. Viewed in this light, an interest in choice
is similar to intangible interests in personal sanctuary that are already
protected by the law.

Constitutional privacy cases often involve medical or medically-related
decisions.[243] These cases, involving birth control,[244] abortion,[245] form of
treatment,[246] and refusal of care at death,[247] stress the importance of individual autonomy. The government interventions that are constitutionally
prohibited in medical privacy cases involve interference with *decisionmaking*, rather than physical intrusion.[248] Constitutional development is often
broadly rooted in common law principles; in this instance the public law
is somewhat in advance of the private.[249] The intangible decisionmaking
focus of the constitutional privacy interest presages the change in private
law proposed here.

As a matter of private law, no explicit extension of a privacy interest to
medical contexts has yet been attempted.[250] But existing tort privacy ac-

---

243. Factually, these cases may involve either a doctor allied with a patient against the intrusions
of the government, *e.g.*, Roe v. Wade, 410 U.S. 113 (1973) (antiabortion laws), or a doctor allied with
the state in seeking to bar a patient's medical choice, *e.g.*, Andrews v. Ballard, 498 F. Supp. 1038
(S.D. Tex. 1980). They do not directly address the allocation of authority as
between the doctor and the patient. Indeed, there is some evidence that the constitutional privacy right
has been vested more in doctors than in patients. Asaro, *Judicial Portrayal of the Physician in Abortion and Sterilization Decisions: The Use and Abuse of Medical Discretion*, 6 HARV. WOMEN'S L.J.
51, 51–52 (1983).
244. Griswold v. Connecticut, 381 U.S. 479 (1965).
245. *Roe*, 410 U.S. 113.
246. *Andrews*, 498 F. Supp. 1038.
247. *See, e.g.*, Bartling v. Superior Ct., 163 Cal. App. 3d 186, 209 Cal. Rptr. 220 (1984); Satz v.
Perlmutter, 362 So. 2d 160 (Fla. Dist. Ct. App. 1978), *aff'd*, 379 So. 2d 359 (Fla. 1980).
248. Some of the constitutional decisions are, like their private law analogues, preoccupied with
degree of physical intrusion as the way to calibrate patient autonomy. *E.g.*, In re Quinlan, 70 N.J.
10, 355 A.2d 647, *cert. denied*, 429 U.S. 922 (1976) (right of permanently noncognitive patient to be
terminated from life support systems). But many involve no physical intrusion, *e.g.*, *Andrews*, 498 F.
Supp. 1038 (patient's right to choose form of treatment), and most emphasize patient autonomy as the
underlying goal, *e.g.*, *Griswold*, 381 U.S. 479 (right to use birth control). A similar transition from
physical to intangible definitions of privacy occurred in Fourth Amendment protection of personal
sanctuary. Katz v. United States, 389 U.S. 347 (1967) (electronic surveillance through phone taps
may violate Fourth Amendment even though there was no physical entrance into area occupied by
petitioner).
249. *Cf.* Rogers v. Okin, 478 F. Supp. 1342 (D. Mass. 1979) (for discussion of case, see *supra*
note 160), *aff'd in part, rev'd in part on other grounds*, 634 F.2d 650 (1st Cir. 1980).
250. In discussing possible expansion of the tort interest in privacy, Prosser observed the potential
connection between constitutional and tort privacy cases. PROSSER & KEETON, *supra* note 18, § 117,
at 866–67. He did not comment specifically on medical applications, however. *Cf.* RESTATEMENT
(SECOND) OF TORTS § 652A comment c (1976) (discussing possible connections between constitu-

The Yale Law Journal   Vol. 95: 219, 1985

tions do protect other interests in intangible personal sanctuary, such as reputation or security, from unwanted publicity.[251] Among presently recognized privacy actions, invasion of a patient's interest in choice somewhat resembles appropriation.[252] The tort of appropriation asserts a kind of property interest in one's likeness and name. An interest in medical choice would assert what amounts to a proprietary interest in information possessed by a doctor concerning one's condition, options and fate. The appropriation at issue in medical cases would be usurpation of the decisional authority that depends upon possession of such information.

The opportunity for maximum feasible control of medical fate would certainly seem to be as important an interest as control of name or likeness, reputation or seclusion. Moreover, although government intrusions on privacy may be justifiable as necessary means to fulfill social goals, a doctor's authority derives only from the patient and should extend no further than the patient decrees. Private usurpation of authority, even with good intentions, is culpable.[253]

The interest in freedom from emotional distress also has much in common with the interest in medical choice. Both interests protect aspects of personal sanctuary. The physical context of health care choice provides an analogue to the physical injury or proximity to physical danger that many jurisdictions require for redress of freestanding emotional distress.[254] In recent years, courts have become less skeptical about the genuineness of freestanding emotional injury.[255] Because objections to recovery for emotional distress paralleled the resistance to stronger protection of patient choice, the increased acceptance of emotional injury claims may ease the way for an interest in medical choice.

Although emotional disturbance is one common consequence of depriva-

tional privacy and tort privacy doctrines).

251. Tort privacy doctrines proscribe invasion of what Professor Fleming calls the "more sophisticated" intangible interests. J. FLEMING, *supra* note 129, at 193.

252. *See id.* at 210–11 (discussing appropriation); PROSSER & KEETON, *supra* note 18, § 117, at 851–54.

253. Some privacy torts require extreme offense or outrage to create a cause of action. RESTATEMENT (SECOND) OF TORTS §§ 652B, 652D, 652E (1976) (intrusion upon seclusion; publicity given to private life; and publicly placing person in a false light). *Cf.* Hirsh, *Current Perspectives on the Tort of Outrage*, 87 CASE & COM., Nov.–Dec. 1982, at 9 (discussing application of action to medical patient's rights). But not all privacy actions require extremely culpable behavior. Thus, appropriation need not involve offensive or outrageous conduct. RESTATEMENT (SECOND) OF TORTS § 652C (1976). Moreover, not all privacy disputes involve unmitigatedly antisocial conduct. News professionals sometimes run afoul of privacy strictures although they, like doctors, are presumptively engaged in a socially legitimate enterprise. Likewise, agents who usurp authority of principals are not excused by their good intentions. RESTATEMENT (SECOND) OF AGENCY § 14 (1958). *See supra* Part III(B)(2).

254. These requirements occur mainly where the action is for negligent infliction, or where the emotional injury is to a bystander. *See, e.g.,* RESTATEMENT (SECOND) OF TORTS §§ 46–48, 312–13 (1976).

255. *See* Molien v. Kaiser Found. Hosp., 27 Cal. 3d 916, 616 P.2d 813, 167 Cal. Rptr. 831 (1980) (recovery of emotional damages for husband of woman negligently informed she had syphilis).

Protecting Patient Choice

tion of choice,[256] leaving injuries to choice to be redressed only as a subset of the emotional distress action would be inappropriate. Such an approach would ignore the frequency and centrality of physical consequences arising from invasions of patient choice. More important, just as analysis of patient choice under traditional informed consent doctrine defines that interest as a particular species of damage rather than as an interest in autonomy per se,[257] subsuming choice under emotional distress would have the same effect. Injury-specific characterizations distort the interest in choice, subjecting it to inappropriate analytic and remedial restraints.[258]

Analogies to present doctrine may also be found if the protection of choice is understood as imposing an affirmative duty. Although the common law does not readily create such duties, it will do so if the defendant's relationship with the plaintiff makes the imposition of such duties appropriate.[259] The medical relationship is founded upon a contract whose substance is caretaking and whose character is fiduciary.[260] There seems little theoretical reason to balk at broadened duties of disclosure to protect patients' interest in an informed choice when other affirmative obligations are already imposed on doctors.[261]

Doctors are universally conceded to be fiduciaries; as such they have special duties to serve their clients' interests. Patients have been redefining their interests in the direction of more active participation in decisionmaking.[262] In the wake of such redefinition, the nature of fiduciary obligation must also change to stress more advising and less deciding. Even if the doctor is conceded to have some authority as an agent, agency doctrine

256. *E.g.*, Berman v. Allan, 80 N.J. 421, 404 A.2d 8 (1979) (recovery of damages for emotional anguish suffered by parents as result of deprivation of opportunity to choose abortion of Down's Syndrome fetus).

257. *See supra* Part II(B).

258. Some limits on recoverable damages for an invasion of choice might be desirable. *See infra* text accompanying notes 294–314.

259. *See* PROSSER & KEETON, *supra* note 18, § 56, at 373–82; RESTATEMENT (SECOND) OF TORTS §§ 314–314B (1976).

260. There are other such relationships to which a duty to enhance choice might theoretically be extended. Lawyers also have contractual and caretaking responsibilities. *See supra* note 240. Yet the underlying concerns of the medical relationship—bodily condition and fate—are ones in which claims to personal autonomy are uniquely compelling. That context seems an appropriate one in which to explore affirmative duties to protect autonomy.

261. Doctors currently may be held liable in tort for several kinds of inaction. Failure to treat can constitute violation of duties of competent care. Failure to disclose risks of treatment may generate liability under informed consent rules. *Cf.* Tresemer v. Barke, 86 Cal. App. 3d 656, 150 Cal. Rptr. 384 (1978) (by virtue of fiduciary relationship doctor obligated to warn former patient about dangers of IUD of which doctor was made aware after treatment of patient).

262. *See* 2 MAKING DECISIONS, *supra* note 2, at 221–25 (96% of patients want to be told about diagnosis of terminal illness; 94% want to be told everything about their medical condition; and in deciding between aggressive and supportive therapy in terminal cases, 79% of public thought decision should be made by patient; only 24% of doctors agreed and only 19% said such decisions actually are made that way).

The Yale Law Journal   Vol. 95: 219, 1985

emphasizes the agent's accountability to the principal's control.[263] Both agency and fiduciary principles require disclosure by the agent-fiduciary as an obligation independent of the substantive fairness (here competence) of the transaction, especially where there is any possible division of loyalty.[264] Particularly with regard to the professions, the call for increased client control over expert-fiduciaries has intensified.[265]

Even commercial actors who are neither fiduciaries nor professionals are increasingly subject to affirmative duties to disclose. In ordinary contract settings, each party is presumed to be acting in her own interest; yet disclosure may be demanded to enable a weaker party to make more informed decisions. Nondisclosure may create a claim for damages or a defense to enforcement of a contract.[266] The trend toward requiring disclosure is strongest when a party has special knowledge or expertise. As imposed in tort law generally, affirmative duties to disclose potential dangers may help to prevent physical injury. But because such duties to warn are not necessarily coupled with a requirement to remove the risk itself, the emphasis on disclosure to enhance plaintiff's choice-making is analogous to the situation here. If a landlord may be required to disclose known crime risks of a neighborhood,[267] or manufacturers the possible hazards of a product,[268] imposing affirmative duties upon doctors to inform their patients' choices seems readily justifiable.

Although the duties proposed here are in some ways broader than these analogous examples,[269] the differences are appropriate. Unlike most product manufacturers and landlords, doctors have a one-to-one relationship with their patients, facilitating personal consultation and discussion. Furthermore, unlike either landlords or manufacturers, doctors have fiduciary and professional responsibility for their patients. Those constraints were traditionally seen as obviating a need for disclosure and deference;[270] they provided a basis for trusting the doctor more than the ordinary contractual

---

263. RESTATEMENT (SECOND) OF AGENCY § 14 (1958).

264. *See supra* note 168.

265. *See supra* note 240.

266. *See, e.g.,* Obde v. Schlemeyer, 56 Wash. 2d 449, 353 P.2d 672 (1960) (basis for claim of damages where seller fails to disclose presence of termites in apartment); Sorrell v. Young, 6 Wash. App. 220, 491 P.2d 1312 (1971) (rescission available where seller knew of defect, buyer was unaware, and defect was not apparent); Slater v. KFC Corp., 621 F.2d 932 (8th Cir. 1980)(duty to disclose where superior knowledge is not within the reasonable reach of less experienced party); *see also* RESTATEMENT (SECOND) OF CONTRACTS § 161(b) (1979).

267. *See, e.g.,* O'Hara v. Western Seven Trees Corp., 75 Cal. App. 3d 798, 142 Cal. Rptr. 487 (1977).

268. *E.g.,* Davis v. Wyeth Laboratories, Inc., 399 F.2d 121 (9th Cir. 1968). For a discussion of a causation standard in relation to product liability warnings, see *supra* note 126.

269. Manufacturers have no duty to tell about alternative products, or landlords about alternative buildings, but only to warn regarding the particular product or building they place on the market.

270. *See* Becker, *supra* note 239, at 27 (discussing code of ethics as guarantee of professionals' trustworthiness and altruism).

Protecting Patient Choice

actor. Increasingly, however, the professional's responsibility is viewed not as a mandate to preempt authority, but as a responsibility to educate, and then defer to, the patient's own decisions. Accordingly, that doctors' affirmative responsibility for disclosure should be greater than that of commercial actors is unsurprising.

B. *How The Interest Would Work*

An interest in medical choice could be administered under either contract or tort doctrine. Either analysis would derive the duty to protect the patient's interest in choice from the doctor-patient relationship—one in order to vindicate reasonable expectations, the other in order to protect the substantive value of autonomy itself.

1. *Contract Analysis*

Because patients have been deemed incapable of individual bargaining about expert services, duties undertaken through a contract for professional care have been given content and specificity through negligence policy rather than through contract analysis. I have argued, however, that although patients may be incapable of supervising the quality and administration of care, they are capable, indeed uniquely so, of balancing ultimate costs and benefits of care decisions. Moreover, they are capable of determining the extent to which they wish to allocate decisionmaking authority to their doctors. Thus, the rationale for adopting a standardized tort analysis does not extend to issues of decisionmaking and allocation of authority; these matters could appropriately be analyzed under contract doctrine. Were such an approach adopted, the entire analytic paradigm would be reversed. Rather than invasion of patient choice being one subtype of injury causation within a professional negligence framework, professionally negligent care would constitute one species of breach of contract.

Explicit agreements concerning the general allocation of authority or about specific care choices will likely be honored under either analytic regime. Traditionally, however, patients have not bargained with their doctors about decisionmaking authority. In the absence of explicit agreement, the problem, contractually, would be to imply a reasonable term. How much delegation of authority should be implied?

Current doctrines show courts to be unwilling to deem decisionmaking authority automatically transferred by the act of hiring a doctor.[271] Be-

---

271. *See supra* note 139. General contract law also frowns on unilateral decisionmaking that results from disparate power or adhesion contracting. *E.g.*, Tunkl v. Regents of Univ. of Cal., 60 Cal. 2d 92, 383 P.2d 441, 32 Cal. Rptr. 33 (1963) (invalidating agreement between hospital and entering

yond the existing rules, both as a matter of expectation and reliance, patients today assume that they will be given the opportunity to make decisions if they wish. Anecdotal and empirical evidence suggest that most patients wish to be informed and to participate more actively in the management of their care.[272] Indeed, patient dissatisfaction with health care frequently centers on doctors' failure to provide sufficient information and dialogue.[273] However, even patients who wish to exercise choice remain dependent on doctors for information. Although public knowledge about medicine has greatly increased, patients still rely on doctors for education and counsel, particularly about their individual condition and options.[274]

By contrast, assuming that payment schemes are adjusted to compensate for time spent, doctors themselves have little, if any, legitimate reliance interest in resisting disclosure or in controlling patients' decisions; they certainly have a less intense interest than do patients. Moreover, doctors are already adapting to patients' growing expectations of involvement, making responsibility to disclose to and consult with patients less foreign than it might once have been.[275] Even if doctors' expectations about authority differ, they have reason to know, and under contract principles therefore to be bound by, the intent of patients.[276] Particularly in their role as fiduciaries, doctors should be held to defer to the expectations and reliance of their patients.

Thus, although express bargaining should be encouraged, where no explicit term is agreed to, patient control of decisionmaking should be the term implied into the contract. Given the tradition of medical paternalism, patients who wish to opt out of such responsibility could easily do so. Those who seek involvement will likely need greater legal protection.[277] A doctor could be expected to bargain explicitly for any other pattern of decisionmaking she wished to require.[278]

---

patient exculpating hospital).

272. *See* 1 MAKING DECISIONS, *supra* note 2, at 17; 2 MAKING DECISIONS, *supra* note 2, at 221–24 (results of empirical survey).

273. *See* Enright, *supra* note 10, at 76, 90 (discussing evidence that high percentage of malpractice suits are in part caused by failure of doctor to establish good communication with patient).

274. *See* J. KATZ, *supra* note 7, at 227 (speaking on doctor's crucial role as teacher) and 78 (noting need for doctors to respond to patients' individual needs for information).

275. *See supra* note 14.

276. *See* RESTATEMENT (SECOND) OF CONTRACTS § 201 (1979).

277. *See* J. KATZ, *supra* note 7, at 1–29 (tracing the history of paternalism in western medicine). For an especially thoughtful series of articles contrasting medical paternalism, legal imperialism, and other alternatives, see Relman, *The Saikewicz Decision: A Medical Viewpoint*, 4 AM. J.L. & MED. 233 (1978); Baron, *Medical Paternalism and the Rule of Law: A Reply to Dr. Relman*, 4 AM. J.L. & MED. 337 (1978); and Buchanan, *Medical Paternalism or Legal Imperialism: Not the Only Alternatives for Handling Saikewicz-type Cases*, 5 AM. J.L. & MED. 97 (1979).

278. The danger that doctors would use their power to insist that patients give them broader decisionmaking authority than the patient might wish would be forestalled by three factors: (1) Contracts would be subject to review under principles governing unconscionability, good faith and adhesion; (2) Doctors may actually be relieved to reduce their responsibility for others' fate; (3) Doctors

Protecting Patient Choice

Once the term governing authority is established, contract analysis would be straightforward, though not simple. A patient explicitly or impliedly contracting for maximum disclosure and choice would be deprived of her expectation if the doctor failed to give material information. To put her where she would have been had the contract been performed, it would be necessary to determine the difference in value between where she would have been had she been given information and choice, and where she is now. Because tort analysis of an interest in choice would also require projection and valuation of what a patient would have chosen, this process would, to a substantial degree, parallel the analysis proposed in the next section.[279]

2. *Tort Analysis*

Although existing tort approaches are seriously deficient, the weight of tradition may cause tort analysis of these issues to be continued. Tort analysis could provide adequate protection if patient choice became an independent and fully protected interest in its own right. Analysis of an independent interest in choice would differ from existing analyses in a number of ways.

Duties involving disclosure of knowledge lend themselves to analyses of intentional conduct. Where a defendant has fiduciary and contractual responsibility to a plaintiff, and has primary access to information essential to the plaintiff's recognition and exercise of choice, the defendant must know that failure to disclose that information is substantially certain to cause invasion of the plaintiff's interest. On the other hand, because the doctor typically claims other justifications for nondisclosure and has no specific intent to harm, the simpler and more punitive assumptions frequently applied to intentional torts seem inappropriate to most situations of medical nondisclosure. Privacy torts encompass both negligent and intentional conduct without being confined to one or the other,[280] and this approach would also be appropriate for patient choice.

A duty to disclose would be triggered by the possession of information

---

are increasingly having to compete for health care dollars. Patients wishing more authority in decisionmaking are likely to have the bargaining power to achieve that goal.

279. In *Gates*, for example, where the patient became blind, she probably would not have lost her sight had she opted for further testing. To assess her loss under contract theory, her expectation should be determined by figuring the value of sight, discounted both by the possibility that she might not have undertaken the additional tests and by the projected outcome of having the tests, offset by any value there is in being blind. Calculation of damages based on prediction of probabilistic outcomes has been undertaken in contracts cases, *e.g.*, Locke v. United States, 283 F.2d 521 (1960) (projected share of business); Rombola v. Cosindas, 351 Mass. 382, 220 N.E.2d 919 (1966) (projected winnings of racehorse). For a discussion of damages under the tort theory, see *infra* text accompanying notes 294–314.

280. *See* RESTATEMENT (SECOND) OF TORTS §§ 652A-652E (1976).

important and relevant to the patient, rather than by a proposal to touch. This approach would reverse the relationship between information and choice that is created under current doctrine. At present, the requirement of consent determines the necessity of disclosure. Because, however, choice arises out of and depends upon knowledge and reflection, the essential point of access must be knowledge itself.[281]

Where disclosure is triggered by touching, occasions for performance of the duty are rather clearly defined. Although a duty to disclose based upon possession of knowledge per se might seem comparatively unbounded,[282] it would not be as unlimited as it might seem. As a function of their existing responsibilities for care, doctors already have the knowledge needed to carry out this proposed new duty.[283] The doctor's duty to know would continue to be regulated in present fashion as a matter of professional competence.[284] At issue in relation to an interest in choice would be what the doctor must disclose of what she does know.

Certainly the duty would not be to disclose all that the doctor knows, but only what is materially relevant to the patient at the time of the disclosure. The doctor should affirmatively offer the following information: (1) material clinical observations or test results that describe the condition of the patient at any stage of care; (2) interpretation of this information by the doctor and her advisers, including material judgments and conclusions based on the data; and (3) material possible responses that the patient might elect in light of the information and the possibilities known to the doctor. In each aspect of the duty, "material"[285] must be understood to

---

281. The importance of proper disclosure of information is heightened by the fact that the same information that would allow the patient to control medical choices would also permit her to make other personal choices that depend on her understanding of her medical condition.

282. Even under the earlier rule, courts worried about imposing a duty that would make it necessary to give patients a medical education. *See, e.g.*, Canterbury v. Spence, 464 F.2d 772, 782 n.27 (D.C. Cir.), *cert. denied*, 409 U.S. 1064 (1972).

283. Because doctors are uniquely (both in the sense of "well" and in the sense of "exclusively") situated to provide information vital to patient choice, the duty to avoid the costs of nondisclosure should be placed on them. *See generally* G. CALABRESI, THE COSTS OF ACCIDENTS (1969) (presenting theory of cheapest cost avoidance as most appropriate method of allocating cost of accidents).

284. Lack of knowledge, however, would be more exposed under the proposed rule than under the present one. *See infra* note 289.

285. Useful work has already been done to define the concept of materiality for purposes of determining the scope of medical disclosure. The concept of materiality under informed consent doctrine inversely relates probability and seriousness: Even relatively remote possibilities may have to be disclosed if their consequences are very serious. *See, e.g.*, Canterbury v. Spence, 464 F.2d at 788. Waltz and Scheuneman originally proposed the test of materiality and attempted to define it. Waltz & Scheuneman, *supra* note 30, at 638–41. *See also* Halligan, *The Standard of Disclosure by Physicians to Patients: Competing Models of Informed Consent*, 41 LA. L. REV. 9 (1980) (discusses tort of deceit as antecedent upon which courts have relied in developing medical disclosure rules); 2 MAKING DECISIONS, *supra* note 2 (gives empirical indications of what public thinks is material). *But see* Epstein, *supra* note 17, at 124 (arguing that there are "no principled limits" to doctrine's requirements for disclosure).

Traditional informed consent doctrine might offer other acceptable methods of narrowing the dis-

Protecting Patient Choice

extend beyond the doctor's certainties.[286] Although some data, judgments and options will be too remote to require mention, disclosure of material *possibilities* in each of the categories is essential. Inappropriate management of uncertainty has been responsible for many of the failures of choice protection analyzed here.[287]

A concept such as "focus of attention" would help to delimit the duty of disclosure. Of the nondisclosures analyzed here as being vital to choice, many occurred where a doctor made an underlying decision not to act.[288] That inaction was not a matter of inadvertance. It was an intentional judgment, the focus of attention and decision, to which liability could have attached had it been incompetent as a matter of professional care. If the relevant knowledge and the decision based upon it were not actually within the doctor's awareness, the issue again becomes whether it should have been—a question of professional competence.[289]

Under a focus of attention approach, information of the type described should be forthcoming with regard to any presenting symptom, problem or condition that has brought the patient to the doctor for care. Material information should also be forthcoming any time the doctor actually has or acquires information as a result of observations made or initiatives undertaken during care, even if the information is not related to the condition that brought the patient to the doctor.[290]

The extent of the duty to disclose general information about possibilities that are not the focus of either the doctor's or the patient's concern at the time of the encounter raises the most difficult issues. Anyone might benefit from a cardiogram to screen for heart problems or a tonometry test to identify glaucoma. Explanations of such possible courses of action and reasons why they should or should not be explored would be endless.

---

closure obligation. Thus, an exception for matters of common knowledge might be employed. In addition, traditional exceptions for mental incapacity, emergency and waiver should apply.

286. J. KATZ, *supra* note 7, at 166–69, 186–89.

287. *E.g.*, Nardone v. Reynolds, 333 So. 2d 25 (Fla. 1976); Hanks v. Doctors Ranson, Swan & Burch, Ltd., 359 So. 2d 1089 (La. Ct. App. 1978); Keogan v. Holy Family Hosp., 95 Wash. 2d 306, 622 P.2d 1246 (1980).

288. *E.g.*, Roark v. Allen, 633 S.W.2d 804 (Tex. 1982) (decision that skull indentations did not require x-ray to determine fracture); Gates v. Jensen, 92 Wash. 2d 246, 595 P.2d 919 (1979) (decision not to test further for glaucoma).

289. Such a rule will create a more precise accountability about knowledge under standards of professional competence. Doctors might find themselves choosing whether to claim they knew but did not disclose (thereby invading the interest in choice), or to admit that they did not know (thereby falling below the threshold for competence).

290. Thus, a patient might come in for an asthma problem, and the doctor might note a skin condition that could be cancerous. Even if the doctor competently concludes it is probably not cancerous, and that no care is necessary, the doctor should disclose the skin condition because it had been a focus of the doctor's attention. If the doctor did not note the condition, the issue would again be one of competence regarding whether she should have. *See also* Ratzan, *Unsolicited Medical Opinion*, 10 J. MED. & PHIL. 147 (1985) (suggesting criteria for and techniques of offering unsolicited medical opinions).

They would threaten what courts have sought to avoid: the obligation to give each patient a medical school education. However, as soon as specific data linking general information to a particular individual is noted, attention is focused and a need to disclose would arise.[291]

Once it is determined that a duty of disclosure applies, breach of that duty ought to be judged not by the standards of expert behavior but by the standards appropriate to protection of patient autonomy. Like the extent of the doctor's knowledge, the accuracy of the doctor's disclosure would still be a question of professional competence, evaluated as it is at present. The occasion for and scope of disclosure, however, would be analyzed in terms of what constitutes reasonable disclosure where one on whom another depends has special access to information relevant to that other's interests, a standard akin to the agent-fiduciary standard. An agent-fiduciary must disclose all information that she knows or should know that the principal would desire to have.[292] Given recent documentation that patients want much more medical disclosure and choice than they currently enjoy,[293] such a duty should extend disclosure well beyond the norms of traditional medical practice.

Once duty and breach are established, sanctioning analysis would also differ if choice were the protected interest. The crucial difficulties stem from the uncertainty regarding what would have happened if the patient's interest in choice had not been invaded. Cooper-Stephenson and Saunders[294] have argued persuasively that an analysis that balances probabilities to achieve an either/or result is appropriate to determinations regarding events that have occurred. Questions of substantive liability are generally of this genre. Those authors urge, however, that a proportional analysis is fairer where a court must assess intrinsically uncertain events. Such events cannot be analyzed as more probable than not because they are inherently unknowable. Most issues of damage valuation are of this type.[295]

---

291. The disclosure required ought to be less extensive with regard to general background information than with regard to its individual application. Such a duty might require the doctor to note briefly the general issue ("Smoking is dangerous to health"), and to provide more extensive information regarding the individual ("Your cough sounds as if you may be having lung problems. We can check it out in the following way . . . ."). Also, the obligation to disclose ought not to recur more than once for a single problem of a single patient unless the doctor acquires relevant new data about the patient or the problem.

292. *See* RESTATEMENT (SECOND) OF AGENCY § 381 (1957).

293. *See supra* note 14.

294. Throughout this section I rely upon K. COOPER-STEPHENSON & I. SAUNDERS, PERSONAL INJURY DAMAGES IN CANADA 83-114 (1981). They present both a theory and a review of the cases with reference to appropriate measurement of damages.

295. Although both Canadian and English law have adopted this approach, courts in the United States have been less enthusiastic. *Id.* at 113. Nevertheless, commentators in the United States have endorsed the proportional approach to such determinations. *E.g.*, King, *supra* note 27, at 1396-97; Tom on Torts, *Kentucky Allows Accident Victim's Recovery for Increased Risk of Future Harm*, 27

Protecting Patient Choice

If one adopts Cooper-Stephenson and Saunders' analysis, a balance of probabilities approach would appropriately serve to determine whether the defendant's nondisclosure more probably than not materially deprived the patient of an interest in choice. Two additional uncertainties would then remain to be assessed in valuing any resulting injury. What would the plaintiff, properly informed, have chosen? What, medically speaking, would have been the result if a different course had been selected? Analysis of these issues should employ what Cooper-Stephenson and Saunders call a simple probability test (proportional), because neither involves events that have actually occurred. Each requires the reconstruction of what would have happened had the defendant not interrupted the chain of events by failing to disclose.

Such interruption, the invasion of choice, results in the loss of an uncertain chance of a preferable outcome. That chance can be valued as a matter of assessing damage.[296] The familiar maxim that courts should not readily allow uncertainty to prevent vindication of an invaded interest comes into play.[297] Damages are adjustable along a monetary continuum. Statistical tools are more readily employed to apportion and value uncertainty for purposes of remedy than to determine substantive liability.[298] Moreover, characterizing the issue as one of valuing injury allows the multiple sub-issues involved in these cases to be resolved in an orderly and sequential manner. The court does not have to compress the sub-issues into a single ultimate question as it must where they are treated as a single question of factual cause.[299] In order to determine the value of the plaintiff's loss of choice, three questions must be answered.

First, how likely is it that an alternative path would have been chosen? The subjectivity of this first branch of uncertainty makes fact-finding with

---

AM. TRIAL LAW. A. L. REP. 302, 302 (Sept. 1984). Some courts have also embraced such a perspective, *e.g.*, Davis v. Graviss, 672 S.W.2d 928, 931–32 (Ky. 1984). *But see* Rosenberg, *The Causal Connection in Mass Exposure Cases: A "Public Law" Vision of the Tort System,* 97 HARV. L. REV. 851, 874 n.99 (1984) (arguing that in sporadic accident cases proportional rule of recovery is less fair than preponderance of evidence rule).

296. *See* King, *supra* note 130, at 1396–97.

The response of the courts to questions of causation and valuation involving preexisting conditions and claims for future consequences has been largely unsatisfactory. Their failure to distinguish between the functions of causation and valuation, or to identify and value rationally the true interests lost, has created a serious gap in the remedial structure. Courts have had difficulty perceiving that a chance of avoiding some adverse result or of achieving some favorable result is a compensable interest in its own right.

Id. at 1354.

297. RESTATEMENT (SECOND) OF TORTS § 912, at 479 (1979).

298. K. COOPER-STEPHENSON & I. SAUNDERS, *supra* note 294, at 83–114.

299. *See* J. FLEMING, *supra* note 132, at 108 (noting problems created by placing "a wide spectrum of inquiries" within "monistic" doctrine of proximate cause). For a discussion of problems arising from courts' tendencies to treat what should be issues of valuation as questions of causation, see King, *supra* note 130, at 1354.

regard to it the most difficult.[300] Although no perfect way of determining an answer exists, as determinations in other circumstances show,[301] the court could derive some probabilistic estimate of alternative courses. The projected decision of this individual, rather than "a reasonable person," should provide the standard; any other standard fails to protect the very autonomy that lies at the heart of the interest.[302]

Subjective states are susceptible of objective proof; they are demonstrable through evidence of conduct or words observable by others.[303] Because the issue here involves a hypothetical rather than an actual event, however, objective evidence will not directly or definitively demonstrate what the individual's choice would have been. Objective evidence, however, could elucidate why this individual might or probably would have chosen a given path.[304]

---

300. The word "subjective" sometimes refers to inner, i.e., mental or emotional, states and sometimes to particularization regarding a given individual. *See* Eisenberg, *The Responsive Model of Contract Law*, 36 STAN. L. REV. 1107 (1984) (discussing these as two main spectra within contract theory). The reconstruction of patient choice actually involves both kinds of subjectivity. In the informed consent caselaw, both types of "subjective" standards have been almost totally rejected as being too unreliable. *See, e.g.*, Canterbury v. Spence, 464 F.2d 772, 790 (D.C. Cir.), *cert. denied*, 409 U.S. 1064 (1972).

301. For instance, where a plaintiff claims damage through reliance on a promise, the court will have to reconstruct what that individual would have done in the absence of the promise, under circumstances in which hindsight and self-interest will taint the evidence. *See, e.g.*, Feinberg v. Pfeiffer Co., 322 S.W.2d 163 (Mo. Ct. App. 1959) (in determining whether plaintiff relied on promised retirement stipend, one issue was whether plaintiff would have quit work if promise had not been made). Like medical choice, reliance involves both reconstruction of what an individual would have chosen to do, and what the outcome of that choice would have been. *See* Eisenberg, *Donative Promises*, 47 U. CHI. L. REV. 1, 18 (1979); *see also infra* note 309; *cf. supra* note 279 (discussing contract cases calculating damages based on prediction of probabilistic outcomes).

302. The approach proposed here parallels Professor Eisenberg's recommendation that most contract law principles should be individualized, and that they may be either objective or subjective, depending upon the circumstances. Eisenberg, *supra* note 300, at 1111. Patient choice cases present more problems both of fairness and of administrability than does the average contract case, but in light of what is at stake, those problems should be manageable. Eisenberg's justification for individualization—that "a major goal of contract law is to facilitate the realization of individual objectives," *id.* at 1111—applies with much greater force here. Bodily fate is a more intense and personal interest than are "highly differentiated goods," and no "cover" at all is possible.

303. *See, e.g.*, Lucy v. Zehmer, 196 Va. 493, 84 S.E.2d 516 (1954) (court used objective words and acts of sellers to determine whether they were joking when they agreed to sale of property); RESTATEMENT (SECOND) OF CONTRACTS § 18 comments a and c, § 19 (1981) (explaining objective standards for evaluating assent to contract); *cf., e.g.*, Lange v. Hoyt, 114 Conn. 590, 159 A. 575 (1932) (Christian Scientists not required to have child undergo surgery to mitigate damages).

304. If, for example, she made her living as a graphic artist or a photographer, she could persuasively claim that she would have gone to more than average lengths to protect her sight. A few courts have allowed consideration of such individual factors under the "in the circumstances" aspect of the reasonable causation standard in informed consent. *See, e.g.*, Steele v. St. Paul Fire & Marine Ins. Co., 371 So. 2d 843 (La. App.), *cert. denied*, 374 So. 2d 658 (La. 1979) (implicitly reflecting special attention courts give to individual choice in procreation cases). Objective information about individuals' hypothetical preferences regarding future medical care has become increasingly available. Several states have adopted provisions allowing individuals to make binding advance statements about care in circumstances of terminal illness. *See, e.g.*, Natural Death Act, CAL. HEALTH & SAFETY CODE §§ 7186-7195 (West Supp. 1985). Legal provisions have been adopted that effectuate clearly stated individual preferences regarding organ donation. *See, e.g.*, Uniform Anatomical Gift Act, CAL. HEALTH

Protecting Patient Choice

Moreover, a requirement to reconstruct the choice of a given individual does not preclude the introduction of non-individualized objective information. Thus, the court would find useful testimony about choices that other people actually make when confronted with similar risks and odds.[305] However, the role of such information should be delimited as bearing only on the credibility of the claim. The individual nature of the ultimate question should be clearly preserved.

The potentially self-serving nature of the plaintiff's testimony should be less worrisome if the court requires and uses objective evidence to determine only a proportional chance that a different path would have been taken. If jury evaluation still seems likely to reflect an excess of sympathy or lack of adequate evaluation of credibility, the court could apply some intermediate protective device. For example, a court could employ a presumption that this individual would have decided as a reasonable person would have, but could then allow the individual to rebut the presumption by showing persuasive objective evidence of individual reasons for deviation.[306]

Second, the jury would have to determine what would have happened if a different choice had been put into effect.[307] Expert testimony would probably be essential here, but again, such testimony should be restricted to assessment of factual medical data. Statistical predictions about outcome odds in a given case would not prove what would actually have happened in the case at bar. But courts routinely use such general data to determine an individual's damages.[308]

Finally, the value of where the plaintiff stands under the actual chain of events would need to be compared with where she would have stood as a result of the alternative course of events, discounted by the appropriate probability assessments. Comparison of values could begin with reasonable averages, but should also factor in objectively demonstrable individual

---

& SAFETY CODE §§ 7150-7157 (West 1970).

305. Such data would be of two kinds: (1) statistics showing what people actually have chosen when faced with comparable decisions; and (2) statistics regarding prospective preferences as established by public opinion polls. *See, e.g.,* 2 MAKING DECISIONS, *supra* note 2, at 136, 244 (percent of public desiring to be informed of condition, including diagnosis of cancer).

306. *Cf.* Cunningham v. Charles Pfizer & Co., 532 P.2d 1377 (Okla. 1975) (presumption plaintiff would have heeded warning on product rebuttable by evidence of what reasonable person would have done).

307. In Gates v. Jensen, the answer would have been relatively easy. Further testing would have had a high probability of discovering the glaucoma. 92 Wash. 2d 246, 250, 595 P.2d 919, 922 (1979). In some cases, however, answers would present more difficulties. For example, if a woman alleges she would have opted for a lumpectomy rather than a radical mastectomy, the jury would have to judge the increased probability of having a recurrence of cancer had she followed the alternative course.

308. Thus, courts awarding damages for wrongful death do not know how long an actual individual would have lived, or how much she would have earned. But they use general actuarial probabilities (which take account of as many individual factors as possible) to render those uncertain projections adequately certain. *See* RESTATEMENT (SECOND) OF TORTS § 92 comments c, d, and e (1976).

The Yale Law Journal   Vol. 95: 219, 1985

variables that affect medical preferences, such as age or occupation, or even personal attitudes or circumstances where those could be established by evidence more probative than the plaintiff's simple assertion.

Applying these proposed techniques would be difficult, but the incentive to resolve the complicated problems associated with the vindication of choice derives from the depth of the concern about patient autonomy. As elsewhere, running some risks with inaccurate damages is preferable to not following the logic of doctrine at all.[309] Moreover, the methods of calculation suggested here should reduce concern about uncertainty and about recoveries being unduly influenced by hindsight.

Issues regarding types of compensable harm would remain. The intangibility of the interest should not obscure the substantial and often physical nature of the consequences flowing from its invasion. As I have demonstrated, the redefinition of interest suggested here would significantly alter the analysis of duty, breach, causation and value in regard to traditional physical injury. Thus, even if courts were to restrict redress for invasions of choice to physical consequences, realignment of the protected interest would significantly increase legal protection of patient choice.

Identification of an intangible interest in choice could also allow recovery for less traditional categories of harm. Courts could evaluate consequences of a substantial but not necessarily "physical" or "injurious" (as socially judged) harm, for example, the birth of an unwanted child or the undesired prolongation of death. Yet, as a matter of sanctioning policy, courts need not deem compensable all consequences of invasions of choice. For example, although emotional distress damages would constitute a particularly likely result of invasions of this interest,[310] courts could restrict such recoveries.[311] However, categorical limits on emotional distress damages in medical contexts seem, if anything, to be eroding.[312]

Under certain conditions, an invasion of choice might not produce any substantial consequences, physical or otherwise. Thus, for instance, if the doctor had not told Ms. Gates of the test indicating possible glaucoma, but she did not, in fact, develop the disease, the doctor would technically have

---

309. For other illustrations of legal redress in conditions of substantial uncertainty, see Davis v. Graviss, 672 S.W.2d 928 (Ky. 1984) (projection of uncertain future injury); Feinberg v. Pfeiffer Co., 322 S.W.2d 163 (Mo. Ct. App. 1959) (reliance on promise); Locke v. United States, 283 F.2d 521 (1960) (value of bargained-for chance); Rombola v. Cosindas, 351 Mass. 382, 220 N.E.2d 919 (1966) (uncertain expectation); RESTATEMENT (SECOND) OF TORTS §§ 910, 924 (1979) (uncertain prospective consequences of present injury).

310. *See, e.g.*, Capron, *supra* note 52, at 639–45.

311. *See, e.g.*, Berman v. Allan, 80 N.J. 421, 404 A.2d 8 (1979). Most courts dealing with wrongful birth actions have allowed emotional distress damages. *See, e.g.*, Jacobs v. Theimer, 519 S.W.2d 846 (Tex. 1975); Naccash v. Burger, 223 Va. 406, 290 S.E.2d 825, 830–31 (1982).

312. *See, e.g.*, Molien v. Kaiser Found. Hosp., 27 Cal. 3d 916, 616 P.2d 813, 167 Cal. Rptr. 831 (1980); Sullivan v. O'Connor, 363 Mass. 579, 587–88, 296 N.E.2d 183, 188–89 (1973); Hirsh, *supra* note 253, at 9–10.

Protecting Patient Choice

violated the interest in information and choice but the consequences here would be mainly intangible and symbolic. Two possible methods of treating such cases emerge. The court could award nominal damages, or it could award general damages, as is done in privacy actions.[313] The latter approach would better redress the purely dignitary element of the new interest. However, because so many demonstrably consequential invasions of patient choice have been ignored under the existing doctrinal scheme, even adoption of the former approach would allow dramatically strengthened protection of patient autonomy. An interest is not delegitimated because in a particular instance its invasion produced little demonstrable harm. Finally, unless the doctor harbored specific or malicious intent to deprive a patient of choice, punitive damages would be inappropriate.[314]

3. *Contract or Tort?*

Several possible grounds for choosing between the two analyses might be suggested. First, the indexing of cases under one or the other doctrinal category may influence the selection of norms and concepts to be used in the analysis. Contract analysis is traditionally rooted in respect for individual choice and might more effectively protect that concern. By contrast, the standard professional negligence action has so dominated tort analysis of medical relationships that it might be difficult for an interest in choice to achieve sufficient independence within the tort domain.

Second, tort has traditionally provided the locus of redress for physical injury. However, both fields have expanded their compass, with contract now recognizing physical and emotional injuries[315] and tort redressing even negligent injuries to economic,[316] emotional,[317] and privacy[318] interests, as well as to more traditional interests in physical well-being and property. There seems little reason to distinguish on this somewhat outmoded basis.

Finally, a tort approach makes a stronger statement about public policy regarding patient autonomy, while contract, deferring to the parties' election, remains more neutral. Under the proposals I make here, however, the outcomes under the two analyses would, in fact, converge. Under my tort analysis, the interest would emanate from public policy but would be subject to individual choice (waiver) by the patient, or with greater diffi-

---

313. *See* W. Prosser, Handbook of the Law of Torts § 117, at 815 (4th ed. 1971); Restatement (Second) of Torts § 904 (1976). These could be based on some standard amount that was more than nominal, or on a jury appraisal of the facts and circumstances.
314. *See* Restatement (Second) of Torts § 908 (1976).
315. *See, e.g.,* Sullivan v. O'Connor, 363 Mass. 579, 296 N.E.2d 183 (1973).
316. *See* Prosser & Keeton, *supra* note 18, § 95A, at 679–81.
317. Restatement (Second) of Torts §§ 46–48, 313 (1976).
318. *Id.* at § 652.

The Yale Law Journal   Vol. 95: 219, 1985

culty, by the doctor if she required waiver as a condition of contracting to provide services. Under the contract analysis, I have proposed that, based both on empirical data about patient expectations and on public policy values, courts should read into the contract, as an implied term, patient control of decisions unless the parties explicitly agree to the contrary. Again, then, the contract would include a term requiring patient control as the background rule, alterable only by the affirmative and mutual decision of the parties.

Under contract analysis there remains some danger that, in implying a term, courts would turn to custom of the trade and supply a term based on traditionally paternalistic medical custom. But the needs and expectations of doctors should not exclusively define what is customary. Moreover, the expectations of both doctors and patients are changing. Public policy points, as it does in other consumer contexts,[319] toward special judicial concern for protection of consumers' (patients') reasonable expectations.

C. Policy Effects

1. Are Patients Capable of Choice?

The interest proposed here would place a great deal of responsibility on patients. Some may fear that many individuals will be unable to discharge the responsibilities that autonomy would impose.[320] Rationality is inevitably limited; motives and wishes are frequently not conscious. Although these are powerful arguments for seeking personal support and expert advice, the same limits apply to the rationality and motives of doctors, relatives or friends. The burden of consequences provides the compelling reason to place final authority with the affected individual rather than with others who advise or care for that individual.

2. Effects on Health Care Outcomes

If patients had more knowledge and control, experts would have less. Would poorer health be the result?[321] Medical decisions involve both uncertainty and conflicts of judgment and value. Neither experts nor society can judge what is best for an individual better than the individual herself. The quality of patient choice will, of course, depend on the quality of

---

319. *See, e.g.*, RESTATEMENT (SECOND) OF CONTRACTS § 211 (1981) (protection against contravention of consumer expectations in standardized agreements).

320. *See* J. KATZ, *supra* note 7, at 26-27. *See generally* R. BURT, *supra* note 5 (discussing complex motives affecting medical choice in a number of specific instances).

321. This is perhaps the core objection to proposals to strengthen patient choice. *See* J. KATZ, *supra* note 7, at 27.

Protecting Patient Choice

information provided by the doctor. But assuming adequate performance of that obligation, patient-made decisions should generally yield outcomes that are preferable as evaluated by the ultimate consumer, the patient.

Moreover, there is evidence that patients who are well-informed progress better than do those who are treated more paternalistically.[322] Such patients implement treatment plans more fully[323] and can aid the doctor's diagnostic process.[324] More debatable, but not to be overlooked, is evidence that the mobilization of patients' psychic resources is critically important in the struggle for health.[325]

3. *Effects on the Distribution of Health Care*

Wealth already buys greater access to health care services.[326] Any system that increased patient autonomy might exacerbate that effect.[327] If choices were more thoroughly subjected to cost-benefit analysis by individ-

---

322. *See* Fiore, *Fighting Cancer—One Patient's Perspective,* 300 New Eng. J. Med. 284 (1979); Mumford, Schlesinger, Glass, Patrick & Curedon, *A New Look at Evidence About Reduced Cost of Medical Utilization Following Mental Health Treatment,* 141 Am. J. Psychiatry 1145 (1984). There is also evidence that information can reduce emotional problems which accompany physical illness. *See* Comment, *When the Truth Can Hurt: Patient-Mediated Informed Consent in Cancer Therapy,* 9 U.C.L.A.-Alaska L. Rev. 143, 151 & n.33, 152 & n.34 (1980).

323. Noncompliance is a serious problem in health care. *See* J. Katz, *supra* note 7, at xiv and sources cited in Introduction n.2; Press, *The Predisposition to File Claims: The Patient's Perspective,* 12 Law, Med. & Health Care 53, 54 (April 1984) (patients' noncompliance reported by some studies as high as 50–60%). Noncompliance likely indicates patients who have "voted with their feet" when they do not feel in control of their treatment. The very term "noncompliance" suggests orders given by the doctor to a passive patient.

324. *See* J. Katz & A. Capron, *supra* note 30, at 89–90. Doctors not providing necessary instruction regarding self-care may be liable for negligent care. *See, e.g.,* Crosby v. Grandview Nursing Home, 290 A.2d 375 (Me. 1972); *see also* LeBlang & King, *supra* note 189, at 24–26.

325. *See* N. Cousins, Anatomy of an Illness as Perceived by the Patient: Reflections on Healing and Regeneration 11, 14–23 (1979); K. Pelletier, Mind as Healer, Mind as Slayer 10–12 (1977); O. Simonton, S. Mathews-Simonton, J. Creighton, Getting Well Again 4–12 (1978).

326. Many people have no health insurance coverage. *See* Bayer, *Justice and Health Care in an Era of Cost Containment,* 9 Soc. Resp.: Journalism, L. Med. 37, 43–47 (1983). For a discussion of the severe problem of access to health care, see 1 President's Comm'n for the Study of Ethical Problems in Medicine and Biomedical and Behavioral Research, Securing Access to Health Care 90–113 (1983) [hereinafter all volumes cited as Securing Access]; Starr, *Medical Care and the Pursuit of Equality in America,* in 2 Securing Access, *supra* at 1–22. For a discussion of the difficulty of access to high cost procedures like organ transplant or renal dialysis, see J. Areen, P. King, S. Goldberg & A. Capron, *supra* note 32, at 852–861; Knox, *Heart Transplants: To Pay or Not to Pay,* 209 Science 570 (1980) (reviewing Department of Health and Human Services criteria for Medicare/Medicaid reimbursement for new technologies), and for relatively low cost procedures such as abortion, see, e.g., Harris v. McRae, 448 U.S. 297, 329–37 (1980) (Brennan, J., dissenting); *id.* at 337–48 (Marshall, J., dissenting).

327. See the discussion of equity concerns under a market controlled system in Havighurst, *Competition in Health Services: Overview, Issues and Answers,* 34 Vand. L. Rev. 1117, 1142–43 (1981). Individual decisionmaking may be less influential because third-party payors play such a central role in access to health care. Congressional Budget Office, Containing Medical Care Costs Through Market Forces 1–2 (1982). *But see* Rushefsky, *A Critique of Market Reform in Health Care: The "Consumer-Choice Health Plan,"* 5 J. Health Pol., Pol'y & L. 720, 726–37 (1981) (suggesting significance of third party reimbursement may have been overestimated).

The Yale Law Journal   Vol. 95: 219, 1985

ual consumers, rather than being made mostly by supposedly wealth-neutral professionals, would comparatively poorer patients end up with even less equitable access to health care than they now have?

Doctor-directed decisionmaking deprives the poor as well as the rich of autonomy and self-determination. Whatever professional ideology would have us believe, professionally competent choice is not in fact immune to economic incentives.[328] The tendency to preempt the choices of poor patients may be significantly greater than it is where wealthy patients are involved.[329] Thus, poor patients may have an even greater stake in strengthened protection for autonomy than do the affluent. The difficulty, however, is that self-determination is a hollow concept to anyone who lacks the resources to implement choice.

The problem of social justice in access to health care is essentially moral and political. Professional expertise cannot and should not provide society with answers about how scarce resources should be distributed any more than it should provide answers about individual utilities regarding medical choice. If there are not enough kidneys to go around, it is disingenuous to pretend that medical expertise can do more than to *advise* regarding some factors that are likely to be relevant in deciding who ought to get one. Expertise can inform those who must make decisions regarding comparative medical risks and benefits. But it should not decide who should receive a transplant any more than it can decide who wants higher levels of certainty. Admittedly, it is politically easier to respond to demands for a "right" to health care by citing the impersonal commands of "medical indication"[330] than it is to articulate and endorse the social, political and economic criteria by which society will determine distribution of health care.[331] Yet offering professional expertise as the source of an-

---

328. Some hospitals and doctors refuse to provide services without advance deposits or proof of insurance. 1 SECURING ACCESS, *supra* note 326, at 100–101.

329. *See* 2 MAKING DECISIONS, *supra* note 2, at 20 (doctors tell less to patients they perceive as being less able to understand, a factor highly correlated with socioeconomic status); Note, *Coerced Sterilization Under Federally Funded Family Planning Programs*, 11 NEW ENG. L. REV. 589, 595 (1976) (describing coercive practices of medical providers in urging sterilization of welfare mothers).

330. *See, e.g.*, Cowan v. Meyers, 3 Civ. 22987 (Cal. Ct. App. filed June 10, 1983) (challenging such restrictions on state-paid health care services). One major effort to introduce the criterion of medical necessity was the Professional Standards Review Organization (PSRO) legislation designed to use peer review to cut costs for Medicare and Medicaid on the basis of whether services were necessary. 42 U.S.C. § 1320(C)(3) (1982). *See* Blumstein, *The Role of PSROs in Hospital Cost Containment*, in HOSPITAL COST CONTAINMENT: SELECTED NOTES FOR FUTURE POLICY 461 (M. Zubkoff, I. Raskin & R. Hanft eds. 1978) (assessing contribution PSROs can make to hospital cost containment). Private insurers also limit their coverage of discretionary services by contract in order to reduce costs. Havighurst, *supra* note 327, at 1127.

331. *See* G. CALABRESI & P. BOBBITT, TRAGIC CHOICES 186–91 (1978); Baily, *"Rationing" and American Health Policy*, 9 J. HEALTH POL., POL'Y & L. 489 (1984) (discussing reluctance of President's Commission to use or explore concept of "rationing" as opposed to "allocation"); Havighurst, *Health Care Cost-Containment Regulation: Prospects and an Alternative*, 3 AM. J.L. & MED. 309, 313–15 (1977) (regarding difficulty of political confrontation with problems of cost con-

Protecting Patient Choice

swers to questions of social justice is at best incomplete and at worst deceitful.

Furthermore, if professional expertise is allowed to regulate the distribution of health care resources, its adequacy as a surrogate for individual choice is further undermined. If doctors allocate care, their loyalty to the best interests of their patients is necessarily diminished, just as it is by other conflicts of interest. A doctor who accepted as optimal a given level of certainty about the presence of glaucoma or about the completeness of an abortion might claim to be acting not only as a rational expert, but also as an implementer of social policy.[332] That doctor could not, however, simultaneously claim to be acting on behalf of a patient who places an unusually high value on her eyesight or on her lifestyle as a nonparent.

The strands of professional competence need to be disentangled from those of social justice, just as they need to be separated more thoroughly from those of individual choice. The question of what limits should be placed upon individual choice by considerations of social justice is beyond the focus of this Article.[333] I have argued only that, in regulating medical decisionmaking, doctrine should maximize individual autonomy rather than decisionmaking by professional experts.

4. *Effects on Consumption and Cost of Health Care*

Increasing demand for medical services is a major cause of rising costs of health care.[334] Increased cost is a problem for individuals, for organizations that finance health care benefits, and for the economy as a whole.[335] Given greater knowledge and control, individuals may increase some kinds of health care consumption. At a minimum, more doctor time would be required to inform and consult with patients regarding their options. Patients who are made aware that additional tests are available to determine, for example, the health of a fetus, the risk of glaucoma, or the possibility of skull fracture might opt for such additional tests.

However, a central premise of much of the current literature on medical cost control is that greater patient choice would yield a significant reduction in health care consumption.[336] Indeed, unless consumers have meaningful control over the implementation of medical recommendations,

---

tainment and cost benefit analysis).

332. For example, by keeping costs down.

333. For a discussion of issues of social justice in health care, see, e.g., 1 SECURING ACCESS, *supra* note 326, at 18–47; Veatch, *What Is a "Just" Health Care Delivery?*, in ETHICS AND HEALTH POLICY 127, 131–42 (R. Veatch and R. Branson eds. 1976).

334. CONGRESSIONAL BUDGET OFFICE, *supra* note 327, at 1.

335. 1 SECURING ACCESS, *supra* note 326, at 184–85.

336. Blumstein & Sloan, *supra* note 154, at 860–61, 894–95; Marmor, Boyer & Greenberg, *Medical Care and Procompetitive Reform*, 34 VAND. L. REV. 1003, 1011–16 (1981).

The Yale Law Journal   Vol. 95: 219, 1985

many cost-control incentives will be ineffective.[337] If fully informed, patients might decline many types of recommended surgery or drugs as being unnecessary or undesirable. For example, there has been much debate about termination of care by patients demanding a right to die, or greater control over the surroundings and conditions under which death or birth will occur.[338] In particular, a deepened knowledge about the value of self-care and prevention, along with a healthier respect for the limits and uncertainties of medicine, would minimize the unrealistic search for absolute protection against danger and mortality.[339]

5. *Effects on Liability Burdens of Doctors*

Recognition of an independent interest in patient information and choice would impose a new or at least a more extensive responsibility, and hence a broadened liability, on doctors. Commentators have expressed concern that liability burdens on doctors are already too great. Yet given what has been said both about patient expectations and about cost control, this new responsibility does not seem inappropriate. Moreover, choice protection would actually reduce doctors' liability in ways that would offset this expansion.

Empirical evidence suggests that even when undesirable medical outcomes occur, the greater the degree to which the patient participates and is informed, the less likely she is to file a malpractice claim.[340] Furthermore, greater protection of patient choice would relieve doctors of some of the responsibility for *decision* risks because more decisions would be made by patients.[341] Sharing authority with patients could, therefore, be both a psychic and a legal relief.

Greater clarity in identifying and protecting an interest in choice might

---

337. Increasing the patient's direct financial responsibility for chosen medical services would also decrease demand. Thus under a regime of increased individual choice, demand could be curtailed by requiring patients who seek levels of care that exceed standards of competent practice to pay a higher share of the cost of such care. Such a scheme might also, however, require a reciprocal program of rebate to those who choose less care than professional norms would recommend.

338. *See, e.g.*, Bartling v. Superior Ct., 163 Cal. App. 3d 186, 209 Cal. Rptr. 220 (1984) (competent adult wished to refuse medical care and be allowed to die); Watchorn, *supra* note 233 (discussing midwifery as desirable and less expensive alternative to hospital birth).

339. Nor would increased protection of choice necessarily promote the practice of defensive medicine. Choice protection does not change standards for what the doctor should know or recommend; it affects only what the doctor should disclose about what she knows. In any case, malpractice suits may be a more limited factor in stimulating defensive medical practice than has been thought. *See* Epstein, *supra* note 17, at 107 n.43.

340. Press, *supra* note 323, at 54 (relationship factors more important than harm *per se* in filing malpractice suits); Enright, *supra* note 10, at 90.

341. Press observes that the myth of medical perfection creates a situation in which "the question of who is in charge is easily converted into a question about who is responsible." Press, *supra* note 323, at 59. *But see* Adams & Zuckerman, *supra* note 35, at 484–85 (informed consent is significantly associated with higher annual rate of malpractice claims after 1976).

Protecting Patient Choice

also reduce unpredictability and irrationality in current malpractice recoveries. Because they receive ambiguous signals from the legal system, doctors have found it difficult to discern meaningful guidelines for conduct.[342] Moreover, growing public anger regarding medical paternalism may sometimes cause juries and even judges to render decisions that are anomalous under established principles, because they feel that patient choice is being inadequately protected by present doctrines. A clear and decisive mandate to disclose information for purposes of patient choice might actually improve predictability and reduce litigation.

Some have suggested that, in dealing with medical accidents generally, no-fault systems are preferable to fault-based analysis under traditional tort approaches.[343] No-fault schemes assume the central issue to be compensation for an irreducible quantum of medical accidents. Such a rationale has force in the context of malpractice but is unpersuasive where the interest is patient autonomy. There is nothing inevitable about the allocation of decisionmaking authority between patients and doctors.[344] Incentives aimed at furthering traditional tort goals of conduct guidance and deterrence are especially appropriate here. Indeed, the whole point of changed standards would be to avoid the very harms occasioned by invasion of choice by altering perceptions both of what is culpable and of what is appropriate with regard to decisionmaking roles.[345]

6. *Effects on the Doctor-Patient Relationship*

Realignment of authority in the doctor-patient relationship raises fears about the quality of that relationship.[346] The spectre of doctor turned puppet is not attractive. Nor are these simply self-serving fears of doctors wishing to retain their uncontrolled authority. There are dangers in rendering either party to a caretaking relationship choiceless.[347]

---

342. 2 MAKING DECISIONS, *supra* note 2, at 25 (only 32% of physicians surveyed agree that the legal requirements of obtaining informed consent are clear and explicit).

343. *See* sources collected in Meisel, *Expansion, supra* note 6, at 143–51; Note, *Comparative Approaches to Liability for Medical Maloccurrences*, 84 YALE L.J. 1141 (1975). Although Epstein argues that consensual principles are generally preferable to strict liability in resolving medical disputes, he undermines his own theory in the context of informed consent by adopting paternalistic medical custom rather than patient expectation as the appropriate measure of disclosure wherever there is no explicit agreement to the contrary. Epstein, *supra* note 17, at 102–07, 120–28.

344. Professor Meisel comments on the conflicting functions of medical accident compensation and informed consent, noting that "[i]t would be ironic if the informed-consent doctrine, which spawned strict liability for medical accidents, were to contain the seeds of its own destruction . . . ." Meisel, *Expansion, supra* note 6, at 151.

345. If the resistance to fault analysis stems from concern about excessive judgments against individual defendants, other forms of control, such as the proportional recovery system proposed here, would be preferable solutions.

346. Fears about the doctor-patient relationship being disrupted by greater patient involvement are mentioned in J. KATZ, *supra* note 7, at 27; Miller, *supra* note 35, at 2100.

347. *See generally* R. BURT, *supra* note 5 (discussing dynamics of doctor-patient relationship and

The Yale Law Journal   Vol. 95: 219, 1985

A broadened obligation to disclose would not make the doctor an impersonal purveyor of technical information. She would remain professionally and personally responsible for recommending and implementing decisions. Nor could she hide behind disclosure of unassimilated information. Rather, she would retain the role of responsible advisor. Accountability for the advising function would have to be carefully monitored, lest the doctor abandon it under the guise of deferring to patient choice.

Patients could not compel a doctor to do something to which the doctor objects as a matter of personal or professional ethics or competence.[348] Given the varied views of doctors, however, patients should usually be able to find someone who has no personal objection to implementing the choice the patient wishes to make.[349]

CONCLUSION

Medical decisionmaking involves the interwoven, overlapping and often competing claims of personal autonomy and professional competence. The challenge of regulating medical decisionmaking is to allocate the proper weight to each of these values. The task is both difficult and important, for the conflict may be between professionally defined "correct" choices in matters ultimately involving life and death, and no less a value than self-determination.

A new model for the allocation of authority between doctors and patients is needed. Existing legal protection for medical patients' autonomy is more limited than has been recognized and more deficient than should be tolerated. Present doctrines falsely equate the protection of autonomy

---

need for both parties to retain power and responsibility).

348. *See, e.g.*, Doe v. Mundy, 378 F. Supp. 731, 736 (E.D. Wis. 1974) (medical personnel not required to perform abortions against personal convictions), *aff'd*, 514 F.2d 1179 (7th Cir. 1975). A right to refuse to perform such services is protected by federal legislation in Title II of The National Research Service Award Act of 1974, Pub. L. No. 93-348, § 214, 88 Stat. 342, 353 (codified at 42 U.S.C. § 300a(b)(2), (c) (1982)). *See* Ruddick, *Doctors' Rights and Work*, 4 J. MED. & PHIL. 192 (1979) (advocating doctors' "bill of rights").

349. *See* 2 MAKING DECISIONS, *supra* note 2, at 23 (36% of patients reported that they have changed doctors because they disagreed with the doctor; 20% report that a doctor has told them to find another doctor if they did not agree with that doctor's advice). A more complete identification of doctor and patient preferences and the development of market-oriented shopping for a doctor whose views are compatible with one's own would be desirable. If no qualified doctor would implement the patient's choice, a difficult conflict occurs. *See* Bouvia v. Riverside County, No. 159780 (Cal. Super. Ct. Dec. 16, 1983). A doctor's autonomy, like a patient's, deserves respect. Common law traditions about omission and commission suggest that it may be worse to force a doctor to act against her values than to deprive the patient of the opportunity to effectuate a desired course of action. The logic of the market also suggests that if no one wishes to provide a service, the patient must go without. Yet the tradition of medical paternalism is so strong that deference to such principles would invite the same weakened protection of patient choice that now exists. Furthermore, access to medical care is widely considered to be one of the most fundamental of necessities. Therefore, in this scenario the presumption of control should be with the patient, and the doctor should carry the burden of showing that there is an unacceptable personal compromise.

Protecting Patient Choice

with control over bodily contact. These doctrines also submerge analysis of the interest in autonomy within the related but divergent framework of redress for professional incompetence. Although courts sometimes provide greater vindication for patient choice where there is a conflict of interest on the part of the doctor or heightened electiveness on the part of the patient, these exceptions are unpredictable and inadequately generalized. Protection of patient autonomy remains derivative rather than direct, episodic rather than systematic. As a result, significant harms to patients' interest in choice go unredressed.

The subtlety of power-sharing in an ideal relationship between doctor and patient must be acknowledged.[350] Even patients who are clearly competent to make decisions will suffer confusion and ambivalence. They will need guidance and support of professionals and loved ones. Moreover, professionals are to a significant degree motivated by caring for others; we need them to continue to be. Respect for patients' autonomy should not cause doctors either to abandon compassion or to shed their responsibility for advising and caring for patients. But medical decisions depend upon moral values, economic considerations and risk preferences, as well as on medical expertise. Because health care decisions affect the patient more directly than anyone else, the patient's choices, educated but not preempted by the doctor's expertise, should be controlling.

The law is not the only relevant tool for achieving such a relationship between doctor and patient. But ultimately the law is about line-drawing, and some basic division of authority is essential both for purposes of norm-setting and of dispute resolution. The fact that practice, time and complexity will embroider nuance and qualification upon the basic structure does not alter the need for such a framework. Patient autonomy should be recognized and protected as a distinct legal interest.

---

350. For a thoughtful discussion of the difficulties and limitations of sharp role delineation both for doctors and patients, see R. Burt, *supra* note 5.

[2]

GERALD ROBERTSON

INFORMED CONSENT TO MEDICAL TREATMENT

THE doctrine of informed consent to therapeutic medical treatment,[1] one of the most controversial issues in American medical law, is now beginning to develop in this country. This article examines the status of the doctrine in English law, against a background of its development in the United States.

I INTRODUCTION

At the outset it is important to define what is meant by the term " informed consent," an exercise which is often overlooked by commentators and judges. As one writer observes [2]:

> In listening to people talk about informed consent I have been struck again and again by their childlike conviction that the phrase has meaning, that it does not require painstaking definition before one can even begin to discuss it.

The need for definition is especially great in this country since the term " informed consent " is not one with which our courts, nor possibly our medical profession, are particularly familiar.[3]

As will be seen below, the concept of informed consent has its roots in a recognition of the patient's right to self-determination. Simply put, the doctrine of informed consent means that a doctor is required to give his patient sufficient information about proposed treatment so as to provide him with the opportunity of making an " informed " or " rational " choice as to whether to undergo the treatment. The use of the terms " rational " and " informed " is obviously vague and arguably question-begging, but the same is true of any general definition of the doctrine of informed consent. It is only when one adds flesh to the skeleton definition that one can begin to understand its meaning. Thus, for example, in one of the

---

[1] In this article, the doctrine of informed consent is discussed in the context of therapeutic treatment, as opposed to non-therapeutic experimentation. Whilst many of the features of the doctrine are common to both situations, additional considerations become relevant when the situation is one of non-therapeutic experimentation. For discussion of the doctrine in this context, see Annas, Glantz and Katz, *Informed Consent to Human Experimentation* (1977).

[2] Katz, " Informed Consent—a Fairy Tale?: Law's Vision " (1977) 39 U.Pitt.L. Rev. 137 at pp. 137–138.

[3] The term " informed consent " appears only to have been used in one reported case in this country — see *Re D. (A Minor)* [1976] Fam. 185. The term is, however, used by a number of writers in English journals; see *e.g.* Skegg, " Informed Consent to Medical Procedures " (1975) 15 Med.Sci. Law 124; Brazier, " Informed Consent to Surgery " (1979) 19 Med.Sci. Law 49. See also the Medical Defence Union booklet, *Consent to Treatment* (1974) at p. 3.

earliest cases involving informed consent, the Supreme Court of Kansas stated that the doctrine required the doctor to make[4]:

> [a] reasonable disclosure ... of the nature and probable consequences of the suggested or recommended ... treatment, and ... a reasonable disclosure of the dangers within his knowledge which are incident to, or possible in, the treatment which he proposes to administer.

Thus it can be seen that the doctrine of informed consent is a legal concept which imposes a duty on the doctor to explain to his patient not only the nature of the proposed treatment, but also the dangers and risks inherent therein. The obvious, and fundamental, question that arises from this is, of course, " how much information and explanation is the doctor required to give "? This will be examined in detail below.

One preliminary point which remains to be discussed is the question of whether there can be said to be a single " doctrine " of informed consent. One leading writer has suggested that[5]:

> The term " informed consent " is seriously misleading when it is used in a way which suggests that there is a single doctrine of informed consent. There is not, for different areas of the law have different requirements, and information which suffices in one area will not necessarily do so in another.

With respect, it is submitted that it *can* be argued that there is a single doctrine of informed consent. It is true, of course, that the amount of information which the doctor is required to disclose to his patient will vary according to the circumstances and, in particular (as will be seen below), according to whether the court regards the non-disclosure of information as relating to the tort of trespass or to the tort of negligence. However, it is submitted that once the law imposes a duty on the doctor to disclose to his patient information relating not only to the general nature and purpose of the proposed treatment, but also to the risks and dangers inherent therein, then, notwithstanding that the amount of required information will vary according to the circumstances, it can be said that a single doctrine of informed consent exists. It will be argued below that English law has now reached this stage.

Since the doctrine of informed consent has its origins in the United States,[6] it is instructive to outline its development in that country,

---

    [4] *Natanson* v. *Kline,* 186 Kan. 393 at p. 410, 350 P. 2d 1093 at p. 1106 (1960).

    [5] Skegg, *supra* note 3, at p. 124.

    [6] The view expressed by some American commentators that the doctrine of informed consent can be traced back to the English decision in *Slater* v. *Baker* (1767) 2 Wils. 359 is at best illusory.

thereby identifying some of the issues with which English courts may have to deal in their application of the doctrine.

II THE EVOLUTION AND DEVELOPMENT OF INFORMED CONSENT
IN THE UNITED STATES

(a) *Pre-1972*

Although there is some indication in American cases prior to 1957 of a concept of informed consent, the decision in that year of the California Court of Appeal in *Salgo* v. *Leland Stanford Jr. University Board of Trustees* [7] is generally regarded as having given birth to the doctrine of informed consent. In that case, the doctor failed to warn his patient of the risk of paralysis inherent in the performance of a translumbar aortography, and as a result of the operation the patient suffered severe paralysis of the lower limbs. His subsequent claim for damages was based, *inter alia*, on the doctor's failure to warn of the risk of paralysis. In the course of its judgment, the court enunciated the following principle [8]:

> [a] physician violates his duty to his patient and subjects himself to liability if he withholds any facts which are necessary to form the basis of an intelligent consent by the patient to the proposed treatment.

Two important points should be noted about this case. First, the court appears to have accepted that, although the doctor was under a duty to disclose information to his patient concerning the inherent risks of the proposed treatment, the question of what risks ought to be disclosed was a matter of medical judgment. Secondly, the court adopted the view that lack of informed consent vitiates the apparent consent which the patient has given, thus rendering the doctor liable in damages for the tort of trespass. The significance of the difference between trespass and negligence, in relation to informed consent, will be discussed later in this section.

The next development was in 1960 in the case of *Natanson* v. *Kline*.[9] The plaintiff suffered injuries as a result of cobalt therapy which was performed to reduce the risk of breast cancer spreading following a mastectomy. She sued the radiologist in negligence for failing to warn her of the risks inherent in the therapy. In the course of its judgment, the Supreme Court of Kansas enunciated the rule set out in the introduction to this article, namely, that the physician is under a duty, *inter alia*, to make a reasonable disclosure to his

---

[7] 154 Cal.App. 2d 560, 317 P. 2d 170 (1957).
[8] *Ibid.* at 578, 317 P. 2d at pp. 180–181.
[9] 186 Kan. 393, 350 P. 2d 1093 (1960).

patient of the risks and dangers incident to the proposed treatment. Unlike the court in *Salgo*, the court in *Natanson* regarded the breach of this duty as constituting negligence, rather than as vitiating apparent consent so as to give rise to a trespass to the person. However, like *Salgo*, the court in *Natanson* regarded the question of what risks ought to be disclosed as being a matter of medical judgment. Thus the doctor was under a duty to make a " reasonable " disclosure of inherent risks, the question of what was " reasonable " in the particular circumstances of the case being decided according to the accepted " reasonable doctor " test, *i.e.* did the defendant act as a reasonable and prudent doctor would have acted in similar circumstances in deciding not to inform the patient of the particular risk?

(b) *Post-1972*

The doctrine of informed consent developed along these lines for the next 12 years, courts accepting that a doctor was under a duty to make a reasonable disclosure to his patient of the inherent risks of the procedure, that failure to make such disclosure related to negligence and not to trespass, and that the question of what constituted " reasonable disclosure " was to be determined by asking what a reasonable doctor would have done in similar circumstances. In effect, this meant that the question of " reasonable disclosure " was determined by the evidence of medical experts in relation to normal medical practice. However, 1972 heralded an attempt to formulate an entirely new, and potentially far-reaching, test for determining what information a doctor was obliged to disclose to his patient in relation to the inherent risks of the proposed treatment. This attempt was made in the case of *Canterbury* v. *Spence*.[10]

The plaintiff in *Canterbury* suffered paralysis as a result of undergoing a laminectomy. His action for damages against the physician was based, *inter alia*, on the allegation that the latter had failed to warn him before the operation of the risk of paralysis therein. In considering the issue of what standard to apply in determining the scope of the physician's duty to disclose such information, the court came to the conclusion that [11]:

> [r]espect for the patient's right of self-determination on a particular therapy demands a standard set by law for a physician rather than one which physicians may or may not impose upon themselves.

The court accepted the view that a physician was under a duty to

[10] 464 F. 2d 772 (D.C.Cir. 1972).
[11] *Ibid*. at 784.

disclose all " material " risks inherent in the proposed treatment. However, whereas courts had previously been content to determine what risks were " material " by asking what risks a reasonable doctor would have disclosed in similar circumstances, the court in *Canterbury* enunciated the " prudent patient " test for determining this issue [12]:

> [A] risk is thus material when a reasonable person in what the physician knows or should know to be the patient's position, would be likely to attach significance to the risk or cluster of risks in determining whether or not to forgo the proposed therapy.

Two reasons, in addition to the patient's right to self-determination, were given by the court to justify this departure from the established view that the meaning of " reasonable disclosure " was a matter for the medical profession to determine. First, it was thought that a standard of disclosure based on the custom of the medical profession could be a façade for non-disclosure. Secondly, the court felt that the question of what risks a person would regard as material was an issue which could be determined without special knowledge of medical science. It is important to note the objective nature of the *Canterbury* test. The test of materiality, and hence disclosure, is not whether the patient himself would have attached significance to the risk, but rather whether a *reasonable person* in the patient's position would have done so.

The court, however, recognised certain exceptions to this duty of disclosure, the most important of which is that of " therapeutic privilege." [13] This exception means that a physician may be entitled to withhold from his patient information concerning the risks of proposed treatment if it can be established, by means of medical evidence, that disclosure of this information would have posed a serious threat of psychological detriment to the patient. This relates to the more general issue of whether a doctor is entitled to withhold information from his patient if he considers this to be in the " best interests of his patient." This is undoubtedly a question which courts in this country will have to face, and for that reason it is examined more fully in Section IV below.

Finally, unlike most pre-1972 decisions on informed consent, the court in *Canterbury* gave full consideration to the question of causation. The relevance of causation in informed consent cases is linked to the difference between trespass and negligence. If one

---

[12] *Ibid.* at 787.

[13] In so doing the court severely undermined its attempt to exclude the " reasonable doctor " standard of care (and the consequent emphasis on expert evidence) from informed consent litigation, since the outcome of the doctor's decision not to disclose information on therapeutic grounds is determined by applying the " reasonable doctor " test. See Katz, *supra* note 2, at pp. 157 *et seq.*

adopts the view, as the early American cases did, that failure by the doctor to disclose necessary information about the proposed treatment vitiates the apparent consent which the patient has given and thus gives rise to the tort of battery, the patient is not required to show that, had this information been given to him, he would have chosen not to undergo the treatment.[14] On the other hand, if one regards failure to disclose information as constituting negligence on the part of the doctor, the basic principles of the tort of negligence dictate that the patient must establish that he would not have chosen to undergo the treatment had he been given the required information. If the patient cannot establish this, he will not succeed in his action in negligence since he will have failed to prove that the injury which he has suffered would not have been sustained had it not been for the negligence of the doctor in withholding the information.

The reason for this important distinction lies in the nature of the plaintiff's claim. If the claim is framed in negligence, the legal wrong of which the plaintiff complains is the failure by the doctor to disclose relevant information and thus, in order to establish the necessary casual link between the legal wrong and the injury suffered, the plaintiff must satisfy the court that he would not have consented to the treatment had he been given the relevant information. However, if the claim is framed in trespass and the court concludes that the failure to disclose information was such as to vitiate the apparent consent given by the plaintiff, the legal wrong of which the plaintiff complains is not the failure itself but rather the performance of medical treatment without consent. It is the latter, and not the former, which in the circumstances constitutes the tort of trespass to the person. Consequently, if the claim is framed in trespass, the plaintiff is not required to show that he would not have consented to the treatment had the information been disclosed to him.

It is evident that, if the plaintiff's claim is based in negligence, difficulties may arise in relation to proof of causation. In dealing with this issue, the court in *Canterbury* once again abandoned a subjective test in favour of an objective one. Thus the court asked, not " would this particular patient have decided against the proposed treatment had he been informed of the material risks," but rather " would a reasonable person in the patient's position have so decided." The reason for adopting this objective test can be seen in the following passage from the judgment in the case of *Cobbs* v. *Grant*,[15] a case which followed the test propounded in *Canterbury*:

---

[14] See *Chatterton* v. *Gerson, The Times,* February 7, 1980, Transcript Judgement at p. 19. It is submitted that the Canadian decision in *Koehler* v. *Cook* (1976) 65 D.L.R. (3d) 766 is incorrect in this respect.

[15] 8 Cal. 3d 229, 104 Cal.Rptr. 505 (1972).

Since at the time of the trial the uncommunicated hazard has materialised, it would be surprising if the patient-plaintiff did not claim that had he been informed of the dangers he would have declined treatment. Subjectively he may believe so with the 20–20 vision of hindsight, but we doubt that justice will be served by placing the physician in jeopardy of the patient's bitterness and disillusionment.

As will be discussed in Section IV below, English courts have preferred a subjective test, rather than an objective one as in *Canterbury,* in relation to the question of causation.

(c) *Present Position*

The present position in the United States is one of contrast between the minority of States which have chosen to follow the lead given by *Canterbury* by adopting the objective " prudent patient " test outlined above, and the majority of States which have been content to adopt the traditional test and determine the question of disclosure of risks by applying the " reasonable doctor " test.[16] One further development should, however, be noted. Since 1975 there has been a growing tendency for individual States to enact legislation which severely curtails the operation of the doctrine of informed consent.[17] For example, some of these enactments go as far as to create as presumption, rebuttable only on proof of fraud, that a patient's signature is conclusive evidence of informed consent having been given. The motive underlying many of these statutes is relevant in relation to the " function " of the doctrine of informed consent, an issue which will now be examined.

III THE FUNCTION OF THE DOCTRINE OF INFORMED CONSENT

The doctrine of informed consent is regarded by most commentators as having two primary functions,[18] namely, to promote individual autonomy and to encourage rational decision making, both of which stem from the basic premise of the patient's right to self-determination.[19] Thus the doctrine can be seen as reflecting two ideals, namely,

---

[16] For a detailed list of the States adopting the majority approach and those adopting the minority approach see Seidelson, " Medical Malpractice: Informed Consent in ' Full-Disclosure ' Jurisdictions " (1976) 14 Duq.L.Rev. 309.

[17] See Annas, Glantz and Katz, *supra* note 1, at pp. 38 *et seq.;* Plante, " The Decline of ' Informed Consent ' " (1978) 35 Wash. & Lee L.Rev. 91.

[18] See, however, the six headings suggested by Katz and Capron, *Catastrophic Diseases: Who Decides What?* (1975) at pp. 82 *et seq.*

[19] See generally Annas, Glantz and Katz, *supra* note 1, at pp. 33 *et seq.*; Strong, " Informed Consent: Theory and Policy " (1979) 5 J.Med. Ethics 196.

(1) that the decision to undergo medical treatment should ulti-
    mately be that of the patient and not that of the doctor; and
(2) that the patient should be given sufficient information to
    provide him with an opportunity of making this decision in a
    rational manner.

It is clear that, in enunciating and developing the doctrine of
informed consent, American courts regarded it as being based on a
recognition of the patient's right to self-determination. Thus, for
example, the court in *Canterbury* declared that [20]:

> The root premise is the concept ... that " every human being of
> adult years and of sound mind has a right to determine what
> shall be done with his own body.... " True consent to what
> happens to one's self is the informed exercise of a choice, and
> that entails an opportunity to evaluate knowledgeably the options
> available and the risks attendant upon each.

However, a closer examination of the evolution and development of
the doctrine of informed consent in the United States indicates that
the promotion of the individual's right to self-determination may not
be the true function of the doctrine. Instead, it can be argued that its
function has been to expand the liability of the medical profession
in order to award compensation to a greater number of victims of
" medical accidents," a theme which has been canvassed by at least
one writer in the United States.[21]

It is beyond doubt that one effect of the recognition of the doctrine
of informed consent is to expand the liability of the medical
profession. The explanation for this is quite simple. Courts, particularly in this country, constantly stress the truism that things can go
wrong in the course of medical treatment without that treatment
having necessarily been performed negligently. Thus, for example,
in the words of Lord Denning in the case of *Hucks* v. *Cole* [22]:

> [w]ith the best will be in the world, things do sometimes go
> amiss in surgical operations or medical treatment.... So a doctor
> is not to be held negligent simply because something goes
> wrong.... He is not liable for mischance or misadventure. Nor
> is he liable for an error of judgment.

This means that a large number of patients who suffer injury in the
course of medical treatment will, under a fault-based system of
compensation such as our own, go without compensation because

---

[20] 464 F. 2d 772 at p. 780 (D.C. Cir 1972) (quoting from *Schloendorff* v. *Society of
New York Hospital*, 211 N.Y. 125 at pp. 129–130 (1914)).
[21] See Meisel, " The Expansion of Liability for Medical Accidents: From
Negligence to Strict Liability by Way of Informed Consent " (1977) 56 Neb.L.Rev.
51.
[22] Court of Appeal Transcript No. 1968/181 at p. 6; *The Times*, 9th May 1968.

they are the victims, not of negligent performance of the treatment, but rather of the risks incident thereto. One way in which to remedy this situation, within the present fault-based framework, is to expand liability by making the doctor answerable in damages for failing to warn the patient of these risks prior to undergoing the treatment. In this way a greater number of medical accident victims receive compensation, by means of extending the liability of the medical profession beyond the bounds of actual negligent performance of treatment. The fact that the doctrine of informed consent leads to this expansion of liability is of fundamental importance in determining, as will be done in Section V, whether or not the doctrine is likely to develop in this country.

However, it can be argued that such expansion of liability was not merely the *effect*, but rather the *purpose*, of the development of the doctrine of informed consent in the United States. As one writer indicates [23]:

> The requirement of informed consent to medical treatment has, for at least the past two decades, been used as the cloth from which courts slowly have begun to fashion a no-fault system for compensating persons who have suffered bad results from medical treatment.

A number of factors support this contention. The doctrine was born at a time when judicial policy in the United States was beginning to turn in favour of the plaintiff in medical malpractice cases. This can be seen, for example, from the development during the same period of a pro-plaintiff attitude in relation to the *res ipsa loquitur* rule of evidence, in an effort to combat the so-called " conspiracy of silence " amongst doctors and to overcome the plaintiff's consequent difficulties in establishing negligence on the part of a doctor.[24] However, before 1972 this judicial policy was not sufficiently strong to lead to an abandonment of the " reasonable doctor " standard in relation to informed consent. By 1972, however, the judicial policy in favour of plaintiffs in medical malpractice litigation had reached such a peak, at least in some States, that desertion of the " reasonable doctor " test in informed consent cases became possible, as can be seen in *Canterbury* and the cases which adopted its reasoning. The real reason underlying the decision in *Canterbury* was not a declaration of faith in the patient's right to self-determination, but, as was outlined in Section II, rather an attempt (arguably unsuccessful) [25] to relieve the plaintiff of the considerable burden of

---

[23] Meisel, *supra* note 21, at p. 77.
[24] See in particular *Salgo* v. *Leland Stanford Jr. University Board of Trustees,* 154 Cal.App. 2d 560, 317 P. 2d 170 at p. 175 (1957).
[25] See *supra,* note 13.

establishing negligence in informed consent cases by means of medical evidence.

Similarly, the recent backlash of legislation restricting the operation of the doctrine of informed consent, outlined in Section II, comes at a time of a recognised " crisis " in relation to medical malpractice litigation in the United States. Once again one can see the doctrine being chartered by the winds of judicial policy in relation to the liability of the medical profession.[26]

Moreover, if the primary purpose of developing a doctrine of informed consent had truly been to promote individual autonomy and to encourage rational decision making, one would expect the courts to have paid at least some attention to the concepts of communication and patient comprehension. This, however, has not been the case. The judicial emphasis has been on the doctor's legal duty to disclose information, with the question of the plaintiff's understanding of such information being almost totally ignored. As the court in *Canterbury* stressed [27] :

> In duty-to-disclose cases, the focus of attention is more properly upon the nature and content of the physician's divulgence than the patient's understanding or consent . . . the vital inquiry on duty to disclose relates to the physician's performance of an obligation, while one of the difficulties with analysis in terms of " informed consent " is its tendency to imply that what is decisive is the degree of the patient's comprehension.

It is wrong to suggest, as some writers have done,[28] that the patient's comprehension of the disclosed information should not be an issue for judicial concern if the function of the doctrine is simply to *encourage* (but not to ensure) rational decision making. The doctrine of informed consent can only become meaningful in terms of the patient's right to self-determination if he actually comprehends the information which is disclosed to him—without such comprehension the patient is not given the opportunity which he requires in order to make a rational decision. Even accepting that the patient's right to self-determination dictates only that he be given a *reasonable* opportunity of making a rational decision as to proposed medical treatment, the extent of the patient's comprehension of the disclosed information should still be a vital issue. The opportunity given may

---

[26] See *e.g.* the case of *Bly* v. *Rhoads,* 216 Va. 645, 222 S.E. 2d 783 (1976) in which the court, commenting on the " prudent patient " rule enunciated in *Canterbury,* observed (at p. 787) that " [s]uch a rule would cause further proliferation of medical malpractice actions in a situation already approaching a national crisis. This is a result which, if at all possible consonant with sound judicial policy, should be avoided".

[27] 464 F. 2d 772 at p. 780 (D.C. Cir. 1972).

[28] See Meisel, *supra* note 21, at p. 117.

be " reasonable " if viewed from the standpoint of the doctor, in terms of the information which he has disclosed, but that opportunity becomes wholly unreasonable for the purpose for which it is given and completely meaningless, if viewed from the patient's standpoint, if he fails to understand the information given to him.

Given that empirical research has shown the inadequacies of doctor-patient communication to be such as to make the giving of truly " informed consent " almost a forlorn hope in practice,[29] it is perhaps not surprising that American courts have tended to overlook the question of patient comprehension and to concentrate instead solely on the doctor's obligation to disclose the information. In so doing, however, they have shown that, in developing the doctrine of informed consent, their primary concern was not the protection of the patient's right to self-determination by means of affording him an opportunity of making a rational decision as to proposed medical treatment. This, in addition to the way in which the inception and development of the doctrine has mirrored judicial policy towards liability of the medical profession, suggest that the doctrine of informed consent is a legal mechanism whose function has simply been to expand the liability of the medical profession in order to compensate a greater number of victims of medical accidents.

IV THE DOCTRINE OF INFORMED CONSENT IN ENGLISH LAW

It is against this background that one can now turn to examine the status of the doctrine of informed consent in English law. At the present time, any writer attempting such an exercise must do so with a considerable degree of caution. Whereas, as has been outlined above, the doctrine has been recognised in American law for over 20 years, its pedigree in English law is far less impressive. There are relatively few cases in this area of English law and thus any conclusions based on such a dearth of authority must of necessity be tentative. This is the main reason for the final section (Section V) in this Article, which attempts to predict how the doctrine of informed consent will develop in this country.

(a) *Consent as to the Nature and Purpose of Proposed Treatment*

It is firmly established in English law that, in the absence of

---

[29] See *e.g.* Cassileth *et al.,* " Informed Consent—Why are Its Goals Imperfectly Realized? " (1980) 302 New Eng.J.Med. 896; Rosenberg, " Informed Consent—A Reappraisal of Patient's Reactions " (1973) 119 Calif. Med. 64; Alfidi, " Informed Consent—A Study of Patient Reaction " (1971) 216 J.A.M.A. 1325; Boyle, " Difference Between Patients' and Doctors' Interpretation of Some Common Medical Terms " [1970] 2 B.M.J. 286.

exceptional circumstances such as an emergency situation,[30] a doctor must obtain the consent of his patient before undertaking treatment involving physical contact with the patient. If he fails to do this, he will be liable in damages for the tort of trespass. The application of this principle can be seen from several cases, for example, *Cull* v. *Butler* [31] (surgeon obtaining consent to curettage but performing hysterectomy) and *Hamilton* v. *Birmingham R.H.B.*[32] (sterilisation operation performed without the consent of the patient).[33]

It is also firmly established that in order for the consent to be valid it must be " real," in the sense that the patient must know what he is consenting to. Thus it follows that, in order to have such knowledge, the patient must be told (and must understand) the general nature and purpose of the proposed treatment. That this proposition is accepted by the medical profession can be seen from the B.M.A. Handbook of Medical Ethics [34] and from the standard consent forms recommended by the Medical Defence Union.[35] Its acceptance in English law can be seen most recently in the case of *Chatterton* v. *Gerson,*[36] in particular from the following dictum of Bristow J.[37]:

> In my judgment once the patient is informed in broad terms of the nature of the procedure which is intended, and gives her consent, that consent is real . . .

However, the apparent clarity of this principle conceals uncertainty. The phrase " the general nature and purpose of the proposed treatment " is one which is often used but seldom explained. What information comes within the ambit of this principle? In particular, can information relating to the inherent risks of proposed treatment ever come within the meaning of the " general nature and purpose " of the treatment, so that failure to disclose such information would vitiate the apparent consent which is given? The answer to this question is significant in that it determines whether a plaintiff who has not been informed of the inherent risks of proposed treatment can sue for damages for trespass to the person. As will be seen

---

[30] See Skegg, " A Justification For Medical Procedures Performed Without Consent " (1974) 90 L.Q.R. 512.

[31] [1932] 1 B.M.J. 1195.

[32] [1969] 2 B.M.J. 456. See also *Devi.* v. *West Midlands R.H.A.* [1980] 7 Current Law 44.

[33] The Annual Reports of the Medical Defence Union contain several references to cases, settled out of court, involving sterilisation operations performed without consent. See 1977 Report at p. 39, 1974 Reports at p. 48.

[34] *The Handbook of Medical Ethics* (1980), para. 1.8.

[35] See M.D.U. booklet, *Consent to Treatment* (1974).

[36] *The Times,* February 7, 1980.

[37] Transcript Judgment, at p. 19.

The writer gratefully acknowledges the assistance of the court in supplying a copy of the judgment in this case.

below, under heading (f), English courts seem intent on answering this question in the negative.

(b) *Disclosure of Risks Inherent in the Proposed Treatment*

Although it is clear that, in order to obtain a valid consent from his patient, a doctor is required to explain the " nature and purpose " of proposed treatment, until recently it was not clear whether the doctor is also under a legal duty (independent of the *validity* of the patient's consent) to inform him of the risks inherent in the treatment, *i.e.* a duty corresponding to the doctrine of informed consent as outlined above. Despite the cautionary note at the beginning of this section, it is submitted that, until the decision of the High Court in *Chatterton* in 1980, there was no English case law to support the existence of such a duty.

There are, however, two cases at first instance which appear to contradict this view and which therefore must be examined. In *Hatcher* v. *Black* [38] the plaintiff, a professional singer, claimed damages from a doctor, alleging that the latter had been negligent in advising her that the proposed treatment (a partial thyroidectomy) involved no risk of damage to her voice. The plaintiff's left vocal chord was paralysed as a result of the operation. Denning L.J. (as he then was), sitting as a judge of first instance,[39] instructed the jury that, although the defendant had admitted telling the plaintiff that the operation involved no risk to her voice, this would not mean that he had been negligent, unless the jury was satisfied that, in giving this advice to the plaintiff, the defendant had fallen below the standard of a reasonably skilful doctor. Denning L.J. also stressed that the decision as to whether to disclose information relating to the risks inherent in the treatment, and even the decision to give the patient false information, were matters for the doctor's own clinical judgment.[40]

It is submitted that this case does not support the proposition that a legal duty is incumbent on the doctor to inform his patient of the risks inherent in proposed treatment. Rather, the approach adopted

---

[38] *The Times*, July 2, 1954.
The text of part of the judge's summing up to the jury is produced in Lord Denning's book *The Discipline of Law* (1979) at pp. 242–244.

[39] " [I]ike a staff officer going back to the regiment for a spell in the line " (Denning, *ibid*. at 242).

[40] A similar approach has been adopted by the Health Service Commissioner in relation to complaints received by him alleging failure on the part of a doctor to inform the patient adequately of the inherent risks of medical treatment. The Commissioner has held that a conscious decision (as opposed to mere forgetfulness) by the doctor not to inform his patient is an exercise of clinical judgment, thereby rendering the complaint outwith the Commissioner's jurisdiction under the National Health Service Act 1977, Sched. 13, para. 19 (1). See Second Report for Session 1979/80 at p. 25; Fourth Report for Session 1979/80, case No. SW. 15/78–79; First Report for Session 1978/79, case No. WW. 6/77–78

in *Hatcher* was to regard the decision as to whether to disclose *any* information as a matter of medical judgment. In other words, *Hatcher* simply reiterates that a doctor is under a legal duty to act in the manner of a reasonably skilful doctor, and the issue of whether this duty encompasses the giving of information relating to risks inherent in the treatment is a question, not of law, but of reasonable medical judgment.

The second case is that of *Bolam* v. *Friern H.M.C.*[41] which involved the doctor's alleged failure to warn his patient of the risk of fractures being sustained in the course of electro-convulsive therapy. In instructing the jury, the judge followed the approach adopted in *Hatcher*, thus reaffirming that the question of whether a doctor should warn his patient of *any* of the risks inherent in the treatment was a matter of medical judgment.[42] It is of interest to note that in both cases the jury returned a verdict in favour of the defendant.

The first sign that English law might recognise a general duty corresponding to the doctrine of informed consent came in 1971 in *Chadwick* v. *Parsons*.[43] In that case the plaintiff suffered severe injuries as a result of undergoing an experimental operation in an effort to cure her deafness. The plaintiff's claim was based, *inter alia*, on the allegation that the doctor had been negligent in failing to warn her of the risk of injury inherent in the operation. The defendant, however, admitted liability and thus the court was denied the opportunity of discussing the doctor's duty in relation to disclosure of information.

As with *Hatcher* and *Bolam*, the case of *O'Malley-Williams* v. *Board of Governors of the National Hospital for Nervous Diseases* in 1974 [44] lends no support to the existence of a doctrine of informed consent in English law. The plaintiff in this case underwent an aortagram, an exploratory procedure involving the insertion of a needle into the patient's arteries. As a result of this procedure, the plaintiff suffered permanent partial paralysis of the right hand, and his resultant claim for damages was based, *inter alia*, on the doctor's alleged failure to inform him of this risk in the procedure. Bridge J. (as he then was) accepted the medical evidence that such injury was a " remote risk " and concluded that failure to warn the patient of

---

[41] [1957] 2 All E.R. 118.

[42] The statement in *Halsbury's Laws of England* (4th ed.), Vol. 30., para. 38, citing *Bolam* and *Hatcher* as authority, should not be read as suggesting that a positive duty to inform the patient of inherent risks exists in English law; the statement merely begs the question by declaring that the doctor " may be liable in damages if he is negligent in failing to inform the patient of the risks involved . . . ."

[43] [1971] 2 Lloyd's Rep. 49 (Q.B.); [1971] 2 Lloyd's Rep. 322 (C.A.).

[44] [1975] 1 B.M.J. 635.

such a risk, where the patient had not himself raised the question with the doctor,[45] did not constitute negligence. This, of course, should not be taken to imply that failure to warn the patient of a risk which is not remote can amount to negligence, an issue on which the court unfortunately chose to remain silent.

Thus it can be seen from the cases discussed above that the courts in this country, while suggesting that there was no positive legal duty incumbent on the doctor to warn his patient of the risks inherent in proposed treatment, at the same time displayed an obvious reluctance to discuss this important issue in anything approaching adequate detail. As the legal correspondent to the British Medical Journal commented, in discussing the *O'Malley-Williams* decision [46]:

> [w]hether there is a positive duty on doctors to keep their patients informed of all aspects of their treatment, even when they pose no queries, is an issue of some importance to the [medical] profession and one that some day will have to be faced head-on.

It was not until the decision of the High Court in *Chatterton* v. *Gerson*[47] in 1980 that the issue was finally " faced head-on," the result being the first enunciation of a positive legal duty corresponding to the doctrine of informed consent.

The plaintiff in *Chatterton* suffered a permanent loss of sensation in her right leg after undergoing two operations, performed by the defendant, to relieve the pain from a post-operative scar in her groin. Her claim for damages for negligence and for trespass was based on the allegation that the defendant had failed to warn her of the inherent risk of loss of sensation. In dismissing the claim in negligence, the court enunciated the following principle [48]:

> In my judgment there is no obligation on the doctor to canvass with the patient anything other than the inherent implications of the particular operation he intends to carry out. He is certainly under no obligation to say that if he operates incompetently he will do damage. The fundamental assumption is that he knows his job and will do it properly. But he ought to warn of what may happen by misfortune however well the operation is done, if there is a real risk of a misfortune inherent in the procedure.

It can be seen from this that the court is imposing a duty on the doctor to disclose to his patient information relating to the risks

---

[45] For discussion of the doctrine of informed consent in relation to questions specifically raised by the patient, see *infra*.

[46] [1975] 1 B.M.J. 635 at p. 636.

[47] *The Times,* February, 7 1980.

[48] Transcript Judgment, at p. 22.

involved in the proposed treatment. However, this duty is restricted
in its scope. Although the first part of the above dictum suggests that
the doctor must disclose all the " inherent implications " of the
operation, it is thought that this will be read in conjunction with what
is said towards the end of the passage, namely, that the duty extends
only to a disclosure of " real " risks.

It is interesting to note the use of the term " real risks." The
adoption of this standard negligence formula in the present context
can be seen to imply that the doctor's duty to disclose the " real
risks " of the operation stems from his overall duty to exercise
reasonable care in the treatment of his patient. The doctor is under
a duty to take reasonable care to avoid exposing his patient to any
foreseeable risk of injury and, as the decided cases indicate,[49]
" forseeable risk " is equated with " real risk." Thus it would follow
that the source of the duty to inform the patient of the " real " risks
inherent in the proposed treatment is simply the overall duty of care
arising from the doctor-patient relationship.

This view, implicit in *Chatterton,* has been expressed by a number
of writers.[50] In one sense this must be correct; if the plaintiff's claim
is based in negligence, it relates to the alleged breach of the doctor's
overall duty of care and it may be seen as artificial to attempt to
itemise individual " duties " so as to distinguish the duty to warn of
inherent risks from the overall duty of care. However, it is submitted
that, although the duty enunciated in *Chatterton* will almost certainly
be seen as stemming from the doctor's overall duty of care, there are
serious dangers implicit in this approach. To regard the obligation
to disclose " real " risks as part of the doctor's overall duty of care
places too much emphasis on the doctor's duty to disclose, and
insufficient emphasis on the patient's right to receive. In other words,
disclosure of the risks inherent in the proposed treatment will be
seen as a product of the doctor's duty of care, rather than as a
product of the patient's right to self-determination. Thus, since the
doctor's duty of care is defined in terms of acting as a reasonable
doctor, there is a danger that in the future, English courts will see
the duty to disclose inherent risks as stemming from the fact that
reasonable doctors disclose such risks (which may be subject to
rebuttal by medical evidence), rather than from the fact that the
patient's right to self-determination demands such disclosure. The
greatest danger in this approach lies in relation to the doctor withholding information in what he considers to be the best interests
of his patient.[51] If, in discussing the doctor's obligation to disclose

---

[49] See *e.g. The Wagon Mound (No. 2)* [1967] 1 A.C. 617 at p. 642.
[50] See *e.g.* Brazier, *supra* note 3, at p. 53.
[51] See *infra,* heading (d).

information, the emphasis is placed on the overall duty of care as its source, rather than on the patient's right to self-determination, there is a danger that the " best interests of the patient " principle will prove to be the exception which erodes the rule.

(c) *The Scope of the Duty to Disclose Risks Inherent in Treatment*

The fundamental question which still has to be discussed in relation to the principle enunciated in *Chatterton* is, of course, how will the courts decide whether or not the particular risk is a " real " one? It is clear that English courts will adopt the test favoured by the majority of States in the United States, namely, that a risk is regarded as a real one if a reasonable doctor in similar circumstances would have disclosed it to his patient. Thus, according to the court in *Chatterton* [52] :

> The duty of the doctor is to explain what he intends to do, and its implications, in the way a careful and responsible doctor in similar circumstances would have done.

Although one writer has expressed the hope that the scope of the duty will not be dictated by evidence of accepted medical practice,[53] *Hatcher, Bolam* and *Chatterton* all suggest that this is likely to be the approach adopted by English courts.

In relation to the extent of the doctor's duty to inform his patient of the risks inherent in proposed treatment, a number of cases have raised the interesting question of whether a distinction should be drawn between the silent patient and the inquiring one. In other words, should the scope of the doctor's duty vary according to whether he is giving the information in response to a question raised by the patient or is merely giving unsolicited advice? An early indication that these two situations might be distinguished came in the case of *Smith v. Auckland Hospital Board,*[54] a decision of the New Zealand Court of Appeal. The court, applying the principle enunciated in *Hedley Byrne & Co. Ltd.* v. *Heller & Partners Ltd.,*[55] held that a doctor must exercise reasonable care in answering a question raised by a patient concerning the risks inherent in proposed treatment, but it declined to discuss whether such a duty arose in the absence of a specific question from the patient. The clearest judicial support for the distinction can be found in the recent Canadian case of *Lepp* v. *Hopp,* in the dissenting judgment of Prowse J.A.[56] :

---

[52] Transcript Judgment, at p. 20.
[53] See Skegg, *supra* note 3, at p. 128.
[54] [1965] N.Z.L.R. 191, reversing [1964] N.Z.L.R. 241.
[55] [1964] A.C. 465.
[56] (1979) 98 D.L.R. (3d) 464 at p. 470.

> In my view, the law draws a distinction between the general
> duty of disclosure imposed upon a surgeon when he is obtaining
> a patient's consent to surgery and the duty of disclosure he is
> under when he responds to specific questions from his patient. . . .
> When specific questions are directed to the surgeon he must
> make a full and fair disclosure in response to them. This duty
> requires a surgeon to disclose risks which are mere possibilities
> if the patient's questions reasonably direct the surgeon's attention
> to risks of that nature and if they are such that the surgeon, in
> all of the circumstances, could reasonably foresee would affect
> the patient's decision.

This dictum highlights the crux of the issue. Following the decision
in *Chatterton*, English law now imposes a duty on the doctor to inform
his patient of the " real " risks inherent in the proposed treatment,
a " real " risk being one which a reasonable doctor would disclose
in similar circumstances. However, what if the patient specifically
asks about a risk which the doctor considers not to be a " real "
one—is the doctor under a duty to give his patient information
concerning that particular risk? There are in fact two aspects to
this issue. First, is the doctor under a duty to say *anything* in
response to such a question, and secondly, if he does decide (or is
obliged) to answer the question, must he do so fully and honestly?

With regard to the first aspect of this issue, the decision in *Smith*
seems to incidate that the doctor is not obliged to answer the
patient's question,[57] a view which is reiterated by a number of
writers.[58] It is submitted that this view is erroneous, it being the
product of misplaced reliance on the principle in *Hedley Byrne*.
Whilst it is true that the House of Lords in *Hedley Byrne* emphasised
that the person whose advice is sought always has the option of
silence, this applies to the situation in which no duty of care exists
before the advice is requested. Thus it is wrong to apply this
principle to the doctor-patient relationship, in which a duty of care
already exists before the question is raised by the patient. It is this
prior existing duty of care which deprives the doctor of the " option
of silence " and which requires him to answer the question with
reasonable care.

Secondly, given that the doctor is obliged to answer the patient's
question concerning specific risks, in so doing must he make a " full
disclosure " of information relating to these risks? The court in
Smith answered this in the negative, suggesting that the doctor is
only obliged to exercise reasonable care in replying to his patient's

---

[57] See [1965] N.Z.L.R. 191, *per* Barrowclough C.J. at p. 198, *per* T. A. Gresson
J. at p. 219.
[58] See Farndale, *Law on Hospital Consent Forms* (1979) at p. 49; *Speller's Law
Relating to Hospitals and Kindred Institutions* (6th ed. 1978) at p. 183.

question, and accepting that this did not necessarily mean that he must give a full, or even an honest, answer.[59] It is thought that English courts would be likely to adopt this approach and to apply the " reasonable doctor " standard enunciated in *Chatterton* to this situation.

Thus it would appear that the law does draw some distinction between the silent patient and the inquiring one. Both are entitled to a reasonable disclosure of the " real " risks inherent in the proposed treatment but, in addition, the inquiring patient is entitled to a reasonable disclosure of information relating to risks about which he has specifically inquired. To hold otherwise would be tantamount to a complete rejection of the patient's right to self-determination. Given that, under the " reasonable doctor " principle enunciated in *Chatterton*, the patient has no say in determining which risks are to be regarded as " real " ones, it is submitted that it is imperative that he should be entitled to a reasonable disclosure of risks about which he specifically inquires. However, it should be stressed that the distinction which the law makes on this issue exists so as to ensure that additional information is given to the inquiring patient and this should in no way prejudice the minimum standard of disclosure to which the silent patient is entitled under the rule in *Chatterton*. It is this minimum standard of disclosure which justifies the distinction which the law makes between those patients who have the self-confidence and articulation to ask questions of their doctor and those patients who do not. The law should seek to ensure that, in relation to disclosure of risks inherent in proposed treatment, the onus lies with the doctor and not with the patient.

(d) *Withholding Information in the Best Interests of the Patient*

As was outlined in Section II, the defence of " therapeutic privilege " has been recognised by courts in the United States as an exception to the doctrine of informed consent. This concept involves the situation where the doctor is of the reasonably held opinion that disclosure of information concerning the risks inherent in the proposed treatment would be likely to cause emotional or psychological distress to his patient. The English cases suggest that possible psychological harm to the patient would be one factor, and probably an important factor, which a reasonable doctor would take into consideration in deciding what information to disclose.[60]

---

[59] [1965] N.Z.L.R. 191, *per* Barrowclough C.J. at p. 198, *per* T. A. Gresson J. at p. 219.

[60] See *e.g. O'Malley-Williams* v. *Board of Governors of the National Hospital for Nervous Diseases* [1975] 1 B.M.J. 635; see also cases involving disclosure of information *after* the performance of an operation, for example, *Waters* v. *Park* [1961] 2 B.M.J. 251; *Daniels* v. *Heskin* [1954] I.R. 73.

However, it is important to examine this in closer detail. There are in fact four reasons why one might argue that information concerning risks should be withheld from the patient if disclosure would be likely to cause psychological distress. First, it could be said that such distress would prevent the patient from making a rational decision and thus would be counter-productive since, as was explained in Section III, the promotion of rational decision-making is seen as one of the functions of the doctrine of informed consent. Secondly, if the patient is being treated for an emotional or psychological complaint, and disclosure of the risks of the treatment would cause such distress and anxiety as to prejudice the chances of the treatment being successful, it may well be that disclosure would be against the best interests of the patient. Thirdly, it could be argued that, if disclosure would be likely to cause serious distress or psychological harm, it would be in the best interests of the patient that the information should not be disclosed. This is accepted by the majority of states in the United States and would undoubtedly find acceptance in English courts, particularly since, as was explained above, the duty to disclose is regarded as merely part of the overall duty of care which the doctor owes his patient.

It is the fourth possible reason for withholding information on the basis of the " best interests of the patient " principle that gives cause for concern. This relates to the situation in which the doctor reasonably believes that the performance of certain medical treatment would be in his patient's best interests. If the doctor suspects that were he to inform his patient of the risks inherent in the treatment the latter would choose not to undergo the treatment, can the doctor use the " best interests of the patient " principle to justify withholding this information? This is a clear example of the concept of paternalism, based on the doctor's opinion of what is best for his patient, over-riding the patient's right to self-determination. There are dicta in the judgments in *O'Malley-Williams* [61] and *Bolam* [62] which indicate support for the withholding of information in this situation, and even the Pearson Commission's Report, in a brief examination of the doctrine of informed consent, states that " A balance has to be maintained between the possible consequences of treatment and

---

[61] Bridge J. observed that disclosing a " remote " risk to a patient might " put him in a position where he feels that he should take the decision, albeit the doctor is obviously much better qualified to weigh up the advantages and the desirability of the proposed operation as against the risks."—[1975] 1 B.M.J. 635 at p. 635.

[62] " [y]ou may well think that when a doctor is dealing with a mentally sick man and has a strong belief that his only hope of cure is submission to electro-convulsive therapy, the doctor cannot be criticised if he does not stress the dangers, which he believes to be minimal, which are involved in that treatment."—[1957] 2 All E.R. 118 at p. 124.

the possible outcome if the treatment is not carried out." [63] The judgment in *Chatterton* is, however, unclear on this issue, the court observing that [64]:

> In what he saws any good doctor has to take into account the personality of the patient, the likelihood of the misfortune, and what in the way of warning is for the particular patient's welfare.

Given that the duty to disclose is regarded as part of the overall duty of care, it seems likely that courts will be willing to accept that a doctor may be justified in withholding information concerning the risks of proposed treatment if he reasonably believes performance of the treatment to be in his patient's best interests and the patient is likely to refuse the treatment if warned of the risks. This is a potentially far-reaching proposition which militates against the basic premise that the decision to undergo medical treatment should ultimately be that of the patient and not that of the doctor. It is hoped that it is a proposition that English courts will accept only in the most exceptional of circumstances.

(e) *Causation*

As was explained in Section II, in a claim for negligence based on the doctor's failure to warn of inherent risks in the proposed treatment, the patient must establish causation, *i.e.* that he would not have consented to the treatment had the risks been disclosed. The English cases suggest that this issue will be determined by asking whether or not the plaintiff himself would have consented to the treatment had he known of the risks,[65] rather than by adopting a purely objective test as in *Canterbury* (See Section II). However, this does not mean that the court is bound by the evidence of the plaintiff that he would not have consented to the treatment had he known of the risks. In testing the plaintiff's credibility, and reliability (since the plaintiff himself may have difficulty in deciding retrospectively whether he would have undergone the treatment despite the risks), the court will have to introduce a certain degree of objectivity. Thus, the extent to which the treatment was truly " elective " and the magnitude and nature of the risk involved are likely to be crucial factors in determining whether or not the patient would have consented to the treatment had he been informed of the risk.

---

[63] *Report of the Royal Commission on Civil Liability and Compensation for Personal Injury* (Cmnd. 7054-I, 1978) Vol. I, para. 1315.

[64] Transcript Judgment, at p. 22.

[65] See *Chatterton* v. *Gerson, The Times,* February 7, 1980, Draft Judgment at p. 23; *Bolam* v. *Friern H.M.C.* [1957] 2 All E.R. 118 at p. 124. See also the analogous case of *McWilliams* v. *Sir William Arrol* [1962] 1 W.L.R. 295.

(f) *Trespass or Negligence?*

As was outlined in Section II, courts in the United States eventually accepted the view that failure to inform the patient of the risks inherent in proposed treatment relates to the tort of negligence and not to the tort of trespass. The position is not so clear in Canada, for example, with courts at present giving conflicting judgments on this issue.[66]

The recent English cases have firmly rejected the view that failure to inform of inherent risks can vitiate consent and give rise to a successful action for battery. For example, the court in *Chatterton*, in dismissing the plaintiff's claim for trespass, observed that [67]:

> [i]t would be very much against the interests of justice if actions which are really based on a failure by the doctor to perform his duty adequately to inform were pleaded in trespass.

A similar policy can be seen in *Wells* v. *Surrey A.H.A.*,[68] a case involving a sterilisation operation performed on the plaintiff. The court held that the doctor had been negligent in failing to give the plaintiff " proper advice " before performing the operation (the question of sterilisation had been first suggested to the plaintiff after she had gone into labour, the operation being performed at the same time as a caesarian section). It is not entirely clear from the report of the case what the court meant by the term " proper advice," but it seems to have involved counselling the plaintiff as to the advisability of being sterilised. The absence of this advice, coupled with the circumstances in which the plaintiff gave her consent, might lead one to conclude that she had not understood the full implications of the operation to which she was consenting. Thus it is somewhat surprising to find that the court concluded that the plaintiff had in fact understood the implications of the operation and had therefore given true consent. It is difficult, in the circumstances of the case, to reconcile this conclusion with the court's finding that the doctor had failed to give his patient proper advice about the implications of the operation. The writer's explanation for this contradiction is that the court was struggling to avoid the conclusion that the doctor was guilty of the tort of battery.

It is submitted that there are two principal reasons for the judicial policy evident in *Chatterton* and *Wells* against trespass claims in informed consent litigation. First, as can be seen from the decisions

---

[66] See generally Picard, " The Tempest of Informed Consent " in *Studies in Canadian Tort Law* (2nd ed. 1977) at p. 129 *et seq.*; *Reibl* v. *Hughes* (1978) 89 D.L.R. (3d) 112 (presently on appeal to the Supreme Court of Canada); *Lepp* v. *Hopp* (1979) 98 D.L.R. (3d) 464.

[67] Transcript Judgment, at pp. 19–20.

[68] *The Times*, July 29, 1978.

in *Fowler* v. *Lanning* [69] and *Letang* v. *Cooper*,[70] judicial policy appears to be in favour of restricting claims in battery to situations involving deliberate, hostile acts, a situation which most judges would regard as foreign to the doctor-patient relationship.[71] Coupled with this is the stigma and damage to professional reputation which courts repeatedly emphasise are an inevitable by-product of a successful claim against a doctor.[72] These consequences are probably seen as even more serious in an action for battery than in an action for negligence. The second reason stems from the view expressed in the concluding section of this article, namely, that courts in this country will attempt to restrict the scope of the doctrine of informed consent, principally by means of the requirement of causation, the use of expert evidence as to accepted medical practice, and emphasis on the " best interests of the patient " principle. Restriction of the doctrine of informed consent in this way would not be possible if it were to be accepted that failure to inform of inherent risks of proposed treatment could ground an action for trespass. As was outlined above, the plaintiff in such an action would not be required to prove, by way of causation, that he would not have consented to the treatment had he been informed of the risks. Similarly, evidence of accepted medical practice has no place in an action for trespass; if failure to disclose a particular risk were to be regarded as vitiating consent, the fact that a reasonable doctor would not have disclosed the risk cannot absolve the defendant from liability for battery. Finally, although the point is not entirely clear,[73] it would seem that a doctor cannot avoid liability for battery simply on the grounds that he was acting in the best interests of his patient. Thus it can be seen that the three principal ways in which the doctrine of informed consent is likely to be restricted would not be available to a court dealing with a case based in trespass.

For these reasons it is thought that English courts will continue to reject the argument that failure on the part of a doctor to inform his patient of the risks inherent in proposed treatment can give rise to an action for trespass to the person.

[69] [1959] 1 Q.B. 426.

[70] [1965] 1 Q.B. 232.

[71] See *e.g.* the sentiments expressed in *Trogun* v. *Fruchtman*, 258 Wis. 2d 569 at p. 599, 207 N.W. 2d 297 at p. 313 (1973) and in *Reibl* v. *Hughes* (1978) 89 D.L.R. (3d) 112 at p. 128.

[72] See *e.g. Whitehouse* v. *Jordan* [1980] 1 All E.R. 650, *per* Lawton L.J. at p. 659; *Fletcher* v. *Bench,* Court of Appeal Transcript No. 1973/313, *per* Megaw L.J. at p. 10; *Hucks* v. *Cole,* Court of Appeal Transcript No. 1968/181, *per* Lord Denning M.R. at p. 6; *Hatcher* v. *Black, The Times,* July 2, 1954.

[73] See Skegg, *supra* note 30. See also *Devi* v. *West Midlands R.H.A.* [1980] 7 *Current Law* 44; *Odam* v. *Young* [1955] 2 B.M.J. 1453.

V THE FUTURE OF THE DOCTRINE OF INFORMED CONSENT IN ENGLISH LAW

This concluding section examines briefly the way in which the doctrine of informed consent is likely to develop in this country in the foreseeable future. It is submitted that the courts will attempt to restrict the scope of the doctrine so as to minimise the extent of the doctor's duty to inform his patient of the risks inherent in proposed treatment. This view is based on the following factors:

(1) As was explained in Section III, the doctrine of informed consent is directly related to judicial policy regarding expansion of the liability of the medical profession. Significant development of the doctrine can only take place in a climate of judicial policy favouring such expansion. As can be seen from many cases on medical negligence in this country—most recently the decision of the House of Lords in *Whitehouse* v. *Jordan* [74]—current judicial policy is clearly against expanding the liability of the medical profession. Until such time as there is a significant change in this judicial policy, the constrained and restricted way in which the doctrine of informed consent has been construed by English courts to date is likely to continue.

(2) The fear that acceptance and development of the doctrine of informed consent might lead to the practice of " defensive medicine," *i.e.* the doctor placing his own interests in not being sued before those of his patient, is likely to find favour amongst many judges.[75] Linked to this is the judicial fear of treading the American pathway to a national " crisis " in relation to medical malpractice litigation, a fear expressed most recently by Lord Denning in *Whitehouse*.[76] Space does not permit a full examination in the present Article of the reasons underlying the fear of a national malpractice " crisis," suffice it to say, in the writer's view, this fear is misplaced.[77] However, given that informed consent is a doctrine of American origin, seen by many, particularly doctors in the United States, as one of the primary causes of the medical malpractice " crisis," it would be surprising if the doctrine were to develop significantly in this country now that the

[74] *The Times*, December 18, 1980, affirming [1980] 1 All E.R. 650.

[75] See *e.g. Smith* v. *Auckland Hospital Board* [1964] N.Z.L.R. 241, *per* Woodhouse J. at p. 251.

[76] [1980] 1 All E.R. 650 at p. 658. See also Denning, *supra* note 38, at p. 244; *Lim* v. *Camden and Islington A.H.A.* [1979] 1 Q.B. 196 at p. 217.

[77] See *e.g. Report of the Royal Commission on Civil Liability and Compensation for Personal Injury* (Cmnd. 7054-I, 1978), Vol. I, paras. 1318–1324.

prospect of an American-style " crisis " has been canvassed by the courts.

(3) The fact that the doctor's duty to disclose the " real " risks inherent in proposed treatment is seen as merely one part of his overall duty of care (thereby shifting emphasis away from the patient's right to self-determination) will restrict development of the doctrine, probably by means of the overriding " best interests of the patient " principle.

(4) Expert evidence as to accepted medical practice is likely to exert considerable influence over the scope of the doctrine, at the same time restricting any expansion of the doctrine in favour of the plaintiff.

(5) A strict application of the requirement of causation is likely to create serious difficulties of proof for plaintiffs in informed consent litigation.

For these reasons it is submitted that the doctrine of informed consent is unlikely to develop in this country and that consequently it will prove to be of limited scope in affording compensation to victims of medical accidents. It is to be regretted that the law should seek to restrict the doctrine of informed consent in this way, since this belies the importance to be attached to the patient's fundamental right to decide whether to undergo proposed medical treatment. The importance of this fundamental right dictates that the doctrine of informed consent ought to be accepted and developed by the courts in this country so as to ensure that patients are given the information which they require to exercise their right to decide whether to undergo proposed medical treatment. For this to happen, much less emphasis would have to be placed on concepts such as " accepted medical practice " and " best interests of the patient " as reasons for excusing non-disclosure. However, regardless of the importance of the patient's right in relation to the decision to undergo medical treatment, one cannot avoid the fact that the doctrine of informed consent, expanding as it does the liability of the medical profession, is the servant of judicial policy regarding such expansion. It is this judicial policy, rather than the importance of the patient's right to determine his own medical treatment, that will dictate the future development of the doctrine of informed consent in this country.

GERALD ROBERTSON *

---

* Lecturer in Law, University of Leicester.

[3]

HISTORICAL EVOLUTION AND MODERN IMPLICATIONS OF CONCEPTS OF CONSENT TO, AND REFUSAL OF, MEDICAL TREATMENT IN THE LAW OF TRESPASS

Danuta Mendelson, Ph.D., LL.M.*

> Many mischiefs arise on the change of a maxim and rule of the Common Law, which those who altered it could not see when they made the change.[1]

INTRODUCTION

It has been suggested that the whole of the private law may be regarded as the law of consent.[2] The law of torts is based on the principle that subject to the law of the land, no one has the right to interfere with another person's physical and economic integrity and freedom without that person's consent.

This article examines the historical and jurisprudential evolution of the concept of consent in the law of trespass to person with an emphasis on issues associated with consent to, and refusal of, medical treatment. Consent to treatment and refusal of treatment have been regarded merely as obverse

---

* Senior Lecturer in Law, Deakin University, School of Law, Burwood, Australia. Address correspondence to Dr. Mendelson at Deakin University, School of Law, 221 Burwood Highway, Burwood, Australia 3125. The author wishes to thank Dr. George Mendelson, Associate Professor at the Faculty of Medicine, Monash University, Melbourne, Australia and Mr. Ian Freckelton, Barrister of the Supreme Court of Victoria and New South Wales, Senior Lecturer at Faculty of Law, Monash University, for their comments and helpful suggestions in the preparation of this article.

[1] E. Coke, 6 Rep. 41. Throughout this article the phrase "common law" is used in its jurisprudential sense to denote the single national customary law, which in the late medieval period displaced the local and the baronial law in England, and to distinguish this system of law from the civil law of continental Europe, and the Scots law.

[2] P. YOUNG, THE LAW OF CONSENT 3 (1986).

1

sides of the same coin.[3] One of the premises of this article is that the law is inconsistent insofar as it considers consent to be a relative value while regarding refusal as an absolute and inalienable right.

For the purposes of this article, the phrase "life-saving treatment" is used to denote medical treatment (antibiotics to treat pneumonia, blood transfusions, certain organ transplants, cardiopulmonary resuscitation, and the like) administered to cure or stabilize a life-threatening but treatable and potentially reversible medical condition, usually in an emergency situation. The phrase also applies to medical treatment undertaken for the purpose of enhancing the quality of life for those patients who suffer from an incurable condition but who are conscious and not hopelessly ill, for instance, patients suffering from chronic renal failure, chronic hepatitis, or chronic lymphatic leukemia. The phrase "life-sustaining treatment" refers to such medical devices as a mechanical ventilator, a catheter, or a feeding tube, which are utilized to keep alive patients who are hopelessly ill because their vital functions are seriously impaired, but who are not terminally ill as, for example, persons in a coma or in a vegetative state.[4]

Medical and legal ramifications of utilizing the legal criterion of "sound mind" as it applies to the issue of consent to, and refusal of, life-saving treatment also will be broached. It is asserted that when assessing the decisional capacity of a patient to refuse life-saving treatment, the traditional notions of "sound mind" should be modified to include modern medical understanding of affective competency.[5] This needs to be done to protect the vulnerable patients whose cognitive capacity may be intact, but whose decisional competency is impaired by illness or systemic disease.

As the title suggests, this article discusses concepts of consent to, and refusal of, medical treatment in the context of the tort of trespass. The tort of negligence is focused on the defendant. Under the law of negligence, one must guard against creating risks that may result in an injury to another when there exists a legal duty of care toward that other person. If a particular risk cannot be eliminated or minimized, then the risk ought to be disclosed to those who may be harmed by it. In cases of negligence relating to the physician-patient relationship, the central question is whether or not the

---

[3] F. ROZOVSKY, CONSENT TO TREATMENT: A PRACTICAL GUIDE 438 (2d ed. 1990).

[4] Mendelson, *Medico-Legal Aspects of the "Right to Die" Legislation in Australia,* 19 MELBOURNE U.L. REV. 112 (1993); A. MEISEL, THE RIGHT TO DIE 94-95 (1989); Jennett, *Treatment of Critical Illness in the Elderly,* 24 HASTINGS CENTER REP. 21 (Sept./Oct. 1994).

[5] "Affect" refers to the immediate emotional experience. Subjective affective sensations such as pleasure, displeasure, irritation, as reported by a patient, are equivalent to symptoms; the observed mood and affective display (anger, joy, sadness, hurt) serve as objective signs. "Mood" refers to a more sustained and less flexible mental state over a longer period of time. In depression or schizophrenia, the affective sensations are often shallow, inadequate, or flattened. Ketai, *Affect, Mood, Emotion and Feeling: Semantic Considerations,* 132 AM. J. PSYCHIATRY 1215 (1975).

defendant medical practitioner has complied with the duty to exercise reasonable care and skill in the provision of diagnosis, advice, and treatment to the patient. The breach of duty may involve a failure to disclose a reasonably foreseeable material risk. However, the patient can only sue in negligence for nondisclosure of the particular risk if the risk actually eventuates, causing an injury.

The issue of consent in negligence is thus relevant insofar as it helps to establish the standard of care expected of a medical practitioner in relation to provision of advice and information. Did the medical practitioner provide enough information to enable the patient to choose between undergoing or not undergoing the risky treatment in question?[6] In the case of *Canterbury v. Spence,*[7] the United States Court of Appeal for the District of Columbia said that the "patient's right to self-decision shapes the boundaries of the duty to reveal."[8] Consequently, the interest in bodily integrity commands "protection, not only against an intentional invasion by an unauthorized operation but also against a negligent invasion by his physician's dereliction of duty to adequately disclose."[9] To paraphrase, the right to decide what should be done to one's body is protected by the torts of trespass and negligence, but in different ways. The tort of trespass protects one's right to decide whether or not to consent to an interference. The tort of negligence protects one's right to be informed about the factors that will be material to that decision.

The law of trespass to person—as further explained below—focuses on the patient's right to be free of any unwanted bodily contacts and the right to decide whether or not such contacts should occur. Therefore, the ultimate issue of the physician's liability in trespass to person has to be determined by reference to the presence or absence of valid consent. In the case of *Reibl v. Hughes,*[10] Chief Justice Laskin of the Canadian Supreme Court noted that he could

> appreciate the temptation to say that the genuineness of consent to medical treatment depends on proper disclosure of the risks which it entails, but . . . unless there has been misrepresentation or fraud to secure consent to the treatment, a failure to disclose the attendant risks, however serious, should go to negligence rather than to battery. Although such a failure relates to an informed choice of submitting to or refusing recommended and appropriate treatment, it arises as the breach of an anterior duty of due care, comparable in legal obligation to the duty

---

[6] The patient's "choice is, in reality, meaningless unless it is made on the basis of relevant information and advice." Rogers v. Whitaker, 175 C.L.R. 479, 490 (1992).

[7] Canterbury v. Spence, 464 F. 2d 772 (D.C. Cir. 1972).

[8] *Id.* at 786.

[9] *Id.* at 793.

[10] Reibl v. Hughes, 114 D.L.R.3d 1 (1980).

4   MENDELSON

of due care in carrying out the particular treatment to which the patient has consented. It is not a test of the validity of the consent.[11]

Likewise, the majority on the High Court of Australia, in the case of
Rogers v. Whitaker,[12] rejected the American doctrine of informed consent in
the context of the law of negligence.[13] The High Court described the phrase
"informed consent" as "somewhat amorphous," and "apt to mislead as it
suggests a test of the validity of a patient's consent."[14] Furthermore, the
High Court commented that the expression "the patient's right to self-
determination" is "perhaps, suitable to cases where the issue is whether a
person has agreed to the general surgical procedure or treatment, but is of
little assistance in the balancing process that is involved in the determination
of whether there has been a breach of the duty of disclosure."[15]

Legal authorities in the United States, Australia, Canada, England, and
New Zealand are drawn upon throughout this article. The decisions cited
may carry merely a persuasive weight in different jurisdictions. However, it
is not the goal of this article to set out authoritatively the law of consent and
refusal in any given jurisdiction, but rather to explore and understand these
concepts with reference to the case law.

I. MODERN LEGAL UNDERSTANDING OF TRESPASS TO PERSON AND THE ROLE OF CONSENT

Consent as a legal concept developed originally within the context of
the law of trespass. Trespass is a generic term that encompasses all kinds of
wrongful direct and intentional interferences with person, land, and chattels
(goods). Trespass to person comprises three separate torts—battery, assault,
and the tort of false (wrongful) imprisonment.[16] This article concentrates on
the concept of consent in relation to the tort of battery.

The modern tort of battery has been defined as an intentional wrong
"which is committed by intentionally bringing about a harmful or offensive
contact with the person of another."[17] This will happen when the direct
offensive contact with the body of another had been desired (purposive) or
known to be substantially certain to result.[18] The tort is based on the prin-

---

[11] *Id.* at 10-11.

[12] *Rogers,* 175 C.L.R. at 490.

[13] In rejecting the American doctrine of informed consent in negligence, the High Court of Australia
followed the majority of the House of Lords in the case of Sidaway v. Governors of Bethlem Royal
Hosp., [1985] A.C. 871.

[14] *Rogers,* 175 C.L.R. at 490.

[15] *Id.*

[16] Although "assault" is a separate tort with its own set of elements, it is often, incorrectly, used as an
appellation for the tort of battery.

[17] J. FLEMING, THE LAW OF TORTS 24 (8th ed. 1992).

[18] *Id.* at 17, 25.

MEDICAL TREATMENT AND THE LAW OF TRESPASS   5

ciple that other persons do not have the right to interfere with the person of another unless he or she validly consents to such an interference.[19] The law considers the tort of trespass to person as safeguarding not only the personal interest in one's physical integrity, but also as protecting the individual against any interference that is offensive to a reasonable sense of dignity and personal autonomy.

The notion of autonomy (from Greek "autos" (self) and "nomos" (rule)) expounds that every individual has the legal right to personal self-determination. In bioethics, the terms "autonomy" and "respect for autonomy" are associated with several ideas, such as privacy, voluntariness, choosing freely, and accepting responsibility for one's choices.[20] In law, the modern doctrine of autonomy is expressed through the rule that each competent individual has the right to noninterference with his or her choices, imposing upon others an obligation not to constrain unnecessarily the autonomous decisions and actions of a competent person.[21]

Generally, in a medical context, the conduct of the treating physician will be intentional, and will have an effect of causing contact with the adult patient's body. The trespassory contact may lose its wrongful character if the physician can provide evidence of valid consent, statutory authorization,[22] or lawful justification,[23] but if there is no evidence on the issue, any medical intervention, no matter how benevolent in motivation, may constitute battery.[24] With respect to medical treatment, Justice McHugh of the High Court of Australia articulated the nature of the modern tort of trespass in the following way:

> It is the central thesis of the common law doctrine of trespass to the person that the voluntary choices and decisions of an adult person of sound mind concerning what is or is not done to his or her body must be respected and accepted, irrespective of what others, including doctors, may think is in the best interests of that particular person.[25]

The courts regard the role of consent in trespass as generally having the effect of transforming what would otherwise be unlawful contact into ac-

---

[19] This principle is also applicable to the torts of assault and false imprisonment.

[20] Beauchamp, *The Four-Principles' Approach,* in PRINCIPLES OF HEALTH CARE ETHICS 6 (R. Gillon ed. 1994).

[21] K. MITCHELL & T. LOVAT, BIOETHICS FOR MEDICAL AND HEALTH PROFESSIONALS 25 (1991).

[22] Mental Health Act (Vic.) of 1986 §§ 12, 13, 73, & 85.

[23] A plea of necessity may provide lawful justification.

[24] "The incision made by the surgeon's scalpel need not be and probably is most unlikely to be hostile, but unless a defence of justification is established it must in my judgement fall within a definition of a trespass to person." T. v. T., [1988] 2 W.L.R. 189, 203 (Wood, J.).

[25] Secretary, Dep't of Health & Community Servs. (NT) v. JWB and SMB (*Marion's Case*), 175 C.L.R. 218, 309 (1992). The case involved the issue of whether parents or the family court should have the power to consent to a sterilization of their profoundly intellectually impaired daughter.

6   MENDELSON

cepted, and acceptable, conduct. Therefore, consensual contact does not, ordinarily, amount to battery.[26] For the purposes of medical practice, the legal function of consent is to "provide those concerned in the treatment with a defence to a criminal charge of assault or battery or a civil claim for damages for trespass to the person."[27]

The patient's right to make decisions about medical treatment has been identified with the legal right to self-determination. For instance, in the case of *In re Conroy*,[28] the New Jersey Supreme Court stated: "On balance, the right to self-determination ordinarily outweighs any countervailing state interests, and competent persons generally are permitted to refuse medical treatment, even at the risk of death."[29]

The right to refuse a life-saving treatment is commonly referred to as the "right to die." Justice Robins of the Ontario Court of Appeal gave the following jurisprudential explanation for the "right to die":

> The right of self-determination which underlies the doctrine of informed consent also obviously encompasses the right to refuse medical treatment. A competent adult is generally entitled to reject a specific treatment or all treatment, or to select an alternate form of treatment, even if the decision may entail risks as serious as death and may appear mistaken in the eyes of the medical profession or of the community. Regardless of the doctor's opinion, it is the patient who has the final say on whether to undergo the treatment.[30]

In the United Kingdom, Lord Goff of Chieveley in the case of *Airedale NHS Trust v. Bland*,[31] defined the patient's right to refuse medical treatment including life-saving treatment in a similar fashion:

> [T]he principle of self-determination requires that respect must be given to the wishes of the patient, so that if an adult patient of sound mind refuses, however unreasonably, to consent to treatment or care by which his life would or might be prolonged, the doctors responsible for his care must give effect to his wishes, even though they do not consider it to be in his best interests to do so.

Hence, the legal status accorded to refusal of medical treatment, including life-saving treatment is formulated in terms of decision-making process, whereby refusal is seen as negatively equipollent with a consent to treatment. But are these two concepts, particularly consent to, and refusal of, life-saving treatment, truly equipollent?

---

[26] *Id.* at 233.

[27] *In re* W (A Minor, Medical Treatment: Court's Jurisdiction), [1992] 3 W.L.R. 758, 765.

[28] 486 A.2d 1209 (N.J. 1985).

[29] *Id.* at 1225.

[30] Malette v. Shulman, 67 D.L.R.4th 321, 328 (1990).

[31] [1993] A.C. 789, 864.

II. HISTORICAL OVERVIEW OF THE CONCEPT OF CONSENT IN THE COMMON LAW OF TORTS

To evaluate whether concepts of consent to, and refusal of, life-saving treatment are equivalent, it is important to understand the origins and the evolution of the law of consent. The common law of trespass developed to provide an alternative remedy to the deeply ingrained custom of blood feud through the law of vengeance—family feud known as "faida"—at the time when customary law was incapable of creating legal institutions that could enforce or maintain civil order within the community. The customary law of vengeance was based upon a highly sensitized understanding of family honor and loyalty combined with the basic instinct to retaliate. It generally was invoked for murder, adultery, violation, or rape of a married woman, violation of the dead, aggravated robbery, and, importantly, any insult to the honor of the family. The law of vengeance was open to all ranks among the Germanic and the Frankish people of the early Middle Ages and neither the Royal authority nor the Church were able to suppress it.[32]

When, in 1252, the Chancery commenced to issue writs[33] of trespass, their primary purpose was to replace the customary laws of faida with the public machinery of legal process manifested by criminal prosecution.[34] The objective behind the original writ of trespass "vi et armis et contra pacem Domini Regis" (with force and arms and contrary to the King's peace) was the punishment of offenders against the royal peace.[35] Procedurally, the allegation in the pleadings that an offense against the royal peace had been committed, was necessary to bring the culprit before the royal courts, and away from the customary and baronial courts. Because forcible trespass involved a breach of the royal peace and so was in itself wrongful, personal damage was not a necessary element of liability.

Under the Salic, Anglo-Saxon, and Anglo-Norman laws, there was a

---

[32] Duels of honor—private combat in the form of consensual revenge for the perceived injury to the participants' honor and reputation—probably were the best known vestiges of "faida."

[33] A "writ" was an order issued by the court in the sovereign's name under the Great Seal, addressed to the sheriff of the county in which the cause of action arose, or where the defendant resided, commanding the sheriff to cause the party complained of to appear in the King's Court on a certain day to answer the complaint. Every writ was founded on a principle of law that gave the plaintiff the legal right to seek a specified remedy.

[34] R. POSNER, LAW AND LITERATURE: A MISUNDERSTOOD RELATION 27 (1988).

[35] There was also an older form of private action—Appeal of Mayhem—an accusation of maiming, that was akin to action in Trespass for recovery of damages. The Appeal of Mayhem was different from the Appeal of Felony whereby a party—a widow or an heir—who had an interest in the person killed prosecuted an accusation of murder either by writ or bill. G. JACOB, NEW LAW DICTIONARY (1756).

8 MENDELSON

procedure in cases involving serious offenses, whereby the guilty party could pay a compensation, "wergeld," (the monetary equivalent of a human life) to the victim of his or her kin in an attempt to preclude the risk of private war. Although the new machinery of justice under the Angevins tended to impose punishments without compensation, in cases of homicide, rape, and wounding, the old custom of wergeld-type compensation survived but was adapted to the new judicial system of royal courts.[36] Until 1694, a defendant found liable in a civil action for trespass, besides being mulcted in damages in favor of the injured plaintiff, also had to pay a fine to the Crown. Thus, even after the civil tort of trespass evolved, it did so without losing its criminal law characteristic of being primarily an offense against the royal or public peace.[37]

Initially, forcible trespass was interpreted literally—with force of arms against the Royal peace. It soon, however, came to be interpreted as meaning any direct and intentional invasion of the plaintiff's rights that may lead to instant retaliation or vengeance, and hence to the breach of the peace.[38] Because consent negates the threat of revenge, the plea of consent generally would have the effect of transforming the otherwise unlawful conduct into legally acceptable conduct. The plea of consent is different from the defense based on the maxim that is today known as "volenti non fit injuria" (no wrong is done to the one who consents),[39] loosely derived from Roman law.[40] The maxim was expressed by Bracton (c 1200-1268) in the *De Exceptionibus* section of his *De Legibus at Consuetudinibus Angliæ*[41] as "cum volenti at scienti non fiat iniuria" (with consent and knowledge no injury is done). Though the word "scienti" was later eliminated, knowledge of the risk of injury being consented to has remained an element of the "volenti" defense, which is based upon the principle that a person should have the right to waive his or her legal rights. Sir Donaldson MR (as he then was), in *Freeman v. Home Office*,[42] pointed out that the maxim of "volenti non fit injuria" provides a bar to enforcing a cause of action; it does not negative the cause of action itself.[43]

Originally, however, the requirement of consent did not indicate the law's concern for the individual's right to self-determination, or even the

[36] Wigmore, *Responsibility for Tortious Acts: Its History*, 7 HARV. L. REV. 315 (1894).
[37] J. FLEMING, *supra* note 17, at 17.
[38] The principle that by being able to obtain compensation under the law of torts, the plaintiff was thereby induced to forgo the right to take revenge was—unsuccessfully—invoked as a basis for liability in Stanley v. Powell, [1891] 1 Q.B. 86.
[39] The spelling of the Latin word "iniuria" as "injuria" is the accepted common-law form of medieval Latin.
[40] Ingman, *A History of the Defence of* Volenti non Fit Injuria, 26 JURIDICAL REV. 1 (1981).
[41] H. BRACTON, DE LEGIBUS AT CONSUETUDINIBUS ANGLIÆ probably was written between 1240 and 1256. *Id.* at 2.
[42] [1984] Q.B. 524 (CA).
[43] *Id.* at 557.

personal right to physical integrity. Rather, the presence of voluntary consent indicated that the plaintiff was willing to forego the right to revenge. Hence, the question of consent was merely a factor in the enforcement of the peace of the realm.

The law looked at consent as an evidentiary factor relating to the issue of non-liability—the denial (in pleading terminology, a traverse) of one of the elements of the cause of action in trespass.[44] For instance, the Nottingham Eyres[45] rolls for 1329 record the pleadings, known as *The Surgeon's Case,* of a patient-plaintiff who complained that the defendant surgeon having undertaken "to cure his eye with herbs and other medicines," instead "put out his eye, so that he lost it, to his damages." According to the Launde, as the plaintiff

> put himself under his [defendant's] medicines and cure, no trespass can be found in him at that time, since he himself submitted to his cure, hence, if he had any action at all it would naturally sound in covenant broken, so we ask judgment whether such bill should be received.[46]

The defendant pleaded that the patient-plaintiff was unable to use the writ of trespass for battery because he had consented to the cure, thus depriving the surgeon's conduct of its trepassory character.[47]

In 1704, Chief Justice Holt, in the case of *Cole v. Turner,*[48] summed up the medieval perception of the cause of action in trespass to person when he said that "the least touching of another in anger is a battery." The concept of consent formed a part of a strictly communitarian system of values and ethics. Therefore, the right to consent to an interference with one's body, though protected by the law through the writ of trespass, was never regarded as an absolute value in itself.

In the *Leviathan or the Matter, Forme and Power of a Commonwealth Ecclesiastical and Civil,*[49] first published in 1651, Thomas Hobbes wrote that no man can be understood to consent to be wounded, chained, or imprisoned. The right of consent was always qualified by the policy considerations of upholding the public order, and was articulated in the rule that

---

[44] H. Luntz & A. Hambly, Torts: Cases and Commentary 681 (1992).

[45] In medieval times, England was divided into areas known as circuits. Nottingham was one such circuit, and it would be visited four times a year by the court to decide all cases that had arisen since the last sitting of the court. Each session of sitting was referred to as an assize.

[46] The Surgeon's Case Nottingham Eyre [AD 1329] Lincoln's Inn, Hale MS 137 (1), f58; Br. Mus. Egerton MS. 2811, f. 218; A. Kirafly, A Source Book of English Law 184 (1957).

[47] The writ of covenant—to secure enforcement of an agreement—was inapplicable because the loss of the eye did not result from a breach of agreement through its nonperformance; it probably was due to the careless or incompetent performance of the agreed procedure.

[48] 6 Mod. 149 (1704).

[49] T. Hobbes, Leviathan ch. XIV (1904).

where "a man license another to beat him, such licence is void as it is against the peace."[50] In the United States, the Superior Court of New Jersey reiterated this rule in the case of *State v. Brown*,[51] when it refused to regard as valid the consent of a wife to being beaten by her husband with his hands "and other objects" if she got drunk. The court reasoned that to allow such a defense would "threaten the dignity, peace, health and security of our country."[52]

From early medieval times, the plea of consent did not suffice to exculpate the defendant from the charge of murder following a premeditated and intentional killing in the course of a fight.[53] Similarly, the law of maims and the crime of malingering are historical examples of the law setting its face against validating the individual's right to consent to what should be done to his or her body in these instances. The reason for the refusal to hold valid consent to self-mutilation or mutilation of the consenting person by another was to ensure that sufficient numbers of able young men were ready to be pressed into service with the Royal army and navy. The primary aim of the law of maims was to prevent the practice of beggary. Coke, in his *Institutes of the Laws of England*,[54] quotes a case where a young and healthy youth asked his friend to maim him, so that he could beg more effectively. Both the young man and his friend were found guilty of mayhem.

The personal right of refusal to an outside interference with one's bodily integrity was protected by law only if the refusal entailed prevention of, or a refusal to participate in, wrongs that were seen as threats to the communitarian principle of preserving public peace. While the institution of serfdom persisted, a serf had no legal right to refuse physical interference with his or her body, for only free men had the right to seek a remedy in the royal courts. Even amongst the free subjects, the two long-lasting exceptions to the tort of battery, namely, the right of the parent or teacher to chastise children and pupils,[55] and the husband's right to beat his wife, have been conspicuous examples of the law's disregard for the individual's right to refuse harmful and demeaning contact.

As civil society developed, jurisprudential emphasis shifted away from the tort of trespass as the primary vehicle for safeguarding the royal peace. The somewhat restricted concept of personal freedom, as developed in classical Greece, was revived in the 17th century to indicate that a person-

---

[50] Matthew v. Ollerton, [1692] Comb. 218, 90 Eng. Rep. 438.

[51] 364 A.2d 27 (N.J. Super. 1976). The husband was charged with the offense of "atrocious assault and battery."

[52] *Brown*, 364 A.2d at 31-32.

[53] Legal duels such as judicial combat, or ordeal by battle, introduced by the Normans constituted exception to the rule that a consensual premeditated killing should constitute murder. Horder, *The Duel and the English Law of Homicide*, 12 OXFORD J. LEGAL STUDIES 419 (1992).

[54] 1 E. COKE, INSTITUTES OF THE LAWS OF ENGLAND 127a & b (1628).

[55] Mansell v. Griffin, [1908] 1 K.B. 947.

MEDICAL TREATMENT AND THE LAW OF TRESPASS   11

ally free individual is a person who is "owner of his own body" in contrast
to the slave who, although a human creature, does not possess such self-
ownership. This articulation of personal freedom is evident in a number of
Periclean funeral orations.[56] In the 17th century, John Locke adopted the
possessory notion of personal self-ownership, as against enslavement of the
self,[57] when he developed the theory of property.[58] Political theories of
personal liberty and proprietary freedom propounded by John Locke and
Thomas Hobbes, in the wake of the English Civil War, and based upon the
notion of self-ownership, became, in the course of the 18th century, a
"deep-seated popular feeling in favour of liberty" at the expense of the
power of the state.[59] The most manifest common law reflection of these
popular feelings was the identification of personal privacy with proprietary
interests and the affirmation of the principle that "by the laws of England,
every invasion of private property, be it ever so minute, is a trespass. No
man can set his foot upon my ground without my licence, but he is liable to
an action, though the damage be nothing."[60]

In the second part of the 18th century, Sir William Blackstone extended the scope of the tort of trespass to person to all nonconsensual
contacts by eliminating the requirement of voilence. Blackstone wrote that
"the law cannot draw the line between different degrees of violence, and
therefore totally prohibits the first and lowest stage of it: every man's person
being sacred, and no other having a right to meddle with it, in any the
slightest manner."[61] For Blackstone, the rationale of the prohibition of all
nonconsensual contacts lay in the sacredness or inviolability of the human
person. He argued that there exists an absolute right to personal security,
vested in each person: "[The] right of personal security consists in a person's legal and uninterrupted enjoyment of his life, his limbs, his body, his
health, and his reputation."[62] As an inviolate legal right, the principle of
sacredness of human person was operative both in public and private
spheres.

---

[56] THUCYDIDES, THE PELOPONNESIAN WAR bk. 2, ch. 4. (R. Warner trans. 1964). For further discussion, see O. PATTERSON, FREEDOM IN THE MAKING OF WESTERN CULTURE 100-01 (1991).

[57] Referring to the Roman concept of personal freedom the "libertas," Cicero called it the "sweetest
of all possessions."

[58] J. LOCKE, THE SECOND TREATISE OF GOVERNMENT § 5.27 (P. Laslett ed. 1970). It was Sir Edward
Coke who stated, admittedly in a somewhat different context, that "the house of everyone is to him
as his castle and fortress as well for his defence against injury and violence as for his repose."
Semayne's Case, 5 Co. Rep. 91a (1604), [1558-1774] All E.R. 62, 63.

[59] 10 W. HOLDSWORTH, A HISTORY OF ENGLISH LAW 658 (1938).

[60] Entick v. Carrington, 2 Wils. K.B. 275, 291, 95 Eng. Rep. 807, 817 (1765) (Lord Camden, C.J.). This
decision was reaffirmed in Australia in Plenty v. Dillon, 171 C.L.R. 635, 639 (1991) (Mason, C.J.,
Brennan & Toohey, J.J.), and in Canada in Colet v. The Queen, 119 D.L.R.3d 521, 526 (1981).

[61] 3 W. BLACKSTONE, COMMENTARIES ON THE LAWS OF ENGLAND 120 (facsimile of the 1st ed. of
1765-1769, 1979).

[62] "Life is the immediate gift of God, a right inherent by nature in every individual." *Id.* vol. 1, at 125,
129-30 & vol. 3, at 119-20.

12   MENDELSON

A. The Emergence of the Concept of Consent Within the Physician-Patient Relationship

The Hippocratic tradition regarded the practice of medicine as art consisting of three components—the disease, the patient, and the physician. The Hippocratic physician was encouraged to aspire to personal virtues of holiness and purity, and to follow professional ethics of compassion, knowledge, and dedication to the patient's welfare, as well as the obligation to transmit medical knowledge. These principles were expressed in the *Hippocratic Oath,*[63] and such other writings of the *Corpus Hippocraticum*[64] as *On the Physician, Precepts, Aphorisms,* and *On Decorum,*[65] which together created the system of medical deontology, based largely on the philosophy of the Pythagorean sect.[66] The Pythagoreans ranked medicine together with music and mantic as supreme sciences, and believed that their pursuit was the best way to express "love for what is truly noble."[67] Deontological principles imposed upon a physician a duty and "the obligatory doing of things because they are, quite simply, the right things to do" in caring for each individual patient.[68]

The deontological system of medicine as presented in *Corpus Hippocraticum,* and in particular the *Hippocratic Oath,*[69] was permeated with Pythagorean philosophy and consequently was not a representative of the classical Greek philosophy as a whole. In fact, the injunction "I will neither give a deadly drug to anybody if asked for it, nor will I make a suggestion to this effect,"[70] was unique to the small Pythagorean sect whose adherents were opposed to suicide believing that there was an inherent value in human life. Because God allocated to humans their position in life as a post to be held and defended, it was a sin to disobey the divine command to live.[71] Ludwig Edelstein, one of the greatest scholars of ancient Greek and Roman medical literature, pointed out that in the eyes of a Hippocratic physician,

---

[63] "In purity and in holiness I will guard my life and my art." L. EDELSTEIN, ANCIENT MEDICINE 6 (1987).

[64] *Corpus Hippocraticum* consists of about 60 treatises, the collection of aphorisms, the Oath, and the Canon. Some of the treatises and aphorisms were written by Hippocrates (460 BCE). However, the *Corpus* as a whole is the work of a large number of medical writers of ancient Greece that was compiled between 430 and 300 BCE, with even later interpolations. HIPPOCRATIC WRITINGS (J. Chadwick & W. Mann trans. 1983).

[65] *On the Physician, Precepts,* and *On Decorum* were written in Hellenistic times.

[66] L. EDELSTEIN, *supra* note 63, at 328-29.

[67] *Id.* at 59.

[68] S. NULAND, DOCTORS: THE BIOGRAPHY OF MEDICINE 24 (1989).

[69] Edelstein, *The Hippocratic Oath,* in LEGACIES IN ETHICS AND MEDICINE 12 (C. Burns ed. 1977).

[70] L. EDELSTEIN, *supra* note 63, at 6.

[71] *Id.* at 17. The Pythagorean approach toward sanctity of life was akin to that of Judaism, which regards the human body not as property of an individual person, but that of the Creator. Individuals are merely custodians or trustees of their bodies, the ownership of which rests with the Creator. In Judaism, every person is charged with a positive duty to preserve health and life.

unless the physician abstained from suggesting or assisting in a patient's suicide, the physician, no less than the patient, was guilty of moral and religious transgression.[72] The Pythagorean view of suicide was opposed to that of Platonists, Cynics, and Stoics, all of whom held suicide permissible for the diseased. Although Aristotelians believed that it was cowardly to succumb to bodily pain, and the Epicureans insisted that people should not be subdued by illness, they condoned suicide in other circumstances.[73] In Roman times, Seneca expressed the Stoic view of suicide in the following terms: "When either nature demands my breath again, or reason bids me dismiss it, I will quit this life, calling all to witness that no one's freedom, my own least of all, has been impaired through me."[74]

One may ask why, in view of its minority status,[75] the Hippocratic school with its life-oriented philosophy, prevailed over the more populous medical schools or sects that were better attuned to the accepted mores of the times.[76] One explanation may be that when it came to the "crunch," patients preferred to seek help from physicians who adhered to a strict code of ethical principles, which prohibited medically assisted suicide. Nevertheless, general tolerance of suicide in Greek and Roman society meant that Hippocratic physicians would have encountered patients who either asked for assistance with suicide, or who, wishing to die, refused to comply with the prescribed therapy. Hippocratic physicians were advised not to undertake treatment of persons in the terminal stages of their disease, nor could they impose therapy upon those who did not want their services. But there also would have been patients who, having sought medical help, refused or were unable to comply with the prescribed therapeutic regime. The Hippocratic physicians stressed the importance of nursing in the healing process. They made frequent visits to their patients, and tended to leave one of their pupils behind to watch over and help with medical care for the sick.[77] They also provided a room in their own homes for treating patients who lived too far away for adequate super-

---

[72] *Id.*

[73] In classical times (5th-3rd century B.C.E.), the Greek City-State of Ceos mandated that people over the age of 60 end their life by drinking hemlock. In the Hellenistic period (3rd-1st century B.C.E.), the political authorities in Thebes and Massalia (modern Marseilles) supplied a free dosage of hemlock on application. Young, *Cross-Cultural Historical Case Against Planned Self-Willed Death and Assisted Suicide*, 39 McGill L. J. 657, 686, 689 (1994).

[74] A. Rogers, A Student's History of Philosophy 148 (1915), *quoted in* D. Klein, A History of Scientific Psychology 116 (1970).

[75] Several medical sects flourished during the Graeco-Roman period, amongst them were the Oulidai at Elea, the Methodists, the Asclepiadeans of Bithynia, the "Sicilian School," and others. Nutton, *Healers in the Medical Market Place: Towards a Social History of Graeco-Roman Medicine*, in Medicine in Society: Historical Essays 15 (A. Wear ed. 1994).

[76] In Roman times, Stoicism often was seen as a spiritual alternative to the national religion. Philosophers were attached to many Roman families in the role of tutors and moral counselors. Thus, a philosopher, along with the physician, would often be present at a deathbed.

[77] *On the Physician* (CMG I: 10, 21; 14,1), *quoted in* L. Edelstein, *supra* note 63, at 99.

vision.[78] The provision of nursing care was not only beneficial to those patients who cooperated with the physician in wishing to get well, but was also helpful in overcoming or mitigating passive refusal or noncompliance with treatment.

It does not appear that seeking an express consent to treatment from the patient constituted an integral part of the Hippocratic tradition, which was based on a covenantal relationship between physician and patient, rather than on the modern principle of consensual partnership. Central to a covenantal relationship is the ethical principle of trust with its corresponding duties and obligations. The Hippocratic physician-patient relationship presupposed that "if the physician [was] going to help, his relationship to his patient must be that of the person in command to the one who obeys."[79] Probably the most famous of the *Hippocratic Aphorisms* affirms that "Life is short, art is long; opportunity is fleeting, experiment is dangerous; judgment is difficult. It is not enough for the physician to do what is necessary, the cooperation of the patient and the attendants must be secured, and circumstances must be favourable."[80]

The relationship in which a patient was expected to cooperate and to put "himself and 'his all' into the hands of the physician" involved a recognition that the patient's trust reposed in the physician encompassed not only the latter's knowledge and skills, but also the person. The principle of the patient's trust imposed upon the physician obligations that included the code of personal ethics prescribed in the *Hippocratic Oath,* and other writings of the *Corpus Hippocraticum.* These writings present the model of a physician as a composite of a person adhering to the ideals of the Pythagorean philosophy[81] with the Aristotelian qualities of a "gentleman" (kindness, self-control, regularity of habits, justness and fairness, a proper and good behavior),[82] as well as the Stoic virtues of wisdom[83] and charity toward all people—free citizens, slaves, and barbarians, including those who are impecunious.[84]

The Hippocratic ideas persisted in an unbroken line following the decline of Roman civilization through the early Middle Ages. Even though

---

[78] Nutton, *supra* note 75, at 49.

[79] L. EDELSTEIN, *supra* note 63, at 98.

[80] 1 THE APHORISMS OF HIPPOCRATES i (Author's rendition) (trans. into Latin and English in T. COAR, THE CLASSICS OF MEDICINE LIBRARY (1982)). *See also* HIPPOCRATIC WRITINGS, *supra* note 64, at 206.

[81] *Hippocratic Oath* reflects the beliefs of the Pythagoreans in the spiritual kinship between the medical teacher and pupil.

[82] L. EDELSTEIN, *supra* note 63, at 329.

[83] Galen (130-201 CE), in an essay entitled *That the Best Physician Is Also a Philosopher,* insisted that a true physician must be an adherent of Platonism, which by then was fused with Aristotelianism and Stoicism. L. EDELSTEIN, *supra* note 63, at 335.

[84] 1 HIPPOCRATES: PRECEPTS 319 (W. Jones trans. 1923).

the Christian Church authorities did not approve of pagan writings, some segments of the *Hippocratic Corpus* were known, and treatises on the ethics and etiquette of medicine written by monks in North European monasteries rendered into a "Christianized" version the pivotal deontological aspects of the *Corpus Hippocraticum*.[85] The essential model of the covenantal physician-patient relationship based on a patient's obedience and trust also was adopted by Moslem and Arabic-speaking Jewish physicians who became the intellectual heirs, custodians, and translators of the works of Hippocrates, Aristotle, and Galen into Hebrew and Arabic.[86] The classical tradition in Europe was revitalized when the scholars of the University of Salerno, which was created as "civitas Hippocratice" at the end of the 9th century, began to translate into medieval Latin, the Hebrew and Arabic manuscripts containing the works of Greek, Roman, and Jewish medical writers.[87] The medieval Latin translations, however, focused upon the practical aspects of medicine, rather than on general theoretical principles.[88]

The absence of any discussion of the issue of consent in the early Middle Ages reflected the feudal law's preoccupation with landed property, the intricacies of the vassalage system, and fiscal privileges. It was only with the advent of the Renaissance and loosening of feudal controls of obligation and privilege that there emerged a philosophical shift toward examination of the rules governing the relationships between individuals—as distinguished from collective rights and duties of the representative "estates," social classes, and industrial guilds. The orientation of the law toward an individual was accelerated by the rediscovery in 1100 in Italy of the *Corpus iuris civilis* of the Emperor Justinian, which was originally compiled between 533 and 556 CE. The opening sentences of the *Institutiones* (*Institutes*) of Justinian: "Iustitia est constans et perpetua voluntas ius suum cuique tribuens" (Justice is the constant and perpetual purpose of giving to each his due), and "Iuris prudentia est divinarum atque humanarum rerum notitia, iusti atque iniusti scientia" (Jurisprudence is the knowledge of things divine and human, the science of just and the unjust)[89] became the foundation of the modern jurisprudence.[90]

---

[85] Kibre, *Hippocratic Writings in the Middle Ages*, 18 BULL. HISTORY MED. 371 (1945); MacKinney, *Medical Ethics and Etiquette in the Early Middle Ages: The Persistence of Hippocratic Ideals*, in LEGACIES, *supra* note 69, at 173.

[86] The Hippocratic Canon was translated into Hebrew by Nathan Hameati of Rome in 1279. Etziony, *The Hebrew-Aramaic Element in Vesalius'* Tabulae Anatomicae Sex, 18 BULL. HISTORY MED. 413 (1945).

[87] Kristeller, *The School of Salerno*, 17 BULL. HISTORY MED. 138 (1945).

[88] *Id.*

[89] Justinian, 1 INSTITUTES 1, § 51 (J. Thomas text & trans. 1985).

[90] The word "ius" has a number of meanings, however, in the context of jurisprudence it was understood as referring to the right of each person. The science, which consisted of knowing the

16   MENDELSON

The principles of the medieval Roman or "civil" law based on the *Corpus Iuris* were taught in all European universities from Salerno and Bologna, to Paris, Oxford, and Cambridge.[91] Late medieval philosophers, many of whom studied Roman law at university, were the first to analyze, though from different perspectives, the internal experiences of man as an individual.[92] These 13th and 14th century thinkers, amongst them Giovanni Bonaventura, Roger Bacon, John Duns Scotus, Johannes Eckhart, and William of Ockham, paved the way for the revival of classical Greek and Roman learning,[93] and a critical re-evaluation of medieval scientific, moral, philosophical, and social dogma in light of the earlier conventions. In a way, the Renaissance rediscovered an individual as a physical being—an object to be studied by anatomists, described by philosophers, and portrayed by artists.

For centuries, midwives, herbalists, gymnastic trainers, "purifiers," and purveyors of charms, incantations, and drugs—as well as physicians— claimed the ability to heal the sick. At the same time, it is known that at least since the beginning of the 15th century, English physicians desired to have standards of entry into their profession regulated. In 1421, the physicians placed before parliament a petition requesting that "no man, of no manner, estate, degree, or condition, practice in Physic, from this time forward, but he have long time used the Schools of Physic within some University, and be graduated in the same."[94] Under the statutes and the common law of medieval England, anyone could practice medicine or surgery with the consent of the patient. However, when the patient died while under the care of a person who was not licensed by the Church, guild, or university to practice medicine or surgery, such a death was held to be a felony.[95]

In the England of the 16th century, medicine was taught as a post-graduate course in the Arts faculties of Oxford and Cambridge and consisted mainly of exposition of classical authorities such as Aristotle and Galen with little scientific instruction or clinical training. When the (Royal) College of Physicians of London was created in 1518 under the Chancellorship of

---

"ius"—the right of each person—was called "ars iuris": the art of law, or the art of what is just. J. HERVADA, NATURAL RIGHT AND NATURAL LAW: A CRITICAL INTRODUCTION 20 (1990).

[91] It was not until mid-19th century that the common law was taught at Oxford and Cambridge.

[92] F. ALEXANDER & S. SELESNICK, THE HISTORY OF PSYCHIATRY 76 (1967).

[93] Galen and Hippocrates were first published in the original Greek in 1525 and 1526 respectively. Etziony, *supra* note 86, at 414.

[94] J. RAACH, A DIRECTORY OF ENGLISH COUNTRY PHYSICIANS 1603-1643, at 8 (1962), *quoted in* Guy, *Episcopal Licensing of Physicians, Surgeons, and Midwives*, 56 BULL. HISTORY MED. 528, 532 (1982).

[95] "If one which is no physician or surgeon . . . will take a cure upon him, and his patient dieth under his hand, this hath been holden to be a felonie." C. MERRET, A COLLECTION OF ACTS OF PARLIA-MENT, CHARTERS, TRIALS AND LAW, AND JUDGES OPINIONS 66 (1660). *See also* IV E. COKE, INSTITUTES OF THE LAWS OF ENGLAND 251 (1648).

Cardinal Wolsey,[96] in the preamble to the College's charter, Henry VIII expressed a desire that the Royal Physicians should promote medical learning through encouragement of the new Italian medical humanism.[97] The primary purpose of the College of Physicians was to control the practice of medicine. At first, however, the influence of the College of Physicians was confined to the metropolitan area extending seven miles from the City of London.[98]

In 1523, the jurisdiction of The Royal College of Physicians extended to the whole of England, and the College was granted judicial powers to regulate educational qualifications and standards of medical practice amongst its members.[99] Yet, for a long time, the powers of the College, particularly outside of London, were more apparent than real. This was because although the Royal College was granted power to adjudicate on the candidate's educational competence to practice medicine, the bishops had retained power to grant the license to practice medicine within their dioceses.[100] Nevertheless, in the course of the following two centuries, ethical codes aiming to lift the standards of medical practice were revised and adapted to the spirit of the nascent Enlightenment with its "quest for immutable laws of nature, of man, and in philosophy."[101] Guided by reason rather than religion and received dogma, the Enlightenment placed at the center of its concerns the nature of individual rights and liberties within civil society.[102]

Physicians, whether members of the College or not, began to critically review contemporary medical practice.[103] In 1556, John Securis published a book entitled *A Detection and Querimonie of the Daily Enormities and Abuses Committed in Physick,* which was aimed at reforming the morality and practice of medicine.[104] In the 17th century, Thomas Sydenham, an

---

[96] Henry VIII granted his letters patent under the Great Seal incorporating the President and College or Commonalty of the faculty of Medicine of London on 23 September 1518. 1 G. CLARK, A HISTORY OF THE ROYAL COLLEGE OF PHYSICIANS OF LONDON 58 (1964).

[97] *Id.* at 56-60.

[98] The College could not compel provincial candidates to come to London for examination. Moreover, throughout the provinces of Canterbury and York, the license that confirmed the physicians' right to practice came from the local diocesan bishop. Guy, *supra* note 94, at 533.

[99] Within its jurisdiction, the officers of the College had the power to imprison and keep at their pleasure those who practiced medicine badly or without a license granted by the College. 14 & 15 Hen. 8, c. 5; 32 Hen. 8, c. 40; 1 Mariæ, St. 2, c. 9. In this respect, the College had the characteristics of a prerogative tribunal.

[100] Guy, *supra* note 94, at 533.

[101] Polani, *The Development of the Concepts and Practice of Patient Consent,* in CONSENT IN MEDICINE CONVERGENCE AND DIVERGENCE IN TRADITION 57, 69 (G. Dunstan & M. Seller eds. 1983).

[102] R. VAN CAENEGEM, AN HISTORICAL INTRODUCTION TO PRIVATE LAW 127 (1988).

[103] MacKinney, *supra* note 85.

[104] Larkey, *The Hippocratic Oath in Elizabethan England,* 4 BULL. HISTORY MED. 201 (1936).

18   MENDELSON

adherent of the new empirical scientific method, known as the "English Hippocrates," stressed that the aim of medicine was to treat the patient, not disease.[105] Subsequently, in 1711, a London physician, Dr. Bernard Mandeville, wrote *A Treatise of the Hypochondriack and Hysterick Passions, Vulgarly Called the Hypo in Men and Vapours in Women,* which was intended for the education of patients as well as physicians.[106]

In his influential *Lectures on the Duties and Qualifications of a Physician,* published in 1772, John Gregory[107] argued that it was the ethical and professional conduct of physicians that enabled the fusion of the two divergent conceptions of the profession of medicine to be sustained, namely the concept of medicine as "an art the most beneficial and important to mankind, or as a trade by which a considerable body of men gain their subsistence."[108] Gregory stressed that the scientific learning and professional skill of every physician must be tempered by "the obligation to humanity, patience, attention, discretion, secrecy, and honour, which he lies under to his patients."[109] Moreover, "it is a physician's duty to do everything in his power that is not morally criminal to save the life of his patient,"[110] though "[e]ven in cases where his skill as a physician can be of no further avail, his presence and assistance as a man and as a friend may be grateful and useful, both to the patient and his nearest relations."[111]

Gregory noted that within the covenantal physician-patient relationship "the government of a physician over his patient should undoubtedly be great, but an absolute government very few patients will submit to."[112] He defined the rights of patients in a covenantal relationship in the following way:

> Every man has the right to speak where his life or his health is concerned, and every man may suggest what he thinks tends to save the life of his friend. It becomes them to interpose with politeness, and deference to the judgment of the physician; it becomes him to hear what they have to say with attention, and to examine it with candour.[113]

The physician must respect his patients' opinions and therapeutic prefer-

---

[105] W. SMITH, THE HIPPOCRATIC TRADITION (1979).

[106] Clark, *Bernard Mandeville, M.D., and Eighteenth Century Ethics,* in LEGACIES, *supra* note 69, at 270.

[107] J. GREGORY, LECTURES ON THE DUTIES AND QUALIFICATIONS OF A PHYSICIAN (printed for W. Strachan & T. Cadell 1772, reprinted in 1992).

[108] *Id.* at 10.

[109] *Id.* at 12.

[110] *Id.* at 39.

[111] *Id.* at 35.

[112] *Id.* at 22-23.

[113] *Id.* at 35.

ences, provided that these preferences are consistent with the patient's safety:

> Sometimes a patient himself, sometimes one of his friends, will propose to the physician a remedy, which, they believe, may do him service. Their proposal may be a good one; it may even suggest to the ablest physician, what, perhaps, till then, might not have occurred to him. It is undoubtedly, therefore, his duty to adopt it.[114]

Consent to medical treatment, as we understand this concept today, was not specifically articulated in the medical treatises, professional codes, and regulations of early modern England.[115] Nevertheless, the notion of patient consent to treatment not only as a legal requirement but also as an ethical construct must have been appreciated, because its legal and ethical significance within the physician-patient relationship was discussed in the 1767 English case of *Slater v. Baker & Stapleton*.[116] This case appears to be a first instance in which the court affirmed the principle that nonconsensual contact in the context of medical treatment ought to be regarded as a legal wrong.[117]

The plaintiff, Slater, sued a surgeon and an apothecary in special action on the case[118] for "ignorantly and unskilfully"—over his protests— refracturing "the callous" (bony material present during healing) of his leg after it was set and placing it in an "extension" instrument thereby causing him an injury. The medical expert witnesses called by the plaintiff testified that it was contrary to the standard practice to refracture a leg unless the bone was setting very badly. They also testified that the use of the extension instrument of the kind employed by the defendants to stretch and straighten the limb during healing was not approved of by the profession. A surgeon expert witness swore "that if the plaintiff was capable of bearing his foot on the ground, he would have disunited the callous if it had been desired by him, but in no case whatsoever without the consent of the patient."[119] The jury awarded the plaintiff £500.

On appeal, the defendants argued that because there was no evidence of ignorance or want of skill (the defendant Baker was apparently the first surgeon in St. Bartholomew's Hospital in London for 20 years), the essence

---

[114] *Id.* at 33.

[115] Larkey, *supra* note 104.

[116] 2 Wils. K.B. 359, 95 E.R. 850 (1767).

[117] For a discussion of this case, see R. FADEN & T. BEAUCHAMP, A HISTORY AND THEORY OF INFORMED CONSENT 116-17 (1986).

[118] In all early cases where the pre-existing relationship precluded an allegation that force of arms had been used, the plaintiffs would use the writ of trespass *sur le cas* (special action on the case) with a count of "ita negligenter" (an adverb designated to indicate the alleged wrongful conduct).

[119] Slater v. Baker & Stapleton, 2 Wils. K.B. 359, 360, 95 E.R. 860, 861 (1767).

of the complaint lay in the fact that the leg "was broke without the plaintiff's consent." Therefore, the appropriate writ was that of trespass "vi at armis" (battery). This was a technical argument designed to defeat the plaintiff's action on the issue of suitability of the writ: if the writ did not fit the facts of the case, it could be quashed, and, in accordance with the maxim "no writ, no remedy," the plaintiff would be left without legal relief. However, the court of the King's Bench rejected the arguments of the defendants. Referring to the evidence about the good character of Baker, the full court noted that "many men skilful in their profession have frequently acted out of the common way for the sake of trying experiments. It seems as if Mr. Baker wanted to try an experiment with this new instrument."[120] As such, his action was rash "and he who acts rashly acts ignorantly."[121] The full court refused to nonsuit the plaintiff on the basis that the proper writ would have been trespass "vi at armis":

> In answer to this, it appears from the evidence of the surgeons that it was improper to disunite the callous without consent; this is the usage and law of surgeons: then it was ignorance and unskilfulness in that very particular, to do contrary to the rule of the profession, what no surgeon ought to have done; and indeed it is reasonable that a patient should be told what is about to be done to him, that he may take courage and put himself in such a situation as to enable him to undergo the operation.[122]

It is interesting to note the 18th century court's disapproval of medical experimentation on human subjects without their consent. The court considered the surgeons' failure to explain the experimental nature of the procedure, and their disregard of the patient's refusal to undergo the operation as an "improper" breach of professional conduct, presumably in violation of the code of the Barber-Surgeon's Company of London.

Rather than elaborating upon strictly legal principles relating to consent, the court explained why it is bad professional practice to keep patients ignorant of the nature of proposed therapy, and to treat them without consent. Two and a quarter centuries after the judgment in *Slater v. Baker & Stapleton,* Lord Donaldson of Lymington MR,[123] provided a very similar description of the clinical purpose of consent to medical treatment. He said that consent of the patient is essential in clinical practice because it encourages the cooperation of the patient and ensures the patient's faith—or at least

---

[120] *Id*. at 862.

[121] "[A]lthough the defendants in general may be as skilful in their respective professions as any two gentlemen in England, yet the Court cannot help saying, that in this particular case they have acted ignorantly and unskilfully, contrary to the known rule and usage of surgeons." *Id*. at 863.

[122] *Id*. at 862.

[123] *In re* W, [1992] 3 W.L.R. 758.

confidence—in the efficacy of the treatment, and thus contributes to the treatment's success.[124]

Because of the nature of the writ under which the plaintiff pursued his cause of action in *Slater,* the question of whether the treating practitioners' failure to explain the nature of the intervention and the disregard of the patient's refusal to undergo the treatment should sound in damages in trespass remained unanswered. The plaintiff's action was essentially to recover damages for the bodily damage he had suffered as a result of the defendants' refracturing the leg and then placing it in an experimental apparatus. The injury to his dignitary interests, as manifest through the surgeons' disregard of his refusal, was treated not as an ultimate issue, but as an evidentiary factor in the determination of the defendants' liability for malpractice.

In Thomas Percival's seminal book on medical ethics,[125] which was originally published in 1803,[126] Percival does not refer specifically to the case of *Slater v. Baker & Stapleton.* Nevertheless, he may have had in mind practices similar to those that gave rise to the lawsuit when he wrote that experimental treatments in medicine and surgery should not be undertaken without proper consultation between all concerned, and only in accordance with sound reasons. Although it has been claimed that research and experimentation are a normal part of clinical practice, in the sense that "every clinical decision ought to involve an experiment,"[127] there is a fundamental distinction between an ordinary therapeutic physician-patient relationship, and a relationship that exists between physician-investigators and patient-subjects. Within the therapeutic physician-patient relationship, the focus of the physician's attention and care is the patient and his or her best interests. When this relationship is altered to accommodate experimental treatment, the physician-investigator has to consider factors that are extraneous to the patient's best interests.[128]

Percival does not discuss the specific issue of consent to, or refusal of, a proposed treatment by a patient. However, he urges respect for the patient's wishes even in circumstances where the treating physician may disagree with them:

> The *feelings* and *emotions* of the patients, under critical circumstances, require to be known and to be attended to, no less than the symptoms of their diseases. Thus,

---

[124] *Id.* at 765.

[125] T. PERCIVAL, MEDICAL ETHICS: OR A CODE OF INSTITUTES AND PRECEPTS, ADAPTED TO THE PROFESSIONAL CONDUCT OF PHYSICIANS AND SURGEONS (1985).

[126] Percival's *Medical Ethics* became the foundation of the American Medical Association's first *Code of Medical Ethics.* AMERICAN MEDICAL ASSOCIATION, CODE OF MEDICAL ETHICS, PROCEEDINGS OF THE NATIONAL MEDICAL CONVENTION (1846-1847).

[127] Wing, *Ethics and Psychiatric Research,* in S. BLOCH & P. CHODOFF, PSYCHIATRIC ETHICS 416 (2d ed. 1991).

[128] This article shall not discuss issues of consent that arise within such a relationship.

extreme *timidity*, with respect to venæsection, contraindicates its use, in certain cases and constitutions. Even the *prejudices* of the sick are not to be contemned [sic], or opposed with harshness.[129]

Likewise, Percival makes the following observations:

The use of *quack medicines* should be discouraged by the faculty, as disgraceful to the profession, injurious to health, and often destructive even of life. Patients, however, under lingering disorders, are sometimes obstinately bent on having recourse to such as they see advertised, or hear recommended, with a boldness and confidence, which no intelligent physician dares to adopt with respect to the means that he prescribes. In these cases, some indulgence seems to be required to a credulity that is insurmountable: And the patient should neither incur the displeasure of the physician, nor be entirely deserted by him. He may be apprised of the fallacy of his expectations, whilst assured, at the same time, that diligent attention should be paid to the process of the experiment he is so unadvisedly making of himself, and the consequent mischiefs, in any, obviated as timely as possible.[130]

Percival adds that "certain active preparations, the nature, composition, and effects of which are well known, ought not to be proscribed as quack medicines."[131] The writing of Gregory and Percival illustrate the core virtues that characterize a humane and benevolent physician of the Enlightenment: scientific approach to evaluation and application of medicinal drugs combined with compassionate care based on nonjudgmental understanding of vulnerabilities, wishes, and needs of those who suffer from illness and disease.

Insofar as Percival was opposed to providing the patient with theoretical reasons for the treatment and the nature of remedies to be prescribed,[132] modern bioethicists would describe his attitude as "paternalistic," based on an assumption that the physician knows better than anyone, including the patient, what is best for the patient. John Gregory, in his *Lecture II,* discussed certain psychological, sociopolitical, and religious considerations why it was wise for the 18th century physician to avoid disclosure to the patient of the properties of medicines and remedies to be employed in the course of therapy.[133] Gregory noted that there were cases "where it may be proper to acquaint a patient with the nature of the remedies, as there are sometimes peculiarities in a constitution, in regard both to the quality and quantity of the medicine, which a physician ought to be informed of before he prescribes it."[134] The decision to forego explanations probably was an

---

[129] T. PERCIVAL, *supra* note 125, at 10-11 (emphasis in original).

[130] *Id.* at 44-45 (emphasis in original).

[131] *Id.*

[132] *Id.* at 169.

[133] J. GREGORY, *supra* note 107, at 60-63.

[134] *Id.* at 63.

expression of professional honesty, for it was often more honest for an 18th century physician—whose practice was guided as much by intuition and clinical experience as by scientific knowledge—to say little or nothing about the benefits and risks involved in a particular course of therapy or medication, than to provide a spurious pseudo-scientific explanation. These considerations, however, did not relieve medical practitioners from an ethical obligation to inform patients that a proposed treatment was novel or experimental.

The term "consent," applying to interpersonal relationships, is absent from the texts of Gregory and Percival. In fact, it was only toward the end of the 18th century that Henry Ballow defined this word in his *Treatise of Equity,* which was published posthumously, in 1793, with annotations by John Fonblanque.[135] The authors were influenced by the theories of Hugo Grotius, who published *De Iure Belli ac Pacis* (on the Law of War and Peace) in 1625, and by Samuel Pufendorf, who built upon the earlier work of Grotius, in authoring two treatises *De Iure Naturae et Gentium Libri VIII* (1672) and *De Officio Hominis et Civis Iuxta Legem Naturalem Libri II* (1673).[136] Grotius and Pufendorf sought to establish a body of certain basic and universal principles that would be binding on all people, irrespective of the time and the place in which they lived.[137] They argued that these principles, like, for example, the obligation to carry out one's promises, had the same certainty and generality as a proposition in mathematics.[138] The body of the basic or axiomatic principles was called natural law, in the sense that they were arrived at by means of rational study and critical observation of human nature and relationships. Concrete rules, which applied to specific areas of law, could be deduced from general concepts and axioms. According to Grotius, the axiomatic principles of natural law were drawn from "the principles of nature, or common consent."[139] In English, this theory of the "law of reason" (*Vernunftrecht*) is referred to as the School of Natural Law. Its legal methodology and ideology were closely linked with the political and philosophical ideas of the Enlightenment.

It is of significance, however, that the legal analysis of the nature of consent as an aspect of interpersonal relationships should have been under-

---

[135] 1 H. BALLOW, A TREATISE OF EQUITY WITH THE ADDITION OF MARGINAL REFERENCES AND NOTES BY JOHN FONBLANQUE (1793, reprinted 1979).

[136] The popularity of Grotius and Pufendorf in England may be gauged by the fact that six editions of the former's *De Iure Belli* were published there before 1750. Between 1682 and 1758, at least nine editions of the Latin version of Pufendorf's *De Officio Hominis et Civis Iuxta Legem Naturalem* had appeared. There were also seven editions of the English translation, and one of the Barbeyrac's French version. P. STEIN, LEGAL EVOLUTION: THE STORY OF AN IDEA 3 (1980).

[137] *Id.*

[138] R. VAN CAENEGEM, *supra* note 102, at 118-19.

[139] The principles of nature were the basis of the law of nature; principles of common consent were the basis of the law of nations. H. GROTIUS, DE IURE BELLI AC PACIS prolegomena § 40 (1623), *quoted in* P. STEIN, *supra* note 136, at 4.

taken first in the context of the developing law of contract refracted through equity jurisprudence. In the late 18th century, the gist of the law of contract was perceived as involving the terms of an agreement made by consenting minds of the contracting parties who were presumed to be equal. The focus of the law of contract was the damage occasioned by the breach of a contractual term. Equity's role was to concentrate upon the persons who are parties to the contract in order to ensure that "no one may be gainer by another's loss,"[140] in the sense that in a relationship in which a transfer of proprietary interests is effected, the stronger party should not be allowed to take advantage of the weaker one. Originally, the law emphasized the consensus of mind by the contracting parties as an indication of true consent. This approach was known as the "subjective theory" of contract. Today the preferred doctrine is the "objective theory," whereby the law is less concerned with the true intentions of the parties and more with outward manifestations of those intentions.[141] Eventually, the nature of consent within the physician-patient relationship would come to be examined in the light of this modern theory.

In the *Treatise of Equity,* Ballow and Fonblanque discussed the nature of consent in the context of the law of agreements pertaining to transfer of property. However, their analysis had wider implications. Grotius, in *De Jure Belli ac Pacis,*[142] defined consent as "an act of reason accompanied with deliberation."[143] Ballow enlarged upon Grotius' definition by suggesting that deliberation indicated "the mind weighing, as in balance, the good and evil on either side."[144] Fonblanque in the annotations, relying on Pufendorf's *De Iure Naturae et Gentium Libri,* explained the constituent elements of consent in the following way: "Every true consent supposes, 1st, a physical power: 2dly, a moral power of consenting; 3dly, a serious and free use of them."[145]

In the United Kingdom, Australia, and Canada, the law considers consent to medical treatment as "real" or "valid" for the purposes of battery if it is given by a competent person who has made the decision voluntarily upon being informed in broad terms of the nature of the procedure that is to be performed.[146] This approach differs from the position adopted by the United States Court of Appeals for the District of Columbia

---

[140] 1 H. BALLOW, *supra* note 135, ch. 1, § 1.

[141] P. YOUNG, *supra* note 2, at 148-49.

[142] H. GROTIUS, *supra* note 139, lib. 2, ch. 11, § 5.

[143] 1 H. BALLOW, *supra* note 135, ch. 2, § 1.

[144] *Id.*

[145] *Id.* § 1, n.(*a*).

[146] Chatterton v. Gerson, [1981] 1 Q.B. 432, 443; Sidaway v. Governors of Bethlem Royal Hospital, [1985] A.C. 871 (Lord Scarman, dissenting); *Marion's Case,* 175 C.L.R. 218 (1992); Malette v. Shulman, 67 D.L.R.4th 321 (1990).

in *Canterbury v. Spence,*[147] which explained that to be valid, the consent has to be "informed": "True consent to what happens to one's self is the *informed exercise* of a choice, and that entails an opportunity to *evaluate knowledgeably* the options available and the risks attendant upon each."[148]

This modern description of the nature of consent may have its source in a first century letter by Pliny the Younger to Catilius Severus. In the letter, Pliny describes the suicide of Titius Aristo who, suffering from protracted illness, called Pliny together with a few intimate friends and told them "to ask the doctors what the outcome of his illness would be, so that if it was to be fatal he could deliberately put an end to his life, though he would carry on with the struggle if it was only to be long and painful . . . ."[149] Pliny commended Titius Aristo for this course of action, and commented that "[m]any people have his impulse and urge to forestall death, but the ability to examine critically the arguments for dying, and to accept or reject the idea of living or not, is a mark of a truly great mind."[150] The original Latin text places more emphasis on the reasoning process, and speaks in terms of "deliberating and weighing one's causes for such decision," and the "counsel of reason."[151]

However, it seems that a more immediate source for the legal notion of informed consent lay in the judicial understanding of the three essential elements of consent to contractual relations originally specified by Ballow, who said that consent must be "an act of reason" involving "deliberation" with the "the mind weighing as in balance the good and evil on either side."[152] Indeed in *Canterbury v. Spence,* the court noted that "one of the difficulties with analysis in terms of 'informed consent' is its tendency to imply that what is decisive is the degree of the patient's *comprehension.*"[153] Both Ballow's definition and the decision in *Canterbury* emphasize the consenting person's cognitive capacity. In today's parlance, consent to medical treatment has to be "an act of reason" in the sense that the consenting person must be shown to have realized that he or she is being asked to make a decision about medical treatment, has understood the information relevant to making this decision, and appreciates how this information would apply to his or her current situation.[154]

---

[147] Canterbury v. Spence, 464 F.2d 772 (D.C. Cir.), *cert. denied,* 409 U.S. 1064 (1972).

[148] *Id.* at 780 (emphasis added).

[149] 1, 22 THE LETTERS OF THE YOUNGER PLINY 56 (B. Radice trans. 1967).

[150] *Id.*

[151] "Nam impetu quodam et instinctu procurrere ad mortem commune cum multis, deliberare vero et causas eius expendere, utque suaserit ratio, vitae mortisque consilium vel suscipere vel ponere ingentis est animi." *See also* Gourevitch, *Suicide Among the Sick in Classical Antiquity,* 43 BULL. HISTORY MED. 501, 514 (1969).

[152] For a discussion of historical definitions of consent, see P. YOUNG, *supra* note 2, at 12-14.

[153] *Canterbury,* 464 F.2d at 780 n.15 (emphasis added).

[154] Culver & Gert, *The Inadequacy of Incompetence,* 68 MILBANK Q. 619, 621 (1990).

B. The Influence of the Philosophical Writings of John Stuart Mill

The Blackstonian principle of the sacredness of the human body helped to extend the focus of the tort of battery from the inviolability of public peace, in which an individual was seen as a component of wider societal structure, to encompass the principle of the right to personal inviolability. However, Blackstone still looked at an individual and the right to personal integrity from the perspective of the communitarian interest of social harmony in the public sphere. Although the principle of personal inviolability or sacredness emphasized the right to be free from physical interference, it did not, automatically, entail the right to personal autonomy. It was philosophers like John Locke, Charles Montesquieu, and John Stuart Mill who helped to invert the viewpoint by introducing the notion of personal liberty based upon delimitation of the power of the state as an expression of communitarian interests in relation to the individual.[155]

In his influential essay *On Liberty*,[156] Mill argued that individuals should be amenable to society and its laws only when their conduct is based on choices that impinge on or concern others. "The only purpose for which power can be rightfully exercised over any member of a civilised community, against his will, is to prevent harm to others. His own good, either physical or moral, is not a sufficient warrant."[157] Mill argued that society has full jurisdiction when an adult person's conduct is "other-regarding," that is, when the person's decisions affect prejudicially the interests of others. When the individual's conduct is "self-regarding" in the sense that it affects the interests of no person besides himself or herself—the individual's freedom to make the choice ought to be absolute because "over himself, over his own body and mind, the individual is sovereign."[158] When the person's conduct has an effect upon the interests of other adults of "ordinary understanding," he or she must seek their "free, voluntary and undeceived consent."[159] In all such cases, according to Mill, "there should be perfect freedom, legal and social, to do the action and stand the consequences."[160]

John Stuart Mill's doctrine that each individual "is the proper guardian of his own health, whether bodily, or mental or spiritual,"[161] has to be read in the context of his discussion of legitimacy of the power of the state. Mill explained that the only legitimate power of the state was that derived from the needs of individuals. The individuals, as he and other philosophers and essayists of that era saw them, seem to have been endowed with the char-

---

[155] M. COWLING, MILL AND LIBERALISM 41 (2d ed. 1990).
[156] J. MILL, ON LIBERTY (1859).
[157] *Id.* at 9.
[158] *Id.*
[159] *Id.* at 11.
[160] *Id.* at 12.
[161] *Id.* at 9.

acteristics of an English gentlemen—they were financially independent,[162] rational, and mature. Mill emphasized that his doctrine of individual liberty was "meant to apply only to human beings in the maturity of their faculties,"[163] as distinct from those

> who are still in a state to require being taken care of by others, [and who] must be protected against their own actions as well as against external injury. For the same reason, we may leave out of consideration those backward states of society in which the race itself may be considered as its nonage.[164]

Hence, the individual sovereignty was not a natural right of all human beings, rather it applied only to certain mature individuals who had the ability to exercise their "higher faculties," and who valued personal freedom to conduct their affairs with other individuals through voluntary agreements based on cooperation, consent, and contract, and without the interference of the state. Such individuals were the exemplars of a "person most interested in his own well-being"[165] and it was to them that Mill accorded the absolute right to decide what to do "with his life for his own benefit."[166]

From the jurisprudential point of view, the notion that the individual alone—rather than society as an institution—has the right to make decisions concerning personal well-being was radical, because it implied that such decisions ought to be accorded legal recognition and protection. Traditionally, the only explicit right of refusal protected by law was the right of refusal by proprietors[167] to part with or to allow strangers to interfere with their proprietary interests without lawful authorization.[168] The implication of Mill's philosophy was that an individual had a personal proprietorship over his or her body and the consequent right to refuse beneficial interference in matters relating to personal well-being:

> He cannot rightfully be compelled to do or forbear because it will be better for him to do so, because it will make him happier, because, in the opinions of others, to do so would be wise, or even right. There are good reasons for remonstrating with

---

[162] Under common-law rules, husbands alone had all the property of the married parties. *Lynch v. Knight*, 9 H.L.C. 577, 599, 131 E.R. 347, 362 (1861).

[163] J. MILL, *supra* note 156, at 9.

[164] *Id.*

[165] *Id.* at 13.

[166] *Id.*

[167] In 1765, Lord Camden, C.J. declared: "Our law holds the property of every man so sacred that no man can set foot upon his neighbour's close without his leave." *Entick v. Carrington*, 19 Howell State Tr. 1029 (1765), 95 E.R. 807, [1558-1774] All E.R. 41.

[168] Rape was a punishable felony not so much because it violated the principle that "every man's person [is] sacred," but because it interfered with the proprietary right that a parent had in his daughter, and husband had in his wife.

28   MENDELSON

him, or reasoning with him, or persuading him, or entreating him, but not for compelling him, or visiting him any evil, in case he do otherwise.[169]

Mill's idea that the individual has an unqualified right to refuse beneficial interference in matters relating to personal well-being appears not to have been based on the principle that all individuals have a natural right to personal liberty. Rather, it was grounded in the utilitarian principle that unless individuals are left free from social pressure when they decide on matters that concern their private interests, including their own well-being, society may find it more difficult to achieve the ends for which it exists.[170] This is a quintessential consequentialist position whereby the choice of the right to appropriate action is determined by the desirability or appropriateness of its consequences.

The utilitarian societal aims and ends espoused by Mill were formulated at the turn of the 19th century by Jeremy Bentham, a close friend of John Stuart's father. Bentham's utilitarian doctrine was founded upon three principles, the first of which states that all human efforts as an organized society should be aimed at maximizing happiness and minimizing suffering in the world. The second principle, known as hedonistic principle, defines the happiness of sentient human beings as the pleasure, or the absence of pain, and suffering as pain, or the absence of pleasure.[171] According to the third principle, the principle of impartiality, pleasures and pains of all sentient beings ought to be taken into consideration when decisions are made. In relation to the actual decision-making process, strict utilitarian philosophy does not permit any favoritism or privileges based upon mutual feelings, family relationships, or shared nationalities.[172]

Mill conceived personal liberty in terms of the classical freedom of action, liberum arbitrium—the freedom of choice between two or more desirable objects or ways of conduct. The notion of liberum arbitrium is predicated upon choice between things equally possible and available to us in statu nascendi as mere potentialities.[173] Actions can be justified only in terms of the outcome that would lead to the greatest utility in the sense of satisfaction or happiness. The relevant choice may be between pain and pleasure or suffering and well-being but it would always be in the context of

---

[169] J. MILL, *supra* note 156, at 9.

[170] M. COWLING, *supra* note 155, at 43-44.

[171] The hedonistic principle of the utilitarian philosophy goes back to the Epicureans who advocated that their followers should decide how to achieve their aspirations to a virtuous life by way of balancing pleasure in the sense of "ataraxia" (a Greek word meaning serenity, tranquility, calmness of mind) against distress, discomfort, or pain.

[172] M. HÄYRY, LIBERAL UTILITARIANISM AND APPLIED ETHICS 3 (1994).

[173] H. ARENDT, THE LIFE OF THE MIND: WILLING 29 (1978). Greek philosophers understood freedom as an objective state of the body rather than as a datum of consciousness or a state of mind—basic freedom was freedom of movement.

survival—death is final, and does not involve any potentiality. For example, St. Augustine (354-430) in *De Libero Arbitrio,*[174] argued that those who believe they chose non-being when they commit suicide are in error because they chose a form of being that will come about one day anyhow, and they chose peace that can exist only as a form or aspect of being.[175] Centuries later, Immanuel Kant in the essay *On Suicide* wrote that "man's freedom cannot subsist except on condition which is immutable. This condition is that man not use his freedom against himself to his destruction."[176]

Whereas the first principle of utilitarianism is vital to the understanding of Mill's philosophical doctrine of personal liberty, the second and third principles of Benthamite utilitarianism have profoundly influenced modern judicial approaches to consent and refusal as legal concepts.

III. THE LAW OF CONSENT IN THE UNITED STATES IN THE FIRST TWO DECADES OF THE 20TH CENTURY

John Stuart Mill's philosophical ideas of personal liberty involving the individual's absolute right to decide what to do "with his life for his own benefit" were reflected in judgments delivered in two cases in the United States. In the 1905 case of *Pratt v. Davis,*[177] a husband placed his wife, Mrs. Davis, in a sanatorium for treatment for epilepsy. The defendant physician found that Mrs. Davis' "uterus was contracted and lacerated, and that the lower portion of the rectum was diseased."[178] He operated for "these difficulties." The patient did not improve, and some 10 weeks later she was returned to the sanatorium, where the physician performed a hysterectomy operation upon her. This operation was performed without the prior consent of Mrs. Davis or her husband.[179] The following extract from the physician's testimony is quoted in the judgment: "I worked her deliberately and systematically, taking chances which she did not realize the full aspect of, deliberately and calmly deceiving the woman; that is I did not tell her the whole truth."[180]

The defense argued that the patient was incompetent to grant consent because she suffered from epilepsy, and that a patient who consults a medical practitioner "gives him implied license to do whatever in the exercise

---

[174] St. Augustine, De Libero Arbitrio, bk. III, v-viii.

[175] H. Arendt, *supra* note 173, at 83.

[176] I. Kant, *On Suicide,* in Lectures on Ethics 148 (L. Enfield trans. 1963).

[177] 118 Ill. App. 161 (1905), *aff'd,* 224 Ill. 300, 79 N.E. 562 (1906).

[178] *Pratt,* 79 N.E. at 563.

[179] Mrs. Davis' physical and mental health deteriorated following the operations and she was declared insane in 1889.

[180] *Pratt,* 79 N.E. at 564.

of his judgment may be necessary.''[181] The judges rejected both arguments, and found that the defendant by acting without consent was liable in trespass. The case before the appellate court was reported in the *Chicago Legal News* in the following way:

> Under a free government at least, the free citizen's first and greatest right, which underlies all others—the right to the inviolability of his person, in other words, his right to himself—is the subject of universal acquiescence, and this right necessarily forbids a physician or surgeon, however skilful [sic] or eminent, who has been asked to examine, diagnose, advise and prescribe (which are at least necessary first steps in treatment and care), to violate without permission the bodily integrity of his patient by a major or capital operation, placing him under an anaesthetic for that purpose, and operating on him without his consent and knowledge.[182]

The Supreme Court of Minnesota cited the above passage with approval when in 1905 it decided the case of *Mohr v. Williams.*[183] In this case, the patient, Anna Mohr, consented to have an operation performed on her right ear. In the course of the procedure, the treating physician decided that it was the patient's left ear that needed the surgery. The physician's non-consensual operation on Ms. Mohr's left ear resulted in serious impairment of her hearing in that ear. She sued the physician for battery. The court affirmed the jury's award of $14,322.50 in damages, holding that the medical practitioner should have obtained Ms. Mohr's express consent before operating on her left ear. In the context of this ruling, the court referred to a passage from section 375 of 1 *Kinkead on Torts,* which articulated the position of the law in relation to consent.

> The patient must be the final arbiter as to whether he will take his chances with the operation, or take his chances of living without it. Such is the natural right of every individual, which the law recognizes as the legal one. Consent, therefore, of an individual must be either expressly or impliedly given before a surgeon may have the right to operate.[184]

The court considered two exceptions to the rule that there must be an express consent to medical treatment.[185] Under the first exception, the law may imply consent in circumstances where a person is injured to the extent of being rendered unconscious and the injuries require prompt medical attention. Under these conditions, ''a physician . . . would be justified in applying such medical or surgical treatment as might reasonably be neces-

---

[181] *Pratt,* 118 Ill. at 166.

[182] Pratt v. Davis, 37 Chic. Legal News 213, 213 (1905).

[183] 104 N.W. 12 (Minn. 1905). The passage also was quoted with approval in Rolater v. Strain, 137 P. 96, 97 (Okla. 1913). Mohr v. Williams was overruled on other grounds in Genzel v. Halvorson, 80 N.W.2d 854, 859 (Minn. 1957).

[184] *Mohr,* 104 N.W. at 14-15.

[185] The Supreme Court of Illinois in *Pratt,* 79 N.E. at 562 also discussed the exception of necessity.

sary for the preservation of [the injured person's] life or limb."[186] The second exception is really a variation of the first—when in the course of an operation to which the patient had consented, "the physician should discover conditions not anticipated before the operation was commenced, and which, if not removed, would endanger the life or health of the patient, he would, though no express consent was obtained or given, be justified in extending the operation to remove and overcome them."[187]

In 1913, the Civil Court of Appeals of Texas in *Rishworth v. Moss*[188] consolidated these two exceptions into a general rule when it stated that "there must be consent in every case, except in an emergency when the delay to obtain consent would endanger the life or health of the patient."[189] In subsequent American cases, as well as in Canada, the United Kingdom, and Australia, the courts upheld the rule that unless the circumstances of emergency apply, a medical or surgical procedure that goes beyond the scope of a patient's express consent should be regarded as trespass, even when there was no evidence of an express prohibition.[190]

The legal justification for the emergency exception to the law of consent when applied to unconscious patients has changed from that of implied consent to the principle of necessity—the medical intervention must be shown to have been necessary "for the protection of the plaintiff's health and possibly his life."[191] The doctrine of necessity, as an exception to the law of consent, allows for provision of nonvoluntary therapy, in circumstances when the patient is not in a position to have or to express any views on the proposed clinical management.[192] This doctrine also applies to patients who are incapable of giving consent by reason of minority, and persons whose state of mind is such as to render their apparent consent invalid.[193]

The common-law doctrine of necessity was developed at the time when palliation was not regarded as an important aspect of medical care, and the study of pain relief was not very well advanced. Pain and suffering were

---

[186] *Mohr*, 104 N.W. at 15.

[187] *Id*.

[188] 159 S.W. 122 (Tex. App. 1913).

[189] *Id*. at 124.

[190] Paulsen v. Gundersen, 260 N.W. 448 (Wis. 1935); Wall v. Brim, 138 F.2d 478 (5th Cir. 1943); Murray v. McMurchy, 2 D.L.R. 442 (1949); T v. T, [1988] 2 W.L.R. 189; Rogers v. Whitaker, 175 C.L.R. 479 (1992).

[191] Marshall v. Curry, 3 D.L.R. 260 (1933).

[192] Airedale NHS Trust v. Bland, [1993] A.C. 789.

[193] J. MASON & R. McCALL SMITH, LAW AND MEDICAL ETHICS 219-20 (4th ed. 1994). The authors distinguish between nonvoluntary therapy and an involuntary treatment, which implies treatment against a competent patient's express wishes. Legal acceptability of involuntary treatment depends upon a balance between the personal interest in autonomy and the interests of life, safety, or welfare of a third party, or of the community. In relation to the enforcement of compulsory vaccination, see Prince v. Massachusetts, 321 U.S. 158 (1944).

accepted as part and parcel of the human condition—one was born in pain, lived in pain, and was expected to die in pain. Modern medicine understands (or ought to understand) that the experience of pain is detrimental to the patient's physical welfare and need not be endured. The aim of multi-modal pain management is to achieve satisfactory pain relief through the administration of adequate dosage and timing of analgesics (including long-acting oral preparations of morphine), palliative radiotherapy, chemotherapy, surgery, hormone therapy, anesthetic and neurosurgical techniques, physical treatment, and psychological support for the patient and his or her family.[194] Yet, palliative medical therapy would not come within the ambit of the defense of necessity because its aim is to prevent harm to the patient's quality of life rather than to protect the patient's life or health in the strict sense.

The facts in both the *Pratt* case and the *Williams* case, involved absence of consent to the particular treatment, rather than an explicit refusal thereof. In the 1913 case of *Rolater v. Strain*,[195] Mattie Inez Strain consented to an operation to drain an infection that developed after she stepped upon a nail which penetrated the big toe of her right foot. In the course of an operation that was performed under an anesthetic, the physician removed the sesamoid bone from her toe. Ms. Strain sued the medical practitioner in trespass, claiming that there was an agreement between them that "no bones should be removed."[196] She was awarded $1000. On appeal, the court upheld the patient's right to refuse certain procedures, and the physician's duty to act within the strict limits imposed by the ambit of consent when it is granted. The problem with the *Rolater* decision, however, is that the Supreme Court of Oklahoma misapplied this jurisprudential principle to the facts before it. The court seemed to persist in a belief that sesamoid bones are an integral part of the human anatomy,[197] when in fact—as the defendant physician rightly pointed out—they are nodules of bone that may be found in certain tendons where they rub over bony surface.[198] The removal of the nodules would have been necessary if they prevented proper drainage of the pus.

When interpreted literally, the principle that physicians will be liable for trespass unless they act within strict limits of the patient's consent, or unless they can avail themselves of the narrow defense of necessity,[199] may

---

[194] R. MOULDS, M. HEMMING, S. ARANDA, R. DAY, A. GLOVER, B. GUTHRIE, R. HELME, K. JACKSON, T. LITTLE, I. MADDOCKS, & G. MENDELSON, 41 ANALGESIC GUIDELINES (1992/93).

[195] 137 P. 96 (Okla. 1913).

[196] *Id.* at 96.

[197] *Id.* at 99.

[198] The sesamoid bone can be found in the tendons of flexor hallucis brevis, the muscle that bends or flexes the big toe. R. SNELL, CLINICAL ANATOMY FOR MEDICAL STUDENTS 38 (4th ed. 1992).

[199] Demers v. Gerety, 515 P.2d 645 (N.M. 1975), *remanded on other grounds*, 520 P.2d 869 (N.M.

lead to absurd results, as illustrated by one recent English case[200] in which a consultant anesthetist was found guilty of an assault (battery) by a suppository. The patient, before having four teeth extracted in a dental clinic, was provided with an explanation about the nature and effects of general anesthesia, but not about procedures that may be undertaken to relieve postoperative pain. She gave her consent to general anesthesia verbally and by implication.[201] While the patient was under the general anesthetic, the anesthetist inserted a diclofenac suppository for postoperative pain.[202] This was done in the presence of the dental surgeon and two female nurses; the patient was informed about the procedure when she regained consciousness. The anesthetist was found guilty of an assault and serious professional misconduct by the professional conduct committee of the General Medical Council,[203] on the grounds that while carrying out the pain-relieving procedure he "inserted the said substance [diclofenac suppository] without the patient's prior valid consent and thus assaulted her."[204] It is arguable that medical contact, which is beneficial to the patient but which is unauthorized due to the physician's genuine mistake as to the ambit of the patient's consent, ought not to be treated as battery with its semi-criminal implications.[205]

The preoccupation with the ambit of the patient's consent predates the jurisprudence of self-determination as a principle of tort, and has at its core the old contractual notion of consent as "an outcome of consenting minds" of the contracting parties.[206] For it was only in 1914 that the idea of a

---

1974). In this case, during the course of an operation under a general anesthetic, the defendant surgeon found that to repair a hernia, which was the authorized procedure, he would have to revise the patient's ileostomy. He did both procedures, and subsequently was sued successfully by the patient. The court determined that a hernia repair was not the kind of surgery undertaken to preserve the patient's health or life, and, because the original procedure could not be carried out without performing the unauthorized procedure, neither operation was permissible.

[200] Mitchell, *A Fundamental Problem of Consent*, 310 BRIT. MED. J. 43 (1995).

[201] The doctrine of implied consent, which is based on the maxim "qui tacet, consetire vedetur" (he who is silent is deemed to have consented), operates in general physician-patient relationships when the patient is lucid, for example, when a person holds up an arm to be vaccinated—it will be taken as a valid assent to the procedure. O'Brien v. Cunard SS Co., 28 N.E. 266 (Mass. Sup. Jud. Ct. 1891).

[202] The suppository was inserted—mistakenly—into the patient's vagina, instead of her rectum.

[203] General Medical Council of the United Kingdom was set up under the Medical Act 1858 (UK). It has regulatory powers, including the power to remove from the Register a practitioner found guilty of infamous conduct in professional respect. As such, it is a prerogative tribunal and a part of the executive arm of the government.

[204] Mitchell, *supra* note 200, at 43. The dental surgeon who had never touched the diclofenac suppository was found guilty of assault and serious professional misconduct by the General Dental Council on the same facts.

[205] McCoid, *A Reappraisal of Liability for Unauthorized Treatment*, 41 MINN. L. REV. 381 (1957).

[206] In Foster v. Wheeler, 36 Ch. C.D. 695, 698 (1887), Kekewich, J. defined contract as "[a]n act in the law whereby two or more persons declare their contract as to any act or thing to be done or forborne by some or one of those persons for the use of the others or other of them." *See also* Cundy v. Lindsay, 3 App. Cas. 459, 465 (1878).

patient's right to self-determination was expressly introduced into the common law. The case was *Schloendorff v. Society of New York Hospital*,[207] and it concerned a surgeon who removed a fibroid tumor in circumstances where the patient had consented to an abdominal examination under anesthesia, but had specifically requested "no operation." The issue before the court was not battery, but the defendant hospital's liability for torts committed by surgeons while using its facilities. In the course of his opinion, Judge Benjamin Cardozo made the often quoted observation that: "Every human being of adult years and sound mind has a right to determine what shall be done with his own body; and a surgeon who performs an operation without his patient's consent commits an assault, for which he is liable in damages."[208] This statement has an important place in the modern jurisprudence—it is relied upon as the basis for the doctrine that the person's right to refuse medical treatment should constitute an absolute personal interest.

The transposition of a utilitarian philosophical idea regarding political rights and commercial freedoms of an individual vis-à-vis the power of a state into the context of individual death-choices in the clinical setting, was filtered through the jurisprudential theory of rights propounded by Ronald Dworkin in a series of articles published in the 1960s and 1970s, the most important of which were collected in 1977 under the title *Taking Rights Seriously*.[209] In his analysis of legal standards that guide the judicial decision-making process, Dworkin made a distinction between policies and principles whereby "principles are propositions that describe rights; policies are propositions that describe goals."[210] Policies set out collective community goals, such as advancement or protection of political aims, economic efficiency, or social welfare.[211] Principles are to be observed because they embody the requirements of justice or fairness or some other dimension of morality, which respect or secure some individual or group right.

Dworkin contended that in civil cases, judicial determinations characteristically are, and should be, generated by principle not policy; and that adjudication of what legal rights people have should be made in the light of an overall political theory that recognizes moral-political background rights (rights that provide a justification for a political decision by the society) as well as those concrete rights against fellow citizens already demarcated by law.[212] Though not without its critics,[213] Dworkin's theory of rights, in

---

[207] 105 N.E. 92 (N.Y. 1914).

[208] *Id.* at 93.

[209] R. DWORKIN, TAKING RIGHTS SERIOUSLY (1977).

[210] *Id.* at 90.

[211] *Id.* at 22, 82.

[212] J. HARRIS, LEGAL PHILOSOPHIES 179 (1986).

[213] D. LYONS, ETHICS AND THE RULE OF LAW (1984); J. STONE, PRECEDENT AND LAW: DYNAMICS OF COMMON LAW GROWTH (1985).

particular, the notion that individual rights are based on two fundamental values—human dignity and political equality—was in harmony with the ideology of the then growing movement of consumerism. Dworkin's emphasis on self as the central tenet of societal values, and the consequent notion of rights that are exclusively centered on the individual, exerted profound influence upon the legal theory and practice in all common-law countries.

IV. THE SANCTITY OF LIFE AND THE SANCTITY OF INDIVIDUAL SELF-DETERMINATION AS COMPETING LEGAL VALUES

Blackstone's principle regarding the absolute right to personal security was predicated upon a more comprehensive principle of sanctity of life—in the sense of inviolability—that he considered fundamental to a civilized society.[214] After the Second World War, this principle was embodied in Article 3 of the *Universal Declaration of Human Rights*. Adopted by the General Assembly of the United Nations in 1948, it declares that "[e]veryone has the right to life, liberty and security of person." In Article 6 of the *International Covenant of Civil and Political Rights* (1966), the principle of sanctity of life has been interpreted as a right not to be deprived of life, except on such grounds as are established by law and consistent with principles of fundamental justice.

The principle of the sanctity of life is common to medicine and to law.[215] In medicine, this principle forms the basis for the prohibition against medically assisted suicide in the *Hippocratic Oath*. In law, the principle of sanctity of life has been expressed in the following way:

> Life and the concept of life, represents a deep-rooted value immanent in our society. Its preservation is a fundamental humanitarian precept providing an ideal which is not only of inherent merit in commanding respect for the worth and dignity of the individual but also exemplifies the finer virtues which are the mark of a civilised order.[216]

At common law, the principle of the sanctity of human life has private and public law aspects. In public law, it has been interpreted by the courts to mean that the state has an interest in the preservation of human life. The

---

[214] 1 W. BLACKSTONE, *supra* note 61, at 129-30.

[215] For a discussion of the concept of autonomy and its interface with the concept of sacredness of life from a religious and a secular perspective, see R. DWORKIN, LIFE'S DOMINION: AN ARGUMENT ABOUT ABORTION, EUTHANASIA, AND INDIVIDUAL FREEDOMS (1993).

[216] Auckland Area Health Bd. v. Attorney-General, [1993] 1 N.Z.L.R. 235, 244 (Thomas, J.).

36   MENDELSON

protection of life remains a primary function of criminal law,[217] and under-lies the state's interest in preventing suicide. The principle of the sanctity of human life also lies at the core of the jurisprudential argument against capital punishment. In private law, the principle is manifested through the tort of battery.

The shift in the hierarchy of values that underpin the tort of battery, namely, from the sanctity of human life, to the sanctity of the human body, to the more recent value of the sanctity of individual self-determination, has been gradual. Neither the *Schloendorff* case, nor any prior case in which the issue of a patient's right to refuse certain medical procedures has been litigated and affirmed by the courts involved refusal of life-saving treatment. In fact, it appears that until *Schloendorff*, the courts still regarded the legal principle of the inviolability of the human body as based essentially upon the communitarian interest in the inviolability of human life. The common point in judgments holding that defendant medical practitioners should be liable for disregarding their patients' instructions, was that such conduct was detrimental to the patients' well-being in the Millsian sense. The approach of the judiciary was in sympathy with the notion that the individual has an unqualified right to refuse beneficial interference in matters connected with his or her personal well-being as a sentient being. This approach excluded death-choices and self-annihilation.

The issue of refusal of therapeutic treatment, when the consequence of the person's choice would bring about death rather than survival, did not arise as a medical legal issue until medicine perfected life-saving and life-sustaining treatment. A procedural difference has emerged as a result of litigation involving the right to refuse life-saving or life-sustaining medical treatment. As noted above, the law of consent focuses on the presence or absence of a valid consent. In trespass, consent can be vitiated by duress, trickery, withholding of information in bad faith, or fraud;[218] therefore, the legal analysis is focused on the past conduct of the defendant-physician. So long as refusal was considered to be merely the obverse of consent for the purposes of establishing whether or not the defendant's conduct should be regarded as wrongful, cases were litigated only after the allegedly noncon-sensual conduct had occurred.

Once the refusal of medical treatment came to be regarded as a separate right, plaintiff-patients began to ask the courts for injunctions and declara-tions to prevent interference with their choice to refuse treatment, including life-saving procedures. Hence, the law of refusal concerns proposed conduct or events, and it tends to focus on the person refusing the life-saving or life-sustaining treatment before it is to be administered. Moreover, because

---

[217] *Id.*
[218] R. v. Willies, [1923] 1 K.B. 340; Hart v. Hernon & Anor., [1984] Aust. Torts Rep. ¶ 80-201.

injunctions and declarations are equitable remedies, the courts asked to grant this kind of relief should be guided not only by the common law but also by the principles of equity.

The seminal cases through which the law of refusal of medical treatment developed concerned the refusal of life-saving blood transfusions by Jehovah's Witnesses. The first successful blood transfusion for therapeutic purposes was carried out by James Blundell in 1829 at Guy's Hospital in London. However, it was only during the Second World War that blood transfusion became a common practice in obstetrics.[219] Jehovah's Witnesses are prohibited by the tenets of their religion to receive blood transfusions.

Application of President & Directors of Georgetown College, Inc.[220] is the leading case on this issue. There, a 25-year-old woman, Jesse E. Jones, who lost approximately two-thirds of her total blood volume due to a ruptured ulcer, was brought to a District of Columbia hospital for emergency care in September of 1963. The attending physicians were of the opinion that the patient would die unless blood transfusions were administered. The patient and her husband were Jehovah's Witnesses and rejected this treatment option. Attorneys for the hospital initially sought a judicial order authorizing a series of blood transfusions and overruling the woman's right to refuse them. When this application was turned down, the attorneys applied to the Court of Appeals for the District of Columbia for an appropriate writ.

During the hearing at the bedside, Mrs. Jones and her husband indicated that while they objected to the blood transfusions on religious grounds, should the court order such procedure, they would not feel morally responsible. Justice Skelly Wright indicated four factors that persuaded him to issue an order authorizing the transfusions. First, the patient was the mother of a seven-month-old child. Consequently, the state had an interest in preserving Mrs. Jones' life; it also had an interest in preventing the abandonment of the child by allowing the mother to die.[221] Second, Justice Wright indicated that Mrs. Jones' religious beliefs were not designed to cause her death: such a result would be only an unfortunate repercussion of these beliefs. By coming to the hospital for treatment, the patient indicated a desire to live.[222] The third factor was a jurisprudential conundrum of whether a patient who exercises the right to refuse life-saving treatment is thereby placing the hospital and the medical personnel in a position of civil and criminal liability for either going ahead with nonconsensual treatment or allowing the patient to die. The judge did not find clear authority for the patient's right to restrict

---

[219] C. SINGER & E. ASHWORTH UNDERWOOD, A SHORT HISTORY OF MEDICINE 699-701 (2d ed. 1962).

[220] 331 F.2d 1000 (D.C. Cir.), *cert. denied*, 377 U.S. 978 (1964).

[221] *Id.* at 1008.

[222] *Id.* at 1009.

the kind of treatment she could receive to the point that death occurred.[223] Justice Wright suggested that the fourth factor was decisive—the life of the patient hung in the balance. Unless he ordered the transfusion "to preserve the status quo,"[224] death would have mooted the entire problem. Rather than not acting, only to learn subsequently that the law required the transfusion to be ordered, the judge erred on the side of life.[225] Each of the four factors discussed by Justice Wright for determining the existence of the right to refuse life-saving treatment has had a jurisprudential sequelae that will be analyzed in the context of subsequent developments.

A. The Interests of the State in Preserving Life and the "Right to Die"

The nature of the balance between the interests of the state and the interest of a patient in exercising the right of self-determination through refusal of life-saving treatment has been considered by United States courts primarily from the perspective of constitutional law.[226] Most of the early cases concerned patients who refused medical treatment forbidden by their religious beliefs, and were argued on the basis of constitutional implications of the first amendment to the United States Constitution as well as the common-law right to self-determination.[227]

In his opinion on the denial of rehearing in *Application of President & Directors of Georgetown College,*[228] Circuit Judge Warren Burger (as he then was) relied on the dissenting opinion of Justice Brandeis in *Olmstead v. United States,*[229] who considered that the fourth amendment to the United States Constitution endeavored to protect "Americans in their beliefs, their thoughts, their emotions and their sensations." It thus "conferred, as against the Government, the right to be left alone—the most comprehensive of rights and the right most valued by civilized man."[230] In a remarkable exercise of mind-reading, Judge Burger determined that

---

[223] *Id.*

[224] *Id.* at 1009-10.

[225] F. ROZOVSKY, *supra* note 3, at 442.

[226] Griswold v. Connecticut, 381 U.S. 479 (1965); Roe v. Wade, 410 U.S. 113, 153 (1973); Cruzan v. Director, Missouri Dep't of Health, 497 U.S. 261 (1990). *See also In re* Quinlan, 355 A.2d 647 (N.J.), *cert. denied,* 429 U.S. 922 (1976). Byrd, *A Right to Die: Can Massachusetts Physicians Withdraw Artificial Nutrition and Hydration from a Persistently Vegetative Patient Following* Cruzan v. Director, Missouri Department of Health?, 26 NEW ENG. L. REV. 199 (1991); Annas, *Nancy Cruzan and the Right to Die,* 323 NEW ENG. J. MED. 670 (1990).

[227] The opening clause of the first amendment to the United States Constitution states that "Congress shall make no law respecting an establishment of religion, or prohibiting the free exercise thereof." The first 10 amendments were ratified in 1791 and form what is known as the American Bill of Rights.

[228] *Georgetown College,* 331 F.2d at 1000.

[229] Olmstead v. United States, 277 U.S. 438 (1928).

[230] *Id.* at 478.

[n]othing in this utterance suggests that Justice Brandeis thought an individual possessed these rights only as to sensible beliefs, valid thoughts, reasonable emotions, or well-founded sensations. I suggest he intended to include a great many foolish, unreasonable and even absurd ideas which do not conform, such as refusing medical treatment even at great risk.[231]

Generally, in the 1970s, cases that involved legal issues associated with the withdrawal of life-sustaining treatment from incompetent patients had at their core the existence of the constitutional right to refuse life-saving or life-sustaining treatment. The incompetent patient's "right" to have life-sustaining treatment withheld or withdrawn was initially interpreted by United States courts as being based on the common-law right to informed consent, "or on both the common-law right and a constitutional privacy right."[232] Although the United States Constitution does not explicitly refer to the right to personal privacy, the courts have found "the unwritten constitutional right of privacy to exist in the penumbra of specific guarantees of the *Bill of Rights*."[233]

Subsequently, in the *Cruzan* case,[234] the United States Supreme Court considered that the "right to die" through refusal of life-sustaining procedures—if it exists[235]—is based not on the right of personal privacy but rather on the "liberty interest" delineated in the fourteenth amendment to the United States Constitution. Section 1 of the fourteenth amendment to the United States Constitution provides that no State shall "deprive any person of life, liberty, or property, without due process of law." The issue before the Supreme Court was whether the fourteenth amendment prohibited the state from requiring clear and convincing evidence of the incompetent person's desire to withdraw or withhold life-sustaining treatment.

Hence, the judicial process employed in these cases entailed balancing state interests against the constitutional rights of the individual. In the case of *Superintendent of Belchertown State School v. Saikewicz*,[236] which involved the application to sanction the withholding of chemotherapy from a profoundly retarded 67-year-old leukemia patient, the Supreme Judicial Court of Massachusetts ruled that four state interests were implicated: (1) the preservation of human life;[237] (2) the protection of innocent third parties who

---

[231] *Georgetown College*, 331 F.2d at 1016-17.

[232] *Cruzan*, 497 U.S. at 271.

[233] *Quinlan*, 355 A.2d at 663.

[234] *Cruzan*, 497 U.S. at 278-80.

[235] The language of the decision in *Cruzan* is ambiguous. However, it is clear from the judgment that the Court—for the purpose of deciding the case—assumed the existence of the right to refuse life-sustaining treatment.

[236] 370 N.E.2d 417 (Mass. 1977).

[237] State interest in the preservation of life is enshrined in the American Declaration of Independence and the Constitution of the United States.

may be adversely affected by the death of the person seeking to exercise his or her "right to die"; (3) the prevention of suicide; and (4) the maintenance of the ethical integrity of the medical profession, including the right of the physician to administer medical treatment to the best of his or her judgment.[238] In *Saikewicz*, the court recognized the interest in preservation of human life as paramount and noted that it was greatest when the affliction was curable.[239]

In the United States, the issue of the right to refuse life-saving treatment tends to be grounded as much in the public constitutional law as in the private law of trespass to person.[240] In Australia and the United Kingdom, neither the interests of the state, as identified by the Supreme Court of the United States in *Saikewicz* and *Cruzan,* including the interest in preservation of life, nor the "liberty interests" of the individual to refuse life-saving treatment have a constitutional foundation. They are grounded in the common law of battery.[241]

Building on Judge Cardozo's statement that "every human being of adult years and sound mind has a right to determine what shall be done with his own body," modern common-law jurisprudence has elevated the principle of inviolability of negative individual decisions regarding one's body above that of the general principle of the sanctity of life.[242] This is because the principle of inviolability of the human body that is seen merely as an expression of the individual interest in personal self-determination, involves, by implication, the right to a death-choice manifested through refusal of life-saving treatment.

In 1986, the California Court of Appeal, in *Bouvia v. Superior Court*,[243] affirmed this doctrine by interpreting the statement of Judge Cardozo as meaning that

> a person of adult years and in sound mind has the right, in the exercise of control over his own body, to determine whether or not to submit to medical treatment. It follows that such a patient has the right to refuse *any* medical treatment even that which may save or prolong her life.[244]

In England, the person's legal right to make a death-choice was succinctly expressed by Lord Goff of Chieveley in the case of *Airedale NHS Trust v.*

---

[238] *Saikewicz,* 370 N.E.2d at 425; *Cruzan,* 497 U.S. at 271.

[239] *Saikewicz,* 370 N.E.2d at 425-26.

[240] Justice Scalia said that his preference would have been for a determination that "the federal courts have no business in this field." *Cruzan,* 497 U.S. at 293 (Scalia, J., concurring).

[241] Mendelson, *Jurisprudential Aspects of Withdrawal of Life Support Systems from Incompetent Patients in Australia,* 69 Australian L.J. 259 (1995).

[242] Malette v. Shulman, 67 D.L.R.4th 321 (1990).

[243] 225 Cal. Rptr. 297 (Cal. App. 1986). Elizabeth Bouvia, a quadriplegic suffering from cerebral palsy, sought injunctive relief to order the High Desert Hospital to accede to her request and remove the nasogastric tube through which nutrition and hydration were supplied to keep her alive. The appellate court granted the injunction. In early 1989, she was still alive with the help of a nasogastric tube. G. Pence, 44 Classic Cases in Medical Ethics (1990).

[244] *Bouvia,* 225 Cal. Rptr. at 300.

Bland,[245] where he stated that "the principle of the sanctity of human life must yield to the principle of self-determination."[246] Thus, the locus of the modern tort of battery has shifted from the sanctity of life to the sanctity of personal choices in relation to one's body and existence.

B. Religious Conviction and the Issue of "Sound Mind" as a Criterion of Decisional Competence

In the *Application of President & Directors of Georgetown College*,[247] Justice Wright's decision took into account the patient's views and religious convictions.[248] Justice Wright noted that Mrs. Jones was a committed Jehovah's Witness—a person whose religious beliefs compelled her to refuse life-saving blood transfusions—but who did not want to die. Her refusal was neither unexpected nor spontaneous. She was an adult who knew about, considered, and accepted the consequences of adhering to the tenets of her religion well before the circumstances that necessitated the blood transfusions arose. As such, her decision fulfilled the three criteria for valid consent as defined by Henry Ballow—it was "an act of reason" and "deliberation" by way of balancing "the good and evil on either side."[249] She also appeared to fulfill the medical requirements of competence, which include the capacity for understanding and communication, the capacity for reasoning and deliberation, and a stable set of values or a conception of what is bad and good.[250] In law, these capacities are subsumed under the legal criterion of "sound mind." The law uses the concept of sound mind to determine decision-making capacity—whether or not the person is, or was, capable of making a decision that ought to be binding on others.

The phrase "sound mind" is not a medical term. The expression denotes a strictly legal concept of competence, which traditionally refers solely to intellectual capacity. The law presumes an adult person to be competent unless the person is shown to be unable to carry out certain mental tasks. Competence, in the sense of cognitive ability to make a contract, to plead, to make a will, to vote in elections or to consent to treatment, is a legal concept and can be determined only by a judge or other duly constituted legal authority, though a psychiatrist or a psychologist may be

---

[245] [1993] A.C. 789.

[246] *Id.* at 864, 826-27 (Hoffman, L.J.).

[247] *Georgetown College*, 331 F.2d at 1009.

[248] *See also In re* Estate of Brooks, 205 N.E.2d 345 (Ill. 1965), where the court said that the patient may elect to pursue religious beliefs by refusing life-saving blood transfusions, provided the decision did not endanger public health, safety, or morals.

[249] 1 H. BALLOW, *supra* note 135, ch. 2, § 1.

[250] A. BUCHANAN & D. BROCK, DECIDING FOR OTHERS: THE ETHICS OF SURROGATE DECISION MAKING 23-25 (1989).

called in to assist in determining the standard of the person's competence.[251]

Although there is no specific case-law definition of "sound mind" for the purposes of the civil law of trespass, this concept has been negatively defined under testamentary law. In the case of *Banks v. Goodfellow*,[252] a legally competent person was described by Sir Alexander Cockburn CJ in the following way:

> [T]o the due exercise of a power . . . involving moral responsibility, the possession of the intellectual and moral faculties common to our nature should be insisted on as an indispensable condition. It is essential to the exercise of such a power that a testator shall understand the nature of the act and its effects; shall understand the extent of the property of which he is disposing; shall be able to comprehend and appreciate the claims to which he ought to give effect; and, with the view to the latter object, that no disorder of his mind shall poison his affections, pervert his sense of right, or prevent the exercise of his natural faculties—that no insane delusion shall influence his will in disposing of his property and bring about a disposal of it which, if the mind had been sound, would not have been made.[253]

In stressing the importance of the dispositor's "natural faculties"—in the sense of his or her cognitive capacity—as an "indispensable" element of "sound mind,"[254] Cockburn CJ was echoing the view of John Stuart Mill when he insisted that the doctrine of individual liberty was "meant to apply only to human beings in the maturity of their faculties."[255]

The language used in the judgment is open to very broad interpretation. It is possible to infer from it that when determining the decision-making competence of any individual, the court may take into consideration any psychiatric condition that may lead to an affective disorder,[256] making him or her unable to understand the moral difference between right and wrong, lead to serious cognitive impairment, or produce a psychotic state. However, in *Banks*, the Court of Queen's Bench chose to interpret the criteria of "sound mind" very narrowly. In this case, the testator was convinced that he was pursued and molested by devils or evil spirits. Nevertheless, he was capable of looking after his financial affairs, and had given clear and rational instructions for his will, which left the greater part of his fortune to the niece

---

[251] P. APPELBAUM & T. GUTHEIL, CLINICAL HANDBOOK OF PSYCHIATRY AND THE LAW (2d ed. 1991).

[252] [1870] 5 Q.B. 549.

[253] *Id.* at 565.

[254] The phrase "natural faculties" has been interpreted in modern testamentary law as including "amongst other things, a comprehension and appreciation of the claims [by relatives, etc.] to which the testator ought to give effect." *In re* Estate of the Late Donald Harold Bonson, slip. op. at 18 (unreported) (Sup. Ct. Northern Territory, Apr. 7, 1995) (Martin, C.J.).

[255] J. MILL, *supra* note 156, at 9.

[256] Major affective disorders are characterized by a prominent and persistent disturbance of mood (depression or mania). The disorder is usually episodic but may be chronic. A PSYCHIATRIC GLOSSARY 87 (A. Werner, R. Campbell, S. Frazier, & E. Stone eds. 5th ed. 1980).

who had looked after him. The court held that the will was valid. For, although the testator was suffering from an insane delusion, it did not influence his testamentary dispositions, because according to Cockburn CJ: "[T]hough mental power may be reduced below the ordinary standard, yet if there be sufficient intelligence to understand and appreciate the testamentary act in its different bearings, the power to make a will remains."[257]

Thus, the juridical test for the purposes of civil law[258] of a person's mental competence—whether or not he or she is of sound mind—is based on the cognitive criteria that measure the person's intellectual capacity to know, including the capacity to understand, weigh, and consider the nature of the proposed course of action.[259] For the purposes of decisional competence, the presumption of sound mind may be negated when the "disorder of the mind" (1) poisons the person's affections; (2) perverts his or her sense of right; (3) prevents the exercise of the person's natural faculties; or (4) where insane delusion influences the person's will.

The test of legal competence as set out in *Banks v. Goodfellow* has been criticized, particularly its reference to the standard of "insane delusion."[260] Yet, even this phrase has been judicially re-defined in terms of cognitive capacity:

> Although made in the light of then existing medical knowledge, his Lordship's statement does not appear to differ, in substance, from the latter-day psychiatrist's test of what is a "delusion," that is, that it is not capable of *rational explanation or amenable to reason,* and that it is not *explicable* by reference to the subject person's education and culture.[261]

In psychiatry, delusions, together with overvalued ideas, are classified under the broad category of impairment of mental function as abnormalities of thought content. Delusions can either be primary or secondary, they may be

---

[257] *Banks,* [1870] 5 Q.B. at 566.

[258] In the Australian and English jurisdictions the rules of criminal insanity in the *McNaghten's Case,* 10 Cl. & F. 200, 8 E.R. 718 (1843), provide the legal test for the insanity defense. Mawson, *Specific Defences to a Criminal Charge: Assessment for Court,* in PRINCIPLES AND PRACTICE OF FORENSIC PSYCHIATRY (R. Bluglass & P. Bowden eds. 1990).

[259] Bursztajn, Hardin, Gutheil, & Brodsky, *Beyond Cognition: The Role of Disordered Affective States in Impairing Competence to Consent to Treatment,* 19 BULL. AM. ACAD. PSYCHIATRY & LAW 383 (1991).

[260] "The reference to an insane delusion is not an invocation of deep medical knowledge." *In Re Crichton,* (unreported) (Sup. Ct. New South Wales, Probate Div., July 22, 1994) (Bryson, J.).

[261] *Re Hodges,* (1988) 14 N.S.W.L.R. 698, 706 (Powell, J.) (emphasis added); applying *Re Crichton,* and *Re Crooks* (unreported) (Sup. Ct. New South Wales, Probate Div., Dec. 4, 1994). *See also* Judge Santow's statement that it is no longer "necessary to find a disorder of the mind in any clinical sense. The delusion must be tested by objective evidence, as to it being fixed, false and incorrigible such as that the testator could not be reasoned out of it. Such delusions or disorders of the mind thus go beyond eccentricity, or vindictiveness, or irrationality, though these may be evidence pointing with other material, to lack of testamentary capacity." Easter v. Griffith, slip. op., at 9 (unreported) (Sup. Ct. New South Wales, Probate Div., June 17, 1994). With due respect, Judge Santow's test while dispensing with the medical explanations, is so vague and broad that it provides no definable standards, and thus endows the court with an untrammelled discretion.

persecutory, grandiose, and alike, or may involve delusions of reference. In patients with schizophrenia, specific delusions of thought broadcasting, and delusions of influence may occur.

The definition of "sound mind" for the purposes of testamentary law must be considered in its context, and in particular, the principle that "the absolute and uncontrolled power of testamentary disposition conceded by law is founded on the assumption that a rational will is a better disposition than any that can be made by the law itself."[262] Nevertheless, the common law in general tends to focus upon the mechanism of the decision-making process rather than the decision itself. Once the procedural criteria as set by the law are satisfied, the actual decision—no matter how irrational and detrimental to the person's well-being—has to be respected. The reason provided by the common law for justifying the line drawn between the decision-making process and the decision is guided by the respect for the dignitary interests of an individual and his or her choices.[263] It would appear that such a complete separation of the decision-making process from the actual decision has its provenance in the dualistic theory of the mind and body dichotomy postulated by the 17th century French mathematician and philosopher René Descartes.[264]

Descartes identified mind, which he defined as a "res cogitans" (thinking thing) or cognition, with the immaterial soul. The experiences of cognition, perception, and emotion were considered by Descartes as the soul's immaterial reactions to some material movement in the blood or spirits of the bodily machine. The feelings, whether of anger, grief, or joy, were not the cause but the consequence of prior material bodily actions and functions.[265] For the purposes of metaphysical inquiry, therefore, all issues related to mind and soul could be separated from the physical body and regarded as the domain of theologians and philosophers. The body, perceived as a complex mechanism with interacting solid and fluid parts, was the province of study by physiologists and physicians. The Cartesian separation of mind and body was challenged from a philosophical point of view already in the 17th century by Baruch Spinoza, who, in the *Principles of Cartesian Philosophy*[266] and the posthumously published trea-

---

[262] *Banks,* [1870] 5 Q.B. at 565.

[263] *In re* Conroy, 486 A.2d at 1225; *Malette,* 67 D.L.R.4th at 328; *Marion's Case,* 175 C.L.R. at 266-68, 272-73, 275, 309-10; *Airedale,* [1993] A.C. at 864-65.

[264] R. DESCARTES, THE PASSIONS OF THE SOUL (1649), *reprinted* in I THE PHILOSOPHICAL WORKS (E. Haladane & D. Ross trans. 1955).

[265] Brown, *Cartesian Dualism and Psychosomatics,* 30 PSYCHOSOMATICS 322 (1989); McCartan, *Monism and Dualism: New Lamps for Old,* 107 J. MENTAL SCI. 809 (1961); Einsenberg, *Disease and Illness,* 1 CULTURE, MED. & PSYCHIATRY 9 (1977); Langley & Brand, *The Mind-Body Issue in Early Twentieth-Century American Medicine,* 46 BULL. HISTORY MED. 171 (1972); D. KLEIN, A HISTORY OF SCIENTIFIC PSYCHOLOGY 339-59 (1970).

[266] B. SPINOZA, PRINCIPLES OF CARTESIAN PHILOSOPHY (1663) (H. Wedeck trans. reprinted 1961).

tise *Ethics*,[267] replaced the Cartesian theory of dualism with the concept of "psychological parallelism" according to which mind and body are inseparable. Mind and body form two aspects of the same entity—the living organism—which experiences its physiological processes psychologically as affects and thoughts. John Locke also repudiated the Cartesian interpretation of res cogitans, and the refusal by Descartes to endorse the old philosophical Latin maxim "nihil est in intellectu, quod non prius fuerit in sensu" (there is nothing in the realm of intellect (understanding) that did not originate from sensory perceptions).[268]

Toward the end of the 18th century in his *Critique of Pure Reason*[269] Immanuel Kant explored the nature of reason in the sense of cognition and the limits of the "knowing" process.[270] Having accepted that all knowledge begins with sensory experience, Kant analyzed how the "sensuous impressions"—intuitions (Anschauung) antecedent to perception—are converted into an experience and then organized by intellect into knowledge. Kant pointed out that "although all our knowledge begins with experience, it does not follow that it arises from experience."[271] Sensory impressions were for Kant occasions for the activation in the mind of the rules of understanding—identified with reason—which through the process of recognition and evaluation as well as categorization, helped the mind to conceptualize the original undifferentiated mass of sensory data into an "organized experience and the unity of consciousness."[272]

In 1858, Rudolf Virchow, in his book *Cellular Pathology Based on Physiological and Pathological Histology*,[273] demonstrated that the causes of the disease process lay in the disturbance of cellular pathology, and not in "invisible ethereal substances" as postulated by the medical followers of Descartes. Accordingly, Virchow suggested that disease could be explained best through changes in physiology and biochemistry of the organism, whereas illness was the subjective experience of suffering.[274] This approach to human homeostasis, which involves the physiological, sensory, and cognitive as well as affective functions, has been widely accepted by modern medicine. Nevertheless, it seems that the legacy of Cartesian separation of

---

[267] B. SPINOZA, ETHICS (W. Hale trans., revised A. Hutchison Stirling, 4th ed. 1937).

[268] D. KLEIN, *supra* note 265, at 357-58. Gottfried Wilhelm Leibnitz (1646-1716) later transformed the maxim by adding "nisi intellectu ipse": there is nothing in the intellect that had not originated in sensory experience, "except for the intellect itself." *Id.* at 375.

[269] I. Kant, *Critique of Pure Reason*, in KANT SELECTIONS (T. Green ed. 1929).

[270] D. KLEIN, *supra* note 265, at 482.

[271] I. KANT, *supra* note 269, at 26.

[272] D. KLEIN, *supra* note 265, at 487.

[273] R. VIRCHOW, DIE CELLULAR-PATHOLOGIE IN IHRER BEGRUNDUNG AUF PHYSIOLOGISCHE UND PATHOLOGISCHE GEWEBELEHRE (1858).

[274] Eisenberg, *supra* note 265; Jennings, *The Confusion Between Disease and Illness in Clinical Medicine*, 135 CAN. MED. A.J. 865 (1986).

mind and body still survives in the courts' analyses of the decision-making process and the decision itself.

It is arguable that the notion of the "sound mind" as legal standard based exclusively on the criterion of cognitive ability of the patient to understand what is being said to him or her, and to make an informed decision in an intellectual sense, is not the most suitable way of ascertaining that person's mental state in the context of a refusal of life-saving treatment, particularly when the decision is made during a medical crisis.[275] The English case of *Re T*[276] illustrates pressures that may impair the decision-making capacity of an adult patient in an emergency situation. Thirty-year-old Ms. T was injured in a car accident when she was 34 weeks pregnant. Though not a Jehovah's Witness herself, Ms. T was brought up by her divorced mother, a fervent member of the sect. The injured woman was admitted to a hospital, where, following diagnosis of pneumonia, she had to be given high doses of antibiotics, oxygen, and pethidine (a narcotic analgesic). After she went into labor, Ms. T was transferred by an ambulance to the labor ward. By that time, Ms. T had had two private conversations with her mother, and subsequently informed the midwife and the physician about her opposition to blood transfusions. The obstetrician assured her that a cesarean section did not usually necessitate a transfusion and, in response to her inquiry, said that other, less effective, procedures also were available. As the physician was leaving, the midwife produced a hospital form of refusal of consent to blood transfusions, which Ms. T signed and the midwife countersigned.[277]

Following an emergency cesarean operation the child was stillborn. Ms. T's condition seriously deteriorated and she was transferred to an intensive care unit. The medical opinion was that Ms. T needed a blood transfusion. She was put on a ventilator and paralyzing medications were administered. Ms. T remained sedated, though in critical condition, while her father, supported by the father of the baby, applied to the court for a declaration that it would not be unlawful for the hospital to administer a blood transfusion in the absence of her consent. Judge Ward granted the declaration, and the appeal from the Official Solicitor as guardian ad litem for Ms. T was dismissed by the Court of Appeal.[278] The court said that at the

---

[275] Gutheil, Bursztajn, Brodsky, & Alexander, *Affective Disorders, Competence, and Decision Making*, in DECISION MAKING IN PSYCHIATRY AND THE LAW (1991).

[276] [1992] 3 W.L.R. 782.

[277] The form was supposed to be countersigned by the medical practitioner, but it was not so signed. Although the form required that its contents and significance be explained to the patient, it was neither read nor explained to Ms. T.

[278] *Re T*, [1992] 3 W.L.R. at 795. The Court of Appeal recognized that apart from the narrow issue of whether Judge Ward's declaration should be affirmed or dismissed, the appeal also had a wider purpose of providing guidance to hospital authorities and to the medical profession on the appropriate response to the refusal by an adult to accept treatment. For a further discussion of this case, see Mendelson, *supra* note 4.

time she signed the hospital refusal of blood transfusion form, the patient was in considerable pain, she was suffering contractions in the first stage of labor, her consciousness was clouded by repeated doses of pethidine, and she was acting under the influence of her mother. In relation to the last factor, outside influences, that may compromise the voluntariness of the patient's decision to refuse life-saving treatment, Master of the Rolls, who delivered the leading judgment, pointed out that

> [t]he real question in each case is: "Does the patient really mean what he says or is he merely saying it for a quiet life, to satisfy someone else or because the advice and persuasion to which he has been subjected is such that he can no longer think and decide for himself?" When considering the effect of outside influences, two aspects can be of crucial importance. First, the strength of the will of the patient. One who is very tired, in pain or depressed will be much less able to resist having his will over-borne than one who is rested, free from pain and cheerful. Second, the relationship of the "persuader" to the patient may be of crucial importance. The influence of parents on their children or of one spouse on the other can be, but is by no means necessarily, much stronger than would be the case in other relationships.[279]

There are a number of reasons why the legal criteria involving the decision-making capacity of seriously medically impaired persons, including those who refuse life-saving treatment, should be different from the traditional approach, which has been developed in relation to determining the validity of consent amongst those who are physically and emotionally well.

The common-law jurisprudence has adopted the third principle of utilitarianism—that of strict impartiality, which precludes from consideration such subjective factors as personal condition, feelings, the effects of kinship, and religious or nationality affiliations—as the touchstone against which all legal standards are traditionally measured.[280] Lord Mustill in *Airedale NHS Trust v. Bland* expressed this rule in the following terms:

> If the patient is capable of making a decision on whether to permit treatment and decides not to permit it his choice must be obeyed, even if on any objective view it is contrary to his best interests. A doctor has no right to proceed in the face of objection, even if it is plain to all, including the patient, that adverse consequences and even death will or may ensue.[281]

Lord Mustill's analysis may be applicable without qualification to Mrs. Jones who, as a member of a particular religious congregation, had made a

---

[279] *Id.* at 797. Lord Donaldson MR added that arguments for refusal of treatment based upon religious beliefs when deployed by someone in a very close relationship with the patient, "should alert the doctors to the possibility—no more—that the patient's capacity or will to decide has been overborne. In other words, the patient may not mean what he says." *Id.*

[280] The utilitarian rule of impartiality fits in well with the common law's set of normative principles known as the rule of law, including the substantive principle of justice, which says that like should be treated alike, and that unfair discrimination should not be sanctioned by law.

[281] *Airedale*, [1993] A.C. at 891.

considered choice to follow the precepts of her creed long before the actual circumstances that necessitated blood transfusion eventuated.[282] However, it is questionable whether such an unqualified rule should be equally applicable to death-choices through refusal of life-saving treatment made by the systemically ill, the febrile, the depressed, those who suffer from psychoses and other mental disorders. The ability of psychiatry to understand human decision-making process has come a long way since Ballow's analysis of the nature of consent and the criteria for determining ''sound mind'' as applied in *Banks v. Goodfellow*. The time has come for reappraisal of these legal concepts in the light of modern medicine.

Medicine, and in particular psychiatry, recognizes that such factors as the patient's personality, affective disorder, medications, external pressures and the setting, may impair clinical competency, leading to a refusal of treatment. Disease is frequently accompanied by stress and/or pain, productive of depression, that may impair the patient's ability to function competently in processing and understanding medical information and making treatment decisions.[283] The prevalence of severe depression among patients who are medically ill has been estimated as being between 10% and 20%, with a prevalence rate of twice that among geriatric patients and those who are severely medically ill.[284] Interviews in the form of psychological or psychiatric autopsy with surviving relatives of suicides have found that a very large proportion (between 50% and 100%) of the deceased had suffered a psychiatric disorder, particularly depressive illness, in the period immediately preceding the suicide.[285] Susan Sorenson observed that ''the elderly, the emotionally stressed, and persons who lack stable connections with others appear to be the most frequent victims of suicide.''[286]

The law presumes that every adult individual is cognitively competent to make all medical decisions until proven otherwise.[287] The case of *In re*

---

[282] *See Malette*, 67 D.L.R.4th at 321, in which the defendant physician who administered blood transfusions to an unconscious card-carrying Jehovah's Witness was held liable for battery. The condition of the patient at the time was critical and transfusion was necessary to preserve her life. The physician argued that he was not satisfied that the card expressed the current view of the plaintiff.

[283] Sprung & Winick, *Informed Consent in Theory and Practice: Legal and Medical Perspectives on the Informed Consent Doctrine and a Proposed Reconceptualisation*, 17 CRIT. CARE MED. 1346 (1989); Winick, *Voluntary Hospitalization after* Zinermon v. Burch, 21 PSYCH. ANNALS 584 (1991).

[284] Meakin, *Screening for Depression in the Medically Ill: The Future of Paper and Pencil Tests*, 160 BRIT. J. PSYCHIATRY 212 (1992).

[285] Persons addicted to drugs or alcohol constituted a substantial minority of those who committed suicide. Levey, *Suicide*, in FORENSIC PSYCHIATRY, *supra* note 258, at 601-02; G. MENDELSON, PSYCHIATRIC ASPECTS OF PERSONAL INJURY CLAIMS (1988); Pokorny, *Prediction of Suicide in Psychiatric Patients*, 40 ARCH. GEN. PSYCHIATRY 249 (1983).

[286] Sorenson, *Suicide among the Elderly: Issues Facing Public Health*, 81 AM. J. PUB. HEALTH 1109, 1110 (1991). From 1980 through 1986, there were 36,798 suicides reported among United States residents over the age of 65 years. Meehan, Saltzman, & Sattin, *Suicides among Older United States Residents: Epidemiologic Characteristics and Trends*, 81 AM. J. PUB. HEALTH 1198, 1198 (1991).

[287] Sullivan & Youngner, *Depression, Competence, and the Right to Refuse Medical Treatment*, 151 AM. J. PSYCHIATRY 971 (1994).

AC^{288} is an example of the application of this legal rule. In this case, a 27-year-old patient, who was 25 weeks pregnant, and who had suffered from a variety of cancers since the age of 13, was admitted to the high-risk unit of the obstetrics department at George Washington University Hospital. The patient, Angela Carder, was diagnosed as being in a terminal stage of an inoperable tumor nearly filling her right lung. At the time the fetus reached 26½ weeks of gestation, its chances of survival were deteriorating, due to the seriousness of Ms. Carder's physical condition. When asked if she still wanted the baby, her answer appeared to be "I don't know; I guess so."[289]

The hospital petitioned for an emergency hearing to be held at the hospital before a judge of the Superior Court of the District of Columbia. The hospital sought a declaration that the cesarean section could be carried out if the patient refused permission. The operation was not intended to save or prolong the mother's life, but to provide a slim possibility of the 50% to 60% chance of survival for the fetus. At the time of the hearing, the judge found that due to heavy sedation and intubation, it was not clear what the patient's wishes were. Nevertheless, he granted the declaration. The baby was born alive, but died within three hours. The patient died of cancer two days later.[290] The District of Columbia Court of Appeals vacated the primary decision.[291] The majority stated that "in virtually all cases," a pregnant woman has the right to decide what is to be done on behalf of herself and the fetus.[292] It is the duty of the court to determine the patient's competency, and, if the patient is found incompetent or otherwise unable to give an informed consent to the proposed therapy, the judge must ascertain her wishes through the process of substituted judgment based on all the evidence.

Medical studies published during the last decade have noted that cognitive disorders are a frequent complication of cancer.[293] These studies show that patients with advanced terminal cancer often experience repeated episodes of cognitive failure[294] as recorded on the Mini-Mental State Question-

---

[288] 573 A.2d 1235 (D.C. App. 1990).

[289] Curran, *Court-Ordered Cesarean Sections Receive Judicial Defeat*, 323 NEW ENG. J. MED. 489, 490 (1990).

[290] The death certificate listed the cesarean section as a "contributing cause" of the patient's death.

[291] *AC*, 573 A.2d at 1248.

[292] *Id.* at 1247. For a discussion of the *AC* case, see Witting, *supra* note 386, at 200.

[293] Coyle, Adelhardt, Foley, & Portenoy, *Character of Terminal Illness in the Advanced Cancer Patient: Pain and Other Symptoms During the Last Four Weeks of Life*, 5 J. PAIN & SYMPTOM MNGMT. 83 (1990); Foley, *The Relationship of Pain and Symptom Management to Patient Requests for a Physician-Assisted Suicide*, 6 J. PAIN & SYMPTOM MNGMT. 289 (1991); Ramsay, *Referral to a Liaison Psychiatrist from a Palliative Care Unit*, 6 PALLIATIVE CARE 54 (1992).

[294] Bruera, Miller, McCallion, Macmillan, Krefting, & Hanson, *Cognitive Failure in Patients with Terminal Cancer: A Prospective Study*, 7 J. PAIN & SYMPTOM MNGMT. 192 (1992).

naire,[295] a screening test used for cognitive assessment.[296] A study using the Abbreviated Mental Test Score (AMTS) and a semistructured application of modified DSM III-R criteria for major depressive illness[297] found that 34% out of 87 terminally ill cancer patients displayed significant cognitive impairment. The principal determinants of cognitive impairment were age and proximity to death.

Cognitive failure in patients with advanced cancer may be caused by medications, sepsis, brain metastases, liver failure, renal failure, hypercalcemia, or hypoglycemia, amongst other possible precipitants. However, in the study by Bruera and colleagues,[298] no cause of cognitive failure could be established in 56% of cancer patients.[299] The available data suggested that cognitive failure was extremely frequent in patients with advanced cancer approximately 16 days before death.[300] Therefore, it has been postulated that cognitive failure may be part of an organic brain syndrome that represents the final stage in many dying patients.[301]

There are only two findings that are open to a tribunal that utilizes the legal standard of ''sound mind''—competence and incompetence. Yet, there are many levels of cognitive impairment. In an acute organic brain syndrome (delirium), the patient develops a global impairment of cognitive functioning, which may be mild and hence easy to overlook. In particular, mild delirium may not be recognized by the clinician if it is associated with only a slight degree of ''clouding of consciousness'' (impaired state of consciousness, which in severe delirium progresses to stupor or coma). Such cognitive failure usually manifests itself as disorientation in relation to time, place, and person. Its particular manifestations also include inability to sequence recent events, odd and inconsistent behavior, irritability, and suspiciousness. A well-developed syndrome may include such features as im-

---

[295] Folstein, Fetting, Lobo, Niaz, & Capozzoli, *Cognitive Assessment of Cancer Patients*, 53 CANCER 2150 (1984); Anthony, LeResche, Niaz, von Korff, & Folstein, *Limits of the ''Mini-Mental State'' as Screening Test for Dementia or Delirium among Hospital Patients*, 12 PSYCHOLOGICAL MED. 397 (1982).

[296] The Mini-Mental State test is specifically designed, through a series of 11 questions, to examine the memory registration and immediate recall, orientation, attention and calculation, short-term memory, and certain aspects of the use of language. The test also evaluates the patient's ability to follow verbal or written commands and his or her constructional ability. The patient's answers are scored, and the level of impairment assessed on the basis of the score out of 30 points. G. MENDELSON, *supra* note 285, at 44.

[297] Power, Kelly, Gilsenan, Kearney, O'Mahony, Walsh, & Coakley, *Suitable Screening Tests for Cognitive Impairment and Depression in the Terminally Ill—A Prospective Prevalence Study*, 7 PALLIATIVE MED. 213 (1993).

[298] Bruera, et al., *supra* note 294.

[299] *Id.* at 194.

[300] More than 80% of cancer patients developed cognitive failure before death in a study reported by Bruera, Fainsinger, Miller, & Kuehn, *The Assessment of Pain Intensity in Patients with Cognitive Failure: A Preliminary Report*, 7 J. PAIN & SYMPTOM MNGMT. 267, 269 (1992).

[301] Bruera, et al., *supra* note 294, at 195.

paired concentration and memory, together with reduced awareness of and responsiveness to the environment.[302] The speech of a person suffering from acute cognitive failure may be characterized by restriction of content, repetition, and perseveration.[303]

Perhaps the most important aspects of acute cognitive failure that need to be considered when a patient is making vital life and death decisions in a clinical setting are the changes that occur with respect to thought content and organic mood changes. These changes may involve impoverishment of intellectual function manifesting itself as concrete thinking—the inability to abstract the sense of what is said from its literal meaning—as well as emotional liability, at times involving a sense of bewilderment that may verge on fear or terror. In extreme cases of delirium, the patient may develop delusions, as well as manifesting cognitive impairment and clouding of consciousness.

In a recent study, Grisso and Appelbaum[304] have investigated decision-making capacity among three groups of hospitalized patients: those with diagnoses of schizophrenia, major depression and ischemic heart disease (angina pectoris), and an equal cohort of community subjects matched on age, race, gender, education, and occupation. Each subject was tested for the ability to (1) express a choice; (2) to ''understand the treatment discourse'' in the sense of understanding information relevant to the decision about treatment; (3) to appreciate the significance of his or her own situation of the information disclosed about the illness and possible treatments (perceptions of the disorder, nonacknowledgment of disorder); and (4) to manipulate the information rationally (or reason about it) in a manner that allows for making comparisons and weighing opinions.[305]

The study found that whereas only a few subjects were unable to express a choice, there were significant differences between the performance of the groups in relation to the three remaining measures. In particular, it is of concern that a substantial number of subjects who performed adequately on one measure revealed impaired performance on another. Thus, of the 72% of subjects with schizophrenia who performed adequately on the understanding measure, 24.1% had impaired performance on appreciation and 14.8% on reasoning.[306] When, in accordance with the legal standard for competency, all measures are compounded, 52% of subjects with schizophrenia would be considered as having impaired capacity to make treatment decisions. Comparable figures for the other groups were

---

[302] W. Fulford, *Organic Psychiatric Disorders*, in ESSENTIAL PSYCHIATRY 110 (N. Rose ed. 1988).

[303] *Id.* at 111.

[304] Grisso & Appelbaum, *Comparison of Standards for Assessing Patients' Capacities to Make Treatment Decisions*, 152 AM. J. PSYCHIATRY 1033 (1995).

[305] *Id.* at 1033.

[306] *Id.* at 1035.

52   MENDELSON

23.9% for patients with major depression, 12.2% for the group with angina
pectoris, and 4% for the three community comparison groups combined.[307]

The law needs to be more attuned to the reality of medical illness as
understood by modern medicine, and to take into account the subtle distinctions in cognitive competency. Moreover, while separating the actual
decision from the cognition-oriented decision-making process may have
some merit, in cases where the choice of life-style is in issue, such separation is inappropriate when applied to cases where the choice is between
life and death. The legal definition of "sound mind" would not exclude a
person with a paranoid disorder, who insists that he or she does not suffer
from the given condition, and is thus quite eager to declare that no treatment
should be undertaken. Yet, as the Grisso and Appelbaum study illustrates,
it is common in paranoid conditions for the person's cognitive functioning
to remain intact. Such a person can appear to have a thorough understanding
of the risks and benefits of the treatment, or of alternative treatments,
without actually being able to interpret these data as relevant in the context
of his or her own situation.[308] It has been claimed that persons suffering from
paranoid conditions,[309] or from serious affective disorders,[310] "constitute the
largest population of treatment refusers."[311]

In the case of *Re T*,[312] Lord Donaldson MR emphasized that the patient's right to choose death should be held paramount only after "a very
careful examination of whether, and if so the way in which"[313] the patient
was exercising that right. "In case of doubt, that doubt falls to be resolved
in favour of preservation of life for if the individual is to override the public
interest, he must do so in clear terms."[314] He expressed the rules pertaining
to the patient's capacity to make legally binding choices concerning medical
treatment in the following way:

> (1) Prima facie every adult has the right and capacity to decide whether or not he
> will accept medical treatment, even if a refusal may risk permanent injury to his
> health or even lead to premature death. Furthermore, it matters not whether the
> reasons for the refusal were rational or irrational, unknown or even non-existent.
> This is so, notwithstanding the very strong public interest in preserving the life and

[307] *Id*. at 1036.

[308] Roth, Appelbaum, Sallee, Reynolds, & Huber, *The Dilemma of Denial in the Assessment of Competency to Refuse Treatment*, 139 AM. J. PSYCHIATRY 910 (1982).

[309] *Id*.

[310] Hoge, Appelbaum, & Lawlor, *A Prospective Multicenter Study of Patients' Refusal of Anti-psychotic
Medication*, 47 ARCH. GEN. PSYCHIATRY 949 (1990).

[311] Bursztajn, et al., *supra* note 259. *See also* Levin, Brekke, & Thomas, *A Controlled Comparison of
Involuntary Hospitalized Medication Refusers and Acceptors*, 19 BULL. AM. ACAD. PSYCHIATRY &
L. 161 (1991) (in some jurisdictions in the United States involuntarily hospitalized psychiatric
patients have the right to refuse medication).

[312] [1992] 3 W.L.R. 782.

[313] *Id*. at 798.

[314] *Id*. at 796.

health of all citizens. However, the presumption of capacity to decide, which stems from the fact that the patient is an adult, is rebuttable. (2) An adult patient may be deprived of his capacity to decide by long-term mental incapacity . . . (3) If an adult patient did not have the capacity to decide at the time of the purported refusal and still does not have that capacity, it is the duty of the doctors to treat him in whatever way they consider, in the exercise of clinical judgment, to be in his best interests. (4) Doctors faced with a refusal of consent have to give very careful and detailed consideration to what was the patient's capacity to decide at the time when the decision was made. It may not be a case of capacity or no capacity. It may be a case of reduced capacity. What matters is whether at that time the patient's capacity was reduced below the level needed in the case of a refusal of that importance, for refusals can vary in importance. Some may involve a risk to life or of irreparable damage to health. Others may not.[315]

These rules apparently were applied by Thorpe J in the 1994 case of *Re C (Adult: Refusal of Treatment)*,[316] when the High Court of England was asked to grant an injunction restraining the hospital from carrying out an amputation without the patient's express written consent. The case involved a 68-year-old man, Mr. C, who was an emigrant to England of Jamaican origin. His passage was paid for by a woman who left him five years after his arrival. A year later he accosted her at work and after an altercation stabbed her. Mr. C was sentenced to a seven-year term of imprisonment, but on being diagnosed as suffering from chronic paranoid schizophrenia, was transferred to a Broadmoor secure hospital. Over the years, he had been treated with medications and ECT. In 1994, Mr. C knocked his left foot in a shower and some three weeks later developed gangrene in that foot.

At a general hospital, the consultant surgeon told Mr. C that unless his leg was amputated below the knee, he would die within a very short time. His prognosis was that at best, Mr. C had a 15% chance of survival without amputation. Mr. C refused to consent to the amputation. However, he was persuaded to agree to a treatment with antibiotics, and then a debridement of the dead tissue under a general anesthetic. Mr. C said he would rather die with two feet than live with one. He expressed grandiose delusions of an international career in medicine during the course of which he had never lost a patient. He affirmed his complete confidence in his ability to survive his present trials aided by God, the "good doctors," and the "good nurses."[317]

Mr. C was seen by three psychiatrists, including Dr. Eastman, a lecturer and a senior consultant in psychiatry at St. George hospital, who explained that schizophrenia is an all-pervasive illness. Features present in Mr. C's case included grandiose and persecutory delusions as well as an incongruity of affect—Mr. C's words did not match the emotions which he

---

[315] *Id.* at 799.
[316] [1994] All E.R. 819.
[317] *Id.* at 822. Mr. C also declared his complete faith in God and, subject to one reservation, in the Bible.

displayed. According to Dr. Eastman, although Mr. C appeared to understand the information about the possible treatments and their outcomes, he did not believe it, and so was unable to weigh the information provided to him, that is, to determine the risks and benefits involved in relation to his own condition. Dr. Eastman considered that Mr. C did not believe in the imminence of his death because of his mental illness. Dr. Eastman indicated that the ultimate conclusion should be reached "by weighing in the scales the preservation of life against the autonomy of the patient. If the patient's capacity to decide is unimpaired, autonomy weighs heavier, but the further capacity is reduced, the lighter the autonomy weighs."[318] The other two psychiatrists agreed with Dr. Eastman's assessment. However, Mr. Rutter, the consultant vascular surgeon, believed in "the sanctity of the individual choice, even if it be wrong"[319] and argued that the amputation should not be performed against the patient's wishes.

Thorpe J of the Family Division of the High Court of England, agreed with Mr. Rutter, and granted an injunction to prevent surgeons from operating on Mr. C's leg without his consent. The judge declared that the presumption in favor of Mr. C's right of self-determination had not been displaced, and his choice not to undergo the amputation had to be respected. In coming to his conclusion, Thorpe J used the legal criterion of "sound mind," which disregards the patient's affective function, including the presence of major functional disorders such as schizophrenia and depression.

There are also some psychopathological conditions in which the individual manifests illness behavior considered to be "abnormal," that is, out of keeping with the objective evidence of disease.[320] A person's illness behavior may be characterized as "abnormal" in cases where there is

> the persistence of an inappropriate or maladaptive mode of perceiving, evaluating or acting in relation to one's own state of health, despite the fact that a doctor (or other appropriate social agent) has offered an accurate and reasonably lucid explanation of the nature of the illness and the appropriate course of management to be followed, based on a thorough examination of all parameters of functioning, and taking into account the individual's age, educational and sociocultural background.[321]

Abnormal illness behavior can take several forms of illness denial.[322] Illness denial may be motivated by a conscious desire to obtain employment, by guilt and shame, by fear of the stigma and discrimination associated with

---

[318] *Id.*

[319] *Id.* at 823.

[320] Pilowsky, *Abnormal Illness Behaviour: A Review of the Concept and Its Implications,* in ILLNESS BEHAVIOUR: A MULTIDISCIPLINARY MODEL 391 (S. McHugh & T. Vallis eds. 1986).

[321] *Id.* at 393.

[322] There are also forms of abnormal illness affirmance, such as Munchausen's Syndrome, factitious disorders, somatoform disorders, hypochondriacal delusions, and the like.

psychiatric symptomatology, or by hope to avoid feared therapies such as chemotherapy and radiotherapy. Sometimes illness denial may have unconscious motivation, such as neurotic noncompliance following myocardial infarction or refusal to accept psychological diagnosis or treatment in the presence of neurotic illness, personality disorder, or drug dependency syndromes. Persons suffering from psychotic depression, manic states, and schizophrenic disorders often present with denial of illness, including somatic pathology. Patients with neuropsychiatric syndromes, such as Korsakoff's psychosis caused by alcohol abuse, also tend to present with confabulatory reactions to illness.[323]

Subtle, or even overt, pressures by family, and sometimes by clinical personnel, may impair the affective function of a patient and morbidly distort his or her view of life leading to refusal of life-saving treatment.[324] Finally, on a sociocultural level, it has been noted that the fundamental shift of traditional values from solicitude and benevolence to patient autonomy and self-fulfilment has had the effect not only of eroding community support for expensive long-term care, but also has affected the self-esteem of the afflicted persons.[325] In this context, one may ponder whether the advocacy of an unqualified right to refuse life-saving treatment is prompted as much by belief in an inalienable right to self-determination as by other, less benevolent, personal and communitarian interests.

The traditional state interest in preservation of life based upon the cost to the community of supporting the family of a person who dies as a result of refusing medical treatment has lost its cogency in the reality of health care economics in the 1990s.[326] For instance, in the United States, approximately 30% of the Medicare budget is spent on medical treatment during the last year of its beneficiaries' lives.[327] The cost of hospital care for an adult patient in a persistent vegetative state for the first three months has been estimated at approximately $149,200, and the costs of long-term care at a nursing facility tend to range from $126,000 to $180,000 per year. Annual cost of home care for children in a persistent vegetative state is estimated at $129,000 for the first year, and $97,000 for subsequent years.[328] While the

---

[323] Pilowsky, *supra* note 320, at 393. Anosognosia, which refers to the apparent unawareness of, or failure to recognize, one's own functional defect (hemiplegia, hemianopia) is a well-known neurological deficit, which also comes within the category of abnormal illness behavior.

[324] Simon, *Silent Suicide in the Elderly*, 17 BULL. AM. ACAD. PSYCHIATRY & L. 83 (1989); Howe, *From the Editor*, 2 J. CLINICAL ETHICS 79 (1991).

[325] Allert, Sponholz, & Baitsch, *Chronic Disease and the Meaning of Old Age*, 24 HASTINGS CENTER REP. 11 (Sept./Oct. 1994).

[326] Malcolm, *Trends in Primary Medical Care Related to Services and Expenditure in New Zealand 1983-1993*, 106 N.Z. MED. J. 470 (1993).

[327] Annas & Miller, *The Empire of Death: How Culture and Economics Affect Informed Consent in the US, the UK, and Japan*, 20 AM. J. L. & MED. 357 (1994).

[328] The Multi-Society Task Force on PVS, *Medical Aspects of Persistent Vegetative State (Part II)*, 330

cost of care for the chronically ill is very high,[329] so is the expense involved
in the provision of certain drugs,[330] and such life-saving treatment as heart,
lung, and liver transplantations.[331] The resurgence of home medical care has
been accompanied by financial and emotional strains on the care providers.[332]

Legislative efforts to facilitate patient refusal of treatment, by way of
such instruments as living wills, advance directives, and their variations[333] is
aimed at furthering the interest in self-determination. However, there is also
an expectation that costs associated with end-of-life medical care will
thereby be substantially contained.[334] The doctrine of the "human capital,"
which is one of the most influential determinants of the nature and the level
of funding of the health care system by governments, measures the strictly
economic costs of disease.[335] The aim of this method of evaluating the value
of life is to "remind the society that the burdens of disease are borne not
only by the sick but by all those who would benefit from the contribution to
society that would be made if the patient were whole again,"[336] or, alter-

---

New Eng. J. Med. 1572 (1994); Arno, Bonuck, & Padgug, *The Economic Impact of High Technology Home Care*, 24 Hastings Center Rep. S15 (Sept./Oct. 1994).

[329] Whereas before World War II most deaths in the United States were caused by infectious diseases
such as tuberculosis and pneumonia, today more than 75% of deaths of people over age 65 result from
chronic degenerative diseases. Link, *Recent American Developments in the Right to Die: The* Cruzan
Case, Living Wills, Durable Powers and Family Consensus Statutes, in Decision-Making and
Problems of Incompetence 219 (A. Grubb ed. 1994).

[330] Richards, Braysher, Gregory, & Rubens, *Advanced Breast Cancer: Use of Resources and Cost
Implications*, 67 Brit. J. Cancer 856 (1993).

[331] Evans, Manninen, & Dong, *An Economic Analysis of Liver Transplantation: Costs, Insurance
Coverage, and Reimbursement*, 22 Gastroenterol. Clin. North. Am. 451 (1993); Evans, Man-
ninen, & Dong, *An Economic Analysis of Heart-Lung Transplantation: Costs, Insurance Coverage,
and Reimbursement*, 105 J. Thorac. Cardiovasc. Surg. 972 (1993); Dodson, Ingraham, Millikan,
Henderson, Ricketts, Galloway, Olson, Caplan, Schoen, & Perlino, *Pediatric Liver Transplantation
in Georgia: A Paradigm for the Health Care Crisis in the United States?*, 60 Am. Surg. 118 (1994);
Loisance & Sailly, *Cost-Effectiveness in Patients Awaiting Transplantation Receiving Intravenous
Inotropic Support*, 8 Eur. J. Anaesthesiol. Supp. 913 (1993).

[332] Arras & Dubler, *Bringing the Hospital Home: Ethical and Social Implications of High-Tech Home
Care*, 24 Hastings Center Rep. S19 (Sept./Oct. 1994); Brakman, *Adult Daughter Caregivers*, 24
Hastings Center Rep. 26 (Sept./Oct. 1994); Snelling, *The Effect of Chronic Pain on the Family
Unit*, 19 J. Adv. Nurs. 543 (1994); Doyal & Wilsher, *Withholding and Withdrawing Life Sustaining
Treatment from Elderly People: Towards Formal Guidelines*, 308 Brit. Med. J. 1689 (1994).

[333] These instruments empower people who anticipate that they may become unconscious while being
under or in need of medical treatment to refuse beforehand administration of life-saving treatment.

[334] The provisions of the Patient Self-Determination Act, 42 U.S.C. § 139cc (f)(1)(A)(i) (Supp. V 1993)
stipulate that every patient being admitted to a health care facility that receives Medicare or Medicaid
funds must be informed about, and provided an opportunity to sign an advance directive. Persels,
Forcing the Issue of Physician-Assisted Suicide, 14 J. Legal Med. 93 (1993); Annas & Miller, *supra*
note 327, at 368. *See also* Emanuel & Emanuel, *The Economics of Dying: The Illusion of Cost
Savings at the End of Life*, 330 New Eng. J. Med. 540 (1994).

[335] Robinson, *Philosophical Origins of the Economic Valuation of Life*, 64 Milbank Q. 133 (1986).

[336] *Id.* at 150.

natively, savings that accrue to the health care system whenever a patient decides to refuse expensive medical treatment, or requests that his or her now "unproductive" life be terminated.[337] It is true that in the context of end-of-life management, provision of high quality palliative care is much more important to the welfare of patients and their families than the employment of life-sustaining "heroic medicine," when its aim merely is to prolong the biological existence of hopelessly ill patients at the cost of their increased suffering. This change in emphasis, however, should not be motivated by the economic concern to save scarce and expensive medical resources. Rather, provision of palliative care should be grounded in the deontological respect for human life regardless of a person's sex, age, creed, or physical or mental status, coupled with acknowledgment that death is an integral and inevitable part of life.[338]

Studies have demonstrated that patients, particularly those with serious injuries, such as spinal cord injury, tend to suffer from depression in the early stages of their treatment, which often manifests itself in an express wish to die.[339] This condition presumably would be compounded when such a patient is also a prisoner. It is imperative that in a civilized society, patients who are prisoners should enjoy rights to self-determination with respect to medical treatment that are no less valuable than those enjoyed by other patients. However, the determination as to whether these patients are truly competent to make life and death choices should not be made on the basis of normative principles, in disregard of their actual affective state and their legal status.

In the United States, in the case of *Thor v. Superior Court of Solano County*,[340] the Supreme Court of California quoted John Stuart Mill's statement that "[o]ver himself, over his own body and mind, the individual is

---

[337] The Northern Territory Rights of the Terminally Ill Act, 1995 (RTIA) received assent on June 16, 1995 in Australia. This law was enacted to "confirm the right of a terminally ill person to request assistance from a medically qualified person to voluntarily terminate his or her life in a humane manner; to allow for such assistance to be given in certain circumstances without legal impediment to the person rendering the assistance," and to provide procedural protection against the possibility of abuse of the rights recognized by the legislation.

[338] Miller, *Denial of Health Care and Informed Consent in English and American Law*, 18 AM. J. L. & MED. 37 (1992); Henry, *Debits and Credits in the Management of Depression*, 20 BRIT. J. PSYCHIATRY SUPP. 33 (1993); Healy, *Psychopharmacology and the Ethics of Resource Allocation*, 162 BRIT. J. PSYCHIATRY 23 (1993); Metcalf, *Is Heart Transplantation a Wise Use of Scarce Health Care Dollars?*, 149 CAN. MED. A.J. 1829 (1993) (editorial); Mehlman & Massey, *The Patient-Physician Relationship and the Allocation of Scarce Resources: A Law and Economic Approach*, 4 KENNEDY INSTIT. ETHICS J. 291 (1994).

[339] Burrows, Judd, Buchanan, & Brown, *Does Depression Negate the Right to Die?*, in THE MAJOR PSYCHOSES AND THE DIVERSITY OF PSYCHIATRY 55-58 (G. Burrows, D. Copolv, B. Singh, & P. Beumont eds. 1986).

[340] 855 P.2d 375 (Cal. 1993).

sovereign''[341] when it decided that Howard Andrews, a prisoner serving a 15-year-to-life sentence for murder, had the right to reject medical treatment, even if it meant that he would die. Andrews became quadriplegic as a result of a jump or a fall from a cell tier at California's Folsom Prison in 1991. At the medical facility at Vacaville, staff psychiatrists who examined Andrews found him "depressed about his quadriplegic condition but mentally competent to understand and appreciate his circumstances."[342] In its brief as an amicus curiae, the California Medical Association argued that the possible inadequacy of medical and other services in prison may compromise the voluntary and rational nature of an inmate's decision. Consequently, when a prisoner refuses life-saving medical treatment, there should be a mandatory judicial hearing to assess the impact of the prison environment on the prisoner's decision-making capacity. In rejecting this suggestion, the court took judicial notice of the presumption that the "medical facilities within prison walls meet the same professional standards as those without,"[343] and of the "constitutional and administrative protections guaranteeing an inmate a proper treatment."[344] The court ruled that a proposal for a mandatory judicial hearing "tends to denigrate the principle of personal autonomy, substituting a species of legal paternalism for the medical paternalism the concept of informed consent seeks to eschew," and declared that " '[r]ationality' is for the patient to determine."[345]

The modern law has been so zealous to secure the individual a right to self-determination that it has lost sight of the wider humanitarian considerations and compassionate principles that play an important part in protecting the vulnerable, the depressed, and the disabled.

C. The Nature of Physician-Patient Relationship

Roscoe Pound pointed out that the legal tradition of common law displays a certain jurisprudential dichotomy. While it focuses upon an individual and zealously guards individual rights, it also tends to impose duties and liabilities upon those standing in certain relations as members of a class rather than upon individuals.[346]

The third factor considered by Justice Skelly Wright in *Application of President & Directors of Georgetown College* was the issue of competing autonomies—the individual autonomy of the patient and the professional autonomy of the attending physicians. The modern jurisprudence has yet to find a clear answer to the problem presented by patients who voluntarily

---

[341] *Id.* at 380 (quoting J. MILL, *supra* note 156, at 13).
[342] *Id.* at 379.
[343] *Id.* at 390.
[344] *Id.*
[345] *Id.* at 389.
[346] R. POUND, THE SPIRIT OF THE COMMON LAW 14 (1921).

come to the hospital but who, once there, choose to exercise their right to refuse life-saving treatment, thereby placing the hospital and medical personnel in a position of potential legal liability for either going ahead with nonconsensual treatment or for allowing the patient to die.[347]

The physician-patient relationship as presented in *Corpus Hippocraticum,* or even in Percival's *Medical Ethics,* has undergone profound changes in the past 200 years.[348] In the Hippocratic tradition, the responsibility for making clinical treatment decisions was delegated to physicians in the belief that their clinical training, a degree of emotional detachment, and the ethical ideals expressed in the Hippocratic Oath,[349] would best qualify them to accurately diagnose and suggest treatment options that were in the best interests of each particular patient.[350] Nevertheless, with regard to the issue of consent, the traditional Hippocratic approach has been modified in accordance with modern social and cultural expectations. Physicians have come to realize that in the necessarily unequal physician-patient relationship, where the medical practitioner has expertise from which the patient hopes to benefit, seeking a consensual approach based upon an adequate disclosure of relevant information goes some way toward ameliorating the ethical dynamics of the relationship. Disclosure of treatment options and discussion of their respective advantages and disadvantages promotes the principle of non-maleficence (discussed below) without derogating from the clinical autonomy of the treating physician. This modified approach presupposes that, insofar as it is practicable, the role and duty of the physician is to work together with the patient toward the therapeutic goals they have arrived at in consultation.

In law, the relationship between patient and physician is today generally regarded as at least partly grounded in the law of contract. Thus, in the English case of *Sidaway v. Board of Governors of the Bethlem Royal Hospital and the Maudsley Hospital*[351] while considering a patient's right to be informed, Lord Templeman observed that "the relationship between doctor and patient is contractual in origin, the doctor performing services in consideration for fees payable by the patient." This notion, though not entirely accurate, presupposes that for a fee, the patient gets the medical practitioner to "service" his or her health. Although unarticulated, the concept of human health as a form of commodity, coupled with the 19th century's principle of freedom of contract, has been as much responsible for affording

---

[347] *Georgetown College,* 331 F.2d at 1009.

[348] A detailed examination of different characterizations of the nature of the physician-patient relationship in law and medicine is too far removed from the main subject of this article.

[349] "I will come for the benefit of the sick, remaining free of all intentional injustice." L. EDELSTEIN, *supra* note 63, at 6.

[350] N. LAOR & J. AGASSI, EPISTEME 15: DIAGNOSIS: PHILOSOPHICAL AND MEDICAL PERSPECTIVES (1990). This kind of approach has been labeled as "paternalistic."

[351] [1985] A.C. 871, 904.

jurisprudential legitimacy to the doctrine that "every human being of adult years and sound mind has a right to determine what shall be done with his own body,"[352] as was the tort-based principle of bodily integrity. Contractual approach, centered as it is on the doctrine of consenting minds, can operate only in circumstances where the wishes of the consenting parties are known. Jurisprudential problems created by the underlying assumption about the contractual nature of the physician-patient relationship are evident in the inability of the law to develop a unified conceptual framework to deal with the issue of withholding or withdrawal of life-sustaining treatment from incompetent persons whose wishes in relation to medical treatment are unknown.[353] The more jurisprudentially satisfactory resolution of this issue can be found within the covenantal model of the physician-patient relationship, based on the best interests standard.

Perhaps due to the perception of health as a commodity, some courts in the United States, Canada, and New Zealand have started to characterize the rights and obligations of medical practitioners and their patients as fiduciary.[354] For instance, in the case of *McInerny v. MacDonald*[355] the Supreme Court of Canada identified the relationship between the physician and the patient with "that which exists in equity between a parent and his child, a man and his wife, an attorney and his client, a confessor and his penitent, and a guardian and his ward" and classified it as "as a fiduciary or trust relationship."[356] The court determined that the fiduciary nature of the relationship obligated the physician "to act with utmost good faith and loyalty and to hold information received from or about a patient in confidence."[357] The characterization of the physician-patient relationship as fiduciary does not accord with the principles of equity. The fiduciary relationship of trust and confidence arises where one party to the relationship assumes the obligation to act in the other's proprietary interests.[358] The adjective "confidential" in a trusting relationship is used to indicate the attribute of "trust and confidence." However, the term "confidential" is

---

[352] *Schloendorff*, 105 N.E. at 93.

[353] Mendelson, *supra* note 241.

[354] Emmett v. Eastern Dispensary and Cas. Hosp., 396 F.2d 931 (D.C. Cir. 1967); Cannell v. Medical & Surgical Clinic, 315 N.E.2d 278 (Ill. App. 1974); Norberg v. Wynrib, 92 D.L.R.4th 449 (1992).

[355] 93 D.L.R.4th 415 (1992).

[356] *Id.* at 423.

[357] *Id.* The fiduciary duty involved not only provision of information concerning the patient's health in the physician's medical records, but extended to "the obligation to grant access to the information the doctor uses in administering treatment." *Id.* at 424.

[358] This kind of trusting relation is characteristic of partnership, agency, trusteeship, the relationship between employer and employee, solicitor and client, as well as companies and directors. A gain derived through breach of a "trusting relationship" may be reversed through equity's gain-stripping remedies. J. GLOVER, COMMERCIAL EQUITY FIDUCIARY RELATIONSHIPS 6 (1995).

used in a different legal sense when it designates a relationship that is formed whenever one party imparts to another private or secret information in reliance upon the express or implied acceptance by the party in the position of a confidant that the communication is for a restricted purpose.[359]

Indeed, in *Sidaway v. Governors of Bethlem Royal Hospital*,[360] Dunn LJ, in the English Court of Appeal, said that the fiduciary rule ''has been confined to cases involving disposition of property, and has never been applied to the nature of the duty which lies upon a doctor . . . .''[361] On appeal, Lord Scarman also rejected the notion that the relationship between patient and physician is of a fiduciary character that would entitle the patient to relief in the event of a breach of fiduciary duty by the medical practitioner.[362] Lord Scarman stated that

> there is no comparison to be made between the relationship of doctor and patient with that of solicitor and client, trustee and cestui qui trust or the other relationships treated in equity as of a fiduciary character. Nevertheless, the relationship of doctor and patient is a very special one, the patient putting his health and his life in the doctor's hands.[363]

Following a thorough examination of the subject in Australia, the majority of the Court of Appeal of the New South Wales Supreme Court[364] approved the reasoning in the judgment of Lord Scarman and rejected the labeling of the physician-patient relationship as fiduciary. Justice Mahoney pointed out that although

> the law requires a doctor to act with the utmost good faith and loyalty to his patient and to hold information given to him by the patient in confidence . . . it is wrong to infer from such obligations that a more general relationship—trustee or fiduciary—exists . . . . A doctor is plainly not a trustee vis-à-vis his patient.[365]

Unless the physician holds in trust for the patient identifiable items of

---

[359] Stephens v. Avery, [1988] 2 All E.R. 477, 482 (Sir Nicholas Browne-Wilkinson). Equity may provide injunctive and restitutionary remedies for breach of the duty of confidentiality.

[360] [1984] 1 Q.B. 493 (C.A.).

[361] *Id.* at 515.

[362] *Sidaway*, [1985] A.C. at 884.

[363] *Id.*

[364] Breen v. Williams (Ct. App. Sup. Ct. New South Wales, Dec. 23, 1994) (unreported) (Kirby, P., Mahoney, and Meagher, JJ.A.). In this case, the plaintiff argued, inter alia, that the fiduciary relationship between a medical practitioner and a patient creates an interest held by the patient in all medical records produced by the physician in relation to the administration of treatment. The physician's fiduciary duty of loyalty and care to the patient obligates the physician to allow the right of physical access to all documents whenever the patient or his or her agent makes a request, rather than through the process of the court's subpoena. The majority of the Court of Appeal rejected this argument.

[365] *Id.*

property, use of such terms as "fiduciary" or "trustee" does not represent accurate statement of the law and consequently "confuses rather than assists proper legal analysis of relationships and of what, in law, results from them."[366] To sum up, a physician patient relationship has some fiducial characteristics, yet, the essential element of a trusteeship over another person's property rights is missing.[367] Therefore, although the relationship between physician and patient is classified as "confidential" and one of dependence, these features alone do not transform it into a "fiduciary" or "trust relationship" as those terms are used in the law of equity.[368] It is more appropriate to use covenantal terminology when referring to a physician-patient relationship.

D. Consent and Clinical Decision-Making

Agreement is an essential element of a covenantal relationship. Lord Donaldson MR originally defined the role of consent to medical treatment in the following way: "Consent by itself creates no obligation to treat. It is merely a key which unlocks the door."[369] In a subsequent judgment he qualified this statement when he said: "On reflection I regret my use in *Re R* of the keyholder analogy, because keys can lock as well as unlock. I now prefer the analogy of a legal 'flak jacket' which protects the doctor from claims by the litigious."[370]

Thus, in the case of *In re J (A Minor)*,[371] the Court of Appeal said that neither a patient nor a court has any statutory or common-law right to insist that a particular treatment or intensive care be provided to the patient when such therapy is not medically indicated.[372] The case involved an 18-month-old child, J, who at the age of one month sustained serious head injuries that rendered him profoundly mentally and physically handicapped, suffering from microcephaly, cerebral palsy, cortical blindness, and severe epilepsy. He was considered unlikely to develop greatly beyond his present state and had an uncertain but shortened life expectancy. J's intermittent convulsive attacks required resuscitative treatment in the hospital, and in December of

---

[366] *Id.* (Mahoney, J.).

[367] United States Surgical Corp. v. Hospital Products Ltd., 157 C.L.R. 41 (1984); Hawkins v. Clayton, 164 C.L.R. 539, 553-54 (1988). In Moore v. Regents of the Univ. of Cal., 221 Cal. Rptr. 146, 150 (Cal. 1990), the Supreme Court of California, pointed out that "a physician is not the patient's financial adviser."

[368] *Cf. Emmett,* 396 F.2d at 931; *Cannell,* 315 N.E.2d at 278; *McInerny,* 93 D.L.R.4th at 415. For an incisive critique of labeling the physician-patient relationship as fiduciary in the judgment of La Forest, J. in *McInerny,* see Breen v. Williams (Sup. Ct. New South Wales, Equity Div. Oct. 10, 1994) (unreported) (Bryson, J.); Breen v. Williams (Ct. App. Sup. Ct. New South Wales, Dec. 23, 1994) (unreported) (Mahoney & Meagher, J.J.). *See also* Mehlman & Massey, *supra* note 338.

[369] *In re R* (A Minor, Wardship: Consent to Treatment), [1992] Fam. 11, 22.

[370] *In re W* (A Minor, Medical Treatment: Court's Jurisdiction), [1992] 3 W.L.R. 758, 767.

[371] [1992] 3 W.L.R. 507, 516.

[372] Id. at 516, 519-20 (Belacombe & Leggatt, L.JJ., concurring).

1991, the consultant pediatrician considered that it was medically inappropriate to use mechanical ventilation procedures for any future resuscitation. Asked to determine whether artificial ventilation and other life-saving treatment should be administered to J, the Court of Appeal held that medical practitioners should not be required to treat patients in a manner contrary to their clinical judgment and professional duty.

In the leading judgment, Lord Donaldson MR presented the following analysis of this issue:

> I have to say that I cannot at present conceive of any circumstances in which this would be other than an abuse of power as directly or indirectly requiring the practitioner to act contrary to the fundamental duty which he owes to the patient. This, subject to obtaining any necessary consent, is to treat the patient in accordance with his own best clinical judgment, notwithstanding that other practitioners who are not called upon to treat the patient may have formed a quite different judgment or that the court, acting on expert evidence, may disagree with him.[373]

Quoting from an earlier decision,[374] the judge explained the legal relationship between physicians and those who have the right to make decisions on behalf of incompetent patients in the following way:

> No one can dictate the treatment to be given to the child—neither court, parents nor doctors. There are checks and balances. The doctors can recommend treatment A in preference to treatment B. They can also refuse to adopt treatment C on the grounds that it is medically contra-indicated or for some reason is a treatment which they could not conscientiously administer. The court or parents for their part can refuse to consent to treatment A or B or both, but cannot insist upon treatment C.[375]

Leggatt LJ noted that the Court of Appeal has not given to physicians any right they did not previously have by ruling that the medical staff should be free, subject to consent not being withdrawn, to treat patients in accordance with their best clinical judgment. The decision "has merely declined to deprive them [physicians] of a power which it is for them alone to exercise."[376] Although the judgments, and therefore the rules, were made with reference to the powers of guardians and courts making treatment decisions for incompetent patients, there is no reason why the same principle of professional autonomy should not apply within a physician-patient relationship when the patient is fully competent. The law sets a limit to the patient's right of self-determination by constraining the patient's capacity to

---

[373] *In re* J, [1992] 3 W.L.R. 507.
[374] *In re* J, [1991] Fam. 33.
[375] *Id.* at 41.
[376] *In re J*, [1992] 3 W.L.R. at 520.

request the kind of treatment that clinical personnel regard as either medically contraindicated or contrary to their conscience.

Clinical decision-making in relation to treatment options involves consideration of the patient's psychological and physical needs, as well as technical and moral aspects which, at times, may be difficult to reconcile. A request by the patient that life-saving treatment be withheld or withdrawn, may involve the physician in having to resolve a conflict between two ethical obligations. The physician's first ethical obligation is to act in accordance with the principle of non-maleficence. This fundamental principle of the Hippocratic tradition in medicine[377] focuses as much on the physician's engagement in the provision of benefit as on the avoidance of harm: "Declare the past, diagnose the present, foretell the future; practice these acts. As to disease, make a habit of two things—to help, or at least to do no harm."[378]

The classical principle of non-maleficence has been understood as tending toward circumspection rather than being action-oriented.[379] It guides the medical practitioner toward rendering help by avoiding conduct that may permit detriment or cause harm to the patient's best interests. The more modern, bioethical principle of beneficence has been defined as

> an obligation to help others further their important and legitimate interests by preventing and removing harms; no less important is the obligation to weigh and balance possible goods against the possible harms of an action. This principle of beneficence potentially demands more than the principle of non-maleficence because it requires positive steps to help others, not merely the omission of harm-causing activities.[380]

Despite their superficial similarity, these two principles are philosophically and ethically separate, and may come into conflict with one another.[381] According to the Hippocratic tradition, in cases of conflict, the moral duty of non-maleficence, other things being equal, has priority. This may require an attempt by the medical practitioner to protect the patient from the harmful consequences of his or her choice when such a choice appears to be due to a major affective disorder, cognitive impairment, or abnormal illness behavior. At the same time, in cases where there exists a conflict between the

---

[377] R. FADEN, *supra* note 117, at 10.

[378] L. EDELSTEIN, *supra* note 63, *Epidemiae*, I, 11, *Hipporatis Opera.*, at 14; 1 W. JONES, HIPPOCRATES 165 (1923-31). Latin maxim *primum* (or *saltem*) *non nocere* [above all, at least do no harm] probably comes from Galen.

[379] K. MITCHELL & T. LOVAT, BIOETHICS FOR MEDICAL AND HEALTH PROFESSIONALS 52 (1991).

[380] Beauchamp, *supra* note 20, at 4-5.

[381] A classic example of the conflict between the principle of non-maleficence and the doctrine of beneficence is that of euthanasia, where the idea of doing good, in the sense of cutting short, or preventing further suffering by annihilating the sufferer, is inimical to the notion of at least doing no harm.

patient and the treating physician, with respect to preference in treatment options, the latter has to be conscious of his or her own psychological responses to a difficult situation and careful not to designate the patient's refusal of treatment as abnormal simply because such refusal is at odds with the physician's views on the issue.[382]

The second, though equally important, obligation of a medical practitioner is to respect the right of patients to make decisions about their own bodies and lives, and to ensure that the medical treatment accords with their wishes. When a legally competent patient appears to make a choice about treatment that is patently contrary to his or her well-being, these two obligations will come into conflict.[383]

Whenever a physician determines that the patient's choice is adversely affected by irrational considerations, be they conscious or unconscious, the physician will attempt to persuade the patient to change or modify that choice but, ultimately, once a legally competent patient has decided to refuse life-saving treatment, legally, the patient's decision must be obeyed. There is a curious anomaly in the legal rules that relate to the right of self-determination in the context of the physician-patient relationship. On the one hand, a medical practitioner has the right to refuse to administer medically contraindicated treatment requested by a competent patient on the ground that submission to such a request would be incompatible with the maintenance of the ethical integrity of the medical profession. On the other hand, the same physician has to respect the patient's right to die through refusal of medical therapy because of respect for the patient's right of self-determination. In both cases, no cause of action in battery will arise so long as the treating physician does nothing and leaves the patient free of uninvited physical contact. Nevertheless, in the first instance, "doing nothing" means noncompliance with the patient's wishes, in as much as the dignitary interests protected by law do not extend to the patient having a right to compel medical personnel to treat him or her in a particular way. In the second instance the physician stays within the law by complying with the patient's wish to die.

E. The Balance of Life and Death and the Refusal of Life-Saving Treatment

The fourth factor, regarded as decisive by Justice Skelly Wright in *Application of President & Directors of Georgetown College*, was the fact that Mrs. Jones' life "hung in the balance."[384] The present common law

---

[382] Pilowsky, *supra* note 320, at 392.
[383] Brock & Wartman, *When Competent Patients Make Irrational Choices*, 322 NEW ENG. J. MED. 1595, 1596 (1990).
[384] *Georgetown College*, 331 F.2d at 1009-10.

regards the right to choose whether or not to undergo life-saving treatment as a manifestation of the individual's inalienable right to self-determination, which has to be respected regardless of the consequences of the decision.[385] Should the applicability of the absolute rule extend to cases where the refusal of life-saving treatment by a pregnant woman will inevitably result in her own death as well as the death of an otherwise viable fetus? In the case of *Re T,* Lord Donaldson MR noted, in obiter dictum, that an absolute right of competent adults to choose whether to consent or to refuse life-saving treatment may be qualified in a case "in which the choice may lead to the death of a viable fetus."[386] However, the Master of the Rolls left this question open.

Sir Stephen Brown P was probably referring to this "open question" when, in a 1992 English case of *Re S (Adult: Refusal of Treatment),*[387] he considered an application by a health authority for a declaration to authorize surgeons and staff of the hospital to carry out an emergency cesarean section operation upon Mrs. S, who was the mother of two young children. She was admitted to the hospital with ruptured membranes and in spontaneous labor, beyond the expected date of birth. By the time the matter came before court, the mother had continued in labor for six days, her situation was extremely serious, and the condition of the fetus was rapidly deteriorating. The position of the fetus was that of "transverse lie," with the elbow projecting through the cervix and the head on the right side of the pelvis. Allowing natural labor to continue was certain to cause rupture of the uterus and the consequent death of the mother and the fetus. Mrs. S, a born-again Christian, refused the operation on religious grounds. Nevertheless, Stephen Brown P granted the declaration authorizing the cesarean section. In the judgment, which was completed within the space of an hour,[388] Stephen Brown P emphasized that the situation was one of "life and death," and the issue had to be determined within "minutes rather than hours."[389] Indeed, the decision came too late for the child, but by acting on the declaration, the physicians

---

[385] *Airedale,* [1993] A.C. at 789; *Re T,* [1992] 3 W.L.R. at 782.

[386] *Re T,* [1992] 3 W.L.R. at 786.

[387] [1992] 4 All E.R. at 671; *Re S* [1993] Fam. 123.

[388] Brown, *Matters of Life and Death: The Law and Medicine,* 62 MEDICO-LEGAL J. 52, 61 (1994).

[389] In the course of his judgment, Stephen Brown, P referred to the decision in the case of *In re* AC, 573 A.2d 1235 (D.C. App. 1990), and suggested the possibility that American courts likely would be in favor of granting a declaration in the case of Mrs. S. It has been asserted that this reference amounted to "a significant reliance upon AC's case." *See* Witting, *Forced Operations on Pregnant Women: In Re S Examined,* 2 TORTS L.J. 193 (1994); I. KENNEDY & A. GRUBB, MEDICAL LAW: TEXT AND MATERIALS 347, 359, 937 (1994). This assertion is incorrect. The circumstances in *Re* AC differed markedly from those in *Re* S. The issue that had to be determined in *Re* AC did not involve life-saving treatment for the mother, but a slim possibility of salvaging the fetus. Moreover, American precedent is at best persuasive in the United Kingdom.

were able to save Mrs. S's life.[390] Believing that ''God was acting through the agency of the gynaecologist,'' Mrs. S soon reconciled herself with the situation and decided against appealing to the Court of Appeal.[391] Nevertheless, Sir Stephen Brown's decision was greeted with at times emotive[392] criticism by lawyers who regarded it as a ''major intrusion into the rights of women.''[393]

The harsh criticism meted out to Stephen Brown P was well grounded in strict legal doctrine, but revealed little in the way of humane understanding. Can a society that calls itself civilized, countenance a situation where a young woman, carrying a viable fetus, dies a cruel, but easily preventable, death from a ruptured uterus? Had the judge refused to grant the declaration, the medical personnel attending Mrs. S, qualified and able to prevent such disaster, would have been constrained from acting by a principle of respect for her autonomy. In *Re S*, Stephen Brown P refused to dogmatically apply an abstract legal doctrine that would have rendered his decision legally unassailable, yet morally and socially indefensible.

Philosophical notions of personal autonomy, which form the foundations of the jurisprudential principles of self-determination were formulated in the context of survival, not annihilation. From a consequentialist point of view, there is a fundamental difference between the outcome of a decision to consent to a life-saving treatment and a decision to refuse such an intervention. Unlike those who make the death choice, persons who consent to life-saving treatment at the very least preserve the status quo, and also, by remaining alive, retain an opportunity to change their mind at a later date. The recent evolution of the law has taken the principle of autonomy to its ultimate conclusion—beyond survival. Therefore, the legal criteria for evaluating the person's capacity to make autonomous choices need to be adapted to take account of that extension. The consequentialist position based upon a simple dichotomy between life and death may be too inflexible to adequately address the variety of circumstances and factors that motivate individual death choices. At the same time, the difference between the consequences of consent to and refusal of life-saving treatment cannot be entirely ignored.

---

[390] Brown, *supra* note 388, at 65.

[391] *Id.* at 63. Mrs. S was urged to appeal by, amongst others, Margaret Puxton, QC who said that ''the decision [of Stephen Brown, P] would probably be overruled by the Court of Appeal,'' and Allan Levy, QC, who expressed a hope that the case would go to appeal because it was ''too important not to go. It should go to the House of Lords.'' Levy added that Mrs. S ''could also bring a civil action for assault if the Appeal Court ruled that the High Court declaration was wrongly made.'' Dyer, *British Court Orders Caesarean Section*, 305 BRIT. MED. J. 978 (1992). One wonders who would be the defendant in Mrs. S's action for battery—because the hospital and the physicians had acted under the authority of the law.

[392] Brown, *supra* note 388, at 65.

[393] Witting, *supra* note 389, at 193.

The law has traditionally adopted a consequentialist approach when it considered communitarian interests, such as the consequences of violent behavior on public order, and disallowed consent to constitute an absolute defense to criminal trespass to person. Reiterating the principle established by Lord Coleridge CJ in 1692 in the case of *Matthew v. Ollerton,*[394] Hawkins J stated in the 1882 case of *R. v. Coney*[395] that "it is not in the power of any man to give an effectual consent to that which amounts to, or has a direct tendency to create, a breach of peace; so as to bar a criminal prosecution." Since the 17th century, the legal efficacy of consent would not extend to the risk of death in duelling.[396]

The common-law rule that consent is no defense to unlawful wounding except in cases of surgery, tattoos, contact sports, and "horse-play"[397] was codified in the United Kingdom in the *Offences Against the Person Act.*[398] Justification for this rule was provided by Lord Lane CJ in 1981 when he declared: "It [is] not in the public interest that people should try to cause or should cause each other bodily harm for no good reason."[399] Lord Lane added that the principle of "public interest" was not intended to "cast doubt upon the accepted legality of . . . reasonable surgical interference."[400] The case concerned two youths who, following a quarrel, agreed to have a fist fight, which resulted in a bloody nose and bruises to the face of one of them.

The rule was affirmed by the majority of the House of Lords in the case of *R. v. Brown*[401] in relation to a group of men who appeared[402] to have consensually engaged in extreme forms of sadomasochistic practices.[403] The House of Lords held that the prosecution does not have to prove lack of consent to infliction of actual harm in the course of sadomasochistic activity.[404] When the consent to bodily interference is provided voluntarily by a

---

[394] [1692] Comb. 218, 90 E.R. 438.

[395] [1882] 8 Q.B.D. 534, 553.

[396] The law—though not necessarily the juries—considered duels of honor involving formal arrangements and the presence of seconds as a premeditated murder, however, the "spur-of-the-moment" duels by chance medley were regarded as unpremeditated, thus amounting to manslaughter. Horder, *supra* note 53.

[397] In R. v. Brown, [1993] 2 W.L.R. 556, 560, 603, respectively, Lord Templeman and Lord Slynn of Hadley added ear-piercing, ritual circumcision, boxing, and chastisement of children to these exceptions.

[398] Offences against the Person Act (U.K.), 1861, §§ 20 & 47.

[399] Attorneys-General Reference (No. 6 of 1980), [1981] 1 Q.B. 715, 719.

[400] *Id.*

[401] [1993] 2 W.L.R. 556.

[402] According to the evidence, alcohol and drugs were employed to encourage consent by some of the participants.

[403] For an in-depth discussion of this case, see Freckelton, *Masochism, Self-Mutilation and the Limits of Consent,* 2 J.L. & MED. 48 (1994).

[404] Although the House of Lords did not cite the United States case of State v. Brown, 364 A.2d 27 (N.J. Super. 1976), its reasoning was not dissimilar. In Canada, in R. v. Jobidon, [1991] 2 S.C.R. 714,

competent person who has balanced the risks and benefits involved, the law distinguishes between operative and inoperative consent taking into consideration the following two factors: (1) the nature of the harm—whether or not the harm consented to is of minor nature, rather than manifesting itself as an actual bodily harm;[405] and (2) the reason for the harm—whether or not the harm was occasioned for a "good reason" or in "public interest."[406]

In cases where the interference cannot be justified on the grounds of "good reason" or "public interest" and the consensual conduct occasions actual, or serious, or grievous bodily harm, the victim's consent will be regarded in law as being of no consequence. In *R. v. Brown,* Lord Templeman rejected the contention that "every person has the right to deal with his body as he pleases."[407] Lord Mustill, in a dissenting judgment, paraphrased John Stuart Mill's words when he said:

> The state should interfere with the rights of an individual to live his or her life as he or she may choose no more than is necessary to ensure a proper balance between the special interests of the individual and the general interests of the individuals who together comprise the populace at large.[408]

Lord Mustill drew the line on the rights of individuals to choose how they may live beyond consent to sadomasochistic practices, but noted that the efficacy of consent does not extend to consensual killing.[409]

The common law's approach to consent is clearly consequential. Its legal efficacy depends entirely on the characterization of the purpose and the outcome of the consensual conduct in question. Consent to interference with one's body as an expression of the right to self-determination may be deemed inoperative when it is "other-oriented," for instance, in the cases of sexual enslavement or sadomasochistic activities.[410] However, the right to self-determination also may be "self-oriented," involving actions directed at one's body, for instance, self-mutilation. Here again, the approach of the

---

the Supreme Court held that consent was ineffective when bodily harm was intended and caused. For the Australian position, see *Marion's Case,* 175 C.L.R. 218 (1992).

[405] Lord Slynn, in the minority decision, considered that the line of availability of consent as a defense should be drawn at the level of the infliction of serious bodily harm.

[406] According to Lord Lowry, "public interest" may include conduct designed for "the enhancement or enjoyment of family life or conducive to the welfare of society." R. v. Brown, [1993] 2 W.L.R. 556, 563.

[407] *Id.* at 564.

[408] *Id.* at 600.

[409] *Cf. Airedale,* [1993] A.C. at 789.

[410] Ian Freckelton has observed that in the context of sadomasochistic activities it was possible to regard the acts in question "as inflicted at the hands in effect of a self-mutilator rather than by another person." Freckelton, *supra* note 403, at 63.

law is consequential—such acts of self-mutilation as ears, nose, and genital piercing tend to be regarded as legally acceptable, but self-mutilation that has the effect of endangering the person's productive capacity or health— cutting off one's hand—may be deemed outside the choices to which an individual has a legal right. A great majority of modern mental health statutes that regulate involuntary commitment stipulate that the certified person's conduct, which was the result of an impaired mental condition, constituted a danger to himself or herself. If the legal validity of consent— whether regarding self, or others—is not considered to be an absolute value but is determined in accordance with the sliding scale of harm, then one may ask why refusal of treatment should be deemed of absolute value irrespective of the harm thereby occasioned?

CONCLUSION

The orientation of the present law of trespass to person has moved too far away from general communitarian considerations implied by the principle that the best way to uphold public peace and social harmony is by effectively safeguarding personal integrity and dignitary interests of all individuals. The notion of an unalienable right to self-determination in matters relating to personal well-being had its origins in the law of contract, which developed under the influence of philosophical theories of social contract and utilitarianism. Transposed into the law of torts, the absolute right to refuse life-saving treatment gives rise to an inference that it is at least in part informed by the economic interest in reducing public health care expenditure. The preoccupation with absolute values is a relatively novel development in common law. Traditionally, the common law tended to be concerned with the individual rights and obligations within the "give and take" principles of community interests rather than with such abstract notions as absolute truth or absolute rights.

Conceptually, the legal right to self-determination is, undoubtedly, a very significant and essential element of modern jurisprudence—people, in general, should be able to exercise control over their bodies in relation to undertaking or cessation of any invasive medical regimen. Nonetheless, there are a number of profound moral and human questions that sit uneasily with the declaratory statements of an ideologically pure notion of personal autonomy. For instance, what are the legal criteria for distinguishing a suicidal refusal of treatment from merely an unreasonable one? At which point should an unreasonable refusal of treatment be treated as an indication of the absence of "sound mind" and the patient considered to be legally incapable of making a decision about treatment choices? Who should decide whether the particular refusal of life-saving treatment amounts to a passive suicide, and whether it is reasonable?

A narrow, cognition-oriented legal standard for valid consent to life-saving medical treatment is sufficient when the consequence of that consent means survival, with the patient still retaining an option to change his or her mind. It is altogether insufficient, however, in cases where the refusal of treatment means death, which allows for no second chances.

There is a danger than an ideological purity of the right to refuse life-saving treatment as an expression of the right to individual self-determination may disguise other considerations. It is much less expensive to uphold the right to die of those who suffer from chronic paranoid schizophrenia, the clinically depressed, the disabled, the systemically ill, and those in pain than to care for them at home, in mental institutions, in prisons, hospitals, and hospices. Unless and until traditional notions of "sound mind" are modified to incorporate the modern medical understanding of affective capacity into the legal standard for valid consent to or valid refusal of life-saving medical treatment, the law will accord greater protection to the hale, the hearty, and the emotionally stable than to the diseased, the mentally ill, and those who are emotionally stressed either through pain or loneliness, or both.

[4]

ALLEN BUCHANAN Medical Paternalism

I

There is evidence to show that among physicians in this country the medical paternalist model is a dominant way of conceiving the physician-patient relationship. I contend that the practice of withholding the truth from the patient or his family, a particular form of medical paternalism, is not adequately supported by the arguments advanced to justify it. Beyond the issue of telling patients the truth is the distinction between "ordinary" and "extraordinary" therapeutic measures, a distinction which, I argue, both expresses and helps to perpetuate the dominance of the medical paternalist model.

There are two main types of arguments against paternalism. First are the arguments that rely upon a theory of moral rights rooted in a conception of personal autonomy. These arguments are more theoretically interesting and perhaps in the end they are the strongest arguments against paternalism. Second are the arguments that meet the paternalist on his own ground and then attempt to cut it from beneath him by showing that his arguments are defective. I shall concentrate on the second type of antipaternalist argument because I wish my arguments to have some practical effect, and I believe that this goal can best be achieved if they are directed against paternalist justifications which are actually employed by the practitioners of medical paternalism. Further, the arguments I advance require a minimum of theoretical baggage. The strength of a rights-based attack on paternalism depends ultimately upon whether a rational founda-

Philosophy & Public Affairs 7, no. 4 © 1978 by Princeton University Press
0048-3915/78/0704-0370$01.05/1

tion for the relevant theory of rights can be produced. It would be unfortunate if successful attacks on medical paternalism had to await
the development and defense of a full-blown theory of moral rights.
By articulating the inadequacy of the justifications which the paternalist himself advances, however, one need rely only upon those
moral views to which the paternalist himself subscribes. My goal,
then, is to present effective criticisms of medical paternalist practices
which rely upon a minimal base of moral agreement between the
paternalist and his critic.

II

Paternalism is usually characterized as interference with a person's
liberty of action, where the alleged justification of the interference is
that it is for the good of the person whose liberty of action is thus
restricted.[1] To focus exclusively on interference with liberty of *action*,
however, is to construe paternalism too narrowly. If a government lies
to the public or withholds information from it, and if the alleged
justification of its policy is that it benefits the public itself, the policy
may properly be called paternalistic.

On the one hand, there may be a direct connection between such a
policy and actual interference with the citizen's freedom to act. In
order to withhold information from the public, agents of the government may physically interfere with the freedom of the press to gather,
print, or distribute the news. Or government officials may misinform
the public in order to restrict its freedom to perform specific acts. The
police, for example, may erect signs bearing the words "Detour: Maintenance Work Ahead" to route unsuspecting motorists around the
wreckage of a truck carrying nerve gas. On the other hand, the connection between withholding of information and actual interference
with freedom of action may be indirect at best. To interfere with the
public's freedom of information the government need not actually
interfere with anyone's freedom to act—it may simply not divulge
certain information. Withholding information may preclude an *informed* decision, and it may interfere with attempts to reach an in-

1. See, for example, G. Dworkin's paper "Paternalism," in S. Gorovitz et al.,
Moral Problems in Medicine (Englewood Cliffs, NJ; Prentice-Hall, 1976), p. 185.

formed decision, without thereby interfering with a person's freedom to decide and to act on his decision. Even if I am deprived of information which I must have if I am to make an informed decision, I may still be free to decide and to act.

Granted the complexity of the relations between information and action, it seems plausible to expand the usual characterization of paternalism as follows: paternalism is interference with a person's freedom of action or freedom of information, or the deliberate dissemination of misinformation, where the alleged justification of interfering or misinforming is that it is for the good of the person who is interfered with or misinformed. The notion of freedom of information is, of course, unsatisfyingly vague, but the political examples sketched above along with the medical examples to follow will make it clearer. We can now turn to a brief consideration of evidence for the claim that medical paternalism is a widespread phenomenon in our society.

III

The evidence for medical paternalism is both direct and indirect. The direct evidence consists of the findings of surveys which systematically report physicians' practices concerning truth-telling and decision-making and of articles and discussions in which physicians and others acknowledge or defend paternalistic medical practices. The indirect evidence is more subtle. One source of indirect evidence for the pervasiveness of medical paternalist attitudes is the language we use to describe physician-patient interactions. Let us now consider some of the direct evidence.

Though there are many ways of classifying cases of medical paternalism, two distinctions are especially important. We can distinguish between the cases in which the patient is legally competent and those in which the patient is legally incompetent; and between those cases in which the intended beneficiary of paternalism is the patient himself and those in which the intended beneficiary is the patient's guardian or one or more members of the patient's family. The first distinction classifies cases according to the *legal status of the patient*, the second according to the *object of paternalism*.

A striking revelation of medical paternalism in dealings with legally competent adults is found in Donald Oken's essay, "What to Tell

Cancer Patients: A Study of Medical Attitudes."[2] The chief conclusion of this study of internists, surgeons, and generalists is that ". . . there is a strong and general tendency to withhold" from the patient the information that he has cancer. Almost 90 percent of the total group surveyed reported that their usual policy is not to tell the patient that he has cancer. Oken also notes that "no one reported a policy of informing every patient." Further, Oken reports that some physicians falsified diagnoses.

> Some physicians avoid even the slightest suggestion of neoplasia and quite specifically substitute another diagnosis. Almost everyone reported resorting to such falsification on at least a few occasions, most notably when the patient was in a far-advanced stage of illness at the time he was seen.[3]

The physicians' justifications for withholding or falsifying diagnostic information were uniformly paternalistic. They assumed that if they told the patient he had cancer they would be depriving him of all hope and that the loss of hope would result in suicidal depression or at least in a serious worsening of the patient's condition.

A recent malpractice case illustrates paternalistic withholding of information of a different sort. As in the Oken study, the object of paternalism was the patient and the patient was a legally competent adult. A bilateral thyroidectomy resulted in permanent paralysis of the patient's vocal cords. The patient's formerly healthy voice became frail and weak. The damage suit was based on the contention that by failing to tell the patient of the known risks to her voice, the physician had violated his duty to obtain informed consent for the operation. The physician's testimony is clearly paternalistic.

> In court the physician was asked "You didn't inform her of any dangers or risks involved? Is that right?" Over his attorney's objections, the physician responded, "Not specifically. . . . I feel that were I to point out all the complications—or even half the complica-

2. In *Moral Problems in Medicine*, p. 112. Oken's study was first published in 1967.
3. Oken, p. 113.

tions—many people would refuse to have anything done, and therefore would be much worse off."[4]

There is also considerable evidence of medical paternalism in the treatment of legally incompetent individuals through the withholding of information from the patients or their guardians or both.[5]

The law maintains that it is the parents who are primarily responsible for decisions concerning the welfare of their minor children.[6] Nonetheless, physicians sometimes assume primary or even total responsibility for the most awesome and morally perplexing decisions affecting the welfare of the child.

The inescapable need to make such decisions arises daily in neonate intensive care units. The most dramatic decisions are whether to initiate or not initiate, or to continue or discontinue life-sustaining therapy. Three broad types of cases are frequently discussed in recent literature. First, there are infants who are in an asphyxiated condition at birth and can be resuscitated but may suffer irreversible brain-damage if they survive. Second, there are infants with Down's syndrome (mongolism) who have potentially fatal but surgically correctable congenital cardiovascular or gastrointestinal defects. Third, there are infants with spina bifida, a congenital condition in which there is an opening in the spine and which may be complicated by paralysis and hydrocephaly. New surgical techniques make it possible to close the spine and drain the fluid from the brain, but a large percentage of the infants thus treated suffer varying degrees of permanent brain-damage and paralysis.

A. Shaw notes that some physicians undertake the responsibility

4. *Malpractice Digest* (St. Paul, MN: The St. Paul Property and Liability Insurance Company, July-August 1977), p. 6.

5. It is interesting to note that according to both the usual and the expanded characterization of paternalism stated above, only a person who has certain physical and mental capacities can be an object of paternalism, since it is only when these capacities are present that it is correct to speak of interfering with that individual's freedom of action, misinforming him, or withholding information from him.

6. For a helpful summary, see J. A. Robertson and N. Frost, "Passive Euthanasia of Defective Newborn Infants: Legal Considerations," *The Journal of Pediatrics* 88, no. 5 (1976): 883-889.

for making decisions about life and death for defective newborns in
order to relieve parents of the trauma and guilt of making a decision.
He cites the following comment as an example of this position.

> At the end it is usually the doctor who has to decide the issue. It is
> . . . cruel to ask the parents whether they want their child to live
> or die. . . .[7]

We have already seen that the information which physicians withhold may be of at least two different sorts. In the cases studied by
Oken, physicians withhold the diagnosis of cancer from their patients.
In the thyroidectomy malpractice case the physician did not withhold
the diagnosis but did withhold information about known risks of an
operation. The growing literature on life or death decisions for defective neonates reveals more complex paternalistic practices. Some
physicians routinely exclude parents from significant participation in
decision-making either by not informing the parents that certain
choices can or must be made, or by describing the child's condition
and the therapeutic options in such a skeletal way as to preclude genuinely informed consent.

A case cited by Shaw is a clear example of a physician withholding
from parents the information that there was a choice to be made.

> Baby A was referred to me at 22 hours of age with a diagnosis of
> esophageal atresia and tracheoesophageal fistula. The infant, the
> firstborn of a professional couple in their early thirties had obvious
> signs of mongolism, about which they were fully informed by the
> referring physician. After explaining the nature of the surgery to
> the distraught father, I offered him the operative consent. His pen
> hesitated briefly above the form and then as he signed, he muttered,
> "I have no choice, do I?" He didn't seem to expect an answer and I
> gave him none. The esophageal anomaly was corrected in routine
> fashion, and the infant was discharged to a state institution for the
> retarded without ever being seen again by either parent.[8]

7. Shaw, "Dilemmas of 'Informed Consent' in Children," *The New England
Journal of Medicine* 289, no. 17 (1973): 886.
   8. Shaw, p. 885.

The following description of practices in a neonate intensive care unit at Yale illustrates how parents may be excluded because of inadequate information about the child's condition or the character of various therapeutic options.

> Parents routinely signed permits for operation though rarely had they seen their children's defects or had the nature of various management plans and their respective prognoses clearly explained to them. Some physicians believed that parents were too upset to understand the nature of the problems and the options for care. Since they believed informed consent had no meaning in these circumstances, they either ignored the parents or simply told them that the child needed an operation on the back as the first step in correcting several defects. As a result, parents often felt completely left out while the activities of care proceeded at a brisk pace.[9]

Not every case in which a physician circumvents or overrides parental decision-making is a case of paternalism toward the parents. In ignoring the parents' primary legal responsibility for the child, the physician may not be attempting to shield the parents from the burdens of responsibility—he may simply be attempting to protect what he perceives to be the interests of the child.

These examples are presented, not as conclusive evidence for the claim that paternalist practices of the sorts discussed above are widespread, but as illustrations of the practical relevance of the justifications for medical paternalism, which I shall now articulate and criticize.

IV

In spite of the apparent pervasiveness of paternalistic practices in medicine, no systematic justification of them is available for scrutiny. Nonetheless, there appear to be at least three main arguments which advocates of paternalism could and sometimes do advance in justification of withholding information or misinforming the patient or his

9. R. Duff and A. Campbell, "Moral and Ethical Dilemmas in the Special-Care Nursery," *The New England Journal of Medicine* 289, no. 17 (1973): p. 893.

family. Since withholding information seems to be more commonly
practiced and advocated than outright falsification, I shall consider
the three arguments only as justifications of the former rather than
the latter. Each of these arguments is sufficiently general to apply to
each of the types of cases distinguished above. For convenience we
can label these three arguments (A) the Prevention of Harm Argument, (B) the Contractual Version of the Prevention of Harm Argument, and (C) the Argument from the Inability to Understand.

The Prevention of Harm Argument is disarmingly simple. It may be
outlined as follows.

1. The physician's duty—to which he is bound by the Oath of Hippocrates—is to prevent or at least to minimize harm to his patient.
2. Giving the patient information X will do great harm to him.
3. (Therefore) It is permissible for the physician to withhold information X from the patient.

Several things should be noted about this argument. First of all, the
conclusion is much weaker than one would expect, granted the first
premise. The first premise states that it is the physician's *duty* to prevent or minimize harm to the patient, not just that it is *permissible*
for him to do so. However, since the weaker conclusion—that withholding information is permissible—seems more intuitively plausible
than the stronger one, I shall concentrate on it.

Second, the argument as it stands is invalid. From the claims that
(1) the physician's duty (or right) is to prevent or minimize harm and
that (2) giving information X will do the patient great harm, it does
not follow that (3) it is permissible for the physician to withhold information X from the patient. At least one other premise is needed:
(2′) giving information X will do greater harm to the patient on balance than withholding the information will.

The addition of (2′) is no quibble. Once (2′) is made explicit we
begin to see the tremendous weight which this paternalist argument
places on the physician's powers of judgment. He must not only determine that giving the information will do harm or even that it will do
great harm. He must also make a complex comparative judgment. He
must judge that withholding the information will result in less harm

on balance than divulging it. Yet neither the physicians interviewed by Oken nor those discussed by Shaw even mention this comparative judgment in their justifications of withholding information. They simply state that telling the truth will result in great harm to the patient or his family. No mention was made of the need to compare this expected harm with harm which might result from withholding the information, and no recognition of the difficulties involved in such a comparison was reported.

Consider two of the cases described above: a terminal cancer case and the thyroidectomy case. In order to justify withholding the diagnosis of terminal cancer from the patient the physician must not only determine that informing the patient would do great harm but that the harm would be greater on balance than whatever harm may result from withholding information. Since the notion of "great harm" here is vague unless a context for comparison is supplied, we can concentrate on the physician's evidence for the judgment that the harm of informing is greater on balance than the harm of withholding. Oken's study showed that the evidential basis for such comparative judgments was remarkably slender.

> It was the exception when a physician could report known examples of the unfavorable consequences of an approach which differed from his own. It was more common to get reports of instances in which different approaches has turned out satisfactorily. Most of the instances in which unhappy results were reported to follow a differing policy turned out to be vague accounts from which no reliable inference could be drawn.

Oken then goes on to focus on the nature of the anticipated harm.

> It has been repeatedly asserted that disclosure is followed by fear and despondency which may progress into overt depressive illness or culminate in suicide. This was the opinion of the physicians in the present study. Quite representative was the surgeon who stated, "I would be afraid to tell and have the patient in a room with a window." When it comes to actually documenting the prevalence of such ontoward reactions, it becomes difficult to find reliable evi-

dence. Instances of depression and profound upsets came quickly to mind when the subject was raised, but no one could report more than a case or two, or a handful at most. . . . The same doctors could remember many instances in which the patient was told and seemed to do well.[10]

It is not simply that these judgments of harm are made on the basis of extremely scanty evidence. The problem goes much deeper than that. To say simply that physicians base such judgments on extremely weak evidence is to overlook three important facts. First, the judgment that telling the truth would result in suicidal depression is an unqualified *psychiatric* generalization. So even if there were adequate evidence for this generalization or, more plausibly, for some highly qualified version of it, it is implausible to maintain that ordinary physicians are in a position to recognize and assess the evidence properly in a given case. Second, it is doubtful that psychiatric specialists are in possession of any such reliable generalization, even in qualified form. Third, the paternalist physician is simply assuming that suicide is not a rational choice for the terminally ill patient.

If we attempt to apply the Prevention of Harm Argument to cases in which the patient's family or guardian is the object of paternalism, other difficulties become apparent. Consider cases of withholding information from the parents of a neonate with Down's syndrome or spina bifida. The most obvious difficulty is that premise (1) states only that the physician has a duty (or a right) to prevent or minimize harm to the patient, not to his family. If this argument is to serve as a justification of paternalism toward the infant patient's family, the advocate of paternalism must advance and support one or the other of two quite controversial premises. He must either add premise (1') or replace premise (1) with premise (1''):

(1') If X is a guardian or parent of a patient Y and Y is the patient of physician Z, then X is thereby a patient of physician Z as well.

(1'') It is the duty of the physician to prevent or minimize harm to his patient and to the guardian or family of his patient.

10. Oken, "What to Tell Cancer Patients," pp. 112, 113.

Since both the law and common sense maintain that one does not become a patient simply by being related to a patient, it seems that the best strategy for the medical paternalist is to rely on (i″) rather than on (i′).

Reliance on (i″), however, only weakens the case for medical paternalism toward parents of defective neonates. For now the medical paternalist must show that he has adequate evidence for psychiatric predictions the complexity of which taxes the imagination. He must first determine all the relevant effects of telling the truth, not just on the parents themselves, but on siblings as well, since whatever anguish or guilt the parents will allegedly feel may have significant effects on their other children. Next he must ascertain the ways in which these siblings—both as individuals and as a peer group—will respond to the predicted anguish and guilt of their parents. Then the physician must determine how the siblings will respond to each other. Next he must consider the possible responses of the parents to the responses of the children. And, of course, once he has accomplished all of this, the physician must look at the other side of the question. He must consider the possible harmful effects of withholding information from patients or of preventing them from taking an active part in decision-making. The conscientious paternalist must consider not only the burdens which the exercise of responsibility will allegedly place upon the parents, and indirectly upon their children, but also the burdens of guilt, self-doubt, and shame which may result from the parents' recognition that they have abdicated their responsibility.

In predicting whether telling the truth or withholding information will cause the least harm for the family as a whole, the physician must first make intrapersonal comparisons of harm and benefit for each member of the family, if the information is divulged. Then he must somehow coalesce these various intrapersonal net harm judgments into an estimate of the total net harm which divulging the information will do to the family as a whole. Then he must make similar intrapersonal and interpersonal net harm judgments about the results of not telling the truth. Finally he must compare these totals and determine which course of action will minimize harm to the family as a whole.

Though the problems of achieving defensible predictions of harm as a basis for paternalism are clearest in the case of defective neonates, they are in no way peculiar to those cases. Consider the case of a person with terminal cancer. To eliminate the complication of interpersonal net harm comparisons, let us suppose that this person has no relatives and is himself legally competent. Suppose that the physician withholds information of the diagnosis because he believes that knowledge of the truth would be more harmful than withholding the truth. I have already indicated that even if we view this judgment of comparative harm as a purely clinical judgment—more specifically a clinical psychiatric judgment—it is difficult to see how the physician could be in a position to make it. But it is crucial to note that the notions of harm and benefit appropriate to these deliberations are not exclusively clinical notions, whether psychiatric or otherwise. In taking it upon himself to determine what will be most beneficial or least harmful to this patient the physician is not simply making ill-founded medical judgments which someday might be confirmed by psychiatric research. He is making *moral* evaluations of the most basic and problematic kind.

The physician must determine whether it will be better for the patient to live his remaining days in the knowledge that his days are few or to live in ignorance of his fate. But again, this is a gross simplification: it assumes that the physician's attempt to deceive the patient will be successful. E. Kübler-Ross claims that in many, if not most, cases the terminally ill patient will guess or learn his fate whether the physician withholds the diagnosis from him or not.[11] Possible harm resulting from the patient's loss of confidence in the physician or from a state of uncertainty over his prospects must be taken into account.

Let us set aside this important complication and try to appreciate what sorts of factors would have to be taken into account in a well-founded judgment that the remainder of a person's life would be better for that person if he did not know that he had a terminal illness than if he did.

Such a judgment would have to be founded on a profound knowledge of the most intimate details of the patient's life history, his characteristic ways of coping with personal crises, his personal and

11. Kübler-Ross, excerpts from *Death and Dying*, quoted in *Moral Problems in Medicine*, p. 122.

vocational commitments and aspirations, his feelings of obligation toward others, and his attitude toward the completeness or incompleteness of his experience. In a society in which the personal physician was an intimate friend who shared the experience of families under his care, it would be somewhat more plausible to claim that the physician might possess such knowledge. Under the present conditions of highly impersonal specialist medical practice it is quite a different matter.

Yet even if the physician could claim such intimate personal knowledge, this would not suffice. For he must not only predict, but also *evaluate*. On the basis of an intimate knowledge of the patient as a person, he must determine which outcome would be *best* for that person. It is crucial to emphasize that the question which the physician must pose and answer is whether ignorance or knowledge will make possible a life that is better *for the patient himself*. The physician must be careful not to confuse this question with the question of whether ignorance or knowledge would make for a better life for the physician if the physician were terminally ill. Nor must he confuse it with the question of whether the patient's life would be a *better life*—a life more valuable to others or to society—if it ended in ignorance rather than in truth. The question, rather, is whether it would be better *for the patient himself* to know or not to know his fate.

To judge that a certain ending of a life would be best for the person whose life it is, is to view that life as a unified process of development and to conclude that that ending is a fitting completion for that process. To view a human life as a unified process of development, however, is to view it selectively. Certain events or patterns of conduct are singled out as especially significant or valuable. To ascertain the best completion of a person's life for that person, then, is to make the most fundamental judgments about the value of that person's activities, aspirations, and experiences.

It might be replied that we do make such value judgments when we decide to end the physiologic life of a permanently comatose individual. In such cases we do make value judgments, but they are not judgments of this sort. On the contrary, we believe that since this individual's experience has ended, his life-process is already completed.

When the decision to withhold information of impending death is understood for what it is, it is difficult to see how anyone could presume to make it. My conjecture is that physicians are tempted to make these decisions in part because of a failure to reflect upon the disparity between two quite different kinds of judgments about what will harm or benefit the patient. Judgments of the first sort fall within the physician's competence as a highly trained medical expert. There is nothing in the physician's training which qualifies him to make judgments of the second sort—to evaluate another human being's life as a whole. Further, once the complexity of these judgments is appreciated and once their evaluative character is understood, it is implausible to hold that the physician is in a better position to make them than the patient or his family. The failure to ask what sorts of harm/benefit judgments may properly be made by the physician in his capacity as a physician is a fundamental feature of medical paternalism.

There is a more sophisticated version of the attempt to justify withholding of information in order to minimize harm to the patient or his family. This is the Contract Version of the Prevention of Harm Argument. The idea is that the physician-patient relationship is contractual and that the terms of this contract are such that the patient authorizes the physician to minimize harm to the patient (or his family) by whatever means he, the physician, deems necessary. Thus if the physician believes that the best way to minimize harm to the patient is to withhold information from him, he may do so without thereby wronging the patient. To wrong the patient the physician would either have to do something he was not authorized to do or fail to do something it was his duty to do and which was in his power to do. But in withholding information from the patient he is doing just what he is authorized to do. So he does the patient no wrong.

First of all, it should be noted that this version is vulnerable to the same objections just raised against the non-contractual Argument from the Prevention of Harm. The most serious of these is that in the cases of paternalism under discussion it is very doubtful that the physician will or even could possess the psychiatric and moral knowledge required for a well-founded judgment about what will be least harmful to the patient. In addition, the Contract Version is vulnerable to other objections. Consider the claim that the patient-physician relationship is a contract in which the patient authorizes the physician to prevent or minimize harm by whatever means the physician deems necessary, including the withholding of information. This claim could be interpreted in either of two ways: as a descriptive generalization about the way physicians and patients actually understand their relationship or as a normative claim about the way the physician-patient relationship should be viewed or may be viewed.

As a descriptive generalization it is certainly implausible—there are many people who do not believe they have authorized their physician to withhold the truth from them, and the legal doctrine of informed consent supports their view. Let us suppose for a moment that some people do view their relationship to their physician as including such an authorization and that there is nothing morally wrong with such a contract so long as both parties entered into it voluntarily and in full knowledge of the terms of the agreement.

Surely the fact that some people are willing to authorize physicians to withhold information from them would not justify the physician in acting toward other patients as if they had done so. The physician can only justify withholding information from a particular patient if this sort of contract was entered into freely and in full knowledge *by this* patient.

What, then, is the physician to do? Surely he cannot simply assume that all of his patients have authorized him to withhold the truth if he deems it necessary. Yet if in each case he inquires as to whether the patient wishes to make such an authorization, he will defeat the purpose of the authorization by undermining the patient's trust.

There is, however, a more serious difficulty. Even the more extreme advocates of medical paternalism must agree that there are some limits on the contractual relationship between physician and patient. Hence the obligations of each party are conditional upon the other party's observing the limits of the contract. The law, the medical profession, and the general public generally recognize that there are such limits. For example, the patient may refuse to undergo a certain treatment, he may seek a second opinion, or he may terminate the relationship altogether. Moreover, it is acknowledged that to decide to do any of these things the patient may—indeed perhaps must—rely on his own judgment. If he is conscientious he will make such decisions on consideration of whether the physician is doing a reasonable job of rendering the services for which he was hired.

There are general constraints on how those services may be rendered. If the treatment is unreasonably slow, if the physician's technique is patently sloppy, or if he employs legally questionable methods, the patient may rightly conclude that the physician has not lived up to the implicit terms of the agreement and terminate the relationship. There are also more special constraints on the contract stemming from the special nature of the problem which led the patient to seek the physician's services in the first place. If you go to a physician for treatment of a skin condition, but he ignores that problem and sets about trying to convince you to have cosmetic nose surgery, you may rightly terminate the relationship. These general and special constraints are limits on the agreement from the patient's point of view.

Now once it is admitted that there are any such terms—that the contract does have some limits and that the patient has the right to terminate the relationship if these limits are not observed by the physician—it must also be admitted that the patient must be in a position to discover *whether* those limits are being observed. But if the patient were to authorize the physician to withhold information, he might deprive himself of information which is relevant to determining whether the physician has observed the limits of the agreement.

I am not concerned to argue that authorizing a physician to withhold information is logically incompatible with the contract being conditional. My point, rather, is that to make such an authorization would show either that (a) one did not view the contract as being conditional or that (b) one did not take seriously the possibility that the conditions of the contract might be violated or that (c) one simply did not care whether the conditions were violated. Since it is unreasonable to expect a patient to make an unconditional contract or to ignore the possibility that conditions of the contract will be violated, and since one typically does care whether these conditions are observed, it is unreasonable to authorize the physician to withhold information when he sees fit. The Contract Version of the Argument from the Prevention of Harm, then, does not appear to be much of an improvement over its simpler predecessor.

There is one paternalist argument in favor of withholding of information which remains to be considered. This may be called the Argument from the Inability to Understand. The main premise is that the physician is justified in withholding information when the patient or his family is unable to understand the information. This argument is often used to justify paternalistic policies toward parents of defective infants in neonate intensive care units. The idea is that either their lack of intelligence or their excited emotional condition prevents parents from giving informed consent because they are incapable of being adequately informed. In such cases, it is said, "the doctrine of informed consent does not apply."[12]

This argument is also vulnerable to several objections. First, it too relies upon dubious and extremely broad psychological generalizations —in this case psychological generalizations about the cognitive powers of parents of defective neonates.

Second, and more importantly, it ignores the crucial question of the character of the institutional context in which parents find themselves. To the extent that paternalist attitudes shape medical institutions, this bleak estimate of the parental capacity for comprehension and rational decision tends to be a self-fulfilling prophecy. In an institution in which parents routinely sign operation permits without even having seen their newborn infants and without having the nature of the therapeutic options clearly explained to them, parents may indeed be incapable of understanding the little that they are told.

Third, it is a mistake to maintain that the legal duty to seek informed consent applies only where the physician can succeed in adequately informing parents. The doctor does not and cannot have a duty to make sure that all the information he conveys is understood by those to whom he conveys it. His duty is to make a reasonable effort to be understood.[13]

Fourth, it is important to ask exactly why it is so important not to tell parents information which they allegedly will not understand. If the reason is that a parental decision based on inadequate understanding will be a decision that is harmful to the *infant*, then the

12. Duff and Campbell, "Moral and Ethical Dilemmas," p. 893.
13. I would like to thank John Dolan for clarifying this point.

Argument from the Inability to Understand is not an argument for paternalism toward *parents*. So if this argument is to provide a justification for withholding information from parents for *their* benefit, then the claim must be that their failure to understand will somehow be harmful to *them*. But why should this be so? If the idea is that the parents will not only fail to understand but become distressed because they realize that they do not understand, then the Argument from the Inability to Understand turns out not to be a new argument at all. Instead, it is just a restatement of the Argument from the Prevention of Harm examined above—and is vulnerable to the same objections. I conclude that none of the three justifications examined provide adequate support for the paternalist practices under consideration. If adequate justification is to be found, the advocate of medical paternalism must marshal more powerful arguments.

V

So far I have examined several specific medical paternalist practices and criticized some general arguments offered in their behalf. Medical paternalism, however, goes much deeper than the specific practices themselves. For this reason I have spoken of "the medical paternalist model," emphasizing that what is at issue is a paradigm, a way of conceiving the physician-patient relationship. Indirect evidence for the pervasiveness of this model is to be found in the very words we use to describe physicians, patients, and their interactions. Simply by way of illustration, I will now examine one widely used distinction which expresses and helps perpetuate the paternalist model: the distinction between "ordinary" and "extraordinary" therapeutic measures.

Many physicians, theologians, ethicists, and judges have relied on this distinction since Pius XII employed it in an address on "The Prolongation of Life" in 1958. In reply to questions concerning conditions under which physicians may discontinue or refrain from initiating the use of artificial respiration devices, Pius first noted that physicians are duty-bound "to take the necessary treatment for the preservation of life and health." He then distinguished between "ordinary" and "extraordinary" means.

> But normally one is held to use only ordinary means—according to circumstances of persons, places, times, and culture—means that do not involve any grave burden for oneself or another.[14]

Though he is not entirely explicit about this, Pius assumes that it is the right of the physician to determine what will count as "ordinary" or "extraordinary" means in any particular case.

In the context of the issue of when a highly trained specialist is to employ sophisticated life-support equipment, it is natural to assume that the distinction between "ordinary" and "extraordinary" means is a distinction between higher and lower degrees of technological sophistication. The Pope's unargued assumption that the medical specialist is to determine what counts as "ordinary" or "extraordinary" reinforces a technological interpretation of the distinction. After all, if the distinction is a technological one, then it is natural to assume that it is the physician who should determine its application since it is he who possesses the requisite technical expertise. In my discussions with physicians, nurses, and hospital administrators I have observed that they tend to treat the distinction as a technological one and then to argue that since it is a technological distinction the physician is the one who should determine in any particular case whether a procedure would involve "ordinary" or "extraordinary" means.[15]

Notice, however, that even though Pius introduced the distinction in the context of the proper use of sophisticated technical devices and even though he assumed that it was to be applied by those who possess the technical skills to use such equipment, it is quite clear that the distinction he explicitly introduced is not itself a technological distinction. Recall that he defines "ordinary" means as those which "do not involve any grave burden for oneself or another." "Extraordinary" means, then, would be those which do involve a grave burden for oneself or for another.

If what counts as "extraordinary" measures depended only upon

14. Pius XII, "The Prolongation of Life," in Reiser et al., *Ethics in Medicine*, (Cambridge, MA: MIT Press, 1977), pp. 501-504.

15. These discussions occurred in the course of my work as a member of committee which drafted ethical guidelines for Children's Hospital of Minneapolis.

what would constitute a "grave burden" to the patient himself, it might be easier to preserve the illusion that the decision is an exercise of medical expertise. But once the evaluation of burdens is extended to the patient's family it becomes obvious that the judgment that a certain therapy would be "extraordinary" is not a technological or even a clinical, but rather a *moral* decision. And it is a moral decision regardless of whether the evaluation is made from the perspective of the patient's own values and preferences or from that of the physician.

Even if one is to evaluate only the burdens for the patient himself, however, it is implausible to maintain that the application of the distinction is an exercise of technological or clinical judgment. For as soon as we ask what would result in "grave burdens" for the patient, we are immediately confronted with the task of making moral distinctions and moral evaluations concerning the quality of the patient's life and his interests as a person.

When pressed for an explanation of how physicians actually apply the distinction between "ordinary" and "extraordinary" therapeutic measures, the director of a neonate intensive care unit explained to me that what counts as "ordinary" or "extraordinary" differs in "different contexts." Surgical correction of a congenital gastrointestinal blockage in the case of an otherwise normal infant would be considered an "ordinary" measure. But the same operation on an infant with Downs' syndrome would be considered extraordinary.

I am not concerned here to criticize the moral decision to refrain from aggressive surgical treatment of infants with Down's syndrome. My purpose in citing this example is simply to point out that this decision *is* a moral decision and that the use of the distinction between "ordinary" and "extraordinary" measures does nothing to help one make the decision. The use of the distinction does accomplish something though: it obscures the fact that the decision *is* a moral decision. Even worse, it is likely to lead one to mistake a very controversial moral decision for a "value-free" technological or clinical decision. More importantly, to even suggest that a complex moral judgment is a clinical or technological judgment is to prejudice the issue of *who* has the right to decide whether life-sustaining measures are to be initiated or continued. Once controversial moral decisions are misperceived as clinical or technological decisions it becomes much easier for the medical paternalist to use the three arguments examined above to justify the withholding of information. For once it is conceded that his medical expertise gives the physician the right to make certain decisions, he can then argue that he may withhold information where this is necessary for the effective exercise of this right. By disguising complex moral judgments as medical judgments, then, the "ordinary/extraordinary" distinction reinforces medical paternalism.

VI

In this paper I have attempted to articulate and challenge some basic features of the medical paternalist model of the physician-patient relationship. I have also given an indication of the powerful influence this model exerts on medical practice and on ways of talking and thinking about medical treatment.

There are now signs that medical paternalism is beginning to be challenged from within the medical profession itself.[16] This, I believe, is all to the good. So far, however, challenges have been fragmentary and unsystematic. If they are to be theoretically and practically fruitful they must be grounded in a systematic understanding of what medical paternalism is and in a critical examination of justifications for medical paternalist practices. The present paper is an attempt to begin the task of such a systematic critique.

16. See, for example, A. Waldman, "Medical Ethics and the Hopelessly Ill Child," *The Journal of Pediatrics* 88, no. 5 (1976): 890-892.

I would like to thank Rolf Sartorius and the editors of *Philosophy & Public Affairs* for several helpful comments on an earlier draft of this paper.

Part II
Reproduction

[5]

Ronald Dworkin

THE
MORALITY OF
ABORTION

Sometimes people who disagree passionately with one another have no clear grasp of what they are disagreeing about, even when the dispute is violent and profound. Most people assume that the great, divisive abortion argument is at bottom an argument about a moral and metaphysical issue: whether even a just-fertilized embryo is already a human creature with rights and interests of its own, a person in the sense I defined in chapter 1, an unborn child, helpless against the abortionist's slaughtering knife. The political rhetoric is explicit that this is the issue in controversy. The "human life" amendment that anti-abortion groups have tried to make part of the United States Constitution declares, "The paramount right to life is vested in each human being from the moment of fertilization without regard to age, health, or conditions of dependency." The "pro-choice" world defends abortion by claiming that an embryo is no more a child than an acorn is an oak. Theological, moral, philosophical, and even sociological discussions of abortion almost all presume that people disagree about abortion because they disagree about whether a fetus is a person with a right to life from the moment of its conception, or becomes a person at some point in pregnancy, or does not become one until birth. And about whether, if a fetus is a person, its right to life must yield in the face of some stronger right held by pregnant women.

I have suggested some preliminary reasons for thinking that this account of the abortion debate, in spite of its great popularity, is fatally misleading. We cannot understand most people's actual moral and political convictions about when abortion is permissible, and what government should do about abortion, in this way. The detailed structure of most conservative opinion about abortion is actually inconsistent with the assumption that a fetus has rights from the moment of conception, and the detailed structure of most liberal opinion cannot be explained only on the supposition that it does not.

Of course, people's opinions about abortion do not come in only two varieties, conservative and liberal. There are degrees of opinion, ranging from extreme to moderate, on both sides, and there are also differences of opinion that cannot be located on a conservative-liberal spectrum at all—neither view about whether a later abortion is worse than an earlier one seems distinctly more liberal or more conservative, for example. Nevertheless, in this part of my argument, I shall suppose that people are spread along a conservative-liberal spectrum because this will make it easier to describe my main points.

We have seen that a great many people who are morally very conservative about abortion—who believe that it is never, or almost never, morally permissible, and who would be appalled if any relative or close friend chose to have one—nevertheless think that the law should leave women free to make decisions about abortion for themselves, that it is wrong for the majority or for the government to impose its view upon them. Even many Catholics take that view: Governor Mario Cuomo of New York among them, as he made explicit in a well-known 1984 speech at Notre Dame University in Indiana.[1]

Some conservatives who take that position base it, as Cuomo did, on the principle that church and state should be separate: they believe that freedom of decision about abortion is part of the freedom people have to make their own religious decisions. Others base their tolerance on a more general notion of privacy and freedom: they believe that the government should not dictate to individuals on any matter of personal morality. But people who really consider a fetus a person with a right to live could not maintain either version. Protecting people from murderous assault—particularly people too weak to protect themselves—is one of government's most central and inescapable duties.

Of course, a great many people who are very conservative about abortion do not take this tolerant view: they believe that governments should ban abortion, and some of them have devoted their lives to achieving that end. But even those conservatives who believe that the law should prohibit abortion recognize some exceptions. It is a very common view, for example, that abortion should be permitted when necessary to save the mother's life.[2] Yet this exception is also inconsistent with any belief that a fetus is a person with a right to live. Some people say that in this case a mother is justified in aborting a fetus as a matter of self-defense; but any safe abortion is carried out by someone else—a doctor—and very few people believe that it is morally justifiable for a third party, even a doctor, to kill one innocent person to save another.

Abortion conservatives often allow further exceptions. Some of them believe that abortion is morally permissible not only to save the mother's life but also when pregnancy is the result of rape or incest.[3] The more such exceptions are allowed, the clearer it becomes that conservative opposition to abortion does not presume that a fetus is a person with a right to live. It would be contradictory to insist that a fetus has a right to live that is strong enough to justify prohibiting abortion even when childbirth would ruin a mother's or a family's life but that ceases to exist when the pregnancy is the result of a sexual crime of which the fetus is, of course, wholly innocent.

On the other side, a parallel story emerges. Liberal views about abortion do not follow simply from denying that a fetus is a person with a right to live; they presuppose some other important value at stake. I exempt here the views of people who think that abortion is never even morally problematic—Peggy Noonan, a White House speech writer in Ronald Reagan's administration, said that when she was in college she "viewed abortion as no more than a surgical procedure"[4]—and that women who have scruples about abortion, or regret or remorse, are silly. Most people who regard themselves as liberal about abortion hold a more moderate, more complex view. I will construct an example of such a view, though I do not mean to suggest that all moderate liberals accept all parts of it.

A paradigm liberal position on abortion has four parts. First, it rejects the extreme opinion that abortion is morally unproblematic, and insists, on the contrary, that abortion is always a grave moral decision, at least from the moment at which the genetic individuality of the fetus is fixed and it has successfully implanted in the womb, normally after about

fourteen days. From that point on, abortion means the extinction of a
human life that has already begun, and for that reason alone involves a
serious moral cost. Abortion is never permissible for a trivial or frivolous
reason; it is never justifiable except to prevent serious damage of some
kind. It would be wrong for a woman to abort her pregnancy because she
would otherwise have to forfeit a long-awaited European trip, or because she would find it more comfortable to be pregnant at a different
time of year, or because she has discovered that her child would be a girl
and she wanted a boy.

Second, abortion is nevertheless morally justified for a variety of
serious reasons. It is justified not only to save the life of the mother and
in cases of rape or incest but also in cases in which a severe fetal
abnormality has been diagnosed—the abnormalities of thalidomide babies, for example, or of Tay-Sachs disease—that makes it likely that the
child, if carried to full term, will have only a brief, painful, and frustrat-
ing life.[5] Indeed, in some cases, when the abnormality is very severe and
the potential life inevitably a cruelly crippled and short one, the paradigm liberal view holds that abortion is not only morally permitted but
may be morally required, that it would be wrong knowingly to bring
such a child into the world.

Third, a woman's concern for her own interests is considered an
adequate justification for abortion if the consequences of childbirth
would be permanent and grave for her or her family's life. Depending
on the circumstances, it may be permissible for her to abort her pregnancy if she would otherwise have to leave school or give up a chance
for a career or a satisfying and independent life. For many women, these
are the most difficult cases, and people who take the paradigm liberal
view would assume that the expectant mother would suffer some regret
if she decided to abort. But they would not condemn the decision as
selfish; on the contrary, they might well suppose that the contrary
decision would be a serious moral mistake.

The fourth component in the liberal view is the political opinion that
I said moral conservatives about abortion sometimes share: that at least
until late in pregnancy, when a fetus is sufficiently developed to have
interests of its own, the state has no business intervening even to prevent
morally impermissible abortions, because the question of whether an
abortion is justifiable is, ultimately, for the woman who carries the fetus
to decide. Others—mate, family, friends, the public—may disapprove,

and they might be right, morally, to do so. The law might, in some circumstances, oblige her to discuss her decision with others. But the state in the end must let her decide for herself; it must not impose other people's moral convictions upon her.

I believe that these four components in the paradigm liberal view represent the moral convictions of many people—at least a very substantial minority in the United States and other Western countries. The liberal view they compose is obviously inconsistent with any assumption that an early-stage fetus is a person with rights and interests of its own. That assumption would, of course, justify the view that abortion is always morally problematic, but it would plainly be incompatible with the fourth component of the package, that the state has no right to protect a fetus's interests through the criminal law, and even more plainly with the third component: if a fetus does have a right to live, a mother's interests in having a fulfilling life could hardly be thought more important than that right. Even the second component, which insists that abortion may be morally permissible when a fetus is seriously deformed, is hard to justify if one assumes that a fetus has a right to remain alive. In cases when a child's physical deformities are so painful or otherwise crippling that we believe it would be in the best interests of the child to die, we might say that abortion, too, would have been in the child's best interests. But that is not so in every case in which the paradigm liberal view allows abortion; even children with quite terrible deformities may form attachments, give and receive love, struggle, and to some degree conquer their handicaps. If their lives are worth a great deal, then, how could it have been better for *them* to have been killed in the womb?

But though the presumption that a fetus has no rights or interests of its own is *necessary* to explain the paradigm liberal view, it is not sufficient because it cannot, alone, explain why abortion is ever morally wrong. Why should abortion raise any moral issue at all if there is no one whom it harms? Why is abortion then *not* like a tonsillectomy? Why should a woman feel any regret after an abortion? Why should she feel more regret than she does after sex with contraception? The truth is that liberal opinion, like the conservative view, presupposes that human life itself has intrinsic moral significance, so that it is in principle wrong to terminate a life even when no one's interests are at stake. Once we see this clearly, then we can explain why liberal and conservative opinions differ in the ways they do.

My discussion so far has emphasized individual moral opinion. But people do not respond to great moral or legal issues only as individuals; on the contrary, many people insist that their views on such important issues reflect and flow from larger, more general commitments or loyalties or associations. They have views, they think, not just as individuals, but as Catholics or Baptists or Jews or protectors of family values or feminists or atheists or socialists or social critics or anarchists or subscribers to some other orthodox or radical view about justice or society. We must consider how far the hypothesis I am now defending—that the abortion debate is about intrinsic value, not about a fetus's rights or interests—helps us better to understand the claims, insights, doctrines, and arguments of these large institutions or movements. I shall raise that question with reference to two of the most prominent groups in the controversy: traditional religions and the women's movement.

RELIGION

Throughout the Western world, even where church and state are normally separated, the battle over abortion has often had the character of a conflict between religious sects. In the United States, opinions about abortion correlate dramatically with religious belief. According to the 1984 American National Election Study, 22 percent of Baptists and fundamentalists, 16 percent of Southern Baptists, and 15 percent of Catholics then believed that abortion should never be permitted. The same survey showed that Lutherans (9 percent of whom would permit no abortions) and Methodists (8 percent) were more liberal denominations, Episcopalians (5 percent) and Jews (4 percent) even more so. Regular churchgoers of all faiths in America are much more likely to hold conservative views about abortion than nonchurchgoers or people who attend church only sporadically. Since religion tends to correlate, at least roughly, with other social divisions in America—with economic class, for example—these divisions may express other influences. But the controversy over abortion in the United States does seem to have a strong religious dimension.[6]

The anti-abortion movement is led by religious groups, uses religious language, invokes God constantly, and often calls for prayer. It embraces members of many religions, as the statistics I just described suggest, including not only fundamentalists but Orthodox Jews, Mormons, and Black Muslims. But Catholics have provided the organizational leadership. In 1980, John Dooling, a federal court judge in New York, declared that the Hyde amendment—which Congress had adopted in 1976 and which prohibited the use of federal medicaid funds to finance abortions—was unconstitutional because it denied people's right to free exercise of religion.[7] In the course of an extraordinarily thorough opinion, Dooling, himself a devout Catholic, said, "Roman Catholic clergy and laity are not alone in the pro-life movement, but the evidence requires the conclusion that it is they who have vitalized the movement, given it organization and direction, and used ecclesiastical channels of communication in its support."[8]

But it is important to note that leaders of many other religious faiths have also spoken out on the subject, including many who hold liberal rather than conservative views, and Dooling cited testimony from a number of them. Many of these statements, both those condemning abortion and those approving it in certain carefully limited circumstances, do not rely on the presumption that a fetus is a person. They all assert the different idea underlying most people's views about abortion: that any instance of human life has an intrinsic, sacred value that one must strive not to sacrifice. Not surprisingly, they all declare or suggest a particular source of that intrinsic, sacred value; they regard human life as the most exalted creation of God.

Dooling quoted, for example, the testimony of Dr. James E. Wood, Jr., executive director of the Baptist Joint Committee on Public Affairs, who reported that Baptists were divided about abortion and that there was no official Baptist position. But Dr. Wood also said that in 1973 the joint committee, reacting to the decision of Catholic bishops to work for a constitutional amendment reversing *Roe* v. *Wade*, objected to a campaign that "would coerce all citizens to accept a moral judgment affirmed by one member of the Body of Christ." Similarly, the 1976 Southern Baptist Convention rejected any "indiscriminate attitude toward abortion, as contrary to the biblical view" but refused to adopt a submitted resolution that declared, "Every decision for an abortion, for whatever reason, must necessarily involve the decision to terminate the life of an innocent human being." Dr. Wood said that in his own opinion, sound Baptist faith condemned abortion for frivolous reasons but recognized it as permissible when pregnancy was involuntary (including pregnancies of very young girls not of an age to consent and of women whose contraceptive devices had failed), cases of fetal deformity, and cases where significant family reasons argued against a pregnancy.[9]

The Reverend John Philip Wagoman, a Methodist minister who in 1980 was dean of the Wesley Theological Seminary in Washington, D.C., and had been president of the American Society of Christian Ethics, testified, in Judge Dooling's words, that "it was a common view among Protestant Christian theologians, and to some extent among other religious bodies, that human personhood—in the sense in which the person receives its maximum value in relation to the Christian faith—does not exist in the earlier stages of pregnancy . . . there is not a fully human person until that stage in development where someone has begun to have experience of reality." But, said Dooling, Dean Wagoman nevertheless insisted that "nearly no aspect of life is more sacred, closer to being human in relation to God, than bringing new life into the world to share in the gift of God's grace. . . . In bringing new life into the world human beings must be sure that the conditions into which the new life is being born will sustain that life in accordance with God's intention for the life to be fulfilled. . . . It matters whether a new life . . . might threaten to undermine the theologically understood fulfillment of already existing human beings." A pregnant woman "responding out of faith and love of God to the love which God has provided to human beings" might decide to have an abortion when the new life would be unlikely to receive the nurture necessary for human fulfillment, either because she is herself only a teenager, for example, or because she is close to menopause or because the existence of a new child would make life much harder for the existing family.[10]

According to the testimony of Rabbi David Feldman, "in Jewish law a fetus is not a person, and no person is in existence until the infant emerges from the womb into the world," so in Jewish law abortion is not murder. (If it were, Rabbi Feldman pointed out, it would not be permissible for a doctor to perform an abortion even to save the mother's life, because that would mean killing one innocent person to save another.)

But Judaism nevertheless holds that abortion is in principle wrong. In the stricter Jewish tradition, Rabbi Feldman said, abortion is objectionable for any reason except to protect the mother's life or sanity or personal well-being; a more liberal tradition, he said, allows more exceptions: protecting a woman from "mental anguish," for example. In both traditions, however, abortion is not merely permissible but mandatory in some cases. In those cases, abortion is required by a woman's sound sense of religious duty, because it is a choice, sanctioned by the Jewish faith, for life in this world as against life in any other. In 1975, the Biennial Convention of the United Synagogues of America declared that abortions, "though serious even in the early stages of pregnancy, are not to be equated with murder, hardly more than is the decision not to become pregnant." It added, "abortions involve very serious psychological, religious, and moral problems, but the welfare of the mother must always be our primary concern." [11]

Each of these declarations insists that any decision about abortion requires reflection about an important value: the intrinsic value of human life. Each interprets that value as resting on God's creative power and love, but each insists that a proper religious attitude must recognize and balance a different sort of threat to the sanctity of life: the threat to a woman's health and well-being that an unwanted pregnancy may pose. To show a proper respect for God's creation, in such cases, requires judgment and balance, not asserting the automatic priority of the biological life of a fetus over the developed life of its mother.

Some conservative theologians and religious leaders have also explicitly said that the crucial question about abortion is not whether a fetus is a person but how best to respect the intrinsic value of human life. The late Professor Paul Ramsey of Princeton, an influential Protestant theologian, was a fierce opponent of abortion. Writing before *Roe* v. *Wade* was decided, he insisted that even the use of intrauterine contraceptive devices, which prevent the implantation of a fertilized egg, was sinful, and he suggested that all young girls be given German measles deliberately to immunize them from that disease so that it would not be necessary to abort any fetuses damaged because a woman contracted the disease in pregnancy. But Ramsey made plain that his strong opinions were based not on the assumption of fetal personhood or rights but on respect for the divine dignity that is "alien" to man but "surrounds" him.

"From this point of view," he said, "it is *relatively* unimportant to say exactly when among the products of human generation we are dealing with an organism that is human and when we are dealing with organic life that is not human. . . . A man's dignity is an overflow from God's dealings with him, and not primarily an anticipation of anything he will ever be by himself alone. . . . The Lord did not set his love upon you, nor choose you because you were already intrinsically more than a blob of tissue in the uterus."[12] Ramsey argued that it is respect for God's creative choice and love of mankind, not any rights of a "blob of tissue in the uterus," that makes abortion sinful.

The Roman Catholic church's condemnation of abortion does seem an important counterexample, however, to my claim that for most people the abortion controversy is not about whether a fetus is a person with a right to live but about the sanctity of life understood in a more impersonal way. The church's present official position about fetal life is set out in its *Instruction on Respect for Human Life in Its Origin and on the Dignity of Procreation,* published in 1987 by the Vatican's Congregation for the Doctrine of the Faith with the consent of the pope. The *Instruction* declares that "every human being" has a "right to life and physical integrity from the moment of conception until death. . . ."[13] But most American Catholics do not seem to accept that view, and it has been the clear official view of the church itself for little more than a century, a fraction of Catholicism's long history. For substantial periods, if there was any reigning opinion within the church hierarchy it was to the contrary: that a fetus becomes a person not at conception but only at a later stage of pregnancy, later than the stage at which almost all abortions now take place. I do not mean that the church ever sanctioned early abortions. Quite the opposite: from its earliest beginnings, the church's condemnation of early as well as late abortion was clear and imperative; it was, as a prominent Catholic layman has put it, a nearly absolute value in the church's history.[14] But it relied not on the derivative claim that a fetus is a person with a right not to be killed, but on the different, detached view that abortion is wrong because it insults God's creative gift of life.

The detached reason for condemning abortion is historically firmer than the view set out in the Vatican's 1987 *Instruction* and also, according to many Catholic philosophers, better grounded in traditional Catholic theology. It also unites the church's opposition to abortion with its other

historical concerns about sexuality, including its opposition to contraception. For many centuries, Catholic theologians stressed these connections, but the claim that a fetus is a person from the moment of
conception dissipates them. The church's official view that abortion is
sinful in nearly all circumstances would not change dramatically if it
were now to abandon the new fetus-is-a-person justification and return
to the older one. That step would have the important advantage, as we
shall see, of changing the nature of the confrontation between the
church and its members in the United States and other countries who
hold strikingly more liberal views about abortion.

Abortion was common in the Greco-Roman world; but early Chris-
tianity condemned it. In the fifth century, St. Augustine called even
married women "in the fashion of harlots" who in order to avoid the
consequences of sex "procure poisons of sterility, and if these do not
work, they extinguish and destroy the fetus in some way in the womb,
preferring that their offspring die before it lives, or if it was already alive
in the womb, to kill it before it was born."[15] None of the early denuncia-
tions of abortion presupposed that a fetus has been ensouled—granted
a soul by God—at the moment of conception. Augustine declared
himself uncertain on that point, and so allowed that in early abortion an
"offspring" may die "before it lives." St. Jerome said that "seeds are
gradually formed in the uterus, and it is not reputed homicide until the
scattered elements received their appearance and members."[16] Catholicism's great thirteenth-century philosopher-saint, Thomas Aquinas,
held firmly that a fetus does not have an intellectual or rational soul at
conception but acquires one only at some later time—forty days in the
case of a male fetus, according to traditional Catholic doctrine, and later
in the case of a female.

Aquinas and almost all later Catholic theologians rejected Plato's
view that a human soul can exist in a wholly independent and disem-
bodied way or can be combined with any sort of substance. Under the
Platonic view, God might combine a human soul with a rock or a tree.
Aquinas accepted instead the Aristotelian doctrine of hylomorphism,
which holds that the human soul is not some independent free-floating
substance that can be combined with anything, but is logically related
to the human body in the same way as the shape or form of any object
is logically related to the raw material out of which it is made. No statue
can have a given form unless *it*—the whole stone, or wood, or wax, or

plaster—has that form. Even God could not bring it about that a huge
unformed block of stone actually had the shape of Michelangelo's
David. By the same token, nothing can embody a human soul, on this
view, unless it already is a human body, which meant, for Aquinas and
later Catholic doctrine, a body with the shape and organs of a human
being. Aquinas therefore denied that a human soul is already instinct in
the embryo that a woman and a man together create through sex. That
initial embryo, he thought, is only the raw material of a human being,
whose growth is directed by a series of souls, each appropriate to the
stage it has reached, and each corrupted and replaced by the next, until
it has finally achieved the necessary development for a distinctly human
soul.

Aquinas's views about fetal development, which he took from Aristotle, were remarkably prescient in some respects. He understood that
an embryo is not an extremely tiny but fully formed child who simply
grows larger until birth, as some later scientists with primitive micro-
scopes decided, but an organism that develops through an essentially
vegetative stage, then a stage at which sensation begins, and, finally, a
stage of intellect and reason. But he was wrong about the biology of
reproduction in two important respects. He believed that the active
power that causes a new human being to grow is what he called the
"generative" soul of the father, acting at a distance through "froth" in the
semen, and that the mother contributes only nourishment sustaining
that growth. Of course, we now know that both parents contribute
chromosomes to the embryo, which has a genetic structure different
from that of either of them. Aquinas also apparently thought that the
fetal brain and other organs necessary to provide the bodily form required for a sentient or intellectual soul are in place by the time of fetal
"quickening" or movement. Modern embryologists believe that the neu-
ral substrate necessary to make any sentience possible has not formed
until much later.[17]

Catholic philosophers are currently engaged in a strenuous debate
about whether Aquinas would have modified his view about when a
fetus is ensouled if he had been aware of what biological science has now
discovered. One group argues that he would then have maintained that
a fetus has a soul from conception: they say that because he believed that
the organic development of a fetus must be directed by a soul, and
because science has shown that this cannot be the soul of the father

acting alone in the way Aquinas supposed, he would have decided that embryological development is directed by the fetus's own soul, which must therefore be present from the start.[18] But this argument seems doubtful. Aquinas thought that the father's soul controlled fetal development at a distance, through some frothy power in the semen. If he had formed his view in the light of modern embryology, he might well have said that the generative souls of both parents direct fetal development together, acting at a distance through the chromosomes each contributes, an opinion that seems much closer to the spirit of his original view than the more radical claim of immediate ensoulment.

The rival group of Catholic philosophers, who argue that Aquinas would not have changed his view, say that his most fundamental reason for denying immediate ensoulment was his hylomorphism—his conviction that a full human soul, which is essentially intellectual, cannot be the form of a creature that has never had the material shape necessary for even the most rudimentary stage of thought or sentience. Joseph Donceel, S.J., puts the point this way: "If form and matter are strictly complementary, as hylomorphism holds, there can be an actual human soul only in a body endowed with the organs required for the spiritual activities of man. We know that the brain, and especially the cortex, are the main organs of those highest sense activities without which no spiritual activity is possible."[19] Donceel and others seem to me right in taking that position (which is the Aristotelian version of the view I defended that a fetus cannot have interests of its own before it has a mental life) to be fundamental to Aquinas's views about ensoulment. But this implies not simply that Aquinas would have continued to deny immediate ensoulment, even if he had had the benefit of modern discoveries, but that he might well have thought that a fetus is ensouled later than he said it was—perhaps not until twenty-six weeks, which is, according to the expert opinion I cited, a cautious choice for a point in fetal development before which sentience is not possible. The combination of traditional Thomist metaphysics and contemporary science might therefore produce a spiritual version of the main distinction drawn in *Roe* v. *Wade:* a fetus has no human soul, and abortion cannot be considered murder, until approximately the end of the second trimester of pregnancy. In any case, however, it is at least problematic whether the now official Catholic view, that a fetus has a full human soul at conception, is consistent with the Thomist tradition.

Nor was that view thought necessary, in the past, to justify the strongest condemnation of even very early abortion. For many centuries, Catholic doctrine, following Aquinas, held that abortion in the early weeks of pregnancy, before the fetus is "formed," is not murder because the soul is not yet present. An instruction manual described as the most influential book of seminary instruction in the nineteenth century still declared, "The fetus, although not ensouled, is directed to the forming of a man; therefore its ejection is anticipated homicide." But though early abortion was not considered murder during this long period, it was certainly considered a grave sin, as the expression "anticipated homicide" insists. Though Jerome did not think an early fetus had a soul, and Augustine was uncertain on the matter, neither of them distinguished between the sinfulness of early and later abortion. Augustine condemned contraception, early abortion—before the fetus "lives"—and later abortion in the same terms. In the Middle Ages, the term "homicide" was sometimes used to name any offense, including contraception, against the natural order of procreation and thus against the sanctity of life conceived as God's divine gift. Decrees of Pope Gregory IX provided that anyone who treated a man or woman "so that he cannot generate, or she conceive, or offspring be born, let it be held as homicide."[20] This expanded conception of homicide, to include not just the killing of an actual human being but any interference with God's creative force, united the church's various concerns with procreation. Masturbation, contraception, and abortion were together seen as offenses against the dignity and sanctity of human life itself. That idea was restated in 1968, in Pope Paul VI's influential encyclical letter about contraception, *Humanae Vitae*.

> Just as man does not have unlimited dominion over his body in general, so also, and with more particular reason, he has no such dominion over his specifically sexual facilities, for these are concerned by their very nature with the generation of life, of which God is the source. For Human life is sacred—all men must recognize that fact, Our Predecessor, Pope John XXIII, recalled, "since from its first beginnings it calls for the creative action of God." Therefore . . . the direct interruption of the generative processes already begun, and, above all, direct abortion, even for therapeutic reasons, are to be absolutely excluded as lawful means of control-

ling the birth of children. Equally to be condemned . . . is direct sterilization, whether of the man or of the woman, whether permanent or temporary. Similarly excluded is an action, which either before, at the moment of, or after sexual intercourse, is specifically intended to prevent procreation—whether as an end or as a means.[21]

For many centuries, this traditional church view—that abortion is wicked because it insults the sanctity of human life even when the fetus killed has not yet been ensouled—was believed capable of sustaining a firm and unwavering moral opposition to early abortion. Even in 1974, when the doctrine that a fetus has a right to life from conception had become fixed in official Catholic doctrine, a declaration by the Sacred Congregation for the Doctrine of the Faith declared that its opposition to abortion did not depend on "questions of the moment when the spiritual soul is infused"—on which, it said, authors are still in disagreement—because even if ensoulment is delayed there is nevertheless a human life preparing for a soul, which is enough to ground a "moral affirmation" that abortion is sinful. The declaration noted that the church's opposition to abortion was just as strong in the long period when this doctrine was denied.[22] Canon and secular law waxed and waned in severity about abortion, but even the severest condemnation of early abortion was thought consistent with denying immediate ensoulment: for a brief period in the sixteenth century, for example, even excommunication was thought a permissible punishment, as it is now, for an early abortion. It is true that the church's present position about abortion is particularly severe by historical standards, not just in the punishment it provides for early abortions but, even more significantly, in the exceptions it refuses to recognize for late ones. In 1930, for example, a papal encyclical made the church's refusal to permit a late-stage abortion to save the life of a mother more rigid; that change had nothing to do with any shift in theological doctrine about ensoulment or the status of an unformed fetus.

It is widely thought that a papal decree in 1869, in which Pius IX declared that even an early abortion is punishable by excommunication, marked the first official rejection of the traditional view that a fetus is ensouled sometime after conception and official adoption of the contemporary immediate-ensoulment view. There is considerable debate among religious historians and philosophers about what prompted the change. Some Catholic philosophers suggest that modern biological discoveries were responsible, but as we saw, these discoveries were at least as likely to lead church leaders to believe that ensoulment takes place not earlier but later than Aquinas thought. Some historians suggest a theological rather than philosophical inspiration for the change in doctrine. In 1854, Pius IX pronounced the dogma of Immaculate Conception, that "the Virgin Mary was, in the first instant of her conception, preserved untouched by any taint of original sin," which seems to presuppose that the Virgin had a soul from that moment. But, as Michael Coughlan has argued, alternate constructions of the dogma are available that suppose that God made an exception in this case, for which there are ample historical precedents.[23]

Though it remains controversial whether any philosophical or doctrinal thesis adequately explains the church's official change of view, there is no doubt that the change gave it a considerable political advantage in its campaign against abortion. Since the eighteenth century, Western democracies had begun to resist explicitly theological arguments in politics. In the United States, the First Amendment to the Constitution provides that Congress has no power to establish any particular religion or to legislate in service of any religion's dogma or metaphysics. By the late nineteenth century, the idea that church and state should be separate was becoming orthodox wisdom in many nations of Europe as well. In a political culture that insists on secular justifications for its criminal law, the detached argument that early abortion is sin because any abortion insults and frustrates God's creative power cannot count as a reason for making abortion a crime. It is revealing that though anti-abortion statutes were enacted throughout the United States in the mid-nineteenth century, religious groups and arguments played almost no part in the campaign, which was conducted largely by doctors newly organized into professional associations. (Some of the campaigning doctors opposed abortion on moral grounds; others wanted to stop competition from nondoctors who performed abortion.)

The Roman Catholic church's change to the doctrine of immediate ensoulment greatly strengthened its political position. People who believe, for whatever reason, that a fetus is a person from the instant of its conception are free to argue that even early abortion is the murder of an unborn child, an argument they cannot make if they believe a fetus acquires a soul or becomes a person only later. In other words, Catholic doctrine now allowed a derivative secular as well as a detached religious argument. Just as any religious body can properly argue, even in a pluralist community that separates church from state, that the rights of children or minorities or the poor should not be neglected, so it can argue that the rights of unborn children must not be sacrificed either. God need not be mentioned in the argument. The declaration by the Sacred Congregation I mentioned, published the year after *Roe* v. *Wade,* emphasized this point. "It is true that it is not the task of the law to choose between points of view or to impose one rather than another. But the life of the child takes precedence over all opinions. One cannot invoke freedom of thought to destroy this life. . . . It is at all times the task of the State to preserve each person's rights and to protect the weakest."[24]

The immediate-ensoulment doctrine had another practical political advantage. The older, traditional doctrine—that early abortion is a sin because it insults the inherent value of God's gift of life—was part of a larger general view of sexuality and creation that condemned abortion, masturbation, and contraception as different manifestations of the sin of disrespect of God and life, all aspects of "homicide" in the broadest sense. The church continues to condemn contraception in the strongest terms; in *Humanae Vitae,* Pope Paul VI denounced as "intrinsically deliberate contraception wrong."[25] But contraception is so firmly a fact of life in many Western countries and has seemed so desirable a part of the attempts made to curb population growth and improve economic life in the nations of the Third World that the church needs a sharp and effective way to distinguish abortion from contraception; in the United States, this became particularly important after the Supreme Court's 1965 decision in *Griswold* v. *Connecticut,* which, together with other decisions in its wake, altogether prohibited states to outlaw contraception. Of course, even according to the traditional view, abortion can be distinguished as much the graver insult to God's creative power, and many deeply religious people plausibly believe that contraception, which frustrates no investment in an actual human life, is no insult at all. But the doctrine of immediate ensoulment makes a more dramatic distinction, because it claims that a conceptus has a divine soul, though a sperm or an ovum does not.

The doctrine has had the conspicuous disadvantage, however, of making official Catholic dogma much more remote from the opinions and practices of most Catholics. In 1992, a Gallup poll reported that 52 percent of American Catholics thought that abortion should be legal in "many or all" circumstances, a further 33 percent in "rare" circumstances, and only 13 percent under no circumstances. It also reported that 15 percent of Catholics believe that abortion is morally acceptable in all circumstances, a further 26 percent in many circumstances, 41 percent in rare circumstances, and only 13 percent in none.[26] As I said, in America, Catholic women are actually no less likely to have an abortion than women generally.

Practicing Catholics could not accept the exceptions that most of them do if they really believed that a fetus is a person with a right to life from the moment of conception. Even in Ireland, a country long dominated by conservative Catholicism, where abortion is constitutionally forbidden, most Catholics apparently reject that view. As I mentioned earlier, when an Irish court forbade a fourteen-year-old rape victim to have an abortion in Britain, the order produced a furor. On appeal, the Irish Supreme Court held that the constitutional ban exempted abortions necessary to save a mother's life, and that because the young woman had threatened to kill herself if forced to bear the child, the exception applied in this case. As Catholic critics pointed out, that opinion would seem to permit abortion not just abroad but in Ireland as well on any occasion on which a pregnant woman threatened to kill herself if abortion was refused and a doctor believed her. But the Irish Supreme Court nevertheless felt compelled by public opinion to find some way of permitting the abortion. The series of events provoked the November 1992 referendum I mentioned, in which a majority refused a constitutional amendment declaring that abortion might be lawful when necessary to save the mother's life, but nevertheless approved constitutional changes allowing Irishwomen to have abortions abroad and information about foreign abortion services to be distributed within Ireland. Though the first of these votes was widely understood as a refusal to liberalize abortion, the law that resulted from the referendum plainly presupposes that a fetus is not a person from conception; if it were, a state would certainly be justified in ordering its citizens not to kill a fetus in a foreign country—indeed, it would be morally obliged to do so. (What if some impoverished country decided to permit infanticide in order to encourage tourism? It would certainly be proper for other countries to forbid their citizens to take unwanted young children there.)

So the Irish people's latest vote is further confirmation that even people who believe, on religious grounds, that the state should prohibit almost all abortions do not actually think that a fetus is a person from the moment of conception. They believe something different but more firmly grounded in Catholic tradition: that abortion is a fierce and rarely justified waste of the divine gift of human life. People who oppose abortion for that reason might well find it acceptable that citizens be permitted to have an abortion abroad. Almost no one is such a moral relativist as to believe that infanticide is morally proper if done where the laws permit it, but many people do think that each nation should be permitted to decide for itself what may be done on its soil, out of respect for fundamental intrinsic values, when no one's rights are violated.

These statistics and events tend to support Gary Wills's strong claim that "most Catholics have concluded that their clerical leaders are unhinged on the subject of sex."[27] If the church were to return to its traditional view about the moral status of a fetus, early and late, it would no longer find itself in such sharp doctrinal confrontation with its own members. According to its present view, Catholics who accept the permissibility of abortion in cases of rape or serious fetal deformity are condoning the murder of innocent persons; official doctrine permits no other description. But in the more traditional view, the differences between hierarchy and laity could be regarded as differences in interpretation of a shared and fundamental commitment—to human life as the gift of God—that all Catholics share. For, of course, Catholics who reject the doctrine of immediate ensoulment and deny that an early abortion is murder may nevertheless agree that early abortion is a very grave act, sinful except in the most pressing circumstances. Joseph Donceel, S.J., does not believe that an early fetus is a person, but he nevertheless insists, "Although a prehuman embryo cannot demand from us the absolute respect which we owe to the human person, it deserves a very great consideration, because it is a living being, endowed with a human finality, on its way to hominization. Therefore it seems to me that only very serious reasons should allow us to terminate its existence."[28] Donceel might well recognize exceptions that more conservative Catholics would not, but the ground of judgment he proposes—whether an exception is permitted by the best understanding of the respect owed to any example of developing human life—encourages conservative and liberal alike to understand their differences as less important than their shared respect for human life as intrinsically and overwhelmingly valuable.

Perhaps Catholic doctrine is already moving in this direction, if not explicitly or self-consciously. One of the most interesting religious developments today is the emergence, among Catholics and Protestants who are firmly opposed to any abortion, of the doctrine some of them call the Consistent Ethic of Life. This doctrine insists that people who oppose abortion must show a consistent respect for human life in their views about other social issues. Joseph Cardinal Bernardin, the archbishop of Chicago, has been a pioneer in developing and defending that thesis. In a series of important essays and speeches, he argues that Catholics who oppose abortion out of respect for human life must, if they are consistent, also oppose the death penalty (at least when its deterrent value is in doubt), work toward a fairer health-care policy for the poor, promote welfare policies that will improve the quality and length of human life, and oppose the legalization of active euthanasia even for terminally ill patients.[29]

Cardinal Bernardin has not, so far as I know, cast any explicit doubt on the official contemporary Catholic view that a fetus is a person from conception. In a recent speech, he urged his listeners to help "save the lives of millions of our unborn sisters and brothers."[30] But his argument—that it is *inconsistent* to support capital punishment or euthanasia while condemning abortion—presupposes that principled opposition to abortion is based on respect for the intrinsic value of life, rather than on any assumption that a fetus is a person with a right to life. For someone who based his condemnation of abortion on the latter ground—that a fetus does have such a right—would *not* be inconsistent in endorsing capital punishment if he also thought (as Bernardin does) that a murderer has forfeited his right to live.[31] Nor would he be inconsistent in supporting euthanasia if he agreed with Bernardin's view about why euthanasia is wrong.

Bernardin explicitly bases his own opposition to euthanasia on a detached, not a derivative, argument. "The grounding principle . . . is found in the Judeo-Christian heritage which has played such an influential role in the formation of our national ethos. In this religious tradition, the meaning of human life is grounded in the fact that it is sacred because God is its origin and its destiny." That principle explains, he says, why it is wrong to judge euthanasia by looking only to the question whether it benefits or injures the patient as an individual, rather than to the deeper question of whether it harms a "social good" which can be in "tension" with "personal rights." It would be inconsistent to oppose abortion and support euthanasia only if opposition to abortion necessarily embraced a parallel detached view: that abortion, too, is wrong not just because a fetus has a right to live, if it does, but because abortion insults the "social good" of respect for life, which it would do even if a fetus had no such right. Of course, I do not mean that Cardinal Bernardin or others drawn to his views cannot also insist that a fetus is indeed a person with rights and interests. But their attractive call for consistency assumes that the case against abortion in no way depends on that view.

FEMINISM

I have been arguing that doctrinal religious opinion about abortion can be better understood as based on the detached assumption that human life has intrinsic value rather than on the derivative idea that a fetus is a person with its own interests and rights. I should like to make an opposite but parallel claim about a large and diverse movement rallying its forces mainly on the "pro-choice" side: I suggest that feminist arguments and studies are grounded not just in denying that a fetus is a person or claiming that abortion is permissible even if it is, but also in positive concerns that recognize the intrinsic value of human life.

Of course, it is a crude mistake to treat all women who regard themselves as feminists, or as part of the women's movement in the general sense, as parties to the same set of convictions. There are serious divisions of opinion within feminism about the best strategies for improving the political, economic, and social position of women—for example, about the ethics and wisdom of censoring literature some feminists find demeaning to women. Feminists also disagree about deeper questions: about the character and roots of sexual and gender discrimination, about whether women are genetically different from men in moral sensibility or perception, and about whether the goal of feminism should be simply to erase formal and informal discrimination or to aim instead at a thoroughly genderless world in which roughly as many fathers are in primary charge of children as mothers and roughly as many women hold top military positions as men. Feminists even disagree about whether abortion should be permitted: there *are* "pro-life" feminists.[32] The feminist views I shall discuss are those that are central to this book, those that are concerned with the special connection between a pregnant woman and the fetus she carries.

In the United States, during the decades before *Roe* v. *Wade,* feminists were leaders in the campaigns to repeal anti-abortion laws in various states: they argued, with an urgency and power unmatched by any other group, for the rights that *Roe* finally recognized. They have since expressed deep disgust with Supreme Court decisions that have allowed states to restrict those rights in various ways,[33] and they have demonstrated in support of their position, risking, in some cases, violent injury at the hands of anti-abortion protesters. Nevertheless, some feminists are among the most savage critics of the arguments Justice Blackmun used in his opinion justifying the *Roe* decision; they insist that the Court reached the right result but for very much the wrong reason. Some of them suggest that the decision may in the end have worked to the detriment rather than the benefit of women.

Blackmun's opinion argued that women have a general constitutional right to privacy and that it follows from that general right that they have the right to an abortion before the end of the second trimester of their pregnancy. Some feminists object that the so-called right to privacy is a dangerous illusion and that a woman's freedom of choice about abortion in contemporary societies, dominated by men, should be defended not by an appeal to privacy but instead as an essential aspect of any genuine attempt to improve sexual equality. It is not surprising that feminists should want to defend abortion rights in as many ways as possible, and certainly not surprising that some should call attention to sexual inequality as part of the reason why women need such rights. But why should they be eager not only to claim an additional argument from equality but actually to reject the right-to-privacy argument on which the Court had relied? Why shouldn't they urge both arguments, and as many others as seem pertinent?

Many of the reasons feminist writers offer to explain their rejection of the right to privacy are indeed unconvincing, but it is important to see *why* in order to identify the illuminating and revealing reasons they also offer. Professor Catharine MacKinnon of the Michigan law school, for example, a prominent feminist lawyer, argues that the right-to-privacy argument presupposes what she regards as a fallacious distinction between matters that are in principle private, like the sexual acts and decisions of couples, which government should not attempt to regulate or supervise, and those that are in principle public, like foreign economic policy, about which government must of course legislate.[34] That distinction, she believes, is mistaken and dangerous for women in several ways. It supposes that women really are free to make decisions for themselves within the private space they occupy, though in fact, she insists, women are often very unfree in the so-called private realm; men often force sexual compliance upon them in private, and this private sexual domination both reflects and helps sustain the political and economic subordination of women in the public community.

Appealing to a right to privacy is dangerous, MacKinnon suggests, in two ways. First, insisting that sex is a private matter implies that the government has no legitimate concern with what happens to women behind the bedroom door, where they may be raped or mauled. Second, the claim that abortion is a private matter seems to imply that government has no responsibility to help finance abortion for poor pregnant women as it helps finance childbirth for them. (Other feminists expand on this point: basing the right to an abortion on a right to privacy seems to suggest, they say, that government does all it needs to do for sexual equality by allowing women this free choice, and ignores the larger truth that any substantial advance toward equality will require considerable public expenditure on welfare and other programs directed to women.) MacKinnon argues that the Supreme Court's 1980 decision in *Harris* v. *McRae*, which reversed Judge John Dooling's decision that the Hyde amendment prohibiting the use of federal funds to finance abortion was unconstitutional, was a direct result of the Court's rhetoric about privacy in *Roe* v. *Wade*.

Is this persuasive? It is certainly true that many women are sexually intimidated and that a presumption of much criminal and civil law—that women who have sexual intercourse have either been raped or have freely and willingly consented—is much too crude, and the American law of sexual harassment has begun slowly to change (in part thanks to MacKinnon's work) to reflect that realization. But there is no evident connection between these facts and MacKinnon's claims about the rhetoric of privacy. The right to privacy that the Court recognized in *Roe v. Wade* in no way assumes that all or even some women are genuinely free agents in sexual decisions. On the contrary, that women are often dominated by men makes it more rather than less important to insist that women should have a constitutionally protected right to control the use of their own bodies. MacKinnon, it is true, disparages the motives of men who favor women's right to abortion. Liberal abortion rules, she says, allow men to use women sexually with no fear of any consequences of paternity; allow them, she says, quoting a feminist colleague, to fill women up, vacuum them out, and fill them up again. But her suspicion of men who are her allies, even if it were well founded, would offer no ground for being more critical of the right-to-privacy argument than of any other argument for liberal abortion rules that men might support.

Nor is the second reason she gives against the right-to-privacy argument—that recognizing privacy in sex means that the law will not protect women from marital rape or help to finance abortions—any more persuasive, for she conflates different senses of "privacy." Sometimes privacy is territorial: people have a right to privacy in the territorial sense when they are entitled to do as they wish in a certain specified space—inside their own home, for example. Sometimes privacy is a matter of confidentiality: we say that people may keep their political convictions private, meaning that they need not disclose how they have voted. Sometimes, however, privacy means something different from either of these senses: it means sovereignty over personal decisions. The Supreme Court has cited, for example, as precedents for the right to privacy in contraception and abortion decisions, its earlier rulings that the Constitution protects the right of parents to send their children to a private school or a school in which a foreign language is taught.[35] That is a matter of sovereignty over a particular parental decision that the Court believed should be protected; it is not a matter of either territorial privacy or secrecy. (It is true that in *Griswold* v. *Connecticut*, the contraception case I described earlier, one justice said that the law must not forbid contraceptives because if it did, policemen would have to search bedrooms. But he alone urged that rationale, and the Court explicitly rejected it in a decision soon after when it held that the right to privacy meant that teen-agers were free to buy contraceptives in drugstores.[36])

The right to privacy that the Court endorsed in *Roe* v. *Wade* is plainly privacy in the sense of sovereignty over particular, specified decisions, and it does not follow, from the government's protecting a woman's sovereignty over the use of her own body for procreation, that it is indifferent to how her partner treats her—or how she treats him—inside her home. On the contrary: a right not to be raped or sexually violated is another example of a right to control how one's body is used. Nor does it follow that the government has no responsibility to assure the economic conditions that make the exercise of the right possible and its possession valuable. On the contrary: recognizing that women have a constitutional right to determine how their own bodies are to be used is a prerequisite, not a barrier, to the further claim that the government must ensure that this right is not illusory.[37]

These explanations that MacKinnon and some other feminists give for their opposition to the language of privacy do not go to the heart of the matter. But other passages in their work suggest a far more compelling explanation: claiming that a right to *privacy* protects a woman's decision whether to abort assimilates pregnancy to other situations that are very unlike it; the effect of that assimilation is to obscure the special meaning of pregnancy for women and to denigrate, by overlooking, its unique character. The claim of privacy, according to these feminists, treats pregnancy as if a woman and her fetus were morally and genetically separate entities. It treats pregnancy, MacKinnon says, as if it were just another case in which two separate entities have either deliberately or accidentally become connected in some way and one party plainly has a "sovereign right" to sever the connection if it wishes. She offers these examples of other such cases: the relationship between an employee and her employer, or between a tenant on short lease and his landlord, or (in a reference to a well-known article about abortion by the philosopher Judith Jarvis Thomson that many feminists dislike) between a sick violinist and a woman who wakes to find that the violinist has been connected by tubes to her body, an attachment that must be maintained for nine months if the violinist is to remain alive. MacKinnon insists that pregnancy is not like those relationships; in a striking passage, she describes what pregnancy is like from the perspective of a woman.

> In my opinion and in the experience of many pregnant women, the fetus is a human form of life. It is alive. . . . More than a body part but less than a person, where it is, is largely what it is. From the

standpoint of the pregnant woman, it is both me and not me. It "is" the pregnant woman in the sense that it is in her and of her and is hers more than anyone's. It "is not" her in the sense that she is not all that is there.[38]

MacKinnon also cites the poet Adrienne Rich's comment, "The child that I carry for nine months can be defined *neither* as me nor as not-me."[39]

By ignoring the unique character of the relationship between pregnant woman and fetus, by neglecting the mother's perspective and assimilating her situation to that of a landlord or a woman strapped to a violinist, the privacy claim obscures, in particular, the special *creative* role of a woman in pregnancy. Her fetus is not merely "in her" as an inanimate object might be, or something alive but alien that has been transplanted into her body. It is "of her and is hers more than anyone's" because it is, more than anyone else's, her creation and her responsibility; it is alive because *she* has made it come alive. She already has an intense physical and emotional investment in it unlike that which any other person, even its father, has; because of these physical and emotional connections it is as wrong to say that the fetus is separate from her as to say that it is not. All these aspects of a pregnant woman's experience—everything special, complex, ironic, and tragic about pregnancy and abortion—is neglected in the liberal explanation that women have a right to abortion because they are entitled to sovereignty over personal decisions, an explanation that would apply with equal force to a woman's right to choose her own clothing.

The most characteristic and fundamental feminist claim is that women's sexual subordination must be made a central feature of the abortion debate. MacKinnon put the point in a particularly striking way: if women were truly equal with men, she said, then the political status of a fetus would be different from what it is now. That seems paradoxical: how can the inequality of women, however unjustified, doom fetuses— half of whom are female—to a lower status, and a lesser right to live, than they would otherwise have? But this objection to MacKinnon's suggestion, like so much else in the public and philosophical debate about abortion, presupposes that the pivotal issue is whether a fetus is a person with interests and rights of its own. The objection would be sound if that were the central issue—if the debate were about a fetus's status in *that* sense. But MacKinnon's point becomes not only sensible but powerful if we take her to be discussing a fetus's status in the detached sense I have distinguished. Then the crucial question is whether and when abortion is an unjustifiable waste of something of intrinsic importance, and MacKinnon's point is the arresting one that the intrinsic importance of a new human life may well depend on the meaning and freedom of the act that created it.

If women were free and equal to men in their sexual relationships, feminists say—if they had a more genuinely equal role in forming the moral, cultural, and economic environment in which children are conceived and raised—then the status of a fetus would be different because it would be more genuinely and unambiguously the woman's own intended and wanted creation rather than something imposed upon her. Abortion would then more plainly be, as of course many women now think it is, a kind of self-destruction, a woman destroying something into which she had mixed herself. Women cannot take that view of abortion now, some feminists argue, because too much sexual intercourse is rape to a degree, and pregnancy is too often the result not of creative achievement but of uncreative subordination, and because the costs of pregnancy and child-rearing are so unfairly distributed, falling so heavily and disproportionately on them.

This argument, at least put in the way I have put it here, may be overstated. It takes no notice of the creative function of the father, for example, and though it shows what is objectionable in relying wholly on the concept of privacy to defend a woman's right to an abortion, it does not prove that the Supreme Court was misguided in relying on that concept in deciding the constitutional issue in *Roe* v. *Wade*. After all, appealing to privacy does not deny the ways in which pregnancy is a unique relationship or the ambivalent and complex character of many pregnant women's attitudes toward the embryos they carry. In fact, the best argument for applying the constitutional right of privacy to abortion, as we shall see in chapter 6, emphasizes the special psychic as well as physical costs of unwanted pregnancies. I do not believe, finally, that even a great and general improvement in gender equality in the United States would either undercut the argument that women have a constitutional right to abortion or obviate the need for such a right.

In spite of these important reservations, the feminist argument has added a very important dimension to the abortion debate. It is true that many women's attitudes toward abortion are affected by a contradictory sense of both identification with and oppression by their pregnancies, and that the sexual, economic, and social subordination of women contributes to that undermining sense of oppression. In a better society, which supported child rearing as enthusiastically as it discourages abortion, the status of a fetus probably would change, because women's sense of pregnancy and motherhood as creative would be more genuine and less compromised, and the inherent value of their own lives less threatened. The feminist arguments reveal another way, then, in which our understanding is cramped and our experience distorted by the one-dimensional idea that the abortion controversy turns only on whether a fetus is a person from the moment of conception. Feminists do not hold that a fetus is a person with moral rights of its own, but they do insist that it is a creature of moral consequence. They emphasize not the woman's right suggested by the rhetoric of privacy, but a woman's responsibility to make a complex decision she is best placed to make.

That is explicitly the message of another prominent feminist lawyer, Professor Robin West, who argues that if the Supreme Court one day overrules *Roe* v. *Wade*, and the battle over abortion shifts from courtrooms to legislatures, women will not succeed in defending abortion rights if they emphasize their right to privacy, which suggests selfish, willful decisions taken behind a veil of immunity from public censure. Instead, she says, women should emphasize responsibility, and she offers what she calls a responsibility-based argument to supplement the right-based claims of *Roe*.

> Women need the freedom to make reproductive decisions not merely to vindicate a right to be left alone, but often to strengthen their ties to others: to plan responsibly and have a family for which they can provide, to pursue professional or work commitments made to the outside world, or to continue supporting their families or communities. At other times the decision to abort is necessitated, not by a murderous urge to end life, but by the harsh reality of a financially irresponsible partner, a society indifferent to the care of children, and a workplace incapable of accommodating or supporting the needs of working parents. . . . Whatever the reason, the

decision to abort is almost invariably made within a web of inter-
locking, competing, and often irreconcilable responsibilities and
commitments.[40]

West is obviously assuming that the audience to which this argument
is addressed has firmly rejected the view that a fetus is a person. If her
claims were interpreted as proposing that a woman may murder another
person in order to "strengthen her ties to others," or because her husband
is financially irresponsible, or because society does not mandate maternity leave, these claims would be politically suicidal for the feminist
cause. West assumes what I have been arguing throughout this chapter:
that most people recognize, even when their rhetoric does not, that the
real argument against abortion is that it is irresponsible to waste human
life without a justification of appropriate importance.

West and other feminists often refer to the research of the sociologist
Professor Carol Gilligan of Harvard University. In a much-cited study,
Gilligan argued that, at least in American society, women characteristically think about moral issues in ways different from men.[41] Women
who are faced with difficult moral decisions, she said, pay less attention
to abstract moral principles than men do, but feel a greater responsibility
to care for and nurture others, and to prevent hurt or pain. She relied
on, among other research studies, interviews with twenty-nine women
contemplating abortion who had been referred to her research program
by counseling services. These women were not typical of all women
considering abortion; although twenty-one of them did have abortions
following the discussions (of the others, four had their babies, two
miscarried, and two could not be reached to learn of their decision), they
were all at least willing to discuss their decisions with a stranger and to
delay their abortions to do so.

One feature of the responses is particularly striking. Though many of
the twenty-nine women in the study were in considerable doubt about
what was the right decision to make, and agonized over it, none of them,
apparently, traced that doubt to any uncertainty or perplexity over the
question of whether a fetus is a person with a right to live. At least
one—a twenty-nine-year-old Catholic nurse—said she believed in the
principle that a fetus is a person and that abortion is murder, but it is
doubtful that she really did believe that, as she also said that she had
come to think that abortion might sometimes be justified because it fell

into "a 'gray' area," just as she now thought, on the basis of her nursing experience, that euthanasia might sometimes be justified in spite of her church's teaching to the contrary. In any case, even she worried, like the others, not about the metaphysical status of the fetus but about a conflict of responsibilities she believed she owed to family, to others, and to herself.

The women in the study did not see this conflict as one between simple self-interest and their responsibilities to others but rather as a conflict between genuine responsibilities on both sides, of having to decide—as a twenty-five-year-old who had already had one abortion put it—how to act in a "decent, human kind of way, one that leaves maybe a slightly shaken but not totally destroyed person." Some of them said that the selfish choice would be to have their babies. One nineteen-year-old felt that "it is a choice of hurting myself [by an abortion] or hurting other people around me. What is more important?" Or, as a seventeen-year-old put it, "What I want to do is to have the baby, but what I feel I should do, which is what I need to do, is have an abortion right now, because sometimes what you want isn't right." When she wanted the child, she said, she wasn't thinking of the responsibilities that go with it, and that was selfish.

All of Gilligan's subjects talked and wondered about responsibility. They sometimes talked of responsibility to the child, but they meant the future hypothetical child, not the existing embryo—they meant that it would be wrong to have a child one could not care for properly. They also worried about other people who would be affected by their decision. One, in her late twenties, said that a right decision depends on awareness of "what it will do to your relationship with the father or how it will affect him emotionally." They talked of responsibility to themselves, but they had in mind not their pleasure, or doing what they wanted now, but their responsibilities to make something of their own lives. One adolescent said, "Abortion, if you do it for the right reasons, is helping you to start over and do different things." A musician in her late twenties said that her choice for abortion was selfish because it was for her "survival," but she meant surviving in her work, which, she said, was "where I derive the meaning of what I am."

Gilligan says, in summary, "Here the conventional feminine voice emerges with great clarity, defining the self and proclaiming its worth on the basis of the ability to care for and protect others." But her subjects talked of another, more abstract, kind of responsibility as well: responsibility to what they called "the world." One said, "I don't need to pay off my imaginary debts to the world through this child, and I don't think that it is right to bring a child into the world and use it for that purpose." Another said that it would be selfish for her to decide to have an abortion because it denied "the survival of the child, another human being," but she did not mean that abortion was murder or that it violated any fetal rights. She put it in very different, more impersonal and abstract terms: "Once a certain life has begun it shouldn't be stopped artificially."

This is a brief but carefully accurate statement of what, beneath all the screaming rhetoric about rights and murder, most people think is the real moral defect in abortion. Abortion wastes the intrinsic value—the sanctity, the inviolability—of a human life and is therefore a grave moral wrong unless the intrinsic value of other human lives would be wasted in a decision *against* abortion. Each of Gilligan's subjects was exploring and reacting to that terrible conflict. Each was trying, above all, to take the measure of her responsibility for the intrinsic value of her *own* life, to locate the awful decision she had to make in that context, to see the decisions about whether to cut off a new life as part of a larger challenge to show respect for all life by living well and responsibly herself. Deciding about abortion is not a unique problem, disconnected from all other decisions, but rather a dramatic and intensely lit example of choices people must make throughout their lives, all of which express convictions about the value of life and the meaning of death.

OTHER NATIONS

In democracies, people's convictions about the nature of the abortion controversy are often reflected not just in their own opinions as individuals and in the positions of groups to which they belong but also in the details of the legal restrictions on abortion that their governments enact. In the United States, since 1973, such legislation has been restricted by the Supreme Court's *Roe* v. *Wade* decision. But there has been a good deal of legislation about abortion in Europe in recent decades, and like the Irish referendum I described it supports the view that most people's concerns about abortion are based on detached rather than derivative reasons.

Professor Mary Ann Glendon of the Harvard Law School wrote an influential book, published in 1987, comparing the American laws of abortion and divorce with those of other Western countries. She argued that the abortion law imposed by *Roe* v. *Wade* is very much out of step with the law of many Western European countries. Some of those nations permit early abortions subject to either few or no practical constraints. But they also, in different ways, recognize and seek to protect the intrinsic value of human life in any form, which Glendon said *Roe* v. *Wade* does not because it unduly emphasizes individual rights and individual liberty, and encourages "autonomy, separation, and isolation in the war of all against all" in contrast with European emphasis on "social solidarity."[42] She suggested that the Supreme Court should revise its holdings so as to permit American states each to reach its own resolution of the abortion dilemma, forbidding only laws that, in the words of an Italian decision she quoted, place "a total and absolute priority" on survival of the fetus. She hoped that a spirit of reasonable compromise would then produce, state by state, compromises along the lines of the European laws she discussed.

I disagree with much of Glendon's analysis. I believe the contrast she draws between "individual rights" and "social solidarity," though now very popular among conservative critics of the liberal tradition, is both simplistic and dangerous. The United States' historical commitment to individual human rights has not proved isolating or Hobbesian, as she and other critics have suggested, nor has it undermined a national sense of community. On the contrary. The United States is a nation of continental size, covering many very different and very large regions, and it is pluralist in almost every possible aspect: racial, ethnic, and cultural. In such a nation, individual rights, to the extent they are recognized and actually enforced, offer the only possibility of genuine community in which all individuals participate as equals. The United States can be a *national* community, moreover, only if the most fundamental rights are national, too, only if the most important principles of freedom recognized in some parts of the country are honored in all others as well. It is true that many of the claims that different groups in America now make about what they are entitled to have by right are inflated and sometimes preposterous. But the possibility of abuse no more refutes the need for genuine individual rights than fascism or communism, each of which has claimed authority in the name of "social solidarity," refutes Glendon's appeals for a greater sense of common goal and purpose.

The European nations that Glendon said have chosen solidarity over rights are increasingly recognizing the poverty and danger of that contrast, moreover. The most distinctive contemporary movement within Western European law is not any communitarian striving to place the virtues of "other important values" above the "values of tolerance," as she recommends.[43] Europe remembers only too well the results of that ordering in its recent past, and is horrified at its return in some parts of Eastern Europe now. No, the most important legal trend is toward constitutionally embedded individual rights adjudicated and enforced by courts—not just national courts, but also the international courts in Luxembourg and Strasbourg, which strive to unite Europe as a community of principle as well as commerce.[44]

Europe is different from America in many ways that make Glendon's hopes that American states will one day follow the European pattern of compromise about abortion seem unrealistic. The United States is much less homogeneous, racially and culturally, than France, Britain, Germany, Spain, Italy, or other European nations, and in some regions of the country, politics are more dominated by religious attitudes and groups than the national politics of many of those countries are.[45] In that respect, parts of America are more like Ireland than they are like Britain, France, Germany, or Italy. As I said, several American states and the territory of Guam, each hoping to persuade the Supreme Court to overrule *Roe v. Wade*, recently adopted very stern anti-abortion statutes—Gaum's did not allow exceptions even for rape—and several other states would be likely to produce such laws if that decision is ever overruled. Nor does it seem likely that either the national Congress or many state legislatures will soon provide the welfare and other support for poor young mothers that is an important part of the European dedication to human life.

Nevertheless, in spite of these important reservations about Glendon's overall argument, I find her comparisons of American law with that of other countries extremely informative and revealing. They confirm, internationally, the hypothesis I have been defending: that the argument over abortion is not well understood as an argument about whether a fetus is a person, but must be reconstructed as an argument of a very different character.

One European country—Ireland, as we have seen—has very strict anti-abortion laws. Five others—Albania, Northern Ireland, Portugal,

Spain, and Switzerland—nominally restrict abortion, even in early pregnancy, to circumstances in which the mother's general health is threatened and, in Spain and Portugal, to cases of rape, incest, or fetal deformity. The remaining Western European countries, including Belgium, Britain, France, Italy, Germany, and the Scandinavian countries, have laws that either explicitly or in practice allow abortion almost on demand in the first stages of pregnancy—during the first three months in most, though until 1991 up to twenty-eight weeks in Britain, which is *beyond* the point at which *Roe* allows American states to prohibit it. Glendon believes that these restrictions do not significantly reduce the level of abortion. The Netherlands, which has one of the most liberal abortion laws, also has one of the lowest rates of abortion, lower than nearly all countries with stricter laws.[46] But, she argues, the European laws nevertheless contrast with *Roe* because whatever their practical effect on the incidence of abortion, they affirm the central communal value of human life and educate people to respect that value.

Glendon points to the French law, which permits abortion in the first ten weeks only if the pregnant woman is "in distress." The law allows a woman to decide herself whether or not she is in distress, and does not require a medical certificate or any other party's approval, though it does require her to accept "counseling." The government pays at least 70 percent of the cost of the abortion, moreover—all of it if the grounds are wholly medical. The practical effect of the French law may therefore be almost the same as if it had explicitly allowed abortion on demand for ten weeks. Any moral condemnation of abortion implicit in the language of the law seems undercut by the nation's willingness to help pay the costs. But Glendon insists on a different point: the language of the law, by requiring that women declare themselves in "distress," instructs that abortion for whimsical reasons or only for convenience is morally wrong.

Professor Laurence Tribe of the Harvard Law School has said that the "French solution, within an Anglo-American legal system . . . seems to teach mostly hypocrisy."[47] The French law would indeed be duplicitous if the French legislature had claimed, as justification for it, that a fetus is a person with a right to live. It would be hypocritical to declare that a woman is free to take the life of another person if she thinks she is "in distress," and even worse to show no collective interest in the good faith or plausibility of her decision. But the statute is not duplicitous but, rather, finely judged if it aims at a detached rather than a derivative goal: that people recognize the moral gravity of a decision about abortion and take personal moral responsibility for it. It lays down an official standard that a woman is expected to interpret and define for herself as an exercise of personal responsibility, and it provides for an occasion of counseling at which the moral gravity of the act can be explored without usurping her own right and duty to make the moral decision for herself.

Glendon rightly calls attention to an important decision of the Federal Republic of Germany's Constitutional Court. In 1974, the West German parliament adopted a liberal abortion statute providing that abortion was permissible for any reason until the twelfth week of pregnancy but illegal after that time except for serious reasons: fetal deformity or a threat to the health of the mother. In 1975, in a complicated and very controversial opinion, the Constitutional Court held that law unconstitutional on the ground that it did not sufficiently value human life.

The court relied, among other provisions, on Article 2(2) of the 1949 West German Basic Law, which declares, "Everyone shall have the right to life and to inviolability of his person." This suggests a derivative ground for the court's decision; it suggests that the court may have believed that even an early fetus has a right to life as powerful as the right of any other person. But the argument the court offered, and the decision it actually reached, are inconsistent with that proposition. The decision can only be understood as resting on the different, detached, ground that any German law of abortion must be drafted so as to acknowledge the intrinsic importance of human life.[48] For the court did not declare that any statute that permitted abortion except, perhaps, to save a mother's life, would be unconstitutional, as it should logically have done if it really meant to declare that every fetus has a guaranteed right to life. Instead, it held that the 1974 statute was invalid because it formally required no reason at all for abortion during the first twelve weeks, and so evidenced no sign of the moral gravity of deliberately ending a human life. The court held that the statute's complete disregard for what, at least after fourteen days of gestation, was plainly a form of human life was inconsistent with the meaning of the 1949 Basic Law, which rests, as the court put it, on "an affirmation of the fundamental value of human life," an affirmation intended wholly to repudiate the utter contempt the Nazis had shown for that value.

The court made plain that it was not ruling out abortions, even on grounds that any conservative would reject as improper. It invited the parliament to adopt a new statute allowing abortion but showing more respect for the intrinsic value of life than the 1974 statute had. By way of illustration, and to ensure that abortion was available for good cause in the interval before a new law was completed, the court drafted and imposed its own "transitional" abortion scheme, which made plain, again, that it did not really affirm a fetal right to life. The transitional rules provided, for example, that abortion was permissible not only in cases of rape, or fetal deformity, or when the mother's health was threatened, but also "in order to avert the danger of a grave emergency" of some other kind to the pregnant woman.

Glendon suggests that the practical differences between these transitional rules the court itself drafted and the law that it had declared unconstitutional were speculative. The real difference, she says, is in the social meaning of the court's declaration that, in principle, abortion is not a matter for whim or caprice but is an issue of moral gravity. In 1976, the West German parliament enacted a new statute whose practical difference from the overruled 1974 law, in terms of what each law in practice prohibits, is even more marginal. The 1976 law provided that abortion is permissible within twelve weeks if continued pregnancy would place a woman in a situation of serious hardship, and up to the twenty-second week if fetal deformity would make it unreasonable to require a woman to continue the pregnancy. It also provided, like the French law, for mandatory counseling before even an early abortion, and for a three-week waiting period between counseling and abortion. As I noted in chapter 1, the unified German parliament adopted a new, even more liberal law in 1992, and the Constitutional Court was expected to rule on the constitutionality of that new law early in 1993.

In 1985, the Spanish Constitutional Court, obviously influenced by the German decision of 1975, considered the constitutionality of new Spanish laws that had repealed old and very strict constraints on abortion and introduced new rules allowing abortion in cases of rape, fetal deformity, and threat to the mother's physical or mental health. The court made the distinction I have been pressing, between the derivative claim that a fetus has rights as a "person" and the detached idea that human life has an intrinsic value that must be recognized and endorsed collectively. It denied that a fetus is a person for purposes of the Spanish constitution, or has the rights of a person, but it said that the Spanish constitution does endorse human life as a value that the nation's laws must respect.⁴⁹ By a close vote, it held the new abortion law unconstitutional but nevertheless set out guidelines for amendment it said would make the law constitutional: that a doctor must certify any claimed threat to the mother's physical and mental health, and that abortion facilities must be licensed.⁵⁰ The Spanish parliament accepted these guidelines and amended the law accordingly. The changes did not, as a practical matter, substantially strengthen restrictions on abortion, but they did signal the collective concern for the gravity of abortion that a majority of the Constitutional Court thought essential.

In 1992, the European Court of Human Rights made an important decision that also presupposed that a fetus is not a person with rights or interests of its own, and that laws prohibiting or regulating abortion can be justified only on the different ground that abortion is thought to jeopardize the inherent value of human life.⁵¹ Before the 1992 referendum, Irish law forbade any organization to supply to a pregnant woman within Ireland the name, address, or telephone number of an abortion clinic in Great Britain, and an Irish court had issued a permanent injunction against two abortion-counseling services that did provide that information. The judge had considered the argument that an injunction would violate a pregnant woman's constitutional right to information, but he had declared that "I am satisfied that no right could constitutionally arise to obtain information the purpose of which was to defeat the constitutional right of the unborn child." The counseling services appealed to the European Court, arguing that the injunction violated the European Convention of Human Rights, to which Ireland is a party. That court did not decide whether the convention guarantees a right to abortion, because it did not need to. But the court did decide that the ban on information violated Article 10 of the Convention, which protects freedom of speech and information. Among other arguments, it said that since information about abortion clinics is available from other sources in Ireland—for example, from British telephone books there—the ban on organizations supplying that information to pregnant women who request it would not prevent enough abortions to justify the constraint on freedom of information. It used, in other words, a test of "proportionality" between the degree to which the ban on information would aid Ireland's policy of protecting fetal life and the degree to which it would harm freedom of speech; it held that the gain to the policy was not significant enough to justify the cost to freedom. But that proportionality test would be bizarre if, as the Irish government argued, a fetus is a person with a right to life: if it is, then a government would be entitled to try to prevent the murder of even one additional fetus, and a ban on direct information about foreign abortion clinics would be appropriate even if most pregnant women had other ways of obtaining that information. The Irish law has now been changed, but the European Court's decision remains important because its proportionality test presupposes that the point of laws banning abortion is not to prevent murder but to protect a public sense of the inherent value of life. It is proper to argue that minor or very marginal gains in achieving *that* goal would not justify substantial abridgments of other rights, including the rights protected by the Convention's Article 10.

THE NEXT STEP

Though this chapter has covered much ground, it has been dedicated mainly to a single claim: that we cannot understand the moral argument now raging around the world—between individuals, within and between religious groups, as conducted by feminist groups, or in the politics of several nations—if we see it as centered on the issue of whether a fetus is a person. Almost everyone shares, explicitly or intuitively, the idea that human life has objective, intrinsic value that is quite independent of its personal value for anyone, and disagreement about the right interpretation of that shared idea is the actual nerve of the great debate about abortion. For that reason, the debate is even more important to most people than an argument about whether a fetus is a person would be, for it goes deeper—into different conceptions of the value and point of human life and of the meaning and character of human death.

I have tried to show the inadequacy of the conventional explanation. But so far I have said little to make the concept of intrinsic value, or of sanctity or inviolability, more precise or to answer the objection that these ideas are too mysterious to figure in a genuine explanation of anything. Nor have I yet explained, except in the most tentative way, how we can make sense of the abortion debate in light of these ideas. These are crucial challenges, and we must confront them at once.

2 *The Morality of Abortion*

1. Mario Cuomo's speech was reprinted in *The New York Review of Books*, October 25, 1984.

2. A *Time*/CNN poll conducted in June 1992 reported that 84 percent of Americans favor abortion when the mother's life is at stake. Public Opinion Online, available in Westlaw, Dialog Library, poll file.

3. The poll described in note 2 also reported that 79 percent of Americans favor abortion in cases of rape or incest.

4. See "She's Come for an Abortion. What Do You Say?" *Harper's* (November 1992): 51–2.

5. The poll described in note 2 also reported that 70 percent of the Americans interviewed favored abortion when the fetus would be born seriously deformed.

6. Though Catholics are less likely to approve of abortion than some other religious groups, they are not less likely to have abortions. According to *Facts in Brief: Abortion in the United States* (New York: The Alan Gutmacher Institute, 1991): "Catholic women are about as likely to obtain an abortion as are all women nationally, while Protestants and Jews are less likely. Catholic women are 30 percent more likely than Protestants to have abortions."

7. *McRae v. Califano*, 491 F. Supp. 630 (1980). The Supreme Court later reversed his decision, *Harris v. McRae*, 448 U.S. 297 (1980). But it did not rule on his claim that the amendment deprived some women of the free exercise of their religion because, it said, none of the plaintiffs had made arguments or alleged facts necessary to raise that issue. 448 U.S. 321.

8. 491 F. Supp. 712.

9. 491 F. Supp. 697–700.

10. 491 F. Supp. 700–702.

11. 491 F. Supp. 696–7.

12. See Paul Ramsey, "The Morality of Abortion," in Robert M. Baird and Stuart E. Rosenbaum, eds., *The Ethics of Abortion* (Buffalo: Prometheus Books, 1989), 61, 66. (italics in original).

13. English translation (London: Catholic Truth Society, 1987).

14. See John Noonan, "A Nearly Absolute Value in History," in John Noonan, ed., *The Morality of Abortion* (Cambridge, Mass.: Harvard University Press, 1970).

15. Augustine, *De nuptias et concupiscentia*, quoted in Noonan, 16.

16. Epistles 121.4, *Corpus Scriptorum Ecclesiasticorum Latinorum*, 56.16.

17. See the discussion of fetal sentience in chapter 1.

18. See, for example, Stephen J. Heaney, "Aquinas and the Presence of the Human Rational Soul in the Early Embryo," *The Thomist* 56 (1992): 19.

19. See Joseph Donceel, S.J., "Immediate Animation and Delayed Hominization," *Theological Studies* 31 (1970): 76, 83.

20. Decretales 5.12.5.

21. English translation, *On Human Life: Encyclical Letter of Pope Paul VI* (London: Catholic Truth Society, 1970), 14–15.

22. *Let Me Live: Declaration by the Sacred Congregation for the Doctrine of the Faith on Procured Abortion, approved and confirmed by Pope Paul VI* (London: Catholic Truth Society, 1974), 5–6.

23. See Michael J. Coughlan, *The Vatican, the Law and the Human Embryo* (Iowa City: University of Iowa Press, 1990), 86–8.

24. *Let Me Live*, 11.

25. *On Human Life*, 16.

26. See "Catholics: 52% Support Abortion in Most Circumstances," *American Political Network* (June 18, 1992); "Catholics' Views Shift on Ordination; Poll Finds Majority Support Women Priests, Abortion Rights," Washington *Post*, June 19, 1992, A4.

27. Wills, *Under God*, 310. Wills cites George Gallup, Jr., and Jim Castelli, *The People's Religion: American Faith in the 90's* (New York: Macmillan, 1989).

28. Joseph F. Donceel, S.J., "A Liberal Catholic's View," in Joel Feinberg, ed., *The Problem of Abortion* (Belmont, Calif.: Wadsworth, 1984), 15.

29. See Joseph Cardinal Bernardin, *The Consistent Ethic of Life* (Kansas City: Sheed & Ward, 1988).

30. See Bernardin, "The Consistent Ethic of Life After *Webster*," Address, Woodstock Theological Center, Georgetown University, March 20, 1990, 9.

31. In an address on "The Death Penalty in Our Time," reprinted in *Consistent Ethic of Life*, 59, Cardinal Bernardin makes plain that the state has the right to execute a murderer, and denies only that it should exercise that right in the circumstances of contemporary society.

32. See Sidney Callahan, "A Moral Obligation," *Sojourners: An Independent Christian Monthly* (November 1989): 18.

33. Some of these decisions, including the *Casey* decision I mentioned in the last chapter, are discussed in chapter 6.

34. See Catharine A. MacKinnon, "Reflections on Sex Equality Under Law," 100 *Yale Law Journal* 1281 (1991).

35. See *Meyer* v. *Nebraska*, 262 U.S. 390 (1923); *Pierce* v. *Society of Sisters*, 268 U.S. 510 (1925).

36. *Carey* v. *Population Services International*, 431 U.S. 678 (1977).

37. In chapter 6 I suggest that the Supreme Court made a mistake in *Harris* v. *McRae*. But its decision was hardly the result of its having previously recognized a right of

privacy in matters of procreation. After all, if women have a privacy right to terminate a pregnancy, they have a privacy right *not* to do so as well, and that fact did not prevent Congress from deciding to help women financially who make that choice. The question raised in *Harris* v. *McRae* was not whether a woman's decision to terminate is a private one, in any sense of privacy, but the very different question of whether Congress may financially support women who make one private choice about pregnancy while refusing to support women who make a different choice that they have an equal constitutional right to make.

38. MacKinnon, "Reflections on Sex Equality Under Law," 1316.
39. See Adrienne Rich, "Of Woman Born," 64 (1976), quoted in MacKinnon, "Reflections on Sex Equality Under Law," 1316 (italics in original).
40. See Robin West, "Taking Freedom Seriously," 104 *Harvard Law Review* 43 (1990): 84–5 (footnotes omitted).
41. See Carol Gilligan, *In a Different Voice* (Cambridge, Mass.: Harvard University Press, 1982).
42. Glendon, *Abortion and Divorce in Western Law,* 58.
43. Ibid., 36.
44. See Anthony Lester, "The Overseas Trade in the American Bill of Rights," 88 *Columbia Law Review* 537 (1988), and Ronald Dworkin, *A Bill of Rights for Britain* (London: Chatto & Windus, 1990).
45. Wills, *Under God.*
46. See Stanley K. Henshaw, "Induced Abortion, A World Review, 1990," *Family Planning Perspectives* 22, no. 2 (March/April 1990): 77–8.
47. Tribe, *Abortion,* 74.
48. In fact, Article 2(2) also provides that the right to life can be abridged by law, and so provides only a dubious argument that the 1974 law, even if it did abridge a right to life, was unconstitutional for that reason. The court also mentioned Article 1(1) of the 1949 constitution, which states, "The dignity of man should be inviolable. To respect and protect it shall be the duty of all state authority." That may be understood as an endorsement of the intrinsic value of human life in the detached form I have been describing, and the court apparently so construed it.
49. The Spanish Supreme Court, which does not have the powers of the Constitutional Court, had said, "Human life in formation is a good that constitutionally merits protection, is a constitutional legal good of the community and not an individual legal good." See Richard Stith, "New Constitutional and Penal Theory in Spanish Abortion Law," in J. Douglas Butler and David F. Walbert, eds., *Abortion, Medicine, and the Law,* 4th ed. (New York: Facts on File, 1992), 368, 375. But the idea that human life is intrinsically valuable, and protected by the Spanish Constitution on that ground, makes more sense, and more sense of the Constitutional Court's opinion, than the odd idea that it is a property belonging to the community as a whole rather than to any individual including itself; if the Constitution meant that odd idea, it is hard to see why the community could not, by liberal abortion legislation, waive its rights to that particular good.
50. A summary of the decision is provided in *Annual Review of Population Law* 12 (1988): 37. A translation of the amended Spanish abortion law appears on page 38.
51. *Case of Open Door and Dublin Well Woman* v. *Ireland, European Court of Human Rights* (October 29, 1992): Volume 246, Series A, Publications of the Court (Köln: Carl Heymanns, Verlag K.G.).

[6]

JOURNAL OF LAW AND SOCIETY
VOLUME 17, NUMBER 1, SPRING 1990
0263-323X $3.00

Abortion Law: Is Consensual Reform Possible?

SHEILA A. M. MCLEAN*

The abortion debate is surely one of the most contentious in the history of law and ethics and its durability is based not merely on the inherent gravity of the issues concerned, but also on the depth of feeling which it generates. There are few areas in which individuals and groups are so firmly convinced of the rightness of their position and of their duty to ensure that their beliefs are translated into law. The recent problems in Canada over the constitutionality of abortion laws shows just how fierce debate can be.[1]

Moreover, the discussion seems never-ending. Even when debate focuses on issues other than abortion, the antagonistic lobbies are not slow to realize the extent to which the outcome has implications for their position. For example, much attention in recent years has focused on the so-called reproductive revolution and questions such as the rights and wrongs of creating 'spare' embryos, their disposal, the use which can be made of them, and so on.[2] The British Government has promised parliamentary time in the next session for a debate on just such matters.[3] But the outcome of these debates is not one which is exclusive to the modern techniques. Evidently, the status accorded to the embryo is of major concern to those who see it either as potential life or merely as a fertilized egg, positions central to the abortion issue.

To offer significant protection to the embryo (or pre-embryo) in respect, say, of research, is to make a step towards recognition of the claim that it is a human life with the rights which are generally attributed to such a status. The implications for the abortion question are obvious and potentially dramatic. Indeed, in the recent decision in Tennessee concerning the disposal of embryos in a divorce action[4] the court made it quite clear that it viewed these pre-embryos as human beings. Their view that life begins at conception (in this case actually at fertilization and not, obviously, at implantation) does not merely affect the decision about what is to be done with these particular embryos, but also had profound implications for the abortion debate. The outcome is a setback for the pro-choice lobby whose case inevitably becomes

*Institute of Law and Ethics in Medicine, University of Glasgow, Stair Building, Glasgow G12 8QQ, Scotland

*I would like to express my gratitude to the following friends and colleagues who have read and commented on early drafts of this article: Elspeth Attwooll, Peter Beharrell, Noreen Burrows, Robin Downie, David Fergus, Ken Mason, and Dorothy Porter.

more difficult every time courts pronounce in this way, particularly so in the United States of America at present given the recent Supreme Court judgment in *Webster*.[5] It is also an important decision for the anti-abortion lobby whose case is strengthened by such legal recognition of its position.

A major hurdle to be overcome if abortion law is to be reformed is the fact, as Luker[6] points out, that both polarized positions in the debate can take the same information and use it to reach diametrically opposed conclusions. Arguing from principle or logic is unlikely to change their conclusions since each group starts with a firm commitment to the underlying morality of their position. For the anti-abortion lobby, all human life is sacred from the moment of conception (perhaps even from fertilization, as is evident from their concern about fertilized but not implanted ova) and therefore is worthy of protection. From this position it is logical to argue that no abortion should ever be conceded, with the possible exception of situations where there is a direct conflict between the mother's right to life and the rights which they would attribute to the embryo or foetus. Equally consistent is the view of the pro-choice lobby, which would argue that women have the right to make decisions about their own bodies, and that women's right to self-determination is critically and irrevocably damaged by state intrusion into their right to choose to terminate a pregnancy.

Whatever position one adopts, it is clear that reconciliation of these extreme opposites is unlikely. If this is the only option, therefore, abortion laws will continue to be the subject of wrangling and jockeying for position between these two opinions, a situation which is likely at best to result in laws which are unsatisfactory for both lobbies. The mistake often made is to presume that logic will ever change this, since there effectively *is* no independent logic which can be applied. The position taken by each side has its own internal logical consistency, but each is value-laden from the beginning. This means that consensual reform is never likely to be achieved if it is based upon an attempt to accommodate these diverse attitudes.

Meanwhile, it is the rest of the interested parties who suffer. It seems likely that the majority of people who think about abortion are not necessarily or inevitably committed to the extreme positions. For the occupants of this 'middle ground' the emotional tugs of part of each position may be considerable and laws which take account of only one position will be unsatisfactory. This paper seeks a way forward, but it does so with a number of warnings which must be borne in mind.

First, it is conceded that the argument presented here also makes certain presumptions. Most importantly, it assumes that there *is* a middle ground which can – perhaps even should – be addressed. It also takes a pragmatic view of rights. No-one, not even the anti-abortion lobby, would deny that women have the rights of citizens, and that these rights include the rights to self-determination and to life. The question of whether or not embryos or foetuses have rights is by no means so easy to answer, and certainly does not command the same consensus. It is also arguably the case that conceding foetal or embryonic rights would have grave consequences for the liberty of others. For example, conceptualizing these rights has led to involuntary, indeed forced, obstetrical interventions in the United States of America,[7] and to attempts to ward foetuses in the United Kingdom.[8] The writer therefore will not concede that embryos or foetuses have 'rights' as such, because the implications of so doing are of great concern. This does not mean that there is no concession to the potential interests of something which could develop into a human being given the appropriate circumstances. To concede more is, in fact, unnecessary in terms of the argument which will be put forward below.

In addition, this discussion should not be taken as offering a panacea, or even as a 'good' idea. Rather, an attempt is being made to test the extent to which there *is* an alternative which, even if it does not command the moral high ground, has the merit of being emotionally more satisfying to those whose views are not extreme, whilst at the same time representing a strategy which could maximize the rights and interests central to the dilemmas raised by the abortion issue. It is, therefore, a potentially practical step forward. More importantly, perhaps, it may serve to rescue the current debate from the swamp into which it seems doomed to sink, given the difficulty – if not impossibility – of radically altering the underlying perspectives of the extremes. It is necessary, therefore, before presenting the argument, to look briefly at the opposing positions. To understand their perspective is helpful, even though this paper is not concerned to opt for one over the other. If the argument is to satisfy the 'middle ground' it must take account of the extremes, perhaps even use some of their ammunition.

THE PROTAGONISTS

There are two very clear and very different views on abortion and its morality. Although there are many shades of grey in between, these tend to set the agenda for debate and to shape the positions adopted by individual politicians in legislative debates. Moreover, in jurisdictions where abortion laws are couched in judicial rather than legislative pronouncements, the relative power (political, economic, and moral) of either side will play a highly significant role in advancing each case. For example, the political colour of the United States Supreme Court is widely recognized as influencing the interpretation of the constitution, as clearly shown in the *Webster* case.[9]

So, what does each of the main protagonists have to say? The extreme anti-abortion lobby has an apparently simple position, namely that all human life is sacred from the moment of conception. Life, in these terms – at least in theory – begins at conception, and therefore anything which interferes with the potential life after that time (including presumably the 'morning after' pill and the intra-uterine device[10]) is unacceptable and contrary to this lobby's moral code. This is usually subject to exceptions, for example the principle of double effect, a doctrine which permits the doing of a 'bad' thing if the overall aim is 'good'. Application of this principle would mean that a pregnant woman who has a uterine tumour can 'morally' have a hysterectomy if the

108

operation will save her life even if it inevitably results in the destruction of an embryo/foetus.

The pro-choice or pro-abortion lobby, on the other hand, argues that all women have the right to choose what happens to their own bodies, including the right to terminate a pregnancy. This position has been argued for on a number of bases, ranging from a person's right to 'self-ownership'[11] to the position that no human being is legally or morally obliged to maintain the life (or, by analogy, potential life) of another.[12]

These positions are apparently irreconcilable. Moral judgements about the significance of conception and potential life dominate the one, whilst existing life and its freedoms dominate the other. For those in the middle, however, there may be problems associated with each. The anti-abortion lobby seems to value the potential for life over the actual life of a woman, whilst the pro-abortion lobby may sometimes seem to give no credence whatsoever to the potential for life, which those fighting for the life of a 'wanted' foetus would strenuously support. Moreover, we have no clear notion of when the moment of conception occurs, nor are we clear when life is truly 'potential'.

It must be said at this point that if consistency of commitment were regarded as sufficient to justify acceptance of one stance over the other, then the pro-choice lobby would win the argument. Even in the face of the relative certainty that their absolutist stance is unlikely to gain political support, they have generally refused to compromise for the sake of political expediency. However, substantial sections of the anti-abortion lobby have done just this, often quite successfully. Of course, absolute consistency may not be a criterion on which to base ultimate agreement or disagreement, but it does inevitably affect the cogency with which any group can argue its case. Both extremes are doubtless aware that it is unlikely that either of their positions will command sufficient support to be translated into law. The question then becomes how far and in what ways they are prepared to modify their position in order that at least *some* of what they wish to achieve will come about. There is nothing necessarily reprehensible in taking cognizance of political and social reality.

An example of such a political compromise is to be found in the recent Abortion Amendment Bill introduced into the British Parliament by David Alton MP.[13] This Bill was the latest in a series of attempts to reduce the maximum time limit at which abortions could lawfully be carried out, and had the enthusiastic support of the anti-abortion lobby. Yet, what would have been the implications of such an amendment? Certainly, it would restrict the availability of later abortions, but it also countenances the certainty of foetal destruction. Given that its protagonists like to call themselves 'pro-life'[14] and that their expressed aim was to protect foetal 'life',[15] it is tempting to ask how it was thought that such an amendment would achieve this. This point will be returned to later, but it raises interesting questions both about the *actual* motivation for change and about the extent to which moral principles can survive political manoeuvering.

It is also worth noting one additional difference between the logic of the two positions – a difference which is important for many. The aim of both lobbies is the translation of their position into law as the mechanism whereby the behaviour which they find offensive may be prohibited, or that which they wish to make permissible may be given social validity. However, the adoption of one position or the other does not have simple consequences. Law may regulate or be permissive, and there is a considerable difference between the two. A law which says 'it is impermissible to do x' demands respect and imposes sanctions, whether or not it has the support of individuals or groups. A law which permits people to do x forces no one to do it, but permits those who wish to, to undertake x. The inevitable outcome of legal adoption of the absolutist position of the anti-abortion lobby would be the restriction of the rights of many whose moral views are in direct opposition to it. In other words, it would be clear restriction of the rights of others to live according to *their* principles. On the other hand, the translation into law of the pro-abortion position, whilst offensive to some, forces them into nothing. No-one would be obliged to avail themselves of legalized abortion.

Arguably, only absolute certainty on the rightness or wrongness of behaviour should permit laws of the former type, and it is clear that there is no such moral or political consensus in respect of the status of embryos or foetuses. Nor, indeed, is there legal consensus. The recent decision that a foetus is not a person for the purposes of section 16 of the Offences Against the Person Act 1861[16] shows no legal agreement exists. An extremist might well say, then, that if we cannot agree that foetuses have the rights, and if the law seems equally uncertain, there is no justification for restrictive legislation in respect of abortion. This is perhaps too legalistic a position to command the support of those who continue to be uneasy about the whole debate. Nonetheless, it is worth bearing in mind in what follows.

Whatever the consistencies or inconsistencies of each position, it seems that, for many people, neither offers a position with which they can be morally comfortable. Some of those who are intuitively closer to the anti-abortion position may nonetheless recognize the need for, or validity of, pregnancy termination in some circumstances. Equally, for those whose preference is for the pro-choice position, this may become problematic when a foetus *could* be saved. The next section of this article will attempt to address these very real dilemmas.

At best it may provide hope that stagnation is not the only option and at worst, it offers another perspective on the debate. It sets out a position likely to be acceptable to many of those described above as occupying the middle ground, for whom neither extreme is acceptable. However, it also hopes to go further, to suggest that there *is* an alternative to the narrow and antagonistic confines within which the debate has hitherto been conducted, and that there are alternative conclusions which can be drawn from them.

AN ALTERNATIVE STRATEGY?

The main issue which differentiates the two main lobbies is their distinctive view of the rights which are at stake. Arguably, however, neither of the extreme stances actually takes full account of the logical conclusions of their position. To take but one example, the attribution of rights to embryos and foetuses places mother and conceptus in direct conflict in a number of possible situations. This is exacerbated by the advances made since the anti-abortion lobby reached its zenith. The moment at which life begins, and the values to be attributed to potential for life, have become, paradoxically, better explicated and simultaneously less certain as medical science progresses. In a sense, therefore, traditional anti-abortion postures are not only challengeable, but also old-fashioned.

They are also potentially more dangerous than they might appear. The insistence on the values of the embryo/foetus which, in the past, would have almost exclusively affected the abortion question, now has wider-ranging implications. To impute rights at this stage of development does not merely provide the logic for denying women abortions. Given the current state of technology, it opens up further opportunities to restrict or scrutinize the behaviour not only of women who are pregnant but also that of all women of child-bearing age. The recent trend in the United States of America[17] – which is spreading to the United Kingdom too[18] – towards coercion of pregnant women would probably be unacceptable to many who would otherwise espouse a position which acknowledged foetal 'rights'. Yet, such an espousal leads inevitably to the conclusion that women of child-bearing age *can*, and perhaps even should, be forced into certain behavioural patterns. Indeed, it is logical that if 'potential' life is to be given equal or similar status to that of real life, then those who have the capacity to carry that life, that is women, should have as great an obligation to care for potential life (even pre-conception) as they do after conception.

On the other hand, the proposition that terminations should lawfully be carried out at all stages in a pregnancy could – depending on its basis – mean that a policy of neonaticide should also be acceptable, and yet many of those who argue for abortion on request would not support this. In fact, it is only the current medical practice of trying to ensure foetal destruction before extrusion that permits the current avoidance of this question.[19]

So, what is the alternative? The argument presented will refer to three parts of pregnancy. This is not because it hinges, as some arguments do, directly on questions of the salvageability of the foetus,[20] but because there can be no doubt that those who are dissatisfied with the extremes *do* see a distinction between the very early stages of a pregnancy and those at which the foetus could be born alive. However logical or illogical this belief may be, it must be taken into account. Neither the extreme pro- nor anti-abortion lobbies would theoretically make such a distinction. Indeed, this may be their only point of agreement.

In the terms of this argument at least, there is the possibility that there may be further points at which agreement in principle could be reached. These points hinge in part on the concessions made by the anti-abortion lobby and in part on a re-evaluation of current practices. To clarify them it is necessary to

111

divide the pregnancy into three parts. Though these stages bear some relationship to those outlined in the landmark American case of *Roe* v *Wade*,[21] this does not mean that the distinctions are made for the same reasons or on the same basis. Rather, they are drawn in part from the public positions of the contesting lobbies and in part from acknowledgement of the emotional or intuitive positions of the 'middle ground'.

It is logical, therefore, to begin with the early stages of a pregnancy. It is here that the public face of the anti-abortion lobby is at its most inconsistent, and therefore that the potential for an (admittedly uneasy) truce is clearest. In the face of political reality and in the interests of making progress towards their desired goal, anti-abortion campaigners have generally conceded that abortion up to a certain stage in pregnancy may (however reluctantly) have to be accepted. The relative complaisance with which many view terminations in the earlier stages of pregnancy, and the cost to human life of our relatively recent experience of outlawing all abortion, make arguing for an absolute ban on abortion a cause which can only be lost. Thus, the lobby has concentrated on narrowing the time during which concessions have to be made.

In the United Kingdom, for example, attempts to amend the Abortion Act 1967 have concentrated on reducing the time limit at which that concession ends. The chosen point usually hinges, in much the same ways as in *Roe* v *Wade*,[22] on the point at which medicine claims that foetuses can be born alive. In other words, a distinction is drawn at the stage of what is commonly referred to as 'viability'. Arguably, by not insisting upon an absolute ban on abortion, the anti-abortion lobby has deviated in a major and highly significant way from its stated moral position. However reluctant that deviation may be, it nonetheless logically means that, in order to achieve *something*, they have conceded early terminations and been prepared not to defend the absolute position which they otherwise claim to hold. These early foetuses, even in their terms, do not attract the same degree of protection as those which are salvageable.

This being the case, there is no logic in arguing against destroying that which nobody is really prepared to argue should be saved. To do so is to ignore, or at best to make serious inroads into, women's rights. And once the concession has been made, the anti-abortion lobby has no remaining moral platform from which to argue that restrictions should be imposed on women's decisions at this stage in their pregnancy. Their manoeuvering, therefore, has two consequences. First, it defeats their own claims to the high moral ground since political expediency is arguably an insufficient argument to justify compromising firmly held beliefs. Second, by making this concession, they lose the right to argue for the imposition of conditions on the exercise of a woman's choice, since the *reason* for termination is irrelevant to the inevitable outcome, which they have already accepted. The conclusion of the first part of the argument, therefore, is that the anti-abortion lobby's public stance cannot serve to defeat women's rights to abortion on request in the early stages of pregnancy. Here, therefore, reform *is* possible. This conclusion is in line with the decision in *Roe* v *Wade*,[23] but not with current law in the United Kingdom, which *does* impose conditions on women seeking terminations, even early ones.[24] The state, therefore, would require to accept that it has no role in regulating early terminations. As an aside, were this to be done, many of the current difficulties about embryo treatment and research would also disappear.

It is, however, at the point at which a foetus, if delivered, realizes its potential for life outside the womb that the moral dilemmas become more difficult to resolve. The use of 'viability' to mark the point at which abortions should cease to be permissible is routinely, and accurately, perceived by pro-abortionists as a major source of restriction on women's right to choose whether or not to terminate a pregnancy. Many of those who would support their claims up until this point part company with them when there is a real and perceived capacity to ensure the survival of a foetus outside the womb. Moreover, the awesome capacities of modern medicine mean that this stage is pushed further and further back. The anti-abortion lobby consistently uses medical opinion to reinforce and validate their arguments for reducing time limits (with the possible exception of situations where the foetus is handicapped).[25] Whether at twenty weeks, twenty-two weeks, or twenty-four weeks, we are told that foetuses can be delivered and kept alive. Not all of them, of course – indeed one suspects rather few of them – but the fact that some more mature foetuses can be saved is a powerful weapon in the argument against the pro-choice lobby. Indeed, even many of those whose preference is for the principles of the pro-choice lobby are instinctively uneasy about the fate of the salvageable but aborted foetus.

Therefore, we must take this point seriously. It is not within the competence of this writer to make judgements about when a foetus *is* salvageable, but it seems clear that medical science is moving closer to the inevitable barrier raised by nature. The time at which this occurs is a mobile one, up to the point at which nature's own limits for development of, for example, lungs, confront the miracles of science. However, given a period of grace, those foetuses at the lower end of this flexible scale may develop sufficiently to become, not *potentially* but *actually* salvageable in greater numbers and with greater frequency. There is little doubt, then, that there is a period of weeks during which the growing foetus is at a very critical stage in its development. Removal from the womb guarantees destruction, whilst retention for a few weeks may lead to a live birth and a sustainable life.

At this point those opposed to abortion become most strident, and many of those who generally favour the rights of women become uneasy. There is in the minds of many a crucial difference between removing from the womb something which could not survive *at that time* and removing something which could. Without needing to specify exact numbers of weeks, it seems that many would concede that termination in these circumstances, unlike in the earlier stages, does require some justification. This is not because foetuses have rights but rather because we have an objection, however logical or illogical, to treating more mature foetuses simply as if they had no parallel with ourselves, perhaps most particularly when they are at a crucially susceptible stage.

So the conclusion could be that at this stage some restriction should be placed on the absolute right to terminate pregnancies. This would mean that some requests for termination might be agreed to and others might not. In those cases where abortion *is* agreed to, there will obviously be foetal destruction since at this stage few foetuses could survive. But, interestingly, the anti-abortion lobby may be said already to have conceded the lives of these foetuses. Even the Alton Bill's supporters were widely reported as being prepared to concede that their chosen eighteen-week time-limit could be flexible in some circumstances, for example, where the foetus was handicapped or where the woman's pregnancy was the result of rape.[26] The first of these concessions equates to what Mason[27] would call foetal grounds – in other words, that termination in these circumstances, even of a 'viable' foetus, is permissible because it is not in the interests of the foetus that it should survive. On the other hand, the second concession takes account of the problems faced by the woman, and is more closely aligned to maternal reasons for termination. But however compassionate, neither of these concessions represents a true commitment to the sanctity of all life.

Thus, even in the arguments of the anti-abortion lobby there is again a concession that the woman's position cannot be entirely ignored. However, it must also be admitted that for many this period, which is crucial to the difference between incapacity for survival and the potential for survival outside the womb, is an important one. The interests of the developing, relatively mature foetus and the rights of the woman who is carrying it are seldom so clearly in conflict.

Resolution, however, may also be possible here. Accepting, as many would, that there is no obvious 'right' position here, might we not satisfy our instincts both to preserve the foetus and to recognize women's rights by placing restrictions on the right to terminate pregnancies? Unlike the first period, it is likely that the 'middle ground' would require some evidence that there is a *reason* for the termination, perhaps a reason similar to those which currently exist under the Abortion Act 1967. Thus, to terminate a pregnancy at this crucial stage in its development, a woman might have to show, for example, that continuing with the pregnancy poses a greater risk to her life or health than terminating it. The period during which such restrictions would apply would only be for the time at which retention in the womb is critical to survival. Since this is not different from the current position adopted during the early stages of pregnancy, it is difficult to see how the anti-abortion lobby's public campaigners could disagree with it. Moreover, unlike the setting of an upper time limit on abortion – the reform currently favoured by that lobby – this option may *save* foetuses rather than result in their inevitable destruction. It can also help to preserve women's rights – at least, it could do so if the third part of the argument is also accepted. Before pursuing this, however, it is worth briefly summarizing where the discussion has taken us so far.

The arguments publicly conceded by the anti-abortion campaign cannot prevent a woman from having an absolute right to terminate a pregnancy where the embryo or foetus cannot at that time be saved. It is, of course, the case that the abortus could, barring unfortunate or unforeseen circumstances, become salvageable if carried to term, but this merely restates the extreme position, and takes no account of the occupants of the middle ground to whom this argument is primarily addressed. In the early stages of a pregnancy there are no demonstrable and unequivocal rights which conflict with those of women *at the time the choice is made*. Assuming that few would deny women *any* rights at this stage, then we should be prepared to agree to abortion on request during this period.

On the other hand, apart from those most firmly wedded to absolute decision-making rights at *all* stages of a pregnancy, many would be prepared to agree that, at the crucial stage at which the unsaveable foetus moves rapidly towards becoming the salvageable foetus, women may have to accept some limitations on their right to choose termination, so long as these restrictions are not disproportionately severe. So, in the first period of a pregnancy, a woman has an absolute right to choose termination, and in this second, relatively brief, period, she has a restricted right. It is at this point that the argument takes a somewhat different turn.

The anti-abortion lobby is consistently prepared to use medical evidence to back its claims. Thus, they argue that a main reason for limiting pregnancy terminations to the very early stages of pregnancy is that, after a certain number of weeks (there is disagreement as to how many) a foetus can now be saved. A foetus – wanted or unwanted – born alive, acquires the rights attributed to all human beings and at that stage becomes a different entity, certainly for legal purposes and, for many, also for moral purposes. Yet, this very information is not logically an argument for *lowering* the time limit for abortions, rather it is an argument for *raising* it. The product of an early termination cannot survive, even with the wizardry at the command of modern medicine, whereas the later termination can.

If viability is a significant watershed for the attitudes of many, and it seems that it is, then how can we reconcile this with women's rights to decide about their own bodies? Some of the most influential pro-choice writers, such as Judith Thompson,[28] are logical and clear but appear to have failed to convince, perhaps by not countering the intuitive response of many to this question. It is, of course, entirely consistent with a pro-choice position not to attempt to do so, but even the internal consistency of these arguments leaves in a real dilemma those whose moral convictions are unrepresented by the extremes.

So, where do we go from here? It seems to be the case that the third stage of pregnancy – that is, the period following salvageability – is a matter of less concern to both lobbies than the first periods are. For the anti-abortion lobby the later stages of pregnancy *are* sacrosanct since the foetus could be born alive and they assume that a cut-off point will have been made considerably before this point is reached. For the pro-choice lobby, no stage in a pregnancy is different from another. If the crucial issue is women's rights, then it remains women's rights. For many, however, such a position is counter-intuitive, however consistent. Is there any way of reconciling these apparently opposed positions in a manner which could satisfy the intuitions of the majority? In order to answer this question it is necessary to challenge two fundamental and routinely made assumptions: that this last period of pregnancy *is* sacrosanct, and that pregnancy termination automatically equates to foetal death.

In fact, these two assumptions are so intimately linked that they may be considered together. What is sacrosanct for many about the final stage of pregnancy is, primarily, the fact that the foetus is recognisably 'human' at this stage, that is, it could be born in the shape of a human baby and kept alive. To anti-abortion protagonists, therefore, the well developed foetus should be saved. At no stage has this lobby argued for any concessions because the anticipated outcome of pregnancy termination at this stage is the destruction of the foetus. Their position on this is, therefore, enormously appealing to many – even those who would not espouse the anti-abortion position at other stages in the pregnancy. On the other hand, the pro-choice lobby, if consistent, would have to argue that pregnancy termination at this stage should be permissible, since the issue is not the development of the foetus but the rights of the woman.

However logical it may be, this last position is counter-intuitive for many people. This is because, as the anti-abortion lobby has stressed, it entails the destruction of something which *at the moment of destruction* could have been saved. Foetuses over a certain age – an age which will vary according to the progress which medicine makes – are able to be born alive and to have an existence independent of their mothers. It matters not whether this existence requires assistance in the first stage, since this would be true of a 'wanted' but premature birth. The argument presented here has not accepted that advances in medical science are necessarily inimical to women's rights, and this situation is another very clear example of a case where the very evidence used by the anti-abortion lobby can facilitate women's rights, without harming the interests of foetuses. In addition, and importantly for the purposes of this argument, the proper use of medical expertise and capacity should satisfy the 'middle ground'.

To date, medical evidence, often introduced by the anti-abortion lobby and also by other concerned individuals, has been said to show that, during the period following the second stage described above, the foetus can be saved. The common reaction, therefore, is that no pregnancy termination should be permitted at this stage because the foetus which could be born alive will be destroyed. But is this inevitable?

If it is true that termination is synonymous with foetal destruction, then the anti-abortion lobby has a powerful emotional case. The woman who, for whatever reason, finds herself seeking a late termination will, even in a more liberal jurisdiction than the United Kingdom, find herself facing grave, if not insurmountable, obstacles. Even those countries which are prepared to admit that women *do* have rights to choose pregnancy termination find it difficult to accept that this is also true in this last stage.[29] The common thread in this reasoning is, not surprisingly, that neither individuals nor states find it easy to adopt a position which effectively ensures the destruction of actually viable life.

However, it is at this point that the argument deviates most significantly from more traditional approaches. If foetal destruction were the only option,

116

then the writer would be forced to adopt one or other of the opposing positions. However, late pregnancy termination is not, and need not be, synonymous with foetal destruction. Indeed, induction, the method commonly used to terminate such pregnancies, is a technique also used in wanted pregnancies. However, other techniques are also used in terminations, designed to ensure as far as possible that the foetus is extruded in such a way that it never has a 'life independent of its mother'. This is, as Skegg[30] succinctly points out, because even a lawful pregnancy termination – that is, one which is within the defences provided by the abortion legislation – does not necessarily mean that the doctor performing the operation will be free from criminal sanction. Charges might still follow from a live birth, even where the reasons for terminating the pregnancy were legally acceptable. It is, therefore, in the interests of the physician that foetuses which are, in theory, salvageable, do not survive.

This is clearly a decision taken in the face of what might be described as a legal anomaly, which forces physicians to protect themselves. It also means that women have no options, and provides – however unwittingly – the fuel for the argument that late pregnancies should always be carried to term. But if these foetuses could be born alive, why should we deliberately destroy them? Some women may seek only termination of their pregnancy, not necessarily the destruction of the foetus.[31] Of course, some may regard the destruction of the foetus as an essential part of pregnancy termination, either because they have no way of knowing that an alternative is available or because that is genuinely what they want. A woman might, after all, simply want to give up maternal rights: this, it might be said, can be done by carrying the foetus to term and making it available for adoption. There would, in that case, be no need to consider the third stage in pregnancy at all. But this is too simplistic.

If we accept that some women (we don't know how many) only want to be relieved of the pregnancy, and that others, who have equated pregnancy termination with foetal destruction might want to be relieved of the pregnancy if an alternative was offered, then this could represent a significant number of women. Those who actually want foetal destruction have a hard case to argue, and would probably not wish to push it too strongly.

On the other hand, the anti-abortionists' position is that their interest is in saving foetal 'life', not in denying women's rights. The position, then *is* soluble. Late pregnancy terminations present no real problems. If the anti-abortion lobby is satisfied by medical evidence that such foetuses could be salvaged, then there is no 'pro-life' reason to deny late terminations, since their own argument is that they could be sustained. The pro-choice position also seems satisfied, since the woman gains the right – hitherto denied – to terminate pregnancies in this later period. In other words, if we *can* save the products of late pregnancy terminations, and we are told that we can, then we need not destroy them. And if this is so, then there is no 'pro-life' reason against late pregnancy terminations.

This is not to deny the inevitable obstacles to this position being accepted. In the United States of America, for example, a requirement that attempts

117

should be made where possible to save 'viable' foetuses in pregnancy terminations was declared unconstitutional,[32] although the grounds for this were as much to do with the terminology of the relevant legislation and the constitution as anything else. There would certainly be no *legal* reason not to make such a requirement in the United Kingdom. But what would such a change actually mean?

It would obviously mean that some women – those who want foetal destruction – would be placed in a difficult position. Arguably, however, they would in one sense be in the same situation as they currently are. That is, at the moment they have no right to make a decision *either* to destroy the foetus *or* not to carry it to term. In another sense they may be better off, since at least part of what they want – that is, to be relieved of the pregnancy – would be feasible. For those who do *not* also seek foetal destruction, there is a considerable gain.

A potential problem arises, however, where the reasons for seeking a late termination are related to the delayed discovery of foetal abnormality. In such cases, it would seem, most commentators have been prepared to agree that termination of pregnancy stands on its own grounds. That is, it is permissible because of the needs of the foetus and not those of the mother. Admittedly, the anti-abortion lobby have to date conceded this only up to the point at which a termination can legally take place. But it is difficult to see how the line can be drawn so arbitrarily. The point is that if we already agree that handicapped foetuses should be destroyed (which is pretty well inevitable in current legal restrictions) then we are saying something about our attitude to handicapped life. Moreover, both British[33] and American courts[34] have been prepared to countenance selective non-treatment decisions on full-term handicapped infants. The distinction between full-term handicapped babies and a late abortus is difficult to see. Whether one agrees with these decisions or not, they are currently accepted by our law and apparently by the majority of our community.

This argument would not insist on the salvaging of the handicapped foetus, since it is not dependent on the sanctity of 'life'. No woman would be forced into a situation of having to deal with a salvaged foetus whose condition was the reason for the pregnancy termination in the first place. The strongest opponents of abortion have already made sufficient concessions for it to be relatively simple to insert into any new legislation an exclusion based on these grounds. In any event, this problem will arise less frequently as science develops tests for handicap which are effective and accurate earlier in pregnancy.

Of course, there are other potential problems associated with legislating for the argument developed here. For example, later terminations may prove to be expensive, since intensive nursing and other care may often be necessary, as they are with spontaneous premature birth. It may even be more expensive to induce birth without poisoning the foetus. But, if we are committed to enhancing both foetal potential and women's rights, these are necessary and worthwhile costs. Equally, it cannot be denied that women may come under pressure to carry the foetus to term, in the interests of even more certain potential for life, but this pressure can and should be resisted. In any event, if women are given *rights*, which they do not currently have at any stage in their pregnancy in the United Kingdom,[35] then they have a better and more convincing platform from which to resist pressure to carry the foetus to term.

It is, of course, the case that there will probably be few circumstances in which this right will be resorted to, but one could without too much difficulty envisage circumstances where its existence could be most valuable. Even without using extreme examples, it should be clear that the abortion decision is not one taken lightly by women, yet imposing strict and early time limits may drive some women into a pressurized – perhaps even hasty – decision in favour of abortion. If that same woman is given time and the option of salvaging the foetus, then decisions may be taken more calmly, and foetal potential may even be saved. This is not to minimize the fact that foetuses are doubtless safer if carried to term, but we cannot have it both ways. If a reason for denying late pregnancy terminations is that we could save that foetus *at that stage*, then we cannot also argue that it cannot be saved.

Thus, any change in the law along the lines suggested would need to take account of these potential difficulties, but none of the problems are insuperable. Lack of funding in the health services cannot be a justification for committing a criminal act (that is, failing to save a foetus born alive) and the resources needed to do so are independent of this discussion. Equally, if we intend to save late abortuses, then we may need to require that late terminations are carried out in ways, and under circumstances, which provide the best potential for saving the abortus. It might also be said that women are put at increased risk in later terminations, and procedural requirements should minimize any increased risk involved. In any event, from the woman's point of view it remains safer and preferable to terminate a pregnancy in the early stages, and most women, given the option, would probably continue to prefer this where possible. But what of the young girl or woman who is either unaware of her pregnancy, or who is too afraid to seek advice on termination? For them, the addition of rights at this stage could be extremely important.

Additional problems may also arise in respect of the woman's obligations and duties in relation to the aborted, but alive, foetus. While these problems do not directly affect this argument, it must be said that there seems little difficulty in resolving them. The position of these women will surely equate with the position of the woman who carries a pregnancy to term with the intention of giving the child up after birth.

CONCLUSIONS

This paper has attempted to identify the main strands in the abortion debate. At the risk of being repetitious, it is useful to restate them at this stage. The anti-abortion lobby would make several claims: (i) all human life is sacred, and therefore all abortion should be outlawed; (ii) but, given political reality, where abortion is permitted, it should be restricted, most particularly in terms of the setting of a (low) upper time limit, beyond which all pregnancy terminations should be unlawful; (iii) the reason for this position is not to attack women, but to protect foetal 'life'.

In terms of the argument presented here, what can be said about these claims? Evidently the first position has the merit of consistency, although it is scarcely in line with at least parts of the second and third claims. In any event, whilst it may represent a valid personal morality, given that it is not shared by everyone it arguably provides a reason only for those who believe it to eschew abortion – it need not limit the rights and freedoms of others who hold this position to be manifestly wrong.

However, it is in the second and third claims that the real problems with the anti-abortion position are evident. The concessions made to political reality result in the question being posed: if all human life is sacred, and this is why one opposes abortion, then why are there defences provided up to a chosen maximum time limit, whatever that is? And, indeed, if the anti-abortion lobby does *not* stick to its extreme position on the sanctity of human life, then what is left of its anti-abortion arguments? That is, what is the source of the remaining opposition? The purported answer may be found in the third claim – namely, that a residual argument against abortion remains in the preservation of foetal life.

Let us look at this claim in the face both of the anti-abortion lobby's own arguments and in the light of the option presented here. In the terms of the former, preserving foetal existence is a fundamental value. Then why permit terminations up to, say eighteen weeks when the absolutely inevitable outcome is foetal destruction? No amount of medical miracles can render the embryo or immature foetus salvageable at this point. If it ever does this it is most likely to be by development outside the womb, however unlikely this currently is. If medicine ever *can* grow embryos to term outside the womb then the current abortion debate becomes obsolete since there is not the same competition between women's right and foetal or embryonic interests. And if medicine develops sufficiently so that extremely premature foetuses can be saved, this still does not constitute an argument against pregnancy termination. In fact, what it does is to make the third strand to the argument presented here even more relevant. There is no reason not to salvage when we can, beyond existing legal constraints which are based on thoroughly out-dated scientific capacity.

In any event, given the state of current knowledge, the anti-abortion campaigners should not, if they are to be consistent, argue the case they currently put forward. Logically, if their aim really is to preserve foetal 'life', they should argue for a *minimum* time for pregnancy termination and not a *maximum*. Their claim to speak for the embryo/foetus is somewhat weakened by the concessions which they have already made.

Let us concede that the second and third aspects to the anti-abortion position are – even despite these inconsistencies – genuine goals. How are they affected by the thesis developed here? Obviously the proposals outlined

120

here relating to the second and third stages of pregnancy enhance the capacity for foetal survival, and if these are genuine aims then they are unchallengeable by an anti-abortion lobby which has already made considerable inroads into its fundamental claim that all human life is sacred. Admittedly, the postulated absolute right to pregnancy termination in the first stage of pregnancy does entail foetal destruction, but then so would all of the proposed amendments to the 1967 Act which have consistently gained the support of anti-abortion groups.

Of course, it might be argued that more pregnancies would be terminated if the current restrictions were lifted, and this may be true. It is equally the case, however, that foetal survival might be enhanced by not forcing women into early – sometimes rushed – decisions, by permitting them the additional option of later pregnancy terminations which do not entail foetal destruction.

And what of the pro-abortion lobby? Their fundamental position would be that of the rights under consideration, those which should be regarded as central to acceptable policy are those of women. The argument presented here would enhance women's rights rather than restrict them. Instead of the need to convince two doctors that she has a case, in the first stage of pregnancy a woman would have an absolute right to terminate a pregnancy. And in the later stages, she would acquire this right. It is admitted that the suggested restrictions in the few weeks crucial to salvageability do make inroads into an absolute right to abortion, but they may be a necessary concession to those whose opinions represent what I have called the middle ground, and they scarcely represent as grave an intrusion into women's rights as does the current position.

What can be concluded, then, from the above? It does seem that some reform may be possible which satisfies those who do not espouse an extreme position. Indeed, some of those who have clung to an anti-abortion approach for lack of an alternative which was morally satisfactory may be persuaded to think again. These would be the people who do not abhor abortion at every stage in a pregnancy, but have joined the anti-abortion approach at the point at which salvageability becomes an issue. The inconsistency of the anti-abortion lobby's views in respect of later terminations may help to convince them that an alternative is plausible.

Both sides to the argument, then, may gain something from the adoption of this approach. Those who gain most, however are those to whom it is addressed – the 'middle ground'. This group may well be able to accept the logic of each opposing position, particularly where they maintain a high level of internal consistency. But they are unable to make the 'leap of faith' to subscribe entirely. An additional benefit of the approach outlined here is that it requires no such leap, but, hopefully, remains internally consistent even in compromise. Certainly it may provide this group – hitherto formally excluded by the pattern of couching the argument in extreme terms – with the beginnings of a platform of their own from which to seek abortion laws which are neither authoritarian on the one hand nor lacking compassion on the other. Indeed, consensual reform of the abortion laws seems to be unlikely without such a platform.

This thesis is not represented as a panacea, but it *is* an alternative. It has the capacity to satisfy some of the demands of both sides of the debate, and thereby to represent a balance between the two extremes. Moreover, it allows the state to maintain an interest in both women's rights and foetal survival, both of which are regarded by most states as important. One problem in the past has been that whilst they are both seen as worthy of protection, they have also been perceived as fundamentally incompatible. The options postulated by this argument suggest that this need not be so. Doubtless much remains to be worked out for this approach to be translated into social and legal reality, but hopefully it provides an alternative basis for discussion of this most enduring and divisive ethical issue.

NOTES AND REFERENCES

1 See, for discussion, *The Observer*, 30 July 1989; *The Observer*, 6 August 1989.

2 For discussion, see *Report of the Committee of Enquiry into Human Fertilization and Embrology* (Warnock Report) (1984; Cmnd. 9314).

3 It should be noted that the same commitment was made last year following the publication of the White Paper, *Human Fertilization and Embryology: A Framework for Legislation* (1987; Cmd. 259). This article was written before the publication and debate on the Human Fertilization and Embryology Bill.

4 See *The Guardian*, 22 September 1989.

5 *Webster* v *Reproductive Health Services*, Supreme Court, 3 July 1989.

6 K. Luker, *Abortion and the Politics of Motherhood* (1984).

7 For discussion, see D. Jonsen, 'A New Threat to Pregnant Women's Autonomy' (1987) 17 *Hastings Center Report* 33: S. A. M. McLean, 'Women, Rights and Reproduction' in *Legal Issues in Human Reproduction*, ed. S. A. M. McLean (1989); U. E. B. Kolder, J. Gallagher, and M. T. Parsons, 'Court-Ordered Obstetrical Interventions' (1987) 316 *New England J. of Medicine* 1192.

8 *D* v *Berkshire County Council* [1987] 1 All E.R. 20; see for discussion, J. E. S. Fortin, 'Legal Protection for the Unborn Child' (1988) *Modern Law Rev.* 54.

9 See above, n. 5.

10 Since both of these work after fertilization.

11 See, for discussion, E. F. Paul and J. Paul 'Self-Ownership, Abortion and Infanticide' (1979) 5 *J. of Medical Ethics* 133.

12 J. J. Thomson, 'A Defence of Abortion' (1971) 1 *Philosophy and Public Affairs* 47.

13 As *The Guardian* noted on 27 October (1987), there were four bills presented at this time seeking to restrict access to abortion, a situation which was described as 'a Parliamentary record for a single issue'.

14 This terminology is also not used here since it represents a highly contentious view of the issues for which this lobby is fighting and those of their opposition.

15 See D. Alton, 'Why the Right to Life must be Paramount' *The Guardian*, 5 October 1987.

16 *Regina* v *Tait*, *The Guardian* 5 May 1989. But see also the unique conviction in Edinburgh Sheriff Court of a man who caused the death of an unborn baby. The child died ninety minutes after being born as a result of an emergency caesarian section *The Guardian* 31 January 1989.

17 See Johnsen, op. cit., n. 7; Kolder et al., op. cit., n. 7.

18 See Fortin, op. cit., n. 8; McLean, op. cit., n. 7.

19 For further discussion of this point, see McLean, op. cit., n. 7; P. D. G. Skegg, *Law, Ethics*

and Medicine (1984). See also Alton, op. cit., n. 15, talking of later pregnancy terminations: 'The baby has either been poisoned or will not survive if born alive. In private clinics the method of dilation and evacuation allows the operating staff to dilate the cervix, crush the child inside the woman and thus facilitate its extraction.' For discussion, see below.

20 The word salvageable is generally used here in preference to 'viable' to distinguish this argument from the traditional framework in which it occurs. Salvageability is taken to mean the capacity for survival if safely delivered.

21 *Roe* v *Wade* 93 S.Ct. 705(1973).

22 id.

23 id.

24 The Abortion Act 1967 provides defences to the criminal offence of abortion – abortion itself remains an offence unless covered by the following exceptions: s. 1 (1) ' . . . a person shall not be guilty of an offence under the law relating to abortion when a pregnancy is terminated by a registered medical practitioner if two registered medical practitioners are of the opinion, formed in good faith (a) that the continuance of the pregnancy would involve risk to the life of the pregnant woman or any existing children of her family, greater than if the pregnancy were terminated; or (b) that there is a substantial risk that if the child were born it would suffer from such physical or mental abnormalities as to be seriously handicapped.'

25 See *The Guardian*, 23 January 1989.

26 See *The Guardian*, 29 January 1988.

27 Compare J. K. Mason, *Medico-Legal Aspects of Reproduction and Parenting* (1989) ch. 5.

28 Thompson, op. cit., n. 12.

29 Even in *Roe* v *Wade* (op. cit., n. 21) the court referred to the state's interest in foetal life in the third trimester as a reason for restricting, if not denying, access to abortion.

30 Skegg, op. cit., n. 19.

31 For discussion, see McLean, op. cit., n. 7.

32 *Thornburgh* v *American College of Obstetricians and Gynaecologists* 106 S.Ct. 2169 (1986).

33 Compare *R* v *Arthur, The Times*, 6 November 1981; *Re B* [1981] 1 W.L.R. 1421; *Re C (a minor) No 2., The Guardian*, 27 April 1989 (C.A.).

34 In 1983 the Department of Health and Human Services promulgated the so called 'Baby Doe' rules under s. 594 of the Rehabilitation Act 1973. The regulations required the posting in maternity and related wards in hospitals of a notice which stated that 'discriminatory failure to feed and care for handicapped infants in this facility is prohibited by federal law' and provided a twenty-four-hour toll-free telephone number to report breaches of this statement. In 1986 the Supreme Court declared these rules to be invalid. In 1984 Congress passed amendments to the Child Abuse and Neglect Prevention and Treatment Act, and following these federal regulations set criteria which each state must meet in order to receive federal grants for its child abuse programme. These require child abuse agencies to establish procedures for responding to reports of medical neglect of infants from whom medically indicated treatment is withheld. The requirements have been taken to mean that all children born with impairments are to receive treatment for life-threatening conditions, whilst infants for whom the immediate prognosis is bad and for whom treatment would be inhumane need not be treated.

35 See the Abortion Act 1967, op. cit., n. 24.

[7]

David W. Meyers

Compulsory Sterilisation and Castration

Compulsory sterilisation is an involuntary or unconsented to[1] surgical operation in present times, rendering the patient or victim – depending on one's characterisation of the practice – sterile or incapable of procreation, though not incapable of coitus.[2]

Castration, the predecessor of surgical sterilisation, was practised in Biblical times and before by the Assyrians, Chinese, Hindus, Egyptians, Greeks, Persians and Romans for various reasons of security, punishment and control of captives, criminals or slaves. In Java, the Malay Peninsula, Australasia and the Amerindians, the aborigines have long practised excision of the sex glands for religious purposes.[3]

De-sexing was introduced into England, primarily as a punitive measure for rapists, by the Normans.[4] However, at common law, private acts of de-sexing were considered to constitute grave demembration. Seton of Pitmedden, expressing the Scottish position in the late seventeenth century, characterised the law dealing with castration in the following terms:

> '*Castratis virilium* is one of the most atrocious demembrations; and when a man does it to himself, he is *sui homicida*. And so punishable with death and confiscation of Goods, And it's equivalent if one suffered himself willingly to be castrated by another.'[5]

Seton understandably does not mention surgical sterilisation, for it did not exist as a medical art in his day and is, in practical terms, a twentieth-century development.[6] Nonetheless, his learned remarks on mutilation seem just as applicable to sterilisation as mutilation in his words was

> 'Cessation and Privation of the Office, and distinct Operation of a Member, albeit no particle of it to be cut off.'[7]

Mackenzie felt that mutilation or the disabling of a member of the body was a capital crime, but Erskine[8] takes exception, saying by Statute Robert II, c. 11, that mutilation was to be punished by the same form of process to be used against a manslayer, but that the punishment was not to be capital.

In his American work, Professor Perkins supports Mackenzie's view with common law authority, stating that the early penalty for mayhem was mutilation, except in the case of castration, where the punishment was death.[9]

Hume, in his *Commentaries* seems to concur with Erskine's discussion of the Statute Robert II. He states that the statute had an intended *in terrorem* effect and that the record in fact showed not a single instance of a capital conviction for the offence of mutilation thereunder. Hume cited 'scourging and banishment forth of Scotland' as the usual penalty.[10]

There is no modern Scottish discussion of compulsory sterilisation and castration. However, Glaister has stated flatly that the only lawful sterilisation is therapeutic sterilisation, the consent of the patient notwithstanding.[11] Gordon, on the other hand, feels that, barring a statute, both consensual sterilisation and castration would be treated as any other surgical operation : lawful if

'recognised by the profession as appropriate and carried out in accordance with proper professional standards.'[12]

Theological Views

The contemporary German theologian, Häring, does not merely denounce the practice of compulsory sterilisation itself as wrong, but condemns participation in any such procedures by the judiciary and the medical profession as sinful. He states:

'More difficult is the case in which the law is not only unjust but actually demands that something sinful in itself be done. We have a sad instance in the laws of those states requiring sterilisation. Even worse would be a law demanding denial of the faith. No judge may co-operate in enforcing or applying these laws – particularly when the law requires the sterilisation of individuals who have never committed the slightest crime, but who are considered "unfit" for marriage or parenthood because of heritage or mental deficiency! What shall we say of the decision of the court which must determine that a certain individual is to be classified as "unfit"? Some writers are inclined to doubt the guilt of a judge who must apply the law by making a decision according to the terms of the law, always provided that he does all in his power to avoid "passing the sentence". However, it seems to me that the official who is primarily responsible for the actual procedure, the physician or other official who makes the "certification" that this innocent individual is fit "only to be a descendant", is guilty of formal co-operation in sin. The law in this instance is no defence, for it requires something unjust, something no one is permitted to do. Obviously, those who actually carry out the law and perform the operation are principals in the crime.'[13]

The Reverend Fletcher pays scant attention to the question of the morality of compulsory sterilisation in his book, *Morals and Medicine*.[14]

Professor Paul Ramsey of Princeton Theological Seminary has expressed the view in his contribution to a recent symposium on 'Morals, Medicine and the Law' that, 'not everyone simply by being has the right to propagate'.[15] He does, however, temper this remark by questioning whether proper safeguards can be established by the law to insure that this type of philosophy does not become subject to 'misuse' by 'errant humanity'.[16]

Ramsey is apparently fearful that man, given the power by laws to deny certain members of society the right to propagate, is not capable of formulating satisfactory criteria for the exercise of such power; that inevitably, such a law would be incapable of fair, impartial administration.

In the same symposium, Rabbi Emanuel Rackman indicates Judaism's general prohibition against sterilisation, subject to the requirement of self-preservation. Discussing state-sponsored eugenic sterilisation, he expresses similar doubts to those of Ramsey:

> 'I dread the extension of the State's police power to include control of the procreative faculties of one person for the benefit of another'.[17]

The American Position

While the lawfulness of voluntary, non-therapeutic sterilisation remains unclear in the United States in the absence of statute,[18] there are twenty-six states with eugenic sterilisation laws, twenty-three of which are of a compulsory nature. All of the various laws designate feeble-minded or mentally retarded persons as within their ambit, all but two include the mentally ill, some fourteen include epileptics and twelve specifically include criminals – most on eugenic grounds, not on punitive grounds.[19]

There are, however, two notable exceptions in the laws of California and Washington. California Penal Code §645[20] provides for sterilisation as a penalty for the crime of carnal abuse of a female under ten years old. Washington has a similar statute.[21]

Seventeen of the state laws apply only to the institutionalised, nine to both. Most of the twenty-three compulsory sterilisation statutes provide for notice, a hearing and judicial appeal, but six states still do not require a hearing and three make no provision for judicial appeal.[22] California makes provision for a formal hearing only if objection is filed by the patient, but it is the practice of the Department of Mental Health to authorise sterilisations only in cases where the inmate 'consents' thereto.[23]

A United States doctor in Pennsylvania claimed to have performed the first sexual sterilisation to prevent procreation in 1889. In Indiana, 600–700 reform school boys were sterilised by Dr Harry C. Sharp, who devised the vasectomy operation even before passage of the State's sterilisation Act in 1907.[24]

In 1897 the first eugenic sterilisation bill was introduced into the Michigan legislature, but defeated. Pennsylvania passed a similar law in 1905, but it was vetoed in a strongly worded message by the governor.[25]

In 1907 the first sterilisation law was successfully enacted in Indiana and, although subsequently declared unconstitutional,[26] was the basis for other laws, which by 1950 had accounted for the sterilisation of over 50,000 persons in America, 20,000 in California alone.[27] By 1964 the cumulative total had reached 63,678. Of these persons, 27,917 were sterilised on grounds of mental illness, 32,374 on grounds of mental deficiency and some 2,387 on other grounds.[28]

Notwithstanding these formidable figures, in recent years the practice of state-inspired sterilisations has come under increasing criticism.[29] In 1963, the figure for California was seventeen sterilisations, Virginia stood second in the nation with thirty-nine, surpassed only by North Carolina with 240 sterilisations performed.[30]

While it is unclear how much of this decrease is a response to outside, public or social pressure and how much is due to a change of belief of those actually administering the eugenic sterilisation laws, several factors may be suggested as accounting for the decrease in yearly sterilisations performed under statutory authority in the United States : a more humanitarian attitude toward the treatment of institutionalised patients, an increasing awareness of the limited state of man's understanding of human genetics and hereditary transmission, and partly as a result, an increasingly unclear and questionable legal basis and support, particularly under the American Constitution, for the practice of state compulsory sterilisation.

The legal decisions regarding sterilisation begin in 1912, shortly after enactment of the first United States statute by Indiana in 1907, and are reported as recently as 1968.[31] (As early as 1872, however, the 8th Amendment's 'cruel and unusual punishment' clause [32] was held to have been enacted to prohibit, among other practices, castration.[33] It should be noted also that of the twelve states with eugenic sterilisation laws specifically applicable to criminals, none authorises castration.[34]) The early cases decided before 1925 struck

30 »   *Compulsory Sterilisation and Castration*

down most of the statutes[35] when they were challenged in the courts
– not in basic principle, but largely for procedural deficiencies
which were held to deny 'due process of law' to the persons involved.[36] One notably different approach, however, which recently
has been receiving some attention,[37] was used by a lower federal
court in *Mickle* v. *Henrichs*,[38] wherein the state of Nevada was restrained from performing a compulsory sterilisation (vasectomy) on
a convicted rapist and probable epileptic, the Court holding it to be
a mutilation which constituted 'cruel or unusual' punishment under
the state constitution.[39] The Court in *Mickle*[40] stated that

> 'Vasectomy in itself is not cruel...but, when resorted to as a punish-
> ment, it is ignominious and degrading, and in that sense it is cruel'.

Because the relevant state clause was in the disjunctive ('or') rather
than in the conjunctive ('and'), as is the federal prohibition, the
usual or unusualness of the punishment was not decisive to the result. In *Davis* v. *Berry*,[41] the federal conjunctive prohibition was held
to be in issue with the state compulsory sterilisation statute which was
applied punitively to recidivistic felons. The Court held:

> 'While it is true that there are differences between the two opera-
> tions of castration and vasectomy, and while it is true that the
> effect upon the man would be different in several aspects, yet the
> fact remains that the purpose and the same shame and humiliation
> and degradation and mental torture are the same in one case as in
> the other. And our conclusion is that the infliction of this penalty
> is in violation of the Constitution, which provides that cruel and
> unusual punishment shall not be inflicted.'

As applied to defectives and the insane for allegedly 'eugenic' rather
than punitive purposes, the courts have not regarded compulsory
sterilisation as a cruel and unusual punishment.[42]

Between 1925 and 1933 a rush of cases involving state sterilisation
schemes – both eugenic and punitive in nature[43] – came before the
courts and were all upheld against various legal attacks. Then, in
1933 the trend showed some sign of shifting and most of the decisions found dealing with compulsory sterilisation since that time
have invalidated the laws and orders involved, thus casting considerable doubt on the continued legality of compulsory sterilisation in
the United States. These cases all merit some discussion.

In 1925, the Michigan Supreme Court upheld the sterilisation of a
sixteen-year-old feeble-minded girl, with the consent of her parents
and after notice and a hearing had been provided.[44] The Court
reasoned as follows:

'There is no element of punishment involved in the sterilisation of feeble-minded persons. In this respect it is analogous to compulsory vaccination [an analogy to be soon after used by Mr Chief Justice Holmes in the landmark U.S. Supreme Court case of *Buck* v. *Bell*, discussed *infra*]. Both are non-punitive. It is therefore plainly apparent that the constitutional [state] inhibition against cruel and unusual punishment has no application to the surgical treatment of feeble-minded persons.'

Mr Justice Wiest filed a vigorous, thoroughgoing dissent in the case, stating bluntly:

'This act violates the Constitution, goes beyond the police power and is void....The bodies of citizens may not, under legislative mandate, be cut into, and the power of procreation destroyed by ligation or mutilation of glands or carving out of organs.'

The *Smith* case set the stage for the most well-known American case dealing with sterilisation, *Buck* v. *Bell*.[45] In *Buck*, Mr Chief Justice Holmes upheld a Virginia statute, under which Carrie Buck, an eighteen-year-old, feeble-minded girl who had shortly before given birth to a feeble-minded child and who herself was the daughter of a feeble-minded mother, was sterilised. The law was challenged on due process grounds, but weathered the attack by providing for notice and a hearing to the subject and by allowing for appeal to the courts. The Virginia statute was more carefully drawn than those earlier state laws which up to *Buck* v. *Bell* had been overturned on due process of law grounds.

The opinion in Buck was remarkably short considering its significance. It finished with the following comments:

'We have seen more than once that the public welfare may call upon the best citizens for their lives. It would be strange if it could not call upon these who already sap the strength of the state for these lesser sacrifices, often not felt to be such by those concerned, in order to prevent our being swamped with incompetence. It is better for all the world, if instead of waiting to execute degenerate offspring for crime, or to let them starve for their imbecility, society can prevent those who are manifestly unfit from continuing their kind. The principle that sustains compulsory vaccination is broad enough to cover cutting the Fallopian tubes. *Jacobson* v. *Massachusetts*, 197 U.S. 11, 25 S.Ct. 338. Three generations of imbeciles are enough.'[46]

Buck has been criticised often, but never overruled, though it may be

32 » *Compulsory Sterilisation and Castration*

during the u.s. Supreme Court's fall 1969 term.[47] Mr Chief Justice Holmes' analogy of compulsory sterilisation to military service is faulty, for the latter involves the country calling on its citizens not for their lives, but only to expose them to the risk of loss of life. In *Jacobsen* the court sustained a $ 5 fine for petitioner's refusal to accept compulsory vaccination; it did not order submission. Furthermore, vaccination has an uncontestedly beneficial effect on the subject and on the society, without depriving the former of any of his capabilities, contrary to compulsory sterilisation.[48]

A number of state court decisions, following in the wake of *Buck* v. *Bell*, upheld various sterilisation (and at least one castration) statutes.[49]

In *State* v. *Schaffer*,[50] compulsory sterilisation of certain state institutionalised inmates was upheld against challenge on grounds it violated due process, was an excessive use of state police (legislative) power and was unfairly discriminatory. In *Davis* v. *Walton*,[51] the compulsory asexualisation (castration) of an 'habital sexual criminal' was upheld against charges that it was cruel and unusual punishment or that it denied the convict 'equal protection of the laws'.[52] *State* v. *Troutman*,[53] held a compulsory sterilisation statute valid, stating that

> '...if there be any natural right for natively mental defectives to beget children, that right must give way to the police power of the state in protecting the common welfare, so far as it can be protected, against this hereditary type of feeble-mindedness.'

The case of *Re Clayton*[54] validated a statutory directive providing that certain feeble-minded and insane inmates or habitual criminals could not be discharged or paroled without first submitting to sterilisation.[55]

Two years later, however, in *Brewer* v. *Valk*,[56] a statute providing for the sterilisation, at public cost, of any mental defective upon petition of his next of kin or legal guardian to specified state authorities was overturned, the court holding it an unconstitutional violation of due process of law for failing to provide the subject with proper notice and a full hearing in order to insure having his position fully and fairly heard. The decision did not question the legality *per se* of the state sterilisation of defectives, but rather limited itself to the inadequate procedural safeguards contained in the statute at issue in the case.

The *Brewer* case did, nevertheless, give ambitious eugenicists in the United States a renewed warning of the scrutiny with which the courts would examine compulsory sterilisation statutes. The year following saw publication of the well-known Brock Committee Report[57] in England. The Report was critical of the limited American experience with compulsory sterilisation[58] and in favour of statutory provision for voluntary sterilisation only.[59] Two years later, a committee of the American Neurological Association, chaired by Dr Abraham Myerson, came out with a similar recommendation that legislation be limited to voluntary sterilisation : careful application of such laws was suggested in certified cases of hereditary-linked diseases, such as schizophrenia, manic-depressive psychosis, feeble-mindedness and possibly epilepsy.[60]

Not long after publication and discussion of these reports, the United States Supreme Court handed down its second opinion dealing with sterilisation. The case, *Skinner* v. *Oklahoma*,[61] reflects a considerable change in the High Court's attitude from the position it had taken fifteen years earlier in *Buck* v. *Bell, supra*. *Skinner* challenged the Oklahoma law, which provided for compulsory sterilisation of 'habitual' criminals, basing his attack on the equal protection of the laws clause of the United States Constitution. The statute at issue defined habitual criminals as those persons convicted two or more times of felonious crimes involving 'moral turpitude'. It then distinguished between larceny and embezzlement, including only the former in its classification as a crime involving the necessary 'moral turpitude', although both were similar and both received the same punishment by state law. Mr Justice Douglas, after opening his majority opinion with the highly appropriate phrase, 'This case touches a sensitive and important area of human rights', went on to invalidate the contested Oklahoma law, relying on the Fourteenth Amendment's equal protection clause. He concluded:

> '...strict scrutiny of the classification which a state makes in a sterilisation law is essential, lest unwittingly or otherwise invidious discriminations are made against groups or types of individuals in violation of the constitutional guaranty of just and equal laws.
>
> When the law lays an unequal hand on those who have committed intrinsically the same quality of offence and sterilises one and not the other, it has made as invidious a discrimination as if it had selected a particular race or nationality for oppressive treatment.'[62]

Mr Justice Jackson, in a separate concurring opinion, chose to emphasise what may well have been the real, unstated foundation of the decision, namely that of bodily integrity and the limits of state-sponsored interference, with, or infringement of, that integrity. He stated succinctly:

HB D

34 » *Compulsory Sterilisation and Castration*

'There are limits to the extent to which a legislatively represented majority may conduct biological experiments at the expense of the dignity and personality and natural powers of a minority – even those who have been guilty of what the majority define as a crime.' [63]

Just what effect *Skinner* has had on *Buck* v. *Bell* is unclear and unstated. No further hints have come from the United States Supreme Court, although state-sponsored sterilisations throughout the country have decreased in the interim. [64] The two cases are not specifically at odds: *Skinner* struck down a compulsory sterilisation statute because it violated the equal protection clause of the Fourteenth Amendment, whereas *Buck* upheld a compulsory sterilisation statute which was contested only on due process grounds under the Fourteenth Amendment. Nonetheless, Mr Justice Jackson's quoted concurring remarks hint at an alternative ground for invalidating such statutes – that of the cruel and unusual punishment clause. [65]

In a case that might have been used to clarify the situation in the United States as regards the constitutionality of requiring sterilisation of a feeble-minded individual as a condition precedent to his release, the United States Supreme Court recently granted *certiorari* in the Nebraska case of *In re Cavitt*. In deciding *Cavitt*, the Nebraska Supreme Court, in a strongly divided opinion, held the state statute allowing for sterilisation of mentally deficient individuals as a prerequisite to parole or release from a state home for such persons was in all respects constitutional and enforceable. The court stated that such a statute denies neither equal protection of the law, due process of the law, nor constitutes a cruel and unusual punishment for crime. Carter, J., in some language reminiscent of that of an earlier day, cites *Buck* v. *Bell* for the proposition that the police power of the state is broad enough to permit sexual sterilisation of mentally deficient inmates where such mental deficiency is hereditary and would 'probably' be inherited by children born to such inmates. Stating that the right of a woman to bear and the right of a man to beget children is a natural and constitutional right, the court in *Cavitt*, nonetheless, went on to state:

'Acting for the public good, the state, in the exercise of its police power, may impose reasonable restrictions upon the natural and constitutional rights of its citizens. Measured by its injurious effect upon society, the state may limit a class of citizens in its right to bear or beget children with an inherited tendency to mental deficiency, including feeble-mindedness, idiocy, or imbecility. It is the function of the legislation and its duty as well, to enact appropriate legislation to protect the public and to preserve the race from the known effects of the procreation of mentally deficient children by the mentally deficient.'[66]

In concluding that the sterilisation of a mentally defective female by salpingectomy is not a cruel and unusual punishment and is in no sense a punishment for crime, the majority in *Cavitt* relied upon several old cases.[67]

With remarkable candour, and relatively little established scientific basis, Carter, J., stated for the court in *Cavitt*,

'It is an established fact that mental deficiency accelerates sexual impulses and any tendencies toward crime to a harmful degree.'[68]

Taking issue with this statement, Smith, J., in his dissenting opinion cites Dr Bernard L. Diamond, prominent psychiatrist and professor, as follows:

'In short, the present state of our scientific knowledge does not justify the widespread use of the sterilisation procedures in mentally ill or mentally deficient persons...it is sometimes proposed that sterilisation is demanded, irrespective of the uncertainties of our knowledge of heredity, in that a mentally ill or feeble-minded person is incapable of providing the emotional and material environment required to raise a normal child. Perhaps this is so, but it raises issues of a sociological and political nature of a very uncertain character and it may be most dangerous to apply such sociological concepts under the guise of a genetic basis that is far from proven and highly uncertain in its application.'[69]

However, the dissenting justices did not challenge the majority's conclusion that the sterilisation law did not constitute cruel and unusual punishment, but rather challenged it on the basis that it denied due process for its vagueness and lack of scientific basis.

The Nebraska Supreme Court had occasion to reconsider its opinion when a motion for rehearing was filed and heard in June of 1968.[70] In denying the motion for rehearing and adhering to its former opinion, the court held that the statute in question was not unconstitutional on the grounds that there was no requirement for a specific finding that offspring of the party to be sterilised would likely be defective. On the rehearing motion, the court once again summarily disposed of the question of cruel and unusual punishment and held that the statute in question satisfied the requirements of due process. Four justices dissented.

In re Cavitt is now before the United States Supreme Court. The Nebraska statute in question has since been repealed, but the State claims this does not moot the case and it may be argued in the fall

36 »   *Compulsory Sterilisation and Castration*

1969 term. It is likely that the decision will be reversed, though whether the basis will be cruel and unusual punishment or denial of due process because the statute failed to impose clear standards for determination of an individual's likely propensity to transmit feeble-mindedness, is unclear. Considering the uncertain scientific basis for the practice of eugenic sterilisation, but nonetheless leaving open the beneficial possibilities of such practice if carefully restricted, it is likely that the United States Supreme Court, if it does in fact invalidate the Nebraska practice in question, will do it on grounds of due process rather than invalidating the entire concept of pseudo-voluntary sterilisation as a cruel and unusual punishment prohibited by the Constitution. Furthermore, while the practice may be 'cruel', it would be difficult to call it 'unusual' in light of its widespread past acceptance by many states. As noted, prior cases in the lower courts have split on the question,[71] but the Supreme Court has recently shown some signs of giving this long-overlooked clause of the Constitution (Eighth Amendment of the 'Bill of Rights') new and wider scope.[72]

Recent academic comment has also suggested that sterilisation is one form of punishment – at least in its punitive if not in its eugenic form – that might well soon be held to contravene protections against cruel and unusual punishment, because it may well in some cases at least be so degrading to the subject, 'as virtually to deny the defendant's humanity'.[73]

Several recent American cases have suggested that a new justification, based on economic considerations, may be sought for compulsory sterilisation laws in the future.

Two judges presiding over probate courts in Ohio have ordered sterilisations despite the absence of any sterilisation law in the state, expressing judicially that such action was warranted to reduce public welfare costs. Beginning with the most notable of their decisions, *In re Simpson*,[74] these two judges have ordered the sterilisation of five mentally retarded females. At least one of the judges has indicated an intention to continue with this practice.[75] *In re Simpson* involved sterilisation of a young imbecile mother, the judge relying on his discretionary interim power at law and in equity to provide for the welfare of incompetents. The case has been severely criticised as an abuse of judicial discretion, but apparently has not been overruled.[76]

In all three of the recent California cases there were no statutory provisions applicable or relied upon by the court, but nonetheless submission to sterilisation was ordered by the judge as a condition of probation. In the first case from Los Angeles County, *Andrada* v. *So. Pasadena Munic. Court*,[77] the defendant decided upon probation after submission to sterilisation rather than a jail sentence when he pleaded guilty to a charge of non-support of his children. Subsequently he regretted his choice and began litigating. Andrada asked and was denied habeas corpus by the California Supreme Court. He asked the United States Supreme Court to review the case and decide if

> 'conditioning probation upon sterilisation constituted cruel and unusual punishment and violated procedural due process'.[78]

The Supreme Court denied *certiorari, In re Andrada*.[79] The trial judge involved has also indicated he will continue to favour such a practice in non-support cases.[80]

In the next case, *People* v. *Tapia*,[81] a couple convicted of welfare fraud were involved. They were offered a reduction of sentence contingent upon filing of a stipulation by counsel or a report from the Santa Barbara County Hospitals that the defendants had 'voluntarily' submitted to the (sterilisation) operations.[82] The matter was not appealed.[83]

Most recently, *In the Matter of Hernandez*,[84] was before the California courts. Here again, a twenty-one-year-old girl was offered the 'choice' between submission to sterilisation and immediate probation, and a six-month jail term, which was the maximum penalty for her offence of being in a room where narcotics were being unlawfully and knowingly used. The subject had two daughters – one illegitimate – on welfare. It was her first offence and her probation report recommended straight probation. The municipal court judge, however, added on the sterilisation requirement at the probation hearing without apparent reason.

On prompt writ of habeas corpus appeal to the Superior Court, the writ was granted, the sterilisation provision was stricken from the probation order and the defendant was released to the custody of her probation officer. The Superior Court held the trial judge had no authority under any state statutes to impose sterilisation as a condition of probation and that in so doing he had abused and exceeded his judicial authority.[85]

In one final case the *New York Times* recently reported that an unwed mother convicted of incinerating her four-day old son agreed to be sterilised on the judge's promise that he would reduce her sentence for murder if she did.[86]

All of these cases indicate that the emphasis in compulsory sterilisation or pseudo-voluntary sterilisation cases may be shifting from a scientific basis grounded on genetics to one grounded simply on social and economic considerations. Iowa's statute is indicative of

38 »   *Compulsory Sterilisation and Castration*

this trend, providing for sterilisation of any persons within the state who would procreate a child likely to '...become a social menace or (economic) ward of the state'.[87] The case of *In re Cavitt* might arguably be justified on economic grounds, by reducing the tax-supported roles in homes for the feeble-minded, but nonetheless preventing such persons, upon release, from procreating offspring likely to subsequently become welfare recipients.

It would seem that the statutory approach of Utah in this area, while highly paternalistic, is superior. Its recent statute provides for compulsory sterilisation of those 'likely' to be incapable of assuming parental responsibilities and only in such cases where the operation would also 'benefit' the subject.[88] At least this approach, though vague, looks to the individual concerned and his welfare, not just to the potential economic burden the state will be saved by sterilisation of the subject. The problem is : by whom and how will his 'benefit' be interpreted.

Legally speaking, this seems to be the unsettled position in which the decreasing practice of compulsory sterilisation finds itself in the United States today. The morality of this situation and the outlook for the future will be discussed after we have had a comparative look at the practice of compulsory sterilisation in other jurisdictions of the world.

The Comparative Position

BRITAIN. There is no modern statutory reference in Britain regarding sterilisation – compulsory or voluntary – or its more severe counterpart, castration.[89] The comprehensive Report of the Departmental Committee on Sterilisation is, however, well worth considering, though its recommendations have never been implemented by legislation.[90] The Committee concluded voluntary sterilisation should be permitted by legislative safeguards in medical cases where recognised opinion thought it would advantage defective couples by removing the fear of procreating more of their kind, where it would allow certain institutionalised patients to be released, where it would prevent such hereditary defects as blindness, deaf-mutism, haemophilia and brachydactyly, shown to be transmissable, and in other cases where family history gave reasonable ground for believing mental defects and disorders likely to be transmitted.[91]

The Committee felt compulsory sterilisation would be an unwarranted intrusion upon personal integrity in the existing state of genetic knowledge and that it would tend to associate mental institutions with compulsory sterilisation rather than with humanitarian treatment.[92]

Again, as recently as 1966, opinion in Britain has called for laws on the subject of voluntary sterilisation.[93]

The Brock Committee Report stressed the importance of clear procedural safeguards if any legislation, even that dealing only with voluntary sterilisation of those in state institutions, was to be enacted. It feared, and rightly so, the unreality or *de facto* involuntary nature of many 'consents' to sterilisation given in circumstances of confinement involving the mentally defective.[94] This is particularly so where reduction in detention period, parole or discharge is to be the result of submission to sterilisation.[95]

It has, in fact, been questioned whether in any circumstances an institutionalised patient or prisoner is really capable of giving free, uncoerced consent.[96] It would appear clear that such circumstances, at least when the patient or prisoner is mentally defective or disordered, give rise to the objectionable inference, in the words of Dr John Marshall, that

> 'one group of individuals is assuming the power to interfere with the bodily integrity of another group who are unable, by reason of their impaired facilities, to meet them on equal terms.'[97]

Glanville Williams has suggested a situation[98] – castration of a sexual psychopath who pleads for the measure to obtain relief from his uncontrollable abnormality – where he feels the voluntary nature of the procedure is clear.[99] In such circumstances, he is of the opinion that the English judges would not regard such a de-sexing operation as unlawful. He draws attention to the recent case of *Cowburn*[100] where the postulated circumstances did, in fact, exist. However, the Court of Criminal Appeal refused to give any assurance that such an operation would be lawful; Williams explains this result as forthcoming because the question was not properly in issue before the Court.[101]

Such a questionable use of voluntary castration is exactly what the West German Ministry of Justice is hoping to enact in a newly-proposed bill.[102] The proposed German bill is to change the present law of Germany as defined by a decision of the German federal court (penal branch) in 1963, in which the court decided that castration is only allowed if it is the *only* means to free a potential delinquent from phases of unconscious criminal conduct and the individual truly consents to the treatment.[103] The castration is to give convicted sex criminals an alternative to incarceration.

Despite Professor Williams' observations, as well as the hoped for effect of the draft German bill, it is contested whether truly voluntary consent can be given in such situations.[104]

DENMARK. Similarly, in Denmark provision is made for voluntary

40 » *Compulsory Sterilisation and Castration*

as well as compulsory castration of sexual offenders and psychotics, but again where release is at least in part dependent on submission to such an operation, its true consensual or voluntary character is missing.[105] Under such laws, Denmark castrated some 600 men between 1929 and 1956.[106] The compulsory castration provisions of the 1935 Danish Act have never been used.[107]

Even with the so-called voluntary castration of sexual offenders, less than ten cases occur annually at Herstedvester.[108] In early 1967 a bill was introduced into the Danish Parliament with the intent to 'amend' the current law relating to compulsory sterilisation and castration by abolishing certain instances of compulsory sterilisation.[109]

HOLLAND. There appears to be only one reported account in Dutch case law on compulsory sterilisation. The Rechtbank (court of first instance) at Roemond convicted a man with homosexual inclinations of a sexual crime (unspecified) and ordered him to submit to curative treatment for an indefinite period while retained in custody. The order, however, was made conditional on defendant's refusal to submit himself to castration. The court rejected the argument that such a serious intrusion into human life could only be warranted by express legislative authority, which did not in fact exist.[110] There was no appeal from the case.[111]

Learned comment[112] has strongly criticised the decision, indicating that express statutory authorisation would have been indispensable for such an order, the preparedness of the patient at the time of trial for castration (as opposed to at the time of operation) being irrelevant.

GERMANY. Germany had compulsory sterilisation laws during the Nazi period from 1933 until 1945, but these laws were abolished by the Allies in 1946.[113] It is interesting to note in this regard that the Nuremburg war trials condemned compulsory eugenic as well as punitive sterilisations carried out in Nazi Germany, but in many instances there was no true distinction in practice between the two.[114] As a result of the abolition of these laws and in the absence of new legislation, the general prohibitions of the criminal law against corporal bodily injury and destruction of one's ability to procreate would prohibit compulsory sterilisation in West Germany today.[115] There has been comment recently in Germany to the effect that even in those situations where sterilisation is allowed at present and is considered to be voluntary in nature, it is actually compulsory owing to subtle pressures or coercions applied or made manifest by family sentiment, mentality or age.[116]

FRANCE. Carbonnier,[117] discussing the French law of natural persons and the inviolability of their bodies, suggests that the state's interest may, in limited situations, warrant restriction of the exercise of individual free will over control of one's body. He mentions only the narrow examples of compulsory vaccination and arrest, giving no mention to sterilisation. Castration is made a felony by the French Penal Code.[118]

BELGIUM. Under the Belgian law there is authority for the viewpoint that sterilisation is only justified when it is performed for therapeutic purposes, 'pour liberer le patient d'une affection physique grave'.[119] It would appear, therefore, that no legal provision is made for compulsory sterilisation in either Belgium or France.

INDIA. In India, the exigencies for compulsory sterilisation are greater, because of the grinding poverty and a burgeoning population. The country's population now stands at about 500 million and is expected to treble in the next forty-six years (during which same period mainland China's population of 710 millions is expected 'only' to double).[120] India has considered compulsory sterilisation of couples with more than three children, but the prospect has now apparently been ruled out because it would violate the 'conscience clause' of the Indian Constitution which ensures religious freedom.[121] However, voluntary sterilisations are carried out on a wide scale on both males and females, with government incentives ranging from a few rupees to transistor radios.[122]

Again, under prevailing conditions of severe poverty and lack of education, do not such inducements make the voluntary characterisations at least questionable? In any event, the decade ending September 1965, saw more than one million Indian citizens sterilised, sixty-eight per cent of them male.[123] In May of 1965 alone, more than 57,000 Indians (eighty per cent males) submitted to sterilisation and government ambitions run to much higher figures.[124] Apart from private clinics, there are over 3,000 hospitals and institutions, and some 'mobile units' equipped for free voluntary sterilisations. By March 1967, at least 2·3 million such operations had been achieved.[125]

ITALY. In Catholic Italy the practice of sterilisation has been punishable as an offence under the Italian Criminal Code. However, in April of last year the Minister of Health recommended abrogation of the offence; it is not clear whether any positive legislative action has been taken on this proposal, but it would seem not.

SOUTH AFRICA. In South Africa there is no provision made for compulsory sterilisation.[126] Recently, a candidate for parliament advocated the compulsory castration of sexual offenders after their second conviction, but his proposal did not receive sympathetic or favourable press coverage and he was soundly defeated in his election bid partly because of it.[127]

42 »   *Compulsory Sterilisation and Castration*

There is, finally, no mention in the Quebec Civil Code of sterilisation and, perhaps indicative of the esteem in which the Louisiana Civil Code holds the subject, it is there discussed only in relation to the castration of bulls.

The Propriety and Morality of Compulsory Sterilisation

EUGENIC. Sir Francis Calton defined eugenics

> '...as the study of agencies under social control which impair or improve the racial qualities of future generations.'[128]

Assuming, for the moment, that man has the right to legislate for the improvement of his race or stock by the use of compulsory sterilisation, genetic science has 'advanced' to the stage today when it is no longer possible to determine those 'manifestly unfit'[129] to procreate because of the assurance they will transmit serious mental, physical or behavioural defect or abnormality. In the words of one physician,

> 'we have made just enough progress in the field of genetics to realise how little we do know and how vast is the uncharted area.'[130]

At the same time, it is probably true enough that

> 'controversial as may be the extent to which mental defectives and certain categories of psychotics contribute to the annual budget of crime, it is beyond doubt that their contribution and that of their offspring considerably exceed the average rate.'[131]

Dr Abraham Myerson, one of the leading authorities in the field, has stated that most so-called subjects for eugenic sterilisation belong rather to the unexplored areas of psychiatric understanding, not to such an 'incipient' science as genetics.[132]

Genetically, it has been learned that nearly all serious, common hereditary ills – for instance, feeble-mindedness, blindness, and the like – are carried by recessive as well as dominant genes, with the result that the person showing no sign of disease or defect may transmit it and he who himself is affected may produce normal offspring. The end result is, for example, that the majority of feeble-minded children are the project of normal, healthy parentage.[133]

Such facts have made it clear that compulsory sterilisation of all sufferers of mental defect or abnormality – regardless of its shown hereditary transmission more often than not – would have only a limited effect on the total incidence of inherited mental defects in the community.[134] Furthermore, estimates indicate that sterilisation of all institutionalised mental patients would only make it possible for the release of between three and five per cent,[135] while at the same time hindering the cause for voluntary institutionalisation by making such confinement at times synonymous with compulsory sterilisation.[136]

These considerations notwithstanding, it can still be argued that a 'slow rate of progress' is better than none when, for example, mental defectives or haemophiliacs are involved.[137] The issue in these types of cases becomes one of whether a desirable but 'slow rate' of progress in eliminating the incidence of these conditions justifies the personal invasion of bodily integrity that unquestionably is also involved.

One eugenic argument for compulsory sterilisation not affected by present lack of genetic understanding is that the feeble-minded are not capable of rearing healthy offspring endowed to them and that society and they themselves would benefit by preventing the bad effects of children being reared in such unhealthy or undesirable environments. Glanville Williams considers this argument alone strong enough to justify eugenic sterilisation, although only in cases which he considers to be voluntary.[138] Taking issue with Professor Williams, another author has cited authority for the proposition that the feeble-minded just as often make good parents as do 'normal' parents.[139] Williams does, however, recognise the *de facto* compulsory nature of sterilisation when offered the inmate as a condition of release, but nonetheless considers this choice between continued institutionalisation and freedom with loss of the right to procreate as the only realistic alternative available in these circumstances.[140]

Catholic dogma is in disagreement with this position. It considers confinement and supervision the less drastic and only moral way to deal with the problem of defectives, even if it is proposed that eugenic sterilisation should be carried out by the state.[141] The right to restrict personal freedom when necessary for protection of the individual concerned or of the state is acknowledged, but it is said not to include interference with the bodily integrity of the subject by mutilation of the physical, God-given ability to procreate.[142]

The Reverend Joseph Hassett, J.S., raises an interesting point in an article, saying that

> 'no person has the moral right to procreate unless he can assume his subsequent obligations with reasonable care.'[143]

Does this mean that a defective, copulating by little other than blind urge, is immoral if his undirected physical urges result in the procreation of offspring he cannot care for? Does the defective or mentally disordered have the necessary mental capacity to act immorally? Reverend Hassett uses the statement to support his view that the state may properly confine certain defectives, when it is necessary to protect them or society from harm.

44 »   *Compulsory Sterilisation and Castration*

Episcopalian Reverend Joseph Fletcher takes issue with the Catholic distinction between confinement and sterilisation, arguing that both, in fact, involve loss of the individual's right to procreate – the former, often, by less humane means. He states: [144]

'The argument that all people regardless of their stature as persons, have a natural-law right to their procreative faculties and that we may not rightfully take them away, is just as fully circumvented by segregation as by sterilisation....There is no difference between compulsory sterilisation and compulsory segregation. The latter quite effectively takes away sexual freedom and destroys procreation.'

That institutionalisation constitutes *de facto* sterilisation for most subjects is probably true. It is not, however, an irreversible situation, as is sterilisation in many instances. Nonetheless, there is something to be said in favour of Reverend Fletcher's viewpoint in that institutional confinement is a gross interference with mental and physical freedom and integrity, while in cases where sterilisation would warrant release only the latter invasion of physical integrity occurs, but only for the benefit of personal freedom from confinement.

The field of eugenics is severely limited by man's lack of genetic understanding, but progress appears to be going forward to a limited extent and some day a really effective correlation between heredity and genetic transmission as compared to behavioural and physiomental abnormalities may be possible. For example, one significant development has appeared in studies carried out by Dr Patricia Jacobs (1965) and Drs Price and Whatmore (1967) in Britain and by Dr Mary Telfer in America (1968), which attempts to relate male chromosomal abnormality (XXY or XYY) with a predisposition to criminal behaviour. These studies, thus far, 'appear to confirm British observations that gross chromosomal errors contribute, in small but consistent numbers, to the pool of antisocial, agressive males who are mentally ill and who become institutionalised for criminal behaviour'. They do not comment on the possibility of hereditary transmission of such chromosomal abnormalities.[145]

The most recent results of research [146] in this interesting area indicate a significant correlation between tallness and anti-social (delinquent, criminal or insane) behaviour and the XYY syndrome, reinforcing the hypothesis of a genetic-behavioural tie, the extra Y chromosome perhaps causing an abnormal accentuation of normal male characteristics of height and social aggressiveness. However, in a recent case where the defence raised the defendant's abnormal XYY chromosomal syndrome as grounds for finding him not mentally

responsible for the homicide at issue, the court held that there was no
clear link between the chromosomal anomaly involved and human
behaviour.[147] The defence in the *Tanner* case had sought to show that,
because the defendant had two Y (male) chromosomes instead of the
usual one, he had ungovernable passions and was therefore legally
insane at the time of the homicidal assault. The judge, while refusing
to 'open a Pandora's box' by allowing the defence based on the
chromosomal abnormality, nonetheless encouraged further research
in this area. It should be noted that during the *Tanner* trial specific
criticism of the above-mentioned Scottish studies on chromosomal
abnormalities and their relation to aggressive behaviour was voiced
by the prosecutor.

In the meantime, it would appear that society can well afford to
wait for a time before legislating against what may be its own potential. One has only to look at a previously proposed eugenic sterilisation statute in the United States to confirm that there is at least some
truth in this observation. The proposed law intended to cover the
following:

> '(1) Feeble-minded; (2) Insane (including the psychopathic); (3)
> Criminal (including the delinquent and wayward); (4) Epileptic;
> (5) Inebriate (including drug-habitués); (6) Diseased (including
> the tuberculous, the syphilitics, the leprous, and others with chro-
> nic, infectious and legally segregable diseases); (7) Blind (inclu-
> ding those with seriously impaired vision); (8) Deaf (including
> those with seriously impaired hearing); (9) Deformed (including
> the crippled); and (10) Dependent (including orphans, ne'er-do-
> wells, the homeless, tramps and paupers).'[148]

The compulsory sterilisation laws already in existence have been accused of this fault by some, being an example of law too quickly
adopting popularised scientific principles without adequate scrutiny
and reflection. The verdict on this accusation against compulsory
sterilisation for eugenic purposes is not yet in. World opinion is still
clearly divided. One of perhaps the best evaluations of the practice
has been succinctly stated by Professor Harry Kalven in the following terms:

> 'The case against sterilisation of the insane then is that there is no
> urgent social problem that will be solved by it, and at present the
> scientific basis for it is too much in controversy to warrant ack-
> nowledging even here so formidable a power in the state. This is
> not to say that some day the scientific predictions may not be so
> high as to outweigh the invasions of personal dignity involved. It
> is to say that they do not yet. We can afford to wait.'[149]

46 » *Compulsory Sterilisation and Castration*

PUNITIVE. Compulsory sterilisation and castration continue as punitive measures in some countries though clearly on a very limited or reduced basis.[150] In the United States, more recent statutes providing for compulsory sterilisation have been careful to avoid any reference to the criminality of the subject, due to the Supreme Court's decision in *Skinner* v. *Oklahoma, supra,* and because of increasing cognizance of the potential effect of constitutional guarantees – both state and federal – against cruel and unusual punishments.[151] As a result, when compulsion is used it is invariably for avowedly 'eugenic' purposes.[152]

Repeated sex offenders are those most commonly proposed as suitable subjects for compulsory sterilisation or castration, And, somewhat surprisingly, the practice has been supported as ethically sound when employed by society to restrain the convicted rapist from procreating.[153] Contrary to oft-stated opinion, neither sterilisation nor castration ensures that the rapist or sexual psychopath will no longer be motivated to commit further sexual offences. Either operation merely removes the sometimes complicating factor of resultant pregnancy in such instances by inducing sterility in the actor, no more. In any event, such operative procedures are attempted physical solutions to a problem basically mental and psychological. The cause of, and answer to, the sexual psychopath's abnormal urges lie in his cranium, not in his scrotum. Castration, like sterilisation, insures neither a reduction in libido nor in sexual act capability.[154] The only certainty of the operation is that its effects are 'very variable'.[155]

Conclusions

Compulsory sterilisation and castration will exist – blatantly and in their cloaked 'voluntary' forms – so long as any given society prefers the concomitant invasion of bodily integrity and dignity (at least when not undertaken freely) to the added social burden and responsibility of confinement and care of those thought to be 'unfit' to procreate. In man's present state of knowledge, it is submitted that such treatment of any individual is only medically and morally justified when carried out pursuant to his free, uncoerced request, once the full implications of the operation have been brought home to him or to those private persons closest to him and responsible for his welfare. As one eminent name in this field has concluded,

> 'There should be no castration; neither of sexual offenders, nor of other categories, neither on a compulsory nor even on a voluntary basis, unless on strictly medical grounds. Moreover, sterilisation should be on a voluntary basis only. It should have no penal character whatsoever; therefore, it should not be applied to law-

breakers as such and should, in particular, not be made a condition of their discharge from a penal institution, great as the temptation may sometimes be to do so.'[156]

In the final analysis, the question is one of the degree to which a particular society is willing to go in insuring and respecting the human dignity and bodily integrity of a certain, less fortunate minority within its midst. In a free society, the question of who is 'fit' to be a parent should not have to be asked. Emphasis should be placed on socialisation, treatment and supervision of individuals who are sexually, mentally or physically defective or disordered, rather than on sterilisation and castration, which make it possible to 'turn them out' into society again with minimum bother or compassion, on the reasoning that they then cannot reproduce their kind and that they have been rendered docile and 'harmless' thanks to the scalpel. As several British commentators have recently observed,

> 'The too ready use of castration could hinder the development of other methods, such as hormone treatment, psychotherapy or institutional regimes. In this country research, and not legislation, is needed....'[157]

There surely must come a point to which medical advances have perhaps already brought us, where society – represented by a legislative majority – no longer has the right to use its knowledge to manipulate and mutilate the bodies of those it feels somehow do not fit the desired social mould.

We know pitifully little about the Mendelian transmission of criminality, mental defectiveness and abnormality, and physical defectiveness. In such circumstances, who is to judge with any certainty those unfit to procreate? What are the criteria? Based on such an insecure foundation, can any compulsory sterilisation law insure against arbitrary and abusive interpretation and implementation at the hands of 'errant humanity?' This danger is too high a price to pay, for

> '...the time has come to question just how far we can safely go in the process of bending the nature of Man for the sake of social comfort and convenience. We need the natural product – warts and all.'[158]

Notes and References

1. The nature or quality of consent that is, or should be, necessary to constitute the operation as truly voluntary rather than involuntary in fact and practice is a difficult problem and will be discussed subsequently in this chapter.
2. See explanation of surgical sterilisation in chapter on Voluntary Sterilisation.
3. Fletcher, *Morals and Medicine*, pp. 143–4.
4. Ibid.
5. Supplement in Sir George Mackenzie, *Laws and Customs of Scotland in Matters Criminal* (1699) p. 16.
6. Fletcher, loc. cit.
7. Mackenzie, op. cit., p. 6 (supp.).
8. *Erskine's Institutes of the Law of Scotland*, Book IV, Title IV (1828) p. 1044 (par. 50).
9. Perkins, *Criminal Law*, p. 146, citing 1 Hawk. P.C. c. 44, §3 (6th ed., 1788). Note that under some American state statutes the penalty for mayhem by castration is death. Ga. Code Ann. c. 26–12 (1953).
10. Hume, *Commentaries* (1884) Vol. 1, p. 331.
11. Glaister, loc. cit.
12. Gordon, op. cit., pp. 774–5.

168 »   *Notes and References*

13. Bernard Häring, C.SS.R., *The Law of Christ*. Cork : The Mercier Press (1963) (translated by Edwin G. Kaiser, C.PP.S.) 510 (From the chapter 'Sins against love of neighbor', sub-chapter 'Cooperation in evil by judges and attorneys').
14. Fletcher, op. cit., pp. 169–71.
15. Ramsey, 'Freedom and responsibility in medical and sex ethics : a protestant view', 31 New York Univ. L.R. 1189, 1199 (1956).
16. Ibid., p. 1200.
17. Rackman, 'Morality in medico-legal problems : a Jewish view' 31 New York Univ. L.R. 1205, 1212 (1956).
18. See chapter on Voluntary Sterilisation.
19. Harry Kalven Jr., 'A special corner of civil liberties : a legal view', 31 New York Univ. L.R. 1223, 1232 (1956).
20. 'Whenever any person shall be adjudged guilty of carnal abuse of a female person under the age of ten years, the court may, in addition to such other punishment or confinement as may be imposed, direct an operation to be performed upon such person, for the prevention of procreation.'
    Cal. Penal Code § 2670 also allows sterilisation of recidivists convicted at least twice of rape, assault with intent to commit rape or seduction, or certain other crimes and who show while inmates that they are 'moral or sexual degenerate or pervert'.
21. Washington Rev. Code Ann. § 9.92.100 (1961).
22. Ferster 'Eliminating the unfit—is sterilization the answer?', 27 Ohio St. L.J. 591, 597 (1966).
23. Calif. Dept. of Men. Health Policy and Operations Manual, § 3520.2, 'Sterilisation will not be authorised in any case unless the patient consents thereto'.
24. Ferster, op. cit., p. 592.
25. Ibid., p. 593.
26. *Williams* v. *Smith*, 190 Ind. 526, 131 N.E. 2 (1921).
27. Williams, *The Sanctity of Life and the Criminal Law*, p. 84.
28. Ferster, op. cit., p. 632.
29. Ibid.
30. Ibid., p. 633.
31. The most recent case, *In re Cavitt*, 157 N.W.2d 171 (Neb., 1968), rehearing, 159 N.W.2d 566 (1968), is now pending in the U.S. Supreme Court on *certiorari*.
32. Quoted at note 39.
33. *Whitten* v. *State* 476 Atl 298, 302 (1872), in 15 Syra L.R. 741 (1964).
34. 15 Syra. L.R. 739 (1964).
35. *State* v. *Feilen* 70 Wash. 65, 126 Pac. 75 (1912), appears to be the only case before 1925 upholding a compulsory sterilisation law. Here it was applied to a man convicted of statutory rape and was held not to constitute cruel punishment.
36. As required by U.S. Constitution, Amendment xiv (and most state constitutions), which asserts that no state can deny a person of 'life, liberty, or property, without due process of law'. This guarantee is essentially one of procedural fairness in the administration and application of government authority.
37. Note : 'The cruel and unusual punishment clause and the substantive criminal law', 79 *Harvard L.R.* 635, 637 (1966).
38. *Mickle* v. *Henrichs*, 262 Fed. 687 (D. Nev. 1918).

Compulsory Sterilisation and Castration   « 169

39. The state constitutional provision being derived from U.S. Constitution Amend. VIII: 'Excessive bail shall not be required, nor excessive fines imposed, nor cruel *and* unusual punishment inflicted.'

40. *Mickle* v. *Henrichs, supra* at 690.

41. *Davis* v. *Berry* 216 Fed. 413 (S.D. Iowa 1914).

42. 15 Syra.L.R. 738, 752 (1964); O'Hara and Sanks, 'Eugenic sterilisation', 45 Geo.L.J. 20, 25 (1956). *In re Cavitt, supra.*

43. Perhaps the use of these terms here should be defined: 'eugenic' sterilisation meaning that performed to prevent the likelihood that some mental or physical defect, disorder or abnormality will be passed to future offspring by hereditary transmission or to prevent those already affected with such conditions from undertaking parenthood; 'punitive' sterilisation meaning that performed for penal reasons, whatever they may be, as for retribution or punishment, or revenge, or deterrence (another penal purpose – that of reformation or rehabilitation of the offender – would appear to be more eugenic than penal in nature, but these fine distinctions are beyond the scope of this study).

44. *Smith* v. *Command* (Mich.) 204 N.W. 140 (1925).

45. *Buck* v. *Bell* 274 U.S. 200, 47 S. Ct. 584 (1927).

46. 274 U.S. 200, at 207.

47. *In re Cavitt*, 183 Neb. 243. 159 N.W.2d 566 (1968) (cert. granted).

48. See 23 *Temple L.Q.* 306 (1950).

49. See annotation on 'Asexualization or sterilization of criminals or defectives' in 87 Albany L.R. 242.

50. *State* v. *Schaffer*, 126 Kan. 607, 270 Pac. 604 (1928).

51. *Davis* v. *Walton*, 74 Utah 80, 276 Pac. 921 (1929).

52. U.S. Constitution, Amend. XIV, no state can deny any person 'equal protection of the laws' (in their enactment, interpretation and enforcement).

53. *State* v. *Troutman*, 50 Idaho 763, 299 Pac, 668 (1931).

54. *Re Clayton,* 120 Neb. 680, 234 N.W. 630 (1931).

55. The same issue is now involved in *In re Cavitt, supra.*

56. *Brewer* v. *Valk*, 204 N.C. 186, 167 S.E. 638 (1933).

57. 1934 Cmd. 4485.

58. Ibid., p. 36.

59. Ibid., p. 37.

60. Abraham Myerson, 'Certain Medical and Legal Phases of Eugenic Sterilisation', 52 *Yale L.J.* 618, 628–31 (1943).

61. *Skinner* v. *Oklahoma* 316 U.S. 535, 62 S. Ct. 1110 (1942).

62. 316 U.S. 535, at 541.

63. 316 U.S. 535, at 546.

64. Birnbaum, 'Eugenic sterilisation: a discussion of certain legal, medical and moral aspects of present practices in our public mental institutions', 175 *J. A. med. Ass.* 951 (1961).

65. Quoted at note 39.

66. *In re Cavitt, supra* at 175.

67. *Re Clayton, supra* (Neb.); *State* v. *Troutman, supra* (id.), *In re Cavitt, supra* at 176.

68. Id. at 177.

69. Id. at 180.

70. 159 N.W.2d 566 (1968).

170 »   *Notes and References*

71. Compare *Mickle* v. *Henrichs, supra*, p. 6, with *State* v. *Feilen, supra*, note 35.

72. *Robinson* v. *California*, 370 U.S. 660 (1962); *Rudolf* v. *Alabama*, 375 U.S. 889 (1963), dissenting opinion of Justices Goldberg, Douglas and Brennan to grant review.

73. 79 Harvard L.R. 635, 637 (1966). In *Trop* v. *Dulles*, 356 U.S. 86 (1958), the USSC indicated that the 8th Amendment required all punishment to be 'within the limits of civilised standards', which the Court defined as those 'evolving standards of decency that mark the progress of a maturing society' (31 Albany L.R. 97, 101 (1967)). This definition of the 'cruel and unusual punishment' clause is broad enough to cover sterilisations, which, while perhaps cruel, because of their widespread practice could not be considered also as unusual within the literal meaning of the 8th Amendment.
     The state court in *Cannon* v. *State*, 196 A 2d 399 (Dela. 1963) refused to uphold a sentence imposing whipping, relying on the 'cruel and unusual punishment' clause, which it stated was to be construed by twentieth-century concepts of severity of punishment.

74. *In re Simpson*, 180 N.E. 2nd 206 (Ohio Probate Court 1962).

75. Ferster, op. cit., p. 607.

76. Note, 61 Michigan L.R. 1359 (1963); 15 Syracuse L.R. 738, 753 (1964).

77. Ferster, op. cit., p. 609.

78. *Andrada* v. *So. Pasadena Munic. Court*, 33 U.S. Law Week 327–8 (1965).

79. *Andrada*, 380 U.S. 953 (1965).

80. Ferster, op. cit., p. 610.

81. *People* v. *Tapia*, Record Case No. 73313, Santa Barbara Superior Court, 7 July 1965.

82. Probation Order, *People* v. *Tapia, supra*, 30 August 1965.

83. Ferster, loc. cit.

84. *In the Matter of Hernandez*, No. 76757 Santa Barbara Superior Court, 8 June 1966.

85. *Ferster*, ibid.; *The Times*, 9 June 1966, p. 10.

86. *N.Y. Times*, 2 June 1966, in Pilpel, 'Birth control and a new birth of freedom', 27 Ohio St. L.J. 679, 682 (1966).

87. Iowa Code Ann. § 145.7 (Amend. 1959), in 31 Albany L.R. 109 (1967). To same effect, Ore. Rev. Stat. § 436,050 (1965), similarly criticised in Pilpel, loc. cit.

88. Utah Code Ann. 64–10–1–64–10–14 (1953) (Amend. by L.1961, chap. 154, § 1), in Albany L.R. 97 (1967).

89. See the 'Introduction and Background' text at pp. 26–7.

90. 1934 Cmd. 4485.

91. Ibid., p. 30–41.

92. Ibid.

93. 'Report of the Council of the Royal College of Obstetricians and Gynaecologists', *Br. med. J.*, 850, 854 (1966).

94. 1934 Cmd. 4485, pp. 37–8. See also, Williams, *The Sanctity of Life and the Criminal Law*, pp. 108–9.

95. See note 78 and accompanying text (p. 37) as a recent example.

96. T. B. Smith, Address, loc. cit.

97. Marshall, op. cit., p. 73.

Compulsory Sterilisation and Castration « 171

98. (1962) Crim. L.R. 154.

99. But as to its effectiveness, see note 154.

100. *The Times*, 12 May 1959; *Lancet* 1090 (1959).

101. [1962] Crim. L.R. 154, 159. See comment on *Cowburn* in (1959) 27 Med.-Leg. J. 136.

102. Wassermann, 'Strafrechtliche Massnahmen zur Verhütung von Triebverbrechen', *Juristische Rundschau* 216–18 (1968).

103. B.G.H.St. 19, 201; Wasserman, *supra*; acknowledgement to Erich Schanze of Frankfurt, Edinburgh, and Harvard Universities for assistance in research and translation of the pertinent German authorities.

104. Gould, 'Castrating into conformity', *New Statesman*, 27 October 1967, 540.

105. Le Maire, 'Danish experiences regarding the castration of sexual offenders', (1956) 47 *J. Crim. Law* 294.

106. Ibid. 295.

107. McWhinnie, 'Denmark—new look at crime'. London : I.S.T.D. (1961) p. 6.

108. Ibid., p. 12.

109. *Berlingske Tidende*, 25 June 1967, p. 7.

110. Decision of 9 September 1947, N.J. 1948, 138.

111. Acknowledgement to Mr J.M.J.Chorus of Leiden and Edinburgh Universities.

112. See Vermeer, *Nederlands Juristenblad* (1948) p. 352.

113. Gesetz no. 11 Kontrollrat (30 January 1946). See comment, Schönke-Schröder, *Strafgesetzbuch Kommentar* (13th ed. 1967), especially § 226a, m.19.

114. See *U.S.* v. *Karl Brandt, et al.*, 1 and 2 Trials of War Criminals, discussed in Donnelly, Goldstein and Schwartz, *Criminal Law*, New York : Glencoe Press (1962) pp. 62 ff.

115. Strafgesetzbuch, §§ 224–5.

116. Wasserman, *supra*; Kohlhass, 'Nach wie vor Rechtsunsicherheit in der Fuge der Sterilisierung', *N.J.W.* 1169–71 (1968).

117. *Droit Civil*, vol. 1, title I (1957).

118. Art. 325.

119. Grosemans, 'Considérations juristiques et déontologiques sur les stérilisations opératoires sur l'homme', 41 *Revue de Droit Pénal* 875, 898 (1961).

120. *The Times*, 6 November 1967, p. 5.

121. *Irish Times*, 30 August, 1967, p. 5. Indian Const., Clause 25(1) : 'Subject to public order, morality and health and to other provisions of this part, all persons are equally entitled to freedom of conscience and the right freely to profess, practise and propagate religion.' Sources consulted by the writer indicate that no fundamental tenets of Hinduism would be contravened by the imposition of compulsory sterilisation in India.

122. Gould, loc. cit.; Blacker and Jackson, 'Voluntary sterilisation for family welfare', *Lancet* 973 (1966).

123. Blacker and Jackson, loc. cit.

124. Ibid.

125. 'The quiet revolution : family planning in India', Embassy of India (1967).

126. Acknowledgement to D. Carey Miller, B.A., LL.B., LL.M. of Natal.

172 » *Notes and References*

Neither Hahlo and Kahn (1960) nor Gardiner and Lansdown (1957) in their respective texts on the South African law discuss the question.

127. Ibid. There is South African authority to the effect that voluntary sterilisation is not illegal by any definite rule of Roman-Dutch law : Gordon, Turner and Price, *Medical Jurisprudence*, p. 68. As to creating grounds for marriage dissolution, see chapter 1.

128. 97 Albany L.R. (1967).

129. Chief Justice Holmes, in *Buck* v. *Bell*, 274, U.S. 200, at 207.

130. Phillips Froham, M.D., 'Vexing problems in forensic medicine : a physician's view', 31 N.Y. Univ. L.R. 1215, 1220 (1956).

131. Mannheim, *Criminal Justice and Social Reconstruction*. London : Kegan Paul, Trench Tribner & Co. (1946) p. 22.

132. Myerson, loc. cit.

133. Williams, *The Sanctity of Life and the Criminal Law*, p. 86 (indicating that some sources put this estimate as high as 89 per cent).

134. According to Carr-Saunders, a fairly substantial reduction in congenital mental deficiency could be expected 'in a century or so' through use of sterilisation. Professor J. B. S. Haldane has said that the sterilisation of all mental defectives could only cut down their general incidence by 10 per cent in the next generation and in some categories no noticeable effect could be expected before thirty or more generations. Mannheim, op. cit., p. 32.

135. St John-Stevas, op. cit., pp. 180–2.

136. 1934 Cmd. 4485. Not so under such acts as the Mental Health (Scotland) Act 1960.

137. Mannheim, loc. cit.

138. Williams, op. cit., pp. 86–9.

139. Bligh, 'Sterilisation and Mental Retardation', 51 *A.B.A.J.* 1059, 1062 (1965), citing Kanner, *Textbook of Feeble-mindedness* 5 (1949).

140. Williams, op. cit., pp. 88–9. The Brock Committee Report points up the need for such a choice in slightly different terms, by saying: '...no person unless conscience bids, ought to be forced to choose between the alternatives of complete abstinence from sexual activity or of risking bringing into the world children whose disabilities will make them a burden to themselves and society' (1934 Cmd. 4485, p. 40).

141. Marshall, op. cit., pp. 72–3; Joseph Hassett, S.J., 'Freedom and order before God : a Catholic view', 31 New York Univ. L.R. 1140, 1181–4 (1956).

142. Ibid.

143. Hassett, op. cit., p. 1183.

144. Fletcher, op. cit., p. 168.

145. See 159 *Science* 1249 (15 March 1968), *The Times*, 19 March 1968 and 24 March 1968, and Price and Whatmore, 'Behaviour disorders and pattern of crime amongst x y y males identified at a maximum security hospital' (Carstairs, Scotland, a paper, 1967).

146. Marinello, Berkson, Edwards and Bannerman, 'A Study of the x y y syndrome in tall men and juvenile delinquents', 208 *J. Am. med. Ass.* 321 (1969); a substantial bibliography is included.

147. *People* v. *Tanner* (Los Angeles Superior Court); *Los Angeles Times*, 7 March 1969, pp. 1, 29.

148. Ferster, op. cit., p. 618, quoted from Laughlin, *Eugenical Sterilisation in the United States*, 446–7 (1922).

149. Kalven, op. cit., pp. 1232–3.

150. McWhinnie, loc. cit.

151. See text at pp. 33–6.

152. Kalven, loc. cit.

153. Fletcher, op. cit., pp. 169–71.

154. William F. Ganong, M.D., *Medical Physiology*, Blackwell Scientific Publications, Oxford and Edinburgh (1967) pp. 190–1. See also Jamieson and Kay, *Surgical Physiology*, Edinburgh : E. and S. Livingstone (1965) p. 735, where the authors state that : 'Castration after puberty is followed by atrophy of the seminal vesicles and prostate, but not of the penis. The extragenital sex characteristics, having developed at normal puberty, do not regress. Sterility is invariable, but desire may persist. Impotence is therefore not invariable, but is common as a result of the psychological disturbance : it could probably be avoided in most cases by sympathetic discussion before operation.'

155. *Br. med. J.* 1, 897 (1955).

156. Mannheim, op. cit., p. 34.

157. (1959) 27 Med.-Leg. J. 136, 138–9.

158. Gould, loc. cit.

[8]

Medical Law Review, 7, Summer 1999, pp. 166–193

REGULATING THE REPRODUCTION BUSINESS?

MARGARET BRAZIER*

I. INTRODUCTION

The Human Fertilisation and Embryology Act 1990[1] sets out to regulate selected parts of reproductive medicine in the United Kingdom. The Act subjects fertility specialists to constraints on their practice and their research quite separate from, and over and above, those legal and ethical constraints generally applicable to all medical practitioners. The Act places limits on what patients seeking certain treatments for infertility may ask for and receive. It creates in the Human Fertilisation and Embryology Authority an apparently powerful regulatory body with powers to control the practice and development of embryology and certain fertility treatments. Reproductive medicine is singled out as special, as a part of medicine of such particular social concern and significance that the state should have a direct stake in its evolution. In singling out reproductive medicine for especial regulatory concern, the United Kingdom is not alone.

This paper seeks to explore some of the issues arising out of the way in which the United Kingdom has tackled developments in reproductive medicine. Some brief comparison with other European jurisdictions is attempted. The potential range of questions which could be addressed is almost endless. Having sketched in the background to the development of what I (somewhat frivolously) designate the 'reproduction business', the paper attempts to address the following questions. What are we regulating, and why? Why interfere with private choices? Is surrogacy special? Why the fuss about donor gametes? Who cares about embryos? What shall we do about cloning? Finally, I consider whether in the context of the reproductive technologies we are today regulating a profession or a business.

I shall seek to demonstrate that the British model of regulating fertility treatment and embryo research has undoubted strengths. It

---

* Professor of Law, University of Manchester. I gratefully acknowledge the stimulus and support of the Commission of the European Communities (DG XII) Biomedical and Health Research programme (BIOMED 2) (Contract No. BMH4–CT 96–1444). I thank all the participants in that programme for their insight and support and I am especially grateful to Sara Fovargue for her comments on an earlier draft of this paper.
[1] See generally, D. Morgan and R.G. Lee, *The Human Fertilisation and Embryology Act 1990* (Blackstone 1991).

ensures a degree of public accountability in the development and delivery both of new treatments and research procedures. It promotes high standards of medical practice and offers those lucky enough to benefit from the advances made in reproductive medicine assurances that their treatment is not likely to be marred by gross misadventure, delivered by maverick doctors, or rank 'amateurs'.[2] Because the British system is built on consensus, regulators, clinicians and scientists work well together. All those strengths benefit patients and promote British reproductive medicine as a success story. The price paid for consensus however is that all too often crucial issues of individual rights, the balance between individual rights and public policy, and issues of conflicting rights are skated over. There is little conceptual depth underpinning British law. The result is that again and again, as new medical developments emerge, we debate the same issues in different disguises. Professor Capron charges the US law in this field '. . . is characterised by incompleteness, contradictions and indefensible policies'.[3] British law too displays contradictions, no single, coherent, philosophy underpins the law's response to reproductive medicine. Yet a regulatory system is in place and perhaps suggests that pragmatism has its advantages?[4]

II. THE BACKGROUND

In July 1999, Louise Brown will celebrated her twenty-first birthday. The revolution in reproductive medicine heralded by her birth as the first child born as a result of *in vitro* fertilisation continues apace. That revolution has profoundly affected the way in which communities within the developed world perceive the age-old process of having children. What was until very recently seen as a couple's private business has become in many cases the business of the state. An area of medicine, treatment of infertility, which was not long ago a 'speciality' which offered little more than minor surgery, advice and tender loving care has grown into a multimillion pound international business. Nor is that business limited to its origins in treatment of infertility. Developments in embryo research and embryology offer radical treatment options for a host of diseases with therapeutic cloning on the horizon perhaps promising to cure diseases such as Parkinson's Disease and consign traditional transplant surgery to history.

Naturally lawyers and philosophers have not stood quietly to one

---

[2] It might be suggested that the 'licensing' of fertility specialists should be seen not as exceptional but as a model for all emerging specialties.

[3] A.M. Capron, 'Issues in US Law on Reproductive Medicine' (1999) SPTL Seminar, King's College, London.

[4] As predicted by *inter alia*, J. Montgomery, 'Rights, Restraints and Pragmatism' (1991) 54 M.L.R. 524; M.A. Jones, 'Human Embryos and the Ethics of Pragmatism' (1985)

1 D N 10

side and simply observed the transformation of reproductive choices from the private to the public arena and the growth of such a profitable new medical business. Reproductive medicine has brought rewards for them too. Committees exploring the legal, social and ethical implications of medical advances abound.[5] Legislation has proliferated across the developed world, and beyond.[6] Litigation has been lively; at least in common law jurisdictions.

For those not intimately involved, one of the delights of the burgeoning reproduction business is the glittering constellation of ethical and legal questions reproductive medicine poses for us. Some of those questions, endlessly debated, are deeply philosophical (and for some of us theological). What is the nature of human life itself? Does possessing human DNA have any moral significance? Others require us to reflect on just what intrinsic rights are involved in procreation. Few might dissent from a rhetorical assertion that men and women have a right to found a family. Begin to debate what that right entails and who enjoys it and dispute resurfaces. Yet other questions are, for the lawyers, delightfully technical as much as morally significant. Before 1979, paternity might on occasion be dubious, but even a rather dim child generally knew his mother.

Within these past two decades of the ascent of the reproduction business, one cry has often (though not universally) united the warring parties—'something must be done'. That 'something' has tended to be the introduction of some form of external regulation of the reproductive technologies. Across Europe, states have elected to implement very different patterns of regulation. Regulation differs both in its extent and in substance. Perhaps a minority of European countries have adopted a scheme attempting a reasonably comprehensive coverage of the reproductive technologies.[7] Others are more selective focusing on particular ethical and legal issues posed by those technologies.[8] For certain countries, the level of disagreement generated by advances in reproductive medicine has meant that, while several attempts have been made to introduce laws regulating the reproductive technologies, only minimal progress has been made in doing so.[9]

---

[5] In France the Braibant and Lenoir Commissions have both addressed the dilemmas of fertility treatments; see M. Latham, 'Regulating the New Reproductive Technologies: A Cross-Channel Comparison' (1998) 3 *Medical Law International* 89. For a European perspective, see J. Glover, *Fertility and the Family*, (the Glover Report on Reproductive Technologies to the European Commission), (Fourth Estate 1989). And see generally, C. MacKellar, (ed.), *Reproductive Medicine and Embryological Research: A European Handbook of Bioethical Legislation* (European Bioethical Research 1998).

[6] In particular, in Egypt and South Africa.

[7] For example, United Kingdom and Spain.

[8] For example, Germany.

[9] For example, Italy.

Whatever the nature or success of national attempts to regulate may be, that regulatory effort has focused almost exclusively on those reproductive technologies which involve either the creation of embryos *ex utero*, or the storage (and use) of donor gametes. Regulation of reproductive medicine remains partial and selective. Whole areas of fertility treatment are not subject to any special regulatory regime, nor are those medical technologies dedicated to the control of fertility. Legislative attention has confined itself to what are still (if somewhat erroneously) described as the *new* reproductive technologies.

The United Kingdom enjoyed perhaps a head start in both the inception of the reproductive business and its subsequent regulation. The Warnock Committee reported in 1984 proposing a comprehensive scheme of regulation for certain of the reproductive technologies.[10] That it took six years for their proposals to be implemented illustrates the difficulty in translating agreement that those technologies should be regulated in some form or other to consensus on what form that regulation should take. Not all Warnock's proposals were implemented in the 1990 Act. Notably their recommendations on surrogacy were only partially accepted by government and then hastily and ham-fistedly hurried through Parliament in the Surrogacy Arrangements Act 1985. Surrogacy in the event neither withered on the vine nor developed fruitfully.

III. WHAT ARE WE REGULATING, AND WHY?

The core of the Human Fertilisation and Embryology Act lies in sections 3 and 4 of the Act. Those sections essentially prohibit the creation of a human embryo outside the human body and the storage of gametes without a licence. Section 3 additionally imposes a series of restrictions on what may, even subject to a licence, be done with human embryos, including what was originally believed to be an absolute ban on human cloning. Subjecting embryo creation and gamete storage to a licensing system confers on the licensing authority (the Human Fertilisation and Embryology Authority—HFEA hereafter) control of a limited sector of reproductive medicine. Virtually all the other provisions of the 1990 Act, which flesh out the rules governing the licensing function of the HFEA, are limited in their impact to procedures involving licensed clinics engaged in either embryo creation or gamete storage.

It is important to recall that the 1990 Act permits three different kinds of licence, all licences to engage in otherwise prohibited activities,

---

[10] *Report of the Committee of Inquiry into Human Fertilisation and Embryology* (Cmnd. 9314 1984) (hereafter the *Warnock Report*).

(1) to provide treatment services, (2) to store embryos and gametes, and, (3) to carry out research on embryos. Once granted a licence, a licence holder must obey both the provisions made within the Act itself, directions of the HFEA and comply with the conditions of the licence.[11] So a *licensed* clinic approached by a single woman seeking donor insemination utilising stored donated gametes must ensure (*inter alia*) that consent to donation was given in the requisite form,[12] must assess whether that woman can adequately provide for the welfare of the child, and must consider the need of the child for a father.[13] A *licensed* clinic providing *in vitro* fertilisation must comply with HFEA guidance not to replace in the woman more than three embryos to minimise the risk of multiple pregnancy.[14] Both sets of constraints have (arguably) their justifications. Donors should give free informed consent. The welfare of future children is, many contend, a matter to be weighed in making reproductive choices. Multiple pregnancy endangers the health of both the pregnant woman and the foetuses she carries. The restrictions on what the licensed clinic may do prevents harms to others.

However, treatments available outside licensed clinics can result in more or less identical harms which escape the long arm of regulation by the HFEA. Artificial insemination using fresh sperm can be achieved on a do-it-yourself basis by couples, or offered with unlicensed medical assistance. The single woman desiring a child can select her own donor and no safeguards protect the future child or monitor the quality of the donor's consent. Moreover, using fresh sperm carries risk to the woman herself via transmission of HIV or some other sexually transmitted disease. In the United Kingdom, GIFT (gamete intra-fallopian transfer) can be provided without a licence albeit the risk of multiple pregnancy is slightly higher with GIFT than with IVF. Fertility drugs to induce supraovulation are accessible without even any requirement for prescription by a fertility specialist and misused such drugs carry the highest risk of multiple pregnancy. Fertility drugs resulted in the tragic conception and stillbirth of Mandy Allwood's octuplets.[15] Paradoxically it seems that procedures more likely to cause harm are beyond the reach of regulation. A select group of fertility treatments only are regulated. The composition of the regulated group is not dictated by the level of risk they pose to the woman being 'treated', the child or any donor.

---

[11] Note that a licensed clinic must comply with the provisions of the 1990 Act and the HFEA Code of Practice in relation to any treatments (including GIFT) provided within the clinic.

[12] Sched. 3, para. 5.

[13] Section 13(5).

[14] *HFEA Code of Practice*, 3rd edn, para. 7.9.

[15] S. Sheldon, 'Multiple Pregnancy and Re(pro)ductive Choice' (1997) 5 *Feminist Legal Studies* 95.

Moreover, fertility treatment itself forms but a small part of what we might style reproductive medicine. Mason's elegant work, *Medico-Legal Aspects of Reproduction and Parenthood*[16] runs to 398 pages. Yet just 100 pages address fertility treatments and embryo research. Of course, the law in the United Kingdom and elsewhere engages with his other concerns, such as contraception, sterilisation and protection of the foetus. But these areas of reproductive medicine are not subjected to regulation by any external public authority analogous to the HFEA. A novel development in contraception such as a contraceptive vaccine or long term implant may have serious social, ethical and medical implications. Consider the proposal by Dr John Guillebaud that, prior to puberty, girls at risk of teenage pregnancy should (with their parents' consent) have a contraceptive implant inserted to be removed only when they were sufficiently mature for motherhood.[17]

So what is the basis for the selection of certain treatments for regulation? The Warnock Report in recommending the creation of the HFEA puts the case thus:[18]

> The protection of the *public*, which we see as the primary objective of regulation, demands the existence of an authority *independent* of Government, health authorities, or *research* institutions. The authority should be specifically charged with responsibility to regulate and monitor practice in relation to those sensitive areas which raise fundamental ethical questions. We therefore recommend the establishment of a new statutory *licensing authority* to regulate *both research* and those infertility services which we have recommended should be subject to control (emphases added)

Elaborating their proposals for a licensing authority, the Warnock Committee stressed that the authority would have two functions, as an advisory body monitoring developments in fertility treatment and embryo research and as a licensing authority for clinics. In its latter, arguably central, function, in the context of fertility treatments, emphasis is placed on ensuring adequate standards of good practice, in relation (*inter alia*) to the qualifications of staff, the screening of gametes, the storage of gametes and embryos. Effectively the authority regulates 'health and safety' or, to use Warnock's words, ensures quality control. In relation to research licences, once again 'quality control' issues are addressed, but so is much more of the substance of

---

[16] J.K. Mason, *Medico-Legal Aspects of Reproduction and Parenthood*, 2nd edn (Ashgate 1998).

[17] 'Doctor calls for schoolgirl birth control implants', *The Times*, 3 February 1999.

[18] *Warnock Report*, para. 13.3.

what might be done with the embryos. It should be clear that the objectives of the research cannot be achieved without the use of human embryos, an indication should be given of the number of embryos to be used, and the researcher should have sought approval from an ethical body in his or her own institution.

Finally, in its key chapter putting the case for regulation, Warnock expressly proposes that the sale or purchase of human embryos be permitted only under licence and subject to conditions prescribed by the licensing authority. What can be gleaned from Warnock, and is it still of relevance today? Two features of their analysis of the case for regulation stand out, first, the pre-eminence given to concern for embryos, and second, the focus on regulating standards. Warnock speaks of the protection of the 'public', and of practice in sensitive areas raising 'fundamental ethical concerns'. The Report ranges over other concerns arising out of the reproductive technologies but again and again the status and consequent fate of the embryo takes centre stage. The creation and use of embryos is arguably what triggers concern. That concern is not so much about the consequences for the woman, whose body will receive such embryos, who with her partner may have fundamental interests at stake, but with society's engagement with the nature of humanity. GIFT (which does not involve the creation of embryos *ex utero*) slips out of sight.

I do not seek to argue that Warnock (or later the HFEA) were indifferent to a host of other questions and in particular the welfare of those receiving treatment. Indeed procedures such as donor insemination only come within the 1990 Act at all because of Warnock's recognition that unregulated practice could endanger patients. And 'quality control' is central to Warnock. What I suggest is this:

(1) Absent the development of procedures opening the door to research on, and manipulation of, embryos, Warnock would never have happened. Embryology, much more than reproductive issues, triggered *public* concern. That focus on embryos endured and largely dominated Parliamentary debate. Unregulated embryo research was simply not an option, paradoxically because Warnock and ultimately the majority in Parliament favoured permitting such research. Regulation was the price for ensuring the 'legitimacy' of such research.[19] Thus to ensure those opposed to embryo research could not undermine that 'legitimacy', any procedure which involved creating an embryo must fall within the jurisdiction of the 'legitimating' authority.

---

[19] As elegantly argued by the current Chairman of the HFEA; see R. Deech, 'Infertility and Ethics' (1997) 5 *Child and Family Law Quarterly* 337.

(2) Warnock deliberated at a very early stage of the 'reproduction revolution'. Neither the science, nor the infrastructure which now underpins the 'reproduction business' was well developed. Examples abounded of fairly crude, even disastrous, practices, for example, storing sperm in the same fridge as the clinic's daily milk supplies. Fears of something going disastrously wrong, two-headed babies and so on, still coloured debate. 'Quality control' was crucial. 'Safety first' has been described as continuing to be the watchword of the HFEA.[20] Consequently the Warnock 'scheme' concentrates on control of what happens in clinics. What happens beyond the clinics is outwith that remit, albeit concerns closely analogous to those raised by clinic-based practice may equally arise in other areas of reproductive medicine.

(3) Almost everything else within the British regulatory framework for embryo research and fertility treatment is consequential. That is not to say it is not important. The framework created for donor consent in relation to gametes is crucial and has provoked a host of legal problems. The provisions relating to payment for gametes,[21] the sections of the Act addressing children's rights of access to information about their genetic parents have profound significance.[22] Section 13(5) of the 1990 Act requiring that clinics consider the welfare of the child, including the child's need for a father, has provoked reams of commentary. All these matters have in practice much occupied the HFEA. Nonetheless because these are all issues not central to Warnock's call for regulation and because Warnock's focus was almost exclusively on *public* policy, with little attention to private rights, the wider implications of embracing such issues within the British regulatory framework were perhaps, with hindsight, insufficiently thought through in the lengthy process which resulted in the 1990 Act.[23]

(4) Albeit it was chaired by a most distinguished moral philosopher, the Warnock Report itself (particularly in comparison to its counterparts elsewhere in Europe) is more of an exercise in pragmatism than an exploration of the philosophy underpinning issues of reproductive choice. Compromise dominates the British regulatory system. Compromise has its benefits. The United Kingdom has had in place for nearly a decade now a regulatory system which ensures patients who receive fertility treatment can be assured of basic

---

[20] Deech, *op. cit.*

[21] Section 12(e).

[22] Subsections 30–2.

[23] Described in M. Brazier, *Medicine, Patients and the Law*, 2nd edn, (Penguin 1992) 259–63.

standards of practice. Charlatans who might use their own sperm to father hundreds of children are excluded from the system. Risks of malpractice are minimised. The United Kingdom has a system which ensures that as scientific developments generate new areas of concern such issues are publicly debated. The HFEA is often used as an 'Aunt Sally', pelted with metaphorical rotten tomatoes for its pronouncements. In its often underrated advisory function, the HFEA promotes a process of public consultation sometimes absent in other jurisdictions. The HFEA is sometimes attacked for its lack of philosophical direction. But was that ever its brief? Britain opted for a limited and pragmatic regulation of research and treatment focusing on ensuring public accountability on the part of both researchers and clinicians, facilitating medical and scientific progress and largely skating over fundamental questions of reproductive choice. Ruth Deech states the question as 'How was the humane treatment of infertile couples and the research appended to it, together with public fear and distrust to be managed?'[24] The answer which has emerged is that *managing* the fertility business and keeping public fears of scientific progress at bay has been the central concern of the HFEA.

IV. WHY INTERFERE WITH PRIVATE CHOICES?

Just one subsection of the 1990 Act directly addresses access to fertility treatment, section 13(5). In a regulatory framework largely focusing on 'quality control' and the need for public control of scientific development, section 13(5) stands out as something of an anomaly. Clinics are licensed, controlled and inspected to assure the public of the quality of the professionals. Section 13(5) addresses the quality of the patients. Up until 1990, clinics offering donor insemination were subject to no conditions as to whom they treated. A clinic's choice to treat (or not to treat) single women, lesbians, or couples where the husband was aged, was unrestricted. Section 13(5) *purports* to restrict access to fertility treatment to extend 'quality control' to users. Developments in reproductive medicine have expanded the scope of section 13(5). Once post menopausal women could be offered treatment, debate focused on should they be. Debate extended well beyond questions such as was treatment safe for the woman, were women fully informed of what the limited chances of success might be and what the additional risks their age entailed. Commentators ask whether any woman beyond the natural age of the menopause should be treated? What about the

---

[24] Deech, *op. cit.*

welfare of a child who in her teens might be cared for by (or caring for) a mother well over seventy?

A number of commentators would answer all the above questions succinctly—'nobody else's business'.[25] The law does not interfere with the reproductive choices of the naturally fertile. What justification is there for interference with the choices of the unfortunately infertile? The Warnock Report rather neatly evades the issue. A relatively mild preference is expressed for the raising of children in conventional two parent families but the Report concludes that the '. . . question of eligibility for treatment is a very difficult one'.[26] Their answer is to accept that doctors may on occasion decline to treat certain patients. Such patients must receive a full explanation of why they are refused treatment. Section 13(5) is not obviously, at least, a translation of Warnock's recognition of a wide margin of clinical discretion. It results from the translation of the process of legitimating fertility treatment to the Parliamentary arena. In the House of Lords a proposal which would have restricted all treatment to married couples was only narrowly defeated.

In the United Kingdom as elsewhere the debate on fertility treatment became in the legislature and in Parliament a debate on family structure, a weapon to attempt to defend conventional families. The justification for doing so was never articulated. It rarely rose or rises above 'two parents good—one parent bad', 'young(ish) mothers good—old mothers bad'. Nor in the United Kingdom is the debate brought to any definitive conclusion. The law requires clinics take into account the welfare of the child and the need of the child for a father. The HFEA in giving guidance to clinics on applying section 13(5) excludes no category of patient from treatment. The Code of Practice sets out what is in effect a wish list of considerations any prospective parent should take into account in seeking to ensure a child to be born enjoys 'a stable and supportive environment'.[27]

Section 13(5) has been described as 'so *imprecise* as to be either all-embracing or meaningless'.[28] The substance of HFEA guidance fleshing out the subsection can be similarly described. Clinics are directed what matters they should consider in making treatment decisions, but as long as the *process* demonstrates that these considerations are addressed,

---

[25] Notably John Harris, see *inter alia*, 'Rights and Reproductive Choice' in J.M. Harris and S. Holm (eds.), *The Future of Reproduction* (OUP 1998) 5–38; R. Bennett and J. Harris, 'Restoring Natural Function: Access to Infertility Treatment and Donated Gametes' (1999) 1 *Human Fertility* (forthcoming).

[26] *Warnock Report*, para. 2.11.

[27] At paras 3.12 to 3.32.

[28] Mason, *op. cit.* at 219.

decisions are left to the clinic's discretion. Giesen[29] has labelled British laws as representing a 'permissive solution' to the dilemmas promoted by reproductive medicine. Legislation permits virtually all principal forms of assisted conception. Only reproductive cloning even now looks·like remaining a totally prohibited area. More importantly the 1990 Act and the HFEA place no absolute restrictions on the kinds of people who may receive treatment. Yet 'permissive' is not how many British commentators regard the criteria governing access to treatment. Accounts abound of the difficulties confronted by groups such as lesbians obtaining licensed treatment. Women at the comparatively early age of 37 are refused treatment because they are 'too old'.[30] How can this apparent paradox be explained?

Two factors help to explain the divergence in judgments as to the 'permissive' nature of access in Britain. First, there is the very obvious point about the distinction between access to NHS treatment and access in the private sector. The very limited availability of NHS treatment forces NHS clinics to operate a rationing policy. Even were the criteria set out by the HFEA to assess whether potential parents can offer the child a stable environment to be treated as a parenting test, NHS clinics would still (at their present resource levels) have to discriminate even between couples scoring near to 100 per cent. NHS clinics opt to solve their resource problems both by including criteria additional to those set out by the HFEA in their assessment of potential parents, and by operating much more rigid exclusionary rules. So, for example, to be treated in the public sector, a couple may both have to be childless. Infertile couples will be rationed to one child only. Patients seeking NHS treatment may face rigid age limits and those who do so outside an established heterosexual relationship often do not fare well. Couples with existing children, women well past NHS age limits, and, in many cases, single women will nonetheless be likely to obtain treatment in the private sector. If one concedes British legislation *allows* 'permissive' access to treatment, the British Treasury restricts such access at public expense.

The discrepancy between ease of access to treatment in the public and the private sectors illustrate the second reason for dispute about 'permissive' legislation. The effect of the general and 'meaningless' admonitions of the 1990 Act and the HFEA's emphasis on the process of decision-making is that clinics enjoy an almost unlimited discretion whom to treat. Their licence will not be at risk unless they can be shown

---

[29] See 'Artificial Reproduction Revisited—Status Problems and the Welfare of the Child— A Comparative View' in C. Bridge (ed.), *Family Law Towards the Millennium* (Butterworths 1997) 235–63.

[30] R. v. *Sheffield Area Health Authority, ex parte Seale* (1994) 25 B.M.L.R. 1.

to have failed to address welfare issues at all. Even within the private sector there is evidence of significant variation in what kinds of patient will or will not be treated. There are (private) clinics who will not treat women over 50. Others will treat women up until 55 or 57. A number of clinics will not touch surrogacy. One or two quite actively promote full surrogacy arrangements, and will assist in partial surrogacy. In this private sector, whether you gain access to treatment very largely depends on *whom* you ask for treatment.

The immediate response to evidence of such variations in access to treatment might be that in creating a fertility lottery British law is weak and inequitable. Comparison with other European jurisdictions promotes reflection. A number of European states have by contrast set out in legislation and in consequent regulatory guidance clear and rigid rules on who may benefit from fertility treatments. They have opted for what Giesen styles a 'prohibitive' solution. Only heterosexual couples may receive treatment. The woman must be of normal childbearing age. Posthumous insemination is unlawful. In France, treatment is available only within a *projet parental*. Nowhere in France could a post-menopausal woman or a lesbian couple lawfully be treated. France at first sight then appears distinctly 'anti-permissive'. Yet in France, unlike in the United Kingdom, couples who fall within the category of patients lawfully entitled to be treated *will* gain access to treatment regardless of their finances. Fertility treatment is publicly funded. Patients denied NHS treatment in the United Kingdom would, as Latham has noted, be better off in 'illiberal' France.[31]

Inequity in access between the public and private sectors in Britain will only disappear by an act of political will. Either, as the government recently promised, greater resources must be committed to fertility treatment within the NHS, or fertility treatment should cease to be publicly funded at all. Neither rational solution is likely to be implemented. Both are politically too risky. Given a continuing state of affairs where fertility treatment is patchily available and partly rationed by postcode, honesty is required. Clinics choosing between patients who meet the basic criteria set out by the HFEA should not be subject to a 'welfare-plus' assessment. Rationing should be overt and not dressed up as a judgment on parenting skills.

Much more fundamental to the question of how effectively British law meets the challenges of the reproductive technologies is the issue of whether the wide discretion entrusted to health professionals in policing access is satisfactory. Professional discretion is attacked from two fronts. 'Liberals' argue that the notion of evaluating parenting ability,

---

[31] M. Latham, 'Regulating the New Reproductive Technologies: A Cross Channel Comparison' (1998) 3 *Medical Law International* 89–177.

the very concern with the welfare of the child, invades areas of private choice and family life. 'Conservatives' maintain that in certain quarters the law is flouted. Assessment of the welfare of the child is a farce. Yet what is the alternative? Equal access to treatment across the spectrum of fertility clinics can only be achieved in two ways. (1) Any discretion to refuse to treat a patient, save on clinical grounds, is withdrawn. If it is technically possible to attempt egg donation and IVF with a single female patient of 61, it must be tried, whatever the qualms of the clinicians. Clinicians become mere technicians.[32] (2) The United Kingdom follows the example of France and Germany and centrally determines what groups of patients may and may not be treated.[33] The HFEA, if you like, answers its own questions. Rather than clinics simply being adjured to bear in mind a couple's (person's) health and age, the HFEA declares that, as in general someone of 65 might find coping with a lively teenager problematic, *no* woman over say 48 should be treated. Imagine the outcry. What about the woman of 50, whose partner is only 35, we would hear. How can you generalise about the effect of ageing?

The central role granted to professionals in British law relating to reproductive medicine is one of its key features. The law grants to doctors powers to make social judgments with the inevitable result that the substance of any 'right' of access to regulated fertility treatments is determined by clinics, by doctors, generally working with ethics committees. The disadvantages of such a system are patent. A group of professionals who gain their position as licence-holders predominantly as a consequence of their scientific and clinical expertise are granted a quite different function. Patients denied treatment will have a sense of grievance and injustice. Yet the system is not without some merits? It allows access decisions to reflect individual circumstances. It avoids arbitrary classifications of 'good' and 'bad' parents. It allows society of the hook from addressing in this context the debate on family structure. All the difficult questions that as a community we have problems in answering are delegated to the professionals. Given the responsibility the law entrusts to them, it is often somewhat unfair to turn round and criticise them however they elect to exercise that responsibility. British law in many respects expressly *professionalises* the day to day control of regulated fertility services. Having done so the law cannot blame all the consequences of professionalisation on the professionals.

---

[32] For an analysis arguing professionals must be recognised as independent moral agents see M. Brazier, *Liberty, Responsibility, Maternity* (1999) *Current Legal Problems* (forthcoming).

[33] For a survey of UK clinics' practice and a cogent proposal for a uniform code of practice, see D. Savas and S. Treece, 'Fertility Clincs: One Code of Practice' (1998) 3 *Medical Law International* 243.

V. IS SURROGACY SPECIAL?

One highly controversial infertility service currently escapes in Britain both most of the regulatory reach of the HFEA, and the professionalisation which so characterises other services. Surrogacy, British style, evolved haphazardly. Perhaps of all the various infertility 'treatments', surrogacy has attracted the greatest critical attention despite the paradox that surrogacy need not involve, in any real sense, treatment. National legal responses to surrogacy have also differed markedly. Many European states have opted for overtly 'prohibitive' solutions. Germany *simply* bans surrogacy, be the arrangement altruistic or commercial. France, Denmark and the Netherlands criminalise any payment for surrogacy services whether made to the surrogate or any third party. Yet, as I understand it, in parts of the USA, surrogacy flourishes as a lawful business.[34] But for good or bad, legislators and judges perceive surrogacy as both special and especially problematic.

'Prohibiting' surrogacy was an option rejected in the United Kingdom by Warnock largely because of that committee's belief no child should be born affected by a 'taint of criminality'.[35] Nonetheless, the majority in Warnock hoped that surrogacy would go away. They sought to achieve this end by proposing that it should become a criminal offence for any third party to assist in a surrogacy arrangement, whether for payment or otherwise. The majority expressly rejected professionalisation of surrogacy. Suggestions put to them that a limited non-profit making surrogacy service should be licensed met with the response that '. . . the existence of such a service would in itself encourage the growth of surrogacy'.

A minority dissent took a rather different view. They doubted that surrogacy would simply disappear and feared the development of risky do-it-yourself arrangements. The minority endorsed regulated surrogacy. The licensing authority responsible for other fertility services should have powers to license surrogacy agencies. Access to a surrogacy agency, and thus surrogacy services, would be exclusively by referral from a gynaecologist.

Had the minority proposals been accepted, surrogacy services too would have been thoroughly professionalised. In the event the Surrogacy Arrangements Act 1985 partially implemented the majority view prohibiting any third party from assisting in the making of a surrogacy arrangement on a *commercial* basis. Altruistic surrogacy, if surrogacy

---

[34] With the consequences graphically described by Alex Capron, *op. cit.*

[35] The debate on surrogacy within the Warnock Committee and thereafter is described in the *Review for Health Ministers of Current Arrangements for Payments and Regulation*, (Cm. 4068)(1998) (hereafter *Surrogacy Review*).

was supposed to be at all, was to be the order of the day in Britain. No criminal penalties attached to couples who paid the surrogate herself (or *vice versa*) but both applications for adoption and for parental orders under section 30 of the 1990 Act prescribed that no more than reasonable expenses should be paid to the surrogate. Surrogacy contracts were made expressly unenforceable.

Surrogacy did not wither on the vine. At least two non-profit making groups, COTS and SPC, established themselves as 'agencies' who introduced surrogates and couples, and advised and assisted with surrogacy arrangements. A number of infertility clinics actively started to engage themselves in helping to establish surrogate pregnancies. Reported payments to surrogates reached, in some instances, levels of £10K to £15K. Despite some favourable media attention, a number of high profile cases emerged where surrogacy had gone disastrously wrong. In July 1997, the British government decided to institute a review of certain aspects of the law pertaining to surrogacy.[36] Essentially, government concern focused on whether some additional degree of regulation of surrogacy was desirable and whether payments to surrogate mothers should be allowed. In this section of the paper, I address primarily the regulation question.

Surrogacy's current freedom from much of the regulatory regime controlling other infertility services has for many of those personally involved in surrogacy arrangements perceived advantages. Where a couple seek a full surrogacy arrangement and must thus resort to IVF in a licensed clinic, they are subject to analogous conditions of assessment designed to address the welfare of the child as any other client of a licensed clinic. Where partial surrogacy suffices, insemination of the surrogate by the male partner can be and, is usually, achieved without medical supervision or assistance. In either case, the nature and progress of the surrogacy arrangement itself is entirely in the hands of the parties themselves with support from a surrogacy agency if desired. Those who truly endorse a *genuinely permissive* approach to infertility treatment might applaud a state of affairs that leaves access to surrogacy so very much in the realm of private choice.

Yet surrogacy involves a multiplicity of risks, risks acknowledged by all those involved in surrogacy. They are well-rehearsed.[37] The surrogate is asked to accept the physical risks and discomfort of pregnancy and childbirth and the unpredictable risks to her psychological well-being if she goes ahead and surrenders the child as agreed. Should the

---

[36] *Ibid.*

[37] See *Surrogacy Review*, Ch. 4. For a critical but at least partially sympathetic analysis of surrogacy see J.K. Mason and A. McCall Smith, *Law and Medical Ethics*, (5th edn.), (Butterworths 1999) 78–88.

arrangement fail, the child's infancy may be clouded by bitter dispute about its future, and the hopes of the couple are devastated. How children as they grow up will respond to knowledge of their origins remains unknown. Surrogacy takes families and society into uncharted waters. Moreover, *three* particular factors about British surrogacy exacerbate concern. (1) Evidence about comparative levels of income and education suggest a significant disparity of bargaining power between surrogate and couple. Most British surrogates are young women living on low incomes or state benefits, with few qualifications and supporting children on their own. (2) The overwhelming incidence of partial surrogacy established via self-insemination occasions danger both of physical risk to the surrogate from disease and emotional risks in that the very ease of the process may preclude time for reflection. (3) In navigating the uncharted waters of surrogacy the principal sources of advice, the voluntary surrogacy agencies, are essentially amateur operations.[38]

I plead guilty to hyperbole, but the current state of the law on surrogacy suggests a scenario in which the most dangerous infertility 'activity' is the least regulated. It is as though the government decided to regulate and license most watersports, including swimming, water aerobics, and springboard diving, yet omitted to regulate high diving.

In evidence submitted to the Surrogacy Review, nearly all respondents favoured some sort of additional regulation.[39] To ensure surrogacy fits neatly into the British regulatory pattern, professionalisation along the lines of the minority proposal in Warnock might appear to be the obvious answer? Before examining why professionalisation (or at least medicalisation) was rejected in the context of surrogacy, a little more needs to be said about why professionalisation failed to take control of surrogacy in 1990. In 1984, when Warnock reported, the medical profession expressed profound opposition to surrogacy arguing that professional involvement in surrogacy was unethical. Prompted originally by the BMA,[40] the profession has undergone a sea-change in attitude. Professional involvement in surrogacy where surrogacy offers the only realistic prospect of overcoming a couple's inability to have a child is now endorsed by the majority of the profession. Certain clinics now regard repeated failed cycles of IVF, particularly in an older woman, as a sufficient indication to suggest resort to surrogacy. Both full and partial surrogacy are available under medical supervision.

---

[38] See *Surrogacy Review*, paras 3.29 to 3.36.
[39] *Surrogacy Review*, Annexes E1 and E2.
[40] *Changing Conceptions of Motherhood: The Practice of Surrogacy in Britain*, (BMA) (1996).

What of course private sector clinics cannot do is involve themselves directly in recruitment of a surrogate.

So why not medicalise surrogacy? The jurisdiction of the HFEA could be extended to license clinics (and associated agencies) to provide comprehensive surrogacy services. The British Fertility Society argued that regulation should make it '... necessary for all surrogacy arrangements, IVF and natural, to go through a proper process of medical assessment counselling and review by an Ethics Committee'.[41] Professionals would ensure physical and psychological risks were addressed. Access to surrogacy would be put on just the same basis as access to IVF and gamete donation, entrusted to the doctors, under guidance from the HFEA, albeit at yet greater cost than other treatments. The British Fertility Society additionally recommended that surrogates should be paid for their service. They echoed a view put strongly by many respondents to the Review. If doctors, nurses and counsellors involved in IVF are paid for their services why should the surrogate not be paid for her reproductive labour?

Those groups currently involved in assisting in surrogacy arrangements also sought regulation, preferably a system which permitted *them* to be licensed and adequately funded. COTS argued eloquently that surrogates should be paid, but also that surrogacy contracts should be enforceable.[42] COTS's case highlights why surrogacy is special and would be difficult to fit neatly into the current framework of professionalisation. COTS advocates a novel variant of professionalisation, the recognition of surrogacy itself as an occupation (if not a profession). Surrogates should be regarded as service providers entitled to the same benefits as other fertility specialists (monetary reward) and subject to the same limitations, external regulation of how they do their 'job' and a contractual obligation to do what they agreed to do.

Thus two variants of professionalisation arrive on the agenda. We could develop and regulate *medical* surrogacy services, or, endorse and regulate *professional* surrogacy. The first option was rejected by the Review team because most of the aspects of surrogacy which make it 'special', which raise social and ethical questions absent in relation to other fertility services, are not *medical* questions. The professional expertise required to advise and assist those contemplating surrogacy is not a clinical expertise. Surrogacy is more closely analogous to adoption than IVF in its problematic areas. Moreover, given surrogacy services within the NHS are limited to one or two rare instances, clinics acting as, or in concert with, agencies would have profound difficulty in acting impartially between couple and surrogate. The couple would be

---

[41] *Surrogacy Review*, para. 6.10.
[42] *Ibid.*, para. 3.34.

their clients and inevitably their prime concern. The second 'solution', *professional surrogacy*, radically challenges both our perceptions of fertility services as an essentially clinical and scientific endeavour, and, society's understanding of motherhood.

To endorse the latter solution, to create in effect a regulated market in motherhood, would take Britain in a markedly different direction from its European partners and well down the road to express recognition of a reproduction business. That road will be further explored in the final section of this paper. The proposals made to the government in the Surrogacy Review Report seek to develop *special* solutions for the *special* problems of surrogacy. Regulation should be implemented by requiring all agencies involved in assisting in surrogacy to be registered with the Department of Health and subject to a Code of Practice. That Code, binding on agencies, would also operate as an advisory document for all surrogacy arrangements, a manual of good practice. Given that the Review also rejects overt payment for a surrogate's services, the number of surrogacy arrangements would be unlikely to grow. Were the Review's proposals to be accepted, a policy of 'containment' might best describe the legal response to surrogacy.

VI. WHY THE FUSS ABOUT DONOR GAMETES?

At least in the context of surrogacy, the potential harms to the surrogate (and indeed to commissioning couples)[43] may be universally recognised, albeit disagreement surfaces about how far the minimisation of such harm is anybody's business but theirs. The various fusses about the use of donor gametes in the nine years since the passing of the 1990 Act may be harder to understand. Warnock's concerns with 'quality control' have largely been met. Protection of the interests of the gamete recipient and her child are adequately addressed. Concerns about long term risks of freezing gametes, especially eggs, problems with poor success rates in unfreezing eggs remain.[44] However, clinicians, scientists and regulators have an adequate framework in which to address problems. Any weakness in this system can not be charged against British laws.

A sharp focus of legal and social concern has in practice turned to questions of control of genetic heritage. How absolute, how rigorously enforced, should an individual's command of his or her genes be? What rights have children to their heritage? When interests in genetic heritage

---

[43] See E. Blyth, '"Not a Primrose Path": Commissioning Parents' Experience of Surrogacy Arrangements in Britain?', (1995) 13 *Journal of Reproductive and Infant Psychology* 185.

[44] See R. Winston, *The IVF Revolution* (Vermilion 1999) 126–7.

conflict with an individual or couple's immediate interest in overcoming infertility, which set of interests takes precedence?

Informed and free consent on the part of gamete donors appears both fundamental and unexceptional, albeit in the Warnock Report itself there is much greater emphasis on the quality of consent of the couple receiving treatment, in particular the person who will ultimately parent a child to whom he or she is not genetically related. Schedule 3 of the 1990 Act nonetheless establishes detailed rules for 'effective consent' to gamete donation. Schedule 3 demands that all donors are offered relevant counselling, provided with all relevant information, and that consent be 'given in writing'! English law imposes no legislative rule requiring that I consent in writing to surgical removal of all my reproductive organs. Yet I must consent in writing to the less invasive procedure of egg retrieval if those eggs are destined for another recipient. Is Schedule 3 be designed to protect my sovereignty over my genetic heritage?

Genetic heritage was at the heart of the Diane Blood controversy. I deal only with this one aspect of the Blood affair. Diane Blood and her husband Stephen had hoped to start a family. Tragically Stephen Blood contracted meningitis and lapsed into a coma. Doctors complied with his wife's request to take sperm from her husband as he lay dying. His sperm was stored at a licensed clinic. The HFEA ruled that treating Mrs Blood with her husband's sperm was unlawful. He had not given an 'effective consent', a consent in writing to storage and use of his sperm. Challenging the Authority's decision by way of an application for judicial review, Mrs Blood argued (*inter alia*) that her husband had expressed to her his wish that, should he die before their planned family arrived, if it was possible, sperm should be taken from him so she could bear their child posthumously. Both the trial judge and the Court of Appeal ruled that treatment in the United Kingdom prohibited use of gametes without the written consent of the donor. The Court of Appeal, of course, did find in Mrs Blood's favour on the issue of whether European Union law should have been considered by the HFEA in their original decision to refuse to allow the stored sperm to be exported so that Mrs Blood could be treated outside the United Kingdom.[45] She was ultimately successfully treated in Belgium and a son born to her late last year. However, the appeal court categorised the taking of the sperm as unlawful, an assault on Mr Blood, and made it clear domestic law

---

[45] *R. v. H.F.E.A. ex parte Diane Blood* [1997] 2 All E.R. 687 (C.A.); discussed elegantly in D. Morgan and R.G. Lee, 'In the Name of the Father? *Ex parte Blood*: Dealing with Novelty and Anomaly' (1997) 60 M.L.R. 840. For a critical analysis of European Community law see T. Hervey, 'Buy Baby: The European Union and Regulation of Human Reproduction' (1998) 18 O.J.L.S. 207–33.

remained unchanged and that the Blood case was a 'one-off' which should never recur.

The principle of sovereignty over genetic heritage remains inviolate then. The donor's interests in his gene pool trump the interests of the infertile individual? Such a position has been challenged as lacking in logic and consistency. Nature affords men no analogous control of their genes? Women have been known to deceive, seduce, entice reluctant partners into parting with their genes. If the principle is sound, should it prevail in private as well as public reproductive activity? In the USA a man is seeking to assert his right to control his genes by suing his former lover for stealing his sperm.[46] That sovereignty over genes however can never truly be absolute is illustrated if we consider our prospective grandchildren. My daughter currently possesses 50 per cent of my gene pool. My interest in my genetic heritage dictates that *I* should have a say in how those genes of mine are utilised by her. Should I seek a declaration that her choice of my grandchildren's father should be subject to my consent?

Diane Blood's battle to have her deceased husband's child provoked a storm of protest. Her plight attracted public sympathy. Calls were made to amend the 1990 Act to allow clinicians discretion to waive the requirements to written consent in deserving cases.[47] The government asked Professor Sheila McLean to review the law relating to removal and use of donor gametes.[48] She recommended retention of the rules arguing that the special status of gametes demanded a high standard of proof of the donor's intent. Control of genetic material was not to be surrendered lightly.

In conceptualising Schedule 3 of the 1990 Act as protecting genetic heritage, do I read too much into the Act? I suspect I may, because elsewhere in the Act the interests of infertile individuals tend to gain priority over competing claims. Consider other provisions of the Act protecting the anonymity of donors and the recent debacle over continued payments of donors. Genetic heritage is not the sole domain of progenitors. *My* interest may be in the future of my genes. My descendants' interests are in the history of *their* genes. An understanding of who they are involves an understanding of who I am. British legislation currently allows access only to non-identifying genetic information. Were I to have acted as an egg donor, my genetic daughter could at 18 apply to the HFEA, discover whether a proposed fiancé might be related

---

[46] 'Seminal case of ownership to go before US judges', *Guardian*, 24 November 1998.

[47] See M. Brazier, 'Hard Cases Make Bad Law?' (1997) 23 *J. Med. Ethics* 341.

[48] *Review of the Common Law Provisions Relating to the Removal of Gametes and the Consent Provisions at the Human Fertilisation and Embryology Act* (Department of Health 1998).

to her and receive such other information as the Authority is by regulations required to give. But if my hypothetical daughter already exists, those regulations cannot include information as to my identity. Access to identifying information can be introduced only from a time when all gamete donors are informed that their anonymity will no longer be protected. Rightly or wrongly it is feared that granting children access to their genetic identity will reduce the supply of donor gametes.

In relation to buying gametes, the HFEA Consultation Paper on payment for gametes, expressed a principled stand against payments yet for the time being payments are to continue. In issuing directions allowing payments to continue, the HFEA reiterated their support for a 'culture of altruism'. They justified continuation of payment because of fears that removing payment 'would seriously jeopardise the supply of sperm donors'.[49]

Mrs Blood would no doubt characterise the British laws on donated gametes as 'prohibitive', contrary to the interests of those seeking treatment. She was unlucky. The framework for supply of donor gametes in British law is deceptive. It appears to centre on protecting the interests of donors. In reality its purposes are often to facilitate the supply of gametes. Donors are 'protected' to encourage donation. They are granted continuing control of their gametes to reassure future donors. Their interest in anonymity is prioritised over their offspring's interest in their genetic heritage to forward the interests of those who seek to benefit from fertility service, and are dependent on an adequate supply of donor gametes.

VII. WHO CARES ABOUT EMBRYOS?

So far this paper has concentrated on fertility services, putting embryo research to one side. Yet I initially asserted that controlling the use of *in vitro* embryos was the engine which drove the Warnock proposals which in turn resulted in the 1990 Act. Warnock was very bothered about embryos. Who cares any more? Embryo research has flourished in the United Kingdom. Within Europe, Britain again stands out as 'permissive' in its regulatory approach to experimentation on embryos. Many of our partners in the European Union either prohibit research outright, as does Germany, or hedge research around within often contradictory restrictions on what kind of research are permitted.[50] In addition to a range of prohibitive controls on research, many European

---

[49] *Directions Given Under the Human Fertilisation and Embryology Act* (Ref. D.1998/1) 7 December 1998.

[50] See M. Latham, 'The French Parliamentary Guidelines of May 1997: Clarification or Fudge' (1998) 3 *Medical Law International* 235.

countries impose other legal constraints on the creation, use and transfer of embryos, notably prohibiting embryo use for commercial or industrial purposes. Trade in embryos is banned.

British legislation permits research under licence from the HFEA for five specific ends.[51] The HFEA may license research to promote advances in infertility treatment, to increase knowledge about the causes of congenital disease, to increase knowledge about the causes of miscarriages, to develop contraceptive treatments, and to develop methods for detecting genetic or chromosomal abnormalities. Additional purposes for which embryo research may be licensed may be specified in secondary legislation. The HFEA (in consultation with the Human Genetics Advisory Commission) recently proposed that two such new purposes should be specified in regulations, developing methods of therapy for mitochondrial diseases and developing methods of therapy for diseased or damaged tissues or organs (i.e. therapeutic cloning).[52]

Embryo use in Britain is certainly controlled, yet the purposes for which human embryos may be used are widely drawn, and the boundaries are set to expand further. No restrictions are placed on the creation of embryos expressly for research purposes. Hundreds of thousands of embryos have in the United Kingdom been the subjects of inevitably destructive research. Are embryos in reality now treated any differently from laboratory artefacts, and treated with caution only because of their tendency to generate moral panic?

Such conceptual basis as there is to British law's approach to embryo status is equivocal. The Warnock Committee declared that 'the embryo of the human species ought to have a special status'.[53] Similarly, in the USA the Ethics Advisory Board adjured that human embryos were entitled to 'profound respect'. Mason robustly dismisses both statements as a nonsense. Embryos are either young humans with rights and interests common to their species or no more in truth than laboratory artefacts.[54] If the latter, protecting or respecting a laboratory artefact would seem indeed a nonsense. Controlling research becomes important not because of any moral claim on behalf of the embryo but solely because of the potential consequences to society of where that research may lead.

Embryo equals artefact is a proposition which is anathema to those (including myself) who opposed allowing experimentation on embryos

---

[51] Sched. 2, para. 3(2).
[52] *Cloning Issues in Reproduction, Science and Medicine,* HGAC and HFEA (1998) (hereafter *Cloning Report*).
[53] *Warnock Report*, para. 11.17.
[54] J.K. Mason, *Human Life and Medical Practice* (Edinburgh University Press 1988) at 94.

at all. However, we lost the war. Does that mean that the regulatory framework for controlling research should now ignore any notion of embryos as special, or at least any more special than human gametes? Anyone opposed to or even uncomfortable with embryo research should simply shut up? I hope not. Attempts to agree some intermediate status for embryos continue. Article 18 of the Council of Europe Convention on Human Rights and Biomedicine demands 'adequate protection of the embryo'. Cries of vacuous may be heard, for the Article begs the question of what is adequate and adequate for what purpose?

To understand concern for embryos *qua* embryos we need to move beyond the scientific disciplines of medicine, law and philosophy and into the more human social sciences particularly social anthropology. Embryos retain symbolic importance.[55] Reflect on the controversy over orphan embryos. Outrage greeted suggestions that where donors could not be traced, embryos should either be donated by the clinics to other infertile couples or used for research. Imagine any other abandoned human body product, for example, several pints of a very rare blood group. No one knows who donated the blood or who first had possession of the supply. Nonetheless screening proves the blood to be A1. If scientists who had control of the blood announced that they would neither release the blood for transfusion into a dying patient nor use it to further their research into blood cancers, that they would simply chuck it away, what public response might be predicted?

British legislation is muddled about embryos no doubt because the society it represents is muddled too. Embryos as laboratory artefacts (whatever the logic of the case) remains an unacceptable resolution of the debate or basis for control of research. Embryos as human beings with independent moral claims on society and the law is (alas) equally unrepresentative of either public judgement or public sentiment. For nine years British regulators have muddled through issues of embryo status. The advent of cloning forces us all to re-evaluate our understanding of embryo status and what controls should be placed on embryo research.

VIII. WHAT SHALL WE DO ABOUT CLONING?

Section 3(3)(d) of the 1990 Act prohibited one form of cloning (properly named nuclear substitution), that is the replacement of the nucleus of an embryo with a nucleus taken from any other person, embryo or development of an embryo. I suspect that legislators believed

---

[55] See S. Bateman-Novaes and T. Salem, 'Embedding the Embryo' in J. Harris and S.Holm (eds.), *The Future of Human Reproduction* (Oxford University Press 1998).

section 3(3)(d) would outlaw the creation of 'carbon copy' clones. Dolly, the sheep who brought cloning into the public arena, was, however, created utilising nuclear substitution into an egg cell, not an embryo. Section 3(3)(d) does not prohibit that form of cloning. The HFEA argue that nonetheless human cloning by whatever means falls within their remit. Section 3(1) requires a licence from the HFEA to bring about the creation of an embryo. But what constitutes an embryo? Section 1 provides that 'embryo means a live human embryo where fertilisation is complete'. When a cell, with its own complete complement of DNA, is taken from an adult fused with an unfertilised egg and cultured to divide and develop, is that process fertilisation? The Department of Health and the HFEA took counsel's opinion and are content that the entity (embryo) created from fusion of egg and alien nucleus is fertilised, and so within the 1990 Act.[56] I cannot agree.

Consider the analogy of plant production. You can reproduce your favourite rose in two ways. Ensure pollination and the creation of seeds resulting in a new rose, and you have a rose resulting from fertilisation. Take a cutting of that rose, root it in compost, and once again you have a new rose. But your second rose is genetically identical to its original and created by propagation not fertilisation. Nuclear substitution constitutes propagation not fertilisation. Consequently I would contend that nuclear substitution into an egg cell is unregulated in the United Kingdom today.

Debate about fertilisation or propagation is more than a lawyer's tiff. Nuclear substitution challenges our understanding of what a human embryo is and what its moral claims may be. Many opponents of embryo research centre their opposition to destruction of embryos on the view that from the creation of a zygote a new genetic person comes into being. From fusion of egg and sperm begins a new human creature, endowed by God with a life separate from her parents. She has a novel genetic identity and, actually or potentially, her own immortal immaterial soul. What then of my clone? 'She' shares my DNA. She is me? Of course, while reproductive human cloning is almost certainly technically feasible, an English academic is unlikely to be able to afford reproductive cloning. More realistically I might look to use *therapeutic* cloning to repair damage to my tissue or organs. Nuclei taken from me could be inserted in (preferably) donated eggs and stem cells cultured to develop whatever cells or tissues I needed. Is an embryo created? I can (as yet) find no way through my own personal dilemma as to the fundamental nature of cloned cell tissue or organs.

What has been the public and legislative response to cloning? Once again a distinction must be drawn between reproductive cloning and

---

[56] *Cloning Report*, para. 3.4.

what has come to be styled therapeutic cloning. Reproductive cloning has met with an almost universal negative response from governmental and official bodies. UNESCO and the Council of Europe have both condemned cloning of human beings as contrary to human dignity. The HFEA and HGAC in the United Kingdom endorses prohibition. Despite their belief that section 3 of the 1990 Act already prevents nuclear substitution into an egg cell without a licence from the HFEA, they state that the UK government '. . . may, nevertheless, consider the possibility of introducing primary or secondary legislation explicitly banning reproductive cloning regardless of the technique used'.[57]

So what is wrong with cloning? The HFEA/HGAC Consultation, albeit endorsing a ban on reproductive cloning, seems lacking in passion in its opposition to reproductive cloning. They express concerns about its safety, yet only trial and error will prove or disprove such concerns. They float scenarios where cloning is used to 'copy' a dead child and argue it would be '. . . morally demeaning and psychologically damaging for someone to learn that the primary reason for their existence lay not in their own value, but in their utility for another purpose, as the substitute for someone else or for the benefit of someone else'. Yet might the same argument not be made in the not uncommon scenario of the landed gentry of England having five, six or more children just to ensure at last the birth of a son and heir.

The august bodies warm a little to cloning as an extreme measure to relieve infertility where nuclear substitution appears to be the only way to produce a genetically related embryo. The 'relief of the pain of infertility is, in general, a good end' we are told. That good, however, is balanced against an 'unbalanced genetic relationship of an entirely unprecedented kind within a family'.[58] The key to the British 'official' stance against reproductive cloning perhaps lies in the following sentence:

> For any type of infertility treatment to function satisfactorily there has to be a degree of social acceptance of the measures being taken. It is quite clear the human reproductive cloning is unacceptable to a substantial majority of the population.[59]

Contemplating the advisory function entrusted to the HFEA, one might have hoped that body would inform public opinion promoting reasoned debate. Alas on this issue for Authority simply submits to a public sentiment uninformed by evidence. Astonishingly virtually none

---

[57] *Cloning Report*, para. 9.2.

[58] For an incisively critical review of the Report, see J.M. Harris, 'Cloning and Balanced Ethics' (forthcoming).

[59] *Cloning Report*, para. 4.8.

of the truly difficult questions ventilated elsewhere by Ruth Deech who chairs the HFEA are addressed in their report.[60]

Therapeutic cloning in contrast is endorsed by the HFEA and HGAC. The endorsement in the United Kingdom (unlike some other European jurisdictions) of the creation of embryos for research is seen as giving the green light to the specific creation of cell nucleus replacement, (cloned embryos), to develop cultured cell lines. Thus people suffering from injury or degenerative disease could provide their own nuclei, which would be replaced in eggs and stem cells would be developed. The resulting tissue (or organ) could be transplanted into the patient with no risk or rejection. The goods of therapeutic cloning outweigh any objections, which in any case the HFEA/HGAC appear to regard as simply rehashing the old debate on embryo use all over again. The only significant concern expressed by the HFEA/HGAC relates to commercialisation of such techniques which begs my final question of just what sort of an enterprise British law now seeks to regulate.

IX. PROFESSION OR MARKET?

The most profound change in regulating reproductive medicine since Warnock is, I would argue, the dramatically increased role of commerce. Warnock based its recommendations in relation to both fertility treatment and research on the supposition that fertility services would be integrated into the NHS and that research was essentially an 'academic' endeavour. The enormous commercial potential of developments in reproductive medicine was hardly foreseen, and opposition to commodification of reproduction was almost a given. Yet debate on commodification and commercialisation is at the forefront of debate today. A fertility 'industry' has developed to provide treatment on a profit-making basis both to British citizens and 'procreative tourists' escaping more prohibitive regimes elsewhere in Europe.[61] Pressure to pay gamete donors and surrogates continue. Accepting HFEA/HGAC proposals to use embryos to develop therapies opens up new vistas for the biotechnology industry. Difficult questions confront regulators. (1) Whatever the pros and cons of recognising a reproduction market, is a covert market more dangerous than an overt market? (2) Given the diversity of regulation worldwide can any single jurisdiction continue to enforce its own rules?

---

[60] R. Deech, 'Family Law and Genetics' in R. Brownsword, W.R. Cornish and M. Llewelyn (eds), *Law and Human Genetics: Regulating a Revolution* (Hart Publishing 1998) 105.
[61] The term used by Linda Nielsen in 'Procreative Tourism, Genetic Testing and the Law' in N. Lowe and G. Douglas (eds.), *Families Across Frontiers* (Kluwer 1996) 831–98.

The reproduction business, even in the United Kingdom, it set to spawn two rather different sorts of market. The first, which effectively exists today, is the market in fertility services. The private sector, involving both private licensed fertility clinics and the companies who will seek to develop both new fertility treatments and therapeutic cloning, necessarily operates on a profit-making basis. They have a vested interest in the expansion of their business. The more treatment cycles a woman undergoes, the more people who seek treatment, the greater the profit to a clinic. In the early years of the reproduction revolution, feminist critics voiced considerable concern about the potential exploitation of women in the name of science.[62] Such criticism has been more muted of late but regulators need to be vigilant to ensure that their stated aim of 'safety first' is comprehensively met by the fertility industry. And 'safety first' must mean more than minimisation of physical risk. It extends to a mission to ensure that individuals are enabled to make their own informed choices of how they spend their money, and when, or if they confront the hazardous enterprise which fertility treatment so often involves.

The second sort of reproduction market, existing only in embryo this side of the Atlantic, involves trade in gametes and uteruses. It is a market which in part derives from the market in fertility services. The argument goes that if Dr Pater can be remunerated for harvesting gametes or establishing a surrogate pregnancy, why should the gamete donor and the surrogate mother not be paid for their services? Reproductive labour should be valued and compensated.

The law in the United Kingdom has long outlawed trade in children. Some proponents of markets in gametes and surrogacy contend paying for gametes, remunerating surrogate mothers does not constitute in any sense buying a child. In the context of surrogacy at least that claim is hard to sustain. Who would be willing to pay for the surrogate's labour unconditionally, to commit themselves to compensate her for her services regardless of whether or not she surrendered the child. Others however have argued eloquently that buying children is not necessarily wrong or dangerous.[63] Objections to markets both in children and in bodily services[64] are based on prejudices or intuitions that profit somehow debases an activity we commend when performed altruistically.[65] Alex Capron argues the case against markets persuasively backed by

---

[62] See S. McLean, *Old Law, New Medicine* (Pandora Press 1999) 25–48.

[63] E. Landes and R. Posner, 'The Economics of the Baby Shortage' (1978) 7 *J. Legal Studies* 323; R. Posner, 'The Regulation of the Market in Adoptions' (1987) 67 *Boston University Law Review* 50–72.

[64] See M.C. Nussbaum, '"Whether from Reason or Prejudice": Taking Money for Bodily Services' (1958) 27 *J. Legal Studies* 693.

[65] N. Duxbury, 'Do Markets Degrade?' (1996) 59 M.L.R. 331.

evidence of the operation of the US reproduction market.[66] The debate in the United Kingdom has only just begun. It needs to be openly articulated. The proponents on markets may commend their advantages, but all concede that markets must be regulated as such. Allowing the development of a market in gametes or surrogacy within a system in no sense designed to police such a market could undermine the good work British regulators have done to far.

Another nightmare awaits the HFEA and its counterparts in Continental Europe. Each national jurisdiction has sought to fashion a scheme of regulation acceptable to its own culture and community. However those wealthy enough to participate in reproduction markets can readily evade their domestic constraints. If I can order sperm on the Internet, or hire a surrogate mother from Bolivia, are British regulators wasting their time? The international ramifications of the reproductive business may prove to be a more stringent test of the strength of British law than all the difficult ethical dilemmas that have gone before.

---

[66] Above at n. 3.

[9]

For ages, medicine has had poor access to the fetus inside the mother's womb. But in relatively recent years, the human body has become transparent. The latest breakthroughs of technology have made it possible, from the very beginning of pregnancy, to consider the fetus as an individual who can be examined and sampled. His or her physician may now establish a diagnosis and prognosis and prescribe a treatment in the same way as in traditional medicine.

— Fernand Daffos[1]

The Maternal-Fetal Dyad
Exploring the Two-Patient Obstetric Model
by Susan S. Mattingly

D evelopments in obstetric medicine during the past ten to twenty years have transformed the clinical status of the fetus.[2] Traditionally physicians have been trained to assess fetal condition by indirect methods: palpating the fetus through the maternal abdominal wall and uterus, measuring hormonal milieu through maternal urine and serum, estimating statistical risks from parental medical histories. While the skillful use of these methods could produce highly reliable clues to fetal health and development, the fetus itself eluded direct examination. Throughout pregnancy the fetus could not be known, but only approached inferentially and probabilistically. Until recently suspected fetal anomalies have been treated indirectly too, by therapeutically managing the maternal environment. Unable to interact with the fetus in clear distinction from its host, physi-

Susan S. Mattingly is associate professor of philosophy at Lincoln University, Jefferson City, Mo.

cians conceptualized the maternal-fetal dyad as one complex patient, the gravid female, of which the fetus was an integral part.

High-resolution ultrasonography and techniques for sampling fetal blood, urine, and other tissue have changed this conceptual scheme. These diagnostic tools penetrate the opaque environment and reveal the fetus to clinical observation in all its anatomical, physiological, and biochemical particularity. When anomalies are detected, *in utero* medical and surgical procedures are already beginning to offer alternatives to therapeutic delivery and neonatal treatment. The biological maternal-fetal relationship has not changed, of course, but the medical model of that relationship has shifted emphasis from unity to duality. Clinicians no longer look to the maternal host for diagnostic data and a therapeutic medium; they look through her to the fetal organism and regard it as a distinct patient in its own right.

What ethical implications flow from

the fetus's transformation from inferred to observed entity? Unfortunately, legal developments have tended to preempt ethical exploration of the new two-patient obstetric model. Some physicians, assuming enhanced rights on the part of the fetal patient, have sought and obtained court orders to perform fetal therapies (notably cesarean deliveries) without maternal consent.[3] Although few in number, these cases raise the possibility of a new standard of clinical practice with far-reaching implications for civil and criminal liabilities to physicians and pregnant women. With legal stakes so high, it is not surprising that ethical inquiry has been displaced. Yet in the absence of independent and thorough ethical analysis one cannot judge whether these developments are compatible with fundamental values of medicine and medical care, and so one cannot know whether physicians have responsibilities, individually or collectively, to promote or resist them.

Well-grounded in law and ethics or

13

Hastings Center Report, January-February 1992

not, cases of court-ordered fetal therapy have set the agenda for debate, focusing attention on the question, What should the physician do when a pregnant woman refuses medical or surgical treatment recommended for the well-being of the newly individuated fetal patient? The two-patient problem for the physician is seen to begin at the point of maternal refusal and is framed as a conflict between values of fetal benefit and maternal autonomy. The medical recommendation precipitating refusal is, presumably, unproblematic. But that presumption requires examination. Inherent in any conceptual shift is the potential for equivocation between the old paradigm and the new. If the physician's recommendation of fetal therapy incorporates one-patient thinking about the maternal-fetal relationship, questions about maternal refusal of that recommendation may be spurious, resting on a logically illicit hybrid of one-patient and two-patient conceptual schemes.

We need, I think, to gain a fresh perspective on this issue by stepping back from the legal debate and considering in a systematic way how ethical guidelines for prenatal medical care are altered by transition to the two-patient obstetric model. How do the familiar principles of beneficence, justice, and autonomy operate within the new model in contrast to the old? Fetal rights and fiduciary responsibilities of professionals, parents, and the state may all be affected by the fetus's newly acquired identity as a second individual patient, but to avoid blurring distinctions among these roles my focus will rest on ethical implications for physicians. After all, elevation of the fetus to patient status has occurred not because of any change in the fetus or in the maternal-fetal relationship but because of a change in physicians—in how they think about and relate to their patients during pregnancy—so it is in the physician-patient relationship that we should expect the ethical repercussions to begin.

For the Patient's Own Good

The ethical principle guiding initial formulations of medical recommendations is beneficence. It directs physicians to recommend that course of therapy most likely to protect and promote patient health, based on estimates of medical benefits relative to burdens for the various treatment options. In making these complex comparisons, physicians are to ignore their own and third-party interests, responding compassionately to patient medical needs alone. For some purposes it is important to distinguish positive duties to offer benefits from negative duties not to inflict burdens. 'Beneficence' then refers more narrowly to the former duties, 'nonmaleficence' to the latter. Nonmaleficence requires that the risks, discomforts, and harms inherent in medical or surgical treatment be offset by proportionate therapeutic gains for the patient. Accordingly, treatment without therapeutic intent is categorically prohibited by the principle of nonmaleficence.

In cases where maternal and fetal burdens associated with fetal therapy are relatively small and prospective benefits to the fetus are substantial, the physician's duty of beneficence on the one-patient obstetric model is clearly to recommend treatment. This is true even if treatment offers *no* medical benefits, only burdens, to the woman in distinction from the fetus. When the maternal-fetal dyad is regarded as an organic whole, what matters is that *combined* maternal-fetal benefits outweigh *combined* maternal-fetal burdens. Distributions of benefits and burdens between fetal and maternal components of the one patient are not ethically relevant.

When fetus and pregnant woman are conceptualized as two individual patients, however, it is no longer appropriate to consider effects of treatment on the two combined. Physicians are to decide what is medically best for each patient considered separately. When fetal benefits outweigh fetal burdens of intervention, beneficence dictates recommending therapy for the fetal patient. But when anomalous fetal conditions pose no threat to maternal health, caring for the fetal patient imposes some degree of discomfort, harm, or risk on the maternal patient with no offsetting therapeutic benefits to her.[4] Maternal medical burdens outweigh maternal medical benefits, such maleficence requires recommending *against* treatment for the maternal patient.

Here is an ethical two-patient problem for the physician that arises well before the point of maternal refusal: treatment medically indicated for one patient is contraindicated for the other, yet both must be treated (or not treated) alike. It is difficult to see a favorable ratio of fetal gains to maternal losses as a problem and not a solution, of course, for we are accustomed to maternal-fetal balancing on the one-patient model. Also, we know that in most cases pregnant women expect to assume reasonable risks to improve the chances of delivering a healthy baby. Willingness to do so is ideally implicit in the choice of pregnancy, and indeed the argument that the pregnant woman increases her responsibility for the fetus's well-being by choosing not to have an abortion is often cited to support the medical duty to provide fetal therapy.[5] Given persistent economic and social obstacles to abortion, not to mention its precarious legality, the degree to which abortion rights increase maternal responsibilities is, I think, dubious, but that is a side issue. The real question is how maternal duties affect professional duties and exactly which duties are affected. Since beneficence considerations are restricted to medical benefits and burdens, it seems clear that maternal morality must be a factor to be weighed against beneficence at a later stage of ethical analysis.

On the two-patient model of the maternal-fetal dyad, a single treatment recommendation for both patients cannot be justified in terms of the beneficence principle alone, for it includes no provision for balancing burdens to one patient against benefits to another. Indeed, tradeoffs *between* patients are expressly prohibited by the exclusion of third-party interests. Beneficence, applying as it does to patients one by one, is logically unequipped to produce a single recommendation for two linked patients with conflicting medical needs.

Mediating the Conflict

Conflicts between duties of beneficence and nonmaleficence to multiple patients are rare in medicine but they do characteristically occur in two areas in addition to obstetrics: live-donor tissue transplantation and nontherapeutic research. In both fields physicians' unusual divided loyalties—to patients in need of medical help and to those put at medical risk to provide that help—have engendered considerable concern and an extensive ethical literature.[6] The resulting codes and practices resist any movement toward a utilitarian ethic whereby imperatives of medical rescue and medical progress would justify imposing relatively small harms and risks on donors and subjects. The rationale for rejecting an approach that trades off benefits against harms between patients hinges on the way medical moral authority is circumscribed. Professional ethical decisions are not generic judgments made from a neutral standpoint preferring always the lesser to the greater harm. They are choices made from the standpoint of the professional as moral agent, hence *causal responsibility* and *motivation* for harm are more significant variables than *quantity* of harm. If physicians do not intervene to help a patient in need of a kidney transplant, the patient suffers harm due to progress of the disease condition, and the physician's choice is at most a contributing factor; if physicians do intervene, the donor suffers harm directly and exclusively from medical intervention. The Hippocratic tradition is shaped by the presumption that moral liability for physician-caused harm to a patient is relieved only by therapeutic intent for that patient, whereas excusing conditions and motivations for failure to benefit a patient are many and varied. Nonmaleficence constrains beneficence and not vice versa.

In transplantation and research ethics, nonmaleficence constraints have been cautiously qualified to permit physicians under narrowly specified conditions to treat some patients nontherapeutically in order to benefit others. First, the medical burdens inflicted must be smaller in relation to anticipated benefits than they are when they accrue to one and the same patient. Second, patients treated nontherapeutically must be volunteers. *Recommending* nontherapeutic treatment remains unethical, although *providing* it is permissible at the subject's or donor's request.

On the one-patient model for obstetric care, conflicts between maternal and fetal needs occur within, not between, patients; they are balanced and resolved by physicians under the principle of beneficence in determining the medically indicated course of therapy. On the two-patient model, however, competing maternal and fetal needs must be settled at a different level, by applying standards of justice. According to these standards, physicians are not at liberty to benefit one patient by inflicting medical harms on another, except under stringently qualified conditions. In most cases, pregnant women, continuing to identify fetal needs and interests with their own, will request treatment to promote fetal health, thereby lifting constraints of nonmaleficence and authorizing physicians to proceed with proportionate fetal therapy. For physicians to recommend fetal therapy as if it were medically indicated for both patients, however, would be misleading and unethical.

The question is whether, having removed fetal needs from the calculus of maternal medical interests and having divided one compound professional-patient obligation into two discrete fiduciary commitments, physicians may discount protective duties owed to the woman as an individual patient in her own right. Is this the stage at which professional duties are altered by maternal duties? In other areas of medicine, the injunction against intentional medical harm is not thought to be affected by patient morality or social role: neither moral debts to society nor obligations of family relationship authorize physicians to take a stronger-than-invitational approach in recruiting research subjects or tissue donors. Indeed, incarcerated felons and other institutionalized populations are virtually off-limits to medical researchers, since distinctions between *inviting, advising,* and *requiring* are difficult to maintain in coercive contexts. More to the point, in transplantation ethics, family pressures on the donor are considered a form of moral coercion, increasing rather than decreasing professional obligations to emphasize the optional nature of the transaction. When alternate volunteers or procedures are unavailable or unlikely to yield successful results, this restrained approach on the part of physicians may result in the loss of significant prospective benefits, including lives that might have been saved. That is the price of role-based limits on professional moral agency. But a professional ethics that allowed treatment recommendations to be based on moral diagnosis of patients and therapeutic intent for others would also exact a price: it would erode the fiduciary character of the physician-patient relationship, undermining the basis for patient trust.

By separating the maternal-fetal dyad conceptually into two individual patients, the new obstetric model bifurcates the process of formulating medical recommendations: physicians should recommend beneficial fetal therapy for the fetal patient, but recommending treatment for the maternal patient contrary to her best medical interests is prohibited by standards for the just resolution of conflicting duties to multiple patients. In two-patient obstetrics, physicians may at most invite and encourage the pregnant woman to submit voluntarily to burdensome treatment for the sake of proportionate fetal benefits. Usually the invitation will be readily accepted, so the distinction between inviting treatment and recommending it will have little practical importance. It is of considerable theoretical importance, however, to the pregnant woman's autonomy.

Honoring the Patient

On the one-patient obstetric model, recommended fetal therapy offers net medical benefits to the pregnant woman, the refusal of which, here as in other medical contexts, should trigger discussion to determine whether her needs and values are in fact incompatible with treatment. Although efforts to encourage consent are appropriate, paternalistic treatment of a competent dissenting patient is unlikely to be justified. In particular, her autonomy cannot be restricted on the grounds that she is causing harm to others, as the pregnant woman on the one-patient model causes harm only to herself.

Rejecting treatment on the two-patient obstetric model is more complicated. The physician's two treatment proposals—the recommendation of therapy for the fetus and the invitation to nontherapeutic maternal treatment as a means to fetal therapy—call for two distinct maternal replies, neither of which is a standard exercise of patient autonomy. First, the recommendation of therapy for the fetus requires a *maternal proxy decision* on behalf of the incompetent fetal patient. Maternal responsi-

Hastings Center Report, January-February 1992

bility for fetal well-being is certainly relevant at this point, and physicians are morally authorized to challenge proxy decisions that are plainly contrary to the patient's best interests. Yet even if an alternate proxy (the father of the future child, for instance, or a court-appointed legal guardian) consents to therapy on behalf of the fetus, another ethical step remains. The physician's second proposal, the invitation to nontherapeutic maternal treatment, requires a *maternal patient decision*. This second step distinguishes fetal therapy from treatment of an infant or child. Treatment of an infant may impose substantial burdens of financial and personal care on parents, but physicians do not directly cause these harms through nontherapeutic practice of the medical art on parents *qua* patients. New technologies notwithstanding, diagnostic and therapeutic interventions on behalf of the fetus do entail medical invasion of the mother, and the proxy *for the fetus* has no ethical standing to consent to this invasion. What if the maternal patient declines treatment of herself?

When a proposed course of treatment is in a patient's medical best interests, refusal raises questions about the professional duty of respect for patient autonomy, because the harm caused by not treating her cannot be justified if the patient's refusal was not fully voluntary. When a patient *requests* treatment contrary to her medical best interests, the situation is the same: the request to donate a kidney, for instance, provokes questions about the duty of respect for patient autonomy because the harm caused by harvesting the kidney cannot be justified if the request was not fully voluntary.

In contrast to both of these cases, refusal of treatment contrary to a patient's medical best interests prompts no such questions about the duty to honor autonomy. When physicians disregard a patient's refusal of harmful treatment, the violation of patient autonomy is the least of their professional wrongs. Since ethical immunity against medical harm is independent of patient autonomy, it is uncompromised by limits on autonomy—incompetence, coercion, harm to others—that sometimes justify paternalism. *Harming* a patient without consent is not medical paternalism but medical maleficence.

A woman's failure to volunteer for fetal therapy may seriously violate her fiduciary responsibilities to the fetus, thus disqualifying her as proxy, but the physician's duties to her as patient remain intact. It is not the woman's moral obligation to consent that authorizes physicians to subject her to harm or risk without therapeutic intent; *consent itself* is necessary—consent that is to the highest degree competent, informed, uncoerced, and harmless to third parties. These exacting standards rule out any attempt to substitute proxy or presumed consent for maternal dissent. As on the one-patient model, physicians would be remiss if they did not make every effort to elicit maternal consent to low-risk, high-gain fetal therapy by providing honest reassurance and encouragement, but in the principles and precedents of medical ethics as applied to the two-patient obstetric model we find no basis for overriding maternal refusals to volunteer for such procedures.

Two-Patient Ethics & the Maternal-Fetal Ecosystem

When the fetus is conceptualized in clinical obstetrics not as an integral part of the pregnant woman (her condition of pregnancy, as it were) but as a second individual patient, the physician's duties to promote fetal well-being are, *prima facie*, increased. Maternal harms no longer weigh against recommendations made for the sake of fetal benefit. Also, the pregnant woman no longer speaks inclusively as maternal-fetal patient; if her decisions are not sufficiently protective of fetal interests an alternate proxy may be sought. But this is only half of the story. The other half is that professional duties to the first patient—the maternal patient—are paradoxically increased as well. Detached conceptually from the fetus, the maternal patient suffers medical harms from fetal therapy that are no longer offset by fetal benefits. Her physician may not recommend fetal therapy for her, and the injunction against harming one patient involuntarily to help another is virtually absolute.

Drawing selectively and equivocally from both models—treating the fetus as an independent patient but continuing to regard the pregnant woman as a compound patient incorporating the fetus—has, I think, caused the physician's ethical dilemma to be misconstrued as a conflict between the duty to benefit the fetus and the duty to respect the woman's autonomy. If maternal refusal of fetal therapy were a standard exercise of patient autonomy, it would be subject to paternalistic review to guard against harms to others. But fetal therapy is beneficial to the pregnant woman only on the old model, where she *includes* the fetus, while fetal harm is harm to another only on the new model, where the fetus is independent and exclusive of the woman. In fact, maternal autonomy plays a peripheral role on the two-patient model: maternal autonomy *qua* proxy may be challenged, and maternal autonomy *qua* patient is redundant, a secondary defense against treatment that may not ethically be recommended for her in the first place. From the standpoint of professional ethics, the obstacle to fetal benefit is not maternal autonomy but maternal nonmaleficence. Newly strengthened duties to help the fetal patient are constrained by stronger duties to do no harm to the individualized maternal patient.

Despite the fetus's new clinical status as a second distinct patient, then, physicians' prerogatives to intervene on its behalf are no greater than before. Whether the maternal-fetal dyad is regarded as one patient or two is less relevant to providing ethical prenatal care than the fact of that dyad's biological unity. Literally, if not conceptually, the pregnant woman incorporates the fetus, so direct medical access to the fetal patient is as remote as ever. Ironically, when the fetus is construed as a second independent patient, physicians' prerogatives to act as fetal advocates are actually diminished. This consequence flows not from any assumed superiority of maternal rights over fetal rights but from differential professional duties to donors and recipients of medical benefits. Two-patient benefit-burden transactions require of physicians a deferential approach to those asked to assume medical risks for others and a readiness to shield reluctant or indecisive patients from involuntary harm. If the example of transplantation ethics is followed in obstetrics, physicians have acquired obligations to neutralize moral pressures on pregnant women arising from family relationships and ensure that any maternal sacrifices to benefit the fetus are strictly voluntary.

But surely our argument has carried us too far. If status as an independent patient affords the fetus relatively *less* protection than its previous state of dependency, instead of revising ethical standards of obstetric care to fit that counterintuitive conclusion one might simply retract the two-patient hypothesis. Perhaps developments in fetal medicine do not require reconceptualizing the obstetric patient after all. Alternatively, since the concept of the fetus as a second patient is already well entrenched in perinatal medical philosophy, one might challenge the orthodox view of the professional-patient relationship, which suppresses dependency relations among patients and posits them as strangers to one another.[7] Deeply ingrained in the Western Hippocratic tradition and in Eastern medical traditions as well, the assumption that physicians should treat patients as generic individuals without regard to social role or status reflects an ideal of egalitarian, compassionate, patient-centered medical care.[8] Can professional obligations be made sensitive to relationships of dependency between patients without detriment to that ideal and without simply making an *ad hoc* exception for the case at hand?

Efforts to reinterpret professional ethical principles to accommodate just such relationships are in fact under way in family practice medicine.[9] Family medicine rejects the reductionist model of illness, which focuses narrowly on proximate causes within the patient as a biological organism, espousing instead a biopsychosocial model of health and disease. It looks beyond organic conditions, even beyond the presenting patient, to family relationships and circumstances that affect and are affected by patient health. For diagnostic and therapeutic purposes, the patient is conceptualized in relation to the family ecosystem. This environmental medical model is not entirely compatible with an individualistic patient-centered professional ethics. Responsibilities of family practice physicians to their patients must be understood expansively to include the family context—guiding patients toward choices that are responsive to their family situations and helping family members fulfill obligations of care to one another.

Adapting the contextual approach of family practice medicine to obstetrics, we might think of the maternal-fetal dyad as an integrated, two-patient ecosystem whose individual components are not conceptually independent. Caring for one implicates the other and the family context. An environmental medical model would remove the specter of dueling specialists vying for medical control of a complicated pregnancy—the *reductio ad absurdum* of the two-patient thesis. It

would counteract any tendency of physicians to discount the impact of fetal treatment on the pregnant woman, now effaced by her clinical transparency, and at the same time legitimize looking beyond the maternal patient to her protective biological and social role. Helping the pregnant woman fulfill her fiduciary duties to the fetus would again, as on the one-patient model, become a primary professional goal.

Once family roles and circumstances are drawn into the purview of patient care decisions, they may not be selectively considered only when they weigh in favor of treatment. Maternal fiduciary duties, for instance, typically extend beyond the fetus to other family members, and standards of family ethics do not always assign highest priority to fetal needs and claims. If the practice of fetal medicine were informed by an environmental maternal-fetal model, family demands would be acknowledged, not dismissed as irrelevant or even illicit conflicts of interest. By assuming obligations to address a wide range of health-related but nonmedical family problems, physicians may make it possible for the woman to accept therapy recommended for the fetus, but sometimes physicians must help patients and proxies make tragic choices forced by limited family circum-

stances, when resources cannot be stretched to meet the basic needs of all.[10] Also, family and medical values will sometimes diverge: increasing the chances for live delivery of a severely damaged fetus, for example, might be a medical value but a family disvalue. A context-sensitive perspective commits physicians to respect a family's well-considered value judgments unless basic family duties are violated.

Not surprisingly, ethical standards evolving in family practice medicine do

---

> Treating the fetus as an independent patient but continuing to regard the pregnant woman as a compound patient incorporating the fetus has caused the physician's ethical dilemma to be misconstrued as a conflict between the duty to benefit the fetus and the duty to respect the woman's autonomy.

---

not sanction doctors' enforcing a duty on the part of family members to sacrifice for each other, although reluctance to volunteer might be considered symptomatic of family dysfunction, to be treated through supportive intervention. In family practice, medical authority is exercised by negotiating medical goals and in collaborative decisionmaking. The physician's last resort in cases of severe and irremediable family problems—petitioning for the temporary or permanent removal to alternate caregivers of dependents at risk—is not available for the fetal dependent, of course, although planning for transfer of the neonate might be considered, but then the social meaning of the maternal-fetal relationship is changed. It reverts to the generic relationship of strangers, so the donor protections of two-person ethics apply: physicians should guard the woman from undue pressures to undergo medical harms for someone else's child.

Maternal-fetal conflicts are interesting out of proportion to their incidence in part because they raise in a compelling way questions about the integration of medical and family ethics, an important and underdeveloped topic. Conceptualizing the maternal-fetal dyad as two unrelated patients is bizarre whether the consequence is to tilt the

Hastings Center Report, January-February 1992

ethical standard toward strongly weighted professional obligations to protect the maternal donor, as I have argued, or in the opposite direction. Yet the integration of family status into the patient role is not a simple or clearcut matter. Patients who voluntarily present assume *prima facie* duties to act in their own medical best interests, but neither medical ethics nor medical education addresses the task of helping patients combine these duties with the imperatives of their family roles. Family responsibilities are lumped together with patients' idiosyncratic preferences and masked by professional respect for individual patient autonomy. But while exclusion of family concerns from medical attention is often unsatisfactory, to select one familial duty that bolsters the case for medical intervention and graft it onto a medical model that otherwise suppresses family relationships clearly will not do.

To expand the medical gaze to encompass family status is to see patients as persons in social systems, and this in turn demands a broader view of professional care than is typical of modern scientific medicine. Family practice medicine is an exception, and a biopsychosocial perspective is implicit, as well, in the traditional medical and ethical values of obstetric care. Recent developments in obstetrics, however, particularly the emergence of a subspecialty in fetology, introduce a narrow focus that sees only the fetus as it survives the pathologies of pregnancy.

Constructing a model of the maternal-fetal dyad as a two-patient ecosystem would restore to medical relevance the relationship of dependence and protection characteristic of the dyad. The effect of such a model would be to join the professional-patient relationships to the two patients almost as closely as if they were a single compound commitment to one compound patient. Protections associated with dependence would be reinstated and the two-patient presumption against maternal medical sacrifice averted. Within a two-patient framework, it is possible, then, to approximate the one-patient standard of obstetric care, but there is no warrant for requiring or permitting physicians to move beyond it toward a stronger posture of fetal protection. One patient or two, independent or dependent, when the various possible models of the maternal-fetal dyad are consistently applied, they converge to reinforce the physician's customary ethical stance—working cooperatively with the pregnant woman for common, linked goals of infant, maternal, and family well-being.

References

1. Fernand Daffos, "Access to the Other Patient," *Seminars in Perinatology* 13, no. 4 (1989): 252.

2. F. A. Manning, "Reflections on Future Directions of Perinatal Medicine," *Seminars in Perinatology* 13, no. 4 (1989): 342-51. In the introductory paragraphs I have relied heavily on Manning's excellent account of the way in which technical innovations in perinatal medicine have brought about subtle but far-reaching changes in underlying philosophy.

3. Veronika E. G. Kolder et al., "Court-Ordered Obstetrical Interventions," *NEJM* 316, no. 19 (1987): 1192-96.

4. Michael R. Harrison et al., "Management of the Fetus with a Correctable Congenital Defect," *JAMA* 246, no. 7 (1981): 774-77.

5. H. Tristram Engelhardt, Jr., "Current Controversies in Obstetrics: Wrongful Life and Forced Fetal Surgical Procedures," *American Journal of Obstetrics and Gynecology* 151 (1985): 313-18. Engelhardt's argument is cited, for example, by Frank A. Chervenak and Laurence B. McCullough, "Ethical Challenges in Perinatal Medicine: The Intrapartum Management of Pregnancy Complicated by Fetal Hydrocephalus with Macrocephaly," *Seminars in Perinatology* 11, no. 3 (1987): 232-39.

6. See, for instance, Gordon Wolstenholme and Maeve O'Connor, eds., *Law & Ethics of Transplantation* (formerly *Ethics in Medical Progress: With Special Reference to Transplantation*) (London: Churchill, 1966); Roberta G. Simmons et al., *Gift of Life: The Social & Psychological Impact of Organ Transplantation* (New York: John Wiley & Sons, 1977); Paul A. Freund, ed., *Experimentation with Human Subjects* (New York: George Braziller, 1970); Robert J. Levine, *Ethics and Regulation of Clinical Research* (Baltimore: Urban and Schwarzenberg, 1981).

7. Informal practice varies widely, but theoretical medical ethics assigns no relevance to family responsibilities in arriving at patient care decisions except to the extent that family members are acknowledged as proxy decisionmakers, and then, perversely, they are to ignore responsibilities they or the patient may have aside from their duty to represent the wishes and interests of the patient. For a different view, see John Hardwig, "What About the Family?" *Hastings Center Report* 20, no. 2 (1990): 5-10.

8. Albert Jonsen, "Do No Harm," in *Cross Cultural Perspectives in Medical Ethics: Readings*, ed. Robert M. Veatch (Boston: Jones and Bartlett, 1989), pp. 199-210.

9. See, for example, Ronald J. Christie and C. Barry Hoffmaster, *Ethical Issues in Family Medicine* (New York: Oxford University Press, 1986).

11. Physicians and parents have distinct fiduciary responsibilities for the fetal patient, reflecting differences of scope between the professional and parental ethical standpoints. I have developed this point more fully in "Fetal Needs, Physicians' Duties," *Midwest Medical Ethics* 7, no. 1 (1991): 8-11.

18

[10]

The Creation of Fetal Rights: Conflicts with Women's Constitutional Rights to Liberty, Privacy, and Equal Protection

Dawn E. Johnsen

Our legal system historically has treated the fetus as part of the woman bearing it and has afforded it no rights as an entity separate from her. A few exceptions to this general rule have been created where necessary to protect the interests of born individuals. In recent years, however, courts and state legislatures have increasingly granted fetuses rights traditionally enjoyed by persons. Some of these recent "fetal rights" differ radically from the initial legal recognition of the fetus in that they view the fetus as an entity independent from the pregnant woman with interests that are potentially hostile to hers. In extreme cases, the state has curtailed the autonomy of women during pregnancy to further what were perceived as adverse fetal interests. For example, women have been compelled to submit to surgery in the form of cesarean sections although they preferred to deliver their children through vaginal childbirth. Similarly, a state court has held that a child may sue her or his mother for injuries resulting from the woman's actions during pregnancy.

The social determination of how the legal system should view the fetus should be informed by a careful consideration of all potential implications.[1] Although the desire to provide legal protection to the fetus often

---

1. This decision is a social one, not dictated by biology. A scientific inquiry reveals only that the fetus is a living entity, as are the egg and the sperm that combine to form the fetus, which has the potential to develop into a recognizable person given approximately nine months of nurturing in the woman's womb. The legal status that society chooses to confer upon the fetus is dependent upon the goals being pursued and the effect of such status on competing values. In the course of defining the word "alive," Professor Arthur Leff offered an insightful and concise discussion of the relevant considerations in determining under what circumstances the fetus should be considered a legal person:

> Important to all these legal problems is the recognition that they *are* legal (and ethical) problems, dependent not on any deceptively 'natural' biological definition of life, but on social and legal decisions. In 'nature,' things just *are*; only people classify. . . . [T]he relevant legal question ought not to be whether a foetus is 'alive' or 'a person' from the moment of conception, or the moment of viability, etc., as if the question were one of natural rather than social decision. A *legal* decision will still have to be made to whom the law ought to give protection and at what cost, paid by who[m] . . . .

Leff, *The Leff Dictionary of Law: A Fragment*, 94 YALE L.J. 1855, 1997 (1985) (emphasis in original).

See also Grobstein, *A Biological Perspective on the Origin of Human Life and Personhood*, in DEFINING HUMAN LIFE: MEDICAL, LEGAL, AND ETHICAL IMPLICATIONS 3, 10–11 (M. Shaw & A. E. Doudera eds. 1983) [hereinafter cited as DEFINING HUMAN LIFE] ("[S]uch matters as social status,

599

The Yale Law Journal   Vol. 95: 599, 1986

reflects a number of important concerns, the recent expansion of fetal rights has not been accompanied by careful consideration of how best to address those concerns. Most ominously, this expansion has ignored the far-reaching implications for women as the bearers of fetuses.

By creating an adversarial relationship between the woman and her fetus, the state provides itself with a powerful means for controlling women's behavior during pregnancy, thereby threatening women's fundamental rights. A woman's right to bodily autonomy in matters concerning reproduction is protected by the constitutional guarantees of liberty and privacy. Furthermore, the Fourteenth Amendment guarantee of equal protection of the laws should be interpreted to prohibit the state from using women's reproductive capability to their detriment. Any legal recognition of the fetus should be scrutinized to ensure that it does not infringe on women's constitutionally protected interests in liberty and equality during pregnancy.

I. THE DEVELOPMENT OF FETAL RIGHTS

A. *Unified Interests: Fetal Rights Contingent Upon Live Birth and Against Third Parties*

Until recently, the law did not recognize the existence of the fetus except for a few very specific purposes. As the Supreme Court stated in 1973 in *Roe v. Wade*,[2] "the unborn have never been recognized in the law

---

rights, and obligations associated with personhood move outside the particular concerns of science and become aspects of social structure and policy, subject to the dynamics of value and legal systems, rational discourse, and political determination."); Wikler, *Concepts of Personhood: A Philosophical Perspective*, in DEFINING HUMAN LIFE, *supra*, at 12, 16 (resolution passed by National Academy of Science states that point at which life begins is "a question to which science can provide no answer"). Legal personhood is a status conferred by the courts or by a legislature and differs greatly from our everyday sense of what personhood signifies. For example, the Supreme Court has held that corporations are "persons" for some legal purposes. *E.g.*, Santa Clara County v. Southern Pac. Ry., 118 U.S. 394 (1886) (corporations protected as legal persons by Fourteenth Amendment). Recognition of these rights is not the result of "some theory that ensoulment occurs at the moment of incorporation" or of the corporation's "startlingly human form." Baron, *The Concept of Person in the Law*, in DEFINING HUMAN LIFE, *supra*, at 121, 125. Rather, justice to the persons connected with the corporation was thought to require a recognition of the corporation as a legal person. Absent such compelling need, however, the Court has denied the corporation status as a legal person. *E.g.*, Bellis v. United States, 417 U.S. 85 (1974) (privilege against compulsory self-incrimination limited to natural persons). The considerations relevant for the question of whether to create fetal personhood obviously are very different from those for corporate personhood; yet in both contexts legal status should be a "function of the different social policies being advanced by different areas of the law." *Id.* at 128.

2. 410 U.S. 113 (1973). The Supreme Court held in *Roe* that a fetus, even when viable, is not a person under the Fourteenth Amendment. *Id.* at 158. It held further that a woman's right to choose, in consultation with her physician, whether or not to terminate her pregnancy is protected by the constitutional right to privacy. *Id.* at 152-53. Although the Court found that the state has a compelling interest in the "potentiality of human life" of the fetus after it reaches viability, it concluded that this interest could not justify prohibiting an abortion even after the point of viability if the abortion is necessary to preserve the life or health of the woman. *Id.* at 162-63.

Women's Rights/Fetal Rights

as persons in the whole sense,"[3] and the law has been reluctant to afford any legal rights to fetuses "except in narrowly defined situations and except when the rights are contingent upon live birth."[4] The limited contexts in which courts first recognized the fetus involved rights that were granted to children. These rights of children were unique in that they required acknowledging a child's prior existence as a fetus in her or his mother's womb. Yet because they contained a live birth requirement, these narrow exceptions were consistent with the prevailing view of the fetus as part of the woman. The fetus was not given any rights independent of its mother; rather, it was only after the fetus became a person at birth that it acquired legal rights as a separate entity.

One of these first instances of legal recognition of the fetus involved the right of inheritance.[5] Where a fetus existed at the time of death of the testator, the fetus was granted the status of a person for the limited purposes of the inheritance, provided that it was subsequently born alive. Fetuses were vested with inheritance rights contingent upon live birth in recognition of parents' presumed desire to provide for children conceived but not yet born at the time of their death.[6]

In another relatively early example of fetal recognition, tort law began looking to the period prior to birth in order to allow a cause of action for prenatal injuries. Before 1946, courts refused to recognize tort claims brought by children for injuries inflicted prior to birth.[7] Today, however, virtually all American jurisdictions allow tort claims for prenatal injuries if the child is subsequently born alive.[8] The purpose of tort law is to provide compensation to victims of tortious conduct and, to a lesser extent,

---

3. *Id.* at 162.

4. *Id.* at 161.

5. *See, e.g.,* Cowles v. Cowles, 56 Conn. 240, 13 A. 414 (1887); Medlock v. Brown, 163 Ga. 520, 136 S.E. 551 (1927); McLain v. Howald, 120 Mich. 274, 79 N.W. 182 (1899); *see also* Uniform Probate Code § 2-108 (1969) ("Relatives of the decedent conceived before his death but born thereafter inherit as if they had been born in the lifetime of the decedent.").

6. *See* Christian v. Carter, 193 N.C. 537, 538, 137 S.E. 596, 597 (1927) (recognition of fetuses "apparently was based upon the presumed oversight or inadvertence of the parent in providing for an existing or a contingent situation"); *see also* Baron, *The Concept of Person in the Law,* in Defining Human Life, *supra* note 1, at 128 ("Prime among the goals of the laws of inheritance is fulfillment of the presumed intentions of the testator.").

This recognition of the fetus has been the exception rather than the rule, even for property law. *See, e.g., In re* Peabody, 5 N.Y.2d 541, 158 N.E.2d 841, 186 N.Y.S.2d 265 (1959) (holding fetus not a person for purposes of § 23 of New York Personal Property Law and distinguishing distinctive purposes served by "fiction" of considering fetus subsequently born alive a person for certain matters of property and tort law).

7. Bonbrest v. Kotz, 65 F. Supp. 138 (D.D.C. 1946) (first case recognizing cause of action by child for injuries received *in utero* after viability). For an example of the law prior to *Bonbrest*, see Dietrich v. Northampton, 138 Mass. 14 (1884) (no cause of action for prenatal injuries).

8. W. P. Keeton, D. Dobbs, R. Keeton & D. Owen, Prosser and Keeton on the Law of Torts § 55, at 368 (5th ed. 1984) [hereinafter cited as Prosser & Keeton].

to deter such harmful acts.[9] It is consistent with these purposes to allow a child to recover against third parties for afflictions she or he presently suffers as a result of tortious conduct inflicted on the pregnant woman. In recognizing born plaintiffs' rights to sue for injuries suffered prenatally, tort law provides a means of compensating children and their parents.[10]

The law of fetal rights in its first phase thus did not afford rights to the fetus *qua* fetus. It did not conceive of the fetus as separate from the woman, but took legal cognizance of the fact that the woman was pregnant. Recognition of the existence of the fetus as part of the pregnant woman was necessary in these instances to protect the interests of born persons, both the subsequently born child and her or his parents. This recognition created no conflicts with the interests of pregnant women.

B. *The Creation of Independent Interests: The Recent Expansion of Fetal Rights*

1. *Erosion of Live Birth Requirement*

Since the *Roe* decision, the law increasingly has recognized the fetus in contexts that are not contingent upon subsequent live birth. A majority of states now consider fetuses that have died *in utero* to be "persons" under wrongful death statutes.[11] Similar developments have occurred in criminal law. According to traditional common law, the destruction of a fetus *in utero* is not a homicide; the alleged victim must have been "born alive."[12] The Supreme Judicial Court of Massachusetts recently became the first American court to break with this long line of precedent. It held that a fetus was a person for purposes of the Massachusetts vehicular homicide statute, and thus a potential homicide victim.[13] In addition, a number of states have adopted legislation imposing criminal sanctions for the destruction of a fetus that are identical to those imposed for the murder of a person.[14]

---

9. *Id.* at § 4.

10. *See* Note, *Live Birth: A Condition Precedent to Recognition of Rights*, 4 HOFSTRA L. REV. 805, 825 (1976) ("The intention in granting recovery in cases of [prenatal injury] is . . . to compensate the postnatal child for the affliction it must bear. Recovery is not, therefore, a recognition that the prenatal child has legal rights.").

11. See PROSSER & KEETON, *supra* note 8, at 370 & n.32 (listing states); Mone v. Greyhound Lines, 368 Mass. 354, 331 N.E.2d 916 (1975) (same); *see also infra* notes 15–17.

12. *See* Commonwealth v. Cass, 467 N.E.2d 1324, 1328 (1984) ("Since at least the fourteenth century, the common law has been that the destruction of a fetus in utero is not a homicide. . . . The rule has been accepted as the established common law in every American jurisdiction that has considered the question.").

13. *Id.*

14. *See, e.g.*, CAL. PENAL CODE § 187 (West Supp. 1986) ("Murder is the unlawful killing of a human being, or a fetus, with malice aforethought."); ILL. ANN. STAT. ch. 38, § 9-1.1 (Smith-Hurd Supp. 1985); IOWA CODE ANN. § 707.7 (West 1979); MICH. COMP. LAWS ANN. § 750.322 (West 1968); MISS. CODE ANN. § 97-3-37 (1973); N.H. REV. STAT. ANN. § 585:13 (1974); OKLA. STAT.

Women's Rights/Fetal Rights

The creation of fetal rights not contingent upon subsequent live birth reflects a legitimate desire to protect the rights of the pregnant woman and the expectant father. Recognizing fetuses in wrongful death actions serves to compensate parents for the loss of their expected child and to protect the interests of a woman who has chosen to carry her pregnancy to term.[15] Such recognition also seeks to deter and punish the tortious conduct.[16] Similarly, feticide laws use the criminal law to protect pregnant women from physical attack and from the harm of having their pregnancies involuntarily and violently terminated by third parties. Holding third parties responsible for the negligent or criminal destruction of fetuses is therefore consistent with, and even enhances, the protection of pregnant women's interests.

Yet the form that this legal recognition often takes creates the potential for the future expansion of fetal rights in ways that conflict with women's interests. By sometimes identifying the fetus rather than the woman as the locus of the right when there is no live birth, recent laws have reflected a dangerous conceptual move.[17] The law no longer recognizes the fetus only

---

ANN. tit. 21, § 713 (West 1983); UTAH CODE ANN. § 76-5-201 (Supp. 1983); WASH. REV. CODE ANN. § 9A.32.060 (1977); WIS. STAT. ANN. § 940.04 (West 1982).

15. As noted by Prosser and Keeton, women traditionally have been allowed to recover damages "for their own injuries caused by miscarriage," but not "for the loss of the child." PROSSER & KEETON, *supra* note 8, at 369 n.30. The Supreme Court has described wrongful death actions for the destruction of a fetus as filling this gap and providing compensation for the loss of a child:

> In a recent development, generally opposed by the commentators, some states permit the parents of a stillborn child to maintain an action for wrongful death because of prenatal injuries. Such an action, however, would appear to be one to vindicate the parents' interest and is thus consistent with the view that the fetus, at most, represents only the potentiality of life.

Roe v. Wade, 410 U.S. 113, 162 (1973).

A number of state courts have recognized wrongful death actions for the destruction of fetuses for the explicit purpose of compensating parents. *E.g.*, Volk v. Baldazo, 103 Idaho 570, 574, 651 P.2d 11, 15 (1982) ("It is clear, therefore, that [the wrongful death statute] confers upon parents a cause of action for the wrongful death of a 'child' and thus protects the rights and interests of the parents, and not those of the decedent child."); Dunn v. Rose Way, Inc., 333 N.W.2d 830, 832-33 (Iowa 1983) (distinguishing between claim by estate of fetus under state's survival statute under which "the wrong is done to the injured person and to that person's estate," and claim by parents for loss of fetus under wrongful death statute under which "the wrong is done to a child's parents," and concluding, "[w]hat is involved here is a right of recovery given to a parent. The parent's loss does not depend on the legal status of the child . . .").

16. *E.g.*, Eich v. Town of Gulf Shores, 293 Ala. 95, 99, 300 So.2d 354, 357 (1974) (allowing suit for wrongful death of fetus "because the punitive nature of our wrongful death statute demands the punishment of the tortfeasor"); Vaillancourt v. Medical Center Hosp., 139 Vt. 138, 142-43, 425 A.2d 92, 95 (1980) ("Under such a rule, there is the absurd result that the greater the harm, the better the chance of immunity, and the tort-feasor could foreclose his own liability.").

17. *E.g.*, *Eich*, 293 Ala. at 99, 300 So.2d at 357 (citing "state's interest and general obligation to protect life"); Danos v. St. Pierre, 402 So.2d 633, 639 (La. 1981) (citing legislative pronouncement that "a human being exists from the moment of fertilization and implantation); Amadio v. Levin, No. 106, slip op. at J-15-9 (Pa. Dec. 4, 1985) ("This Court's former view that the real objective of these lawsuits was to compensate the parents of their deceased children . . . is not only incorrect, but if accepted, merely perpetuates the notion that a child is inseparable from its mother while en ventre sa mere."); *Vaillancourt*, 139 Vt. at 142, 425 A.2d at 94 ("A viable unborn child, is, in fact, biologically speaking, a presently existing person and a living human being . . . ."); Baldwin v. Butcher, 155 W.

603

The Yale Law Journal   Vol. 95: 599, 1986

in those cases where it is necessary to protect the interests of the subsequently born child and her or his parents. Rather, the law has conferred rights upon the fetus *qua* fetus. Conceptualizing the fetus as an entity with legal rights independent of the pregnant woman has made possible the future creation of fetal rights that could be used against the pregnant woman. In some instances, this potential has already been realized.

2. Fetal Rights Against Pregnant Women

a. Existing Rights

In one such case, a Michigan court held that a child could sue his mother for taking tetracycline during her pregnancy, allegedly resulting in the discoloration of the child's teeth.[18] The court stated that the appropriate standard for liability was that of the "reasonable" pregnant woman.[19] Another court has suggested that a woman may be sued by her child for not preventing its birth if she had prior knowledge of the probability of its being born "defective."[20] In some states, a woman can be deprived of custody of her child even before its birth if the state feels that her actions during pregnancy endanger the fetus.[21] In Michigan, a state whose laws do not expressly extend to "prenatal abuse," a court held that evidence of a woman's prenatal "abuse" or "neglect" could be considered during proceedings instituted by the state to deprive her of custody of her newborn child.[22] The court further held that this evidence could be obtained by reviewing the woman's medical records without her consent, records whose confidentiality was protected by both federal and state statutes. California's criminal child abuse statute, which requires a parent "to furnish necessary food, clothing, shelter or medical attendance," extends to fetuses and imposes a criminal penalty of up to one year in jail and a two

---

Va. 431, 438–39, 184 S.E.2d 428, 432 (1971) (holding fetus is a person for wrongful death statute is "technically correct in view of the fact that 'biologically speaking' such a child is, in fact, a presently existing person, a living human being") (quoting Panagopoulous v. Martin, 295 F. Supp. 220, 226 (S.D. W. Va. 1969)).

  18. Grodin v. Grodin, 102 Mich. App. 396, 301 N.W.2d 869 (1980).
  19. *Id.* at 400–02, 301 N.W.2d at 870–71.
  20. The court saw "no sound public policy which should protect those parents from being answerable for the pain, suffering, and misery which they have wrought upon their offspring." Curlender v. Bio-Science Laboratories, 106 Cal. App. 3d 811, 829, 165 Cal. Rptr. 477, 488 (1980) (dictum).
  21. *See, e.g.,* N.J. STAT. ANN. § 30:4C–11 (West 1981):
      Whenever it shall appear that any child within this State is of such circumstances that his welfare will be endangered unless proper care or custody is provided, an application . . . may be filed . . . seeking that the Bureau of Childrens Services accept and provide such care or custody of such child as the circumstances may require . . . . The provisions of this section shall be deemed to include an application on behalf of an unborn child . . . .
  22. *In re* Baby X, 97 Mich. App. 111, 293 N.W.2d 736 (1980) (within twenty-four hours of birth, child began exhibiting signs of drug withdrawal).

Women's Rights/Fetal Rights

thousand dollar fine.[23] Perhaps most alarmingly, states have taken direct injunctive action against pregnant women. Courts have seized custody of fetuses (i.e., of pregnant women) in order to enjoin women from taking drugs that are potentially harmful to fetuses.[24] They have ordered women to submit to blood transfusions to benefit the fetus,[25] and have even compelled women against their wishes to undergo cesarean sections instead of vaginal delivery.[26]

b. *Potential Expansion*

The creation of fetal rights that can be used to the detriment of pregnant women is a very recent phenomenon, and thus far has occurred in only a relatively small number of cases. Yet, absent an increased awareness of the costs to women's autonomy, these rights will almost certainly continue to expand.[27] Given the fetus's complete physical dependence on

23. CAL. PENAL CODE § 270 (West Supp. 1986) ("A child conceived but not yet born is to be deemed an existing person insofar as this section is concerned.").

24. *See* Chicago Trib., Apr. 9, 1984, at 1, col. 4 (reporting Champaign County judge's order designating fetus ward of state as result of "abuse" by its mother in form of her heroin habit); *see also* Reyes v. State, 75 Cal. App. 3d 214, 141 Cal. Rptr. 912 (1977) (criminal charge brought against woman for endangering fetus by using heroin during pregnancy; court held relevant statute applied only to children, not fetuses); Boston Globe, Apr. 27, 1983, at 8, col. 1 (reporting physician's request for court to order testing of pregnant woman for drug abuse and to take "what steps are necessary to insure the fetus's proper development").

25. Raleigh Fitkin-Paul Morgan Memorial Hosp. v. Anderson, 42 N.J. 421, 201 A.2d 537, *cert. denied*, 377 U.S. 985 (1964) (woman objected to blood transfusion on religious grounds). This case, however, was decided prior to the Court's establishment of the constitutional right to privacy in reproductive matters. *See* Griswold v. Connecticut, 381 U.S. 479 (1965); *infra* note 75 (citing cases).

26. Jefferson v. Griffin Spalding County Hosp., 247 Ga. 86, 274 S.E.2d 457 (1981) (per curiam) (woman objected to surgery on religious grounds); Annas, *Forced Cesareans: The Most Unkindest Cut of All*, HASTINGS CENTER REP., June 1982, at 16 (reporting two additional cases in which women were ordered to undergo cesarean sections).

27. Strong forces are currently encouraging this expansion and are not balanced by a consideration of the competing values. Several amendments to the U.S. Constitution have been proposed that would explicitly grant fetuses rights as "persons" under the Constitution. *E.g.*, S.J. Res. 17, 97th Cong., 1st Sess. (1981); H.R.J. Res. 62, 97th Cong., 1st Sess. (1981) ("Section 1. With respect to the right to life the word 'person' as used in this article and in the fifth and fourteenth articles of amendment to the Constitution of the United States applies to all human beings . . . including their unborn offspring at every stage of their biological development."). Similar statutes have been introduced by which Congress, without amending the Constitution, would attempt to define "person" as including fetuses for purposes of the Fourteenth Amendment. *E.g.*, S. 158, 97th Cong., 1st Sess., 127 CONG. REC. 24,141–42 (1981) ("Section 1. (a) The Congress finds that the life of each human being begins at conception. (b) The Congress further finds that the fourteenth amendment to the Constitution of the United States protects all human beings."). For further examples of this type of legislation, see Westfall, *Beyond Abortion: The Potential Reach of a Human Life Amendment*, 8 AM. J.L. & MED. 97, 97–102 (1982); Hyde, *The Human Life Bill: Some Issues and Answers*, 27 N.Y.L. SCH. L. REV. 1077, 1077–78 (1982). Senator Orrin Hatch has recently proposed an amendment to the Civil Rights Act of 1964 that would extend its coverage to fetuses, thereby providing them with civil rights. S. 522, 99th Cong., 1st Sess., 131 CONG. REC. S2262–64 (daily ed. Feb. 27, 1985). Statutes creating "fetal personhood" under the law have also been proposed in a number of state legislatures. *See, e.g.*, Memo from Sandra Kurjiaka, ACLU of Arkansas, to Leadership of Pro-Choice Organizations, Emergency Assistance to Defeat the Arkansas Unborn Child Amendment (Aug. 16, 1984) (on file with author).

Furthermore, a number of legal commentators have recently called for an expansion of fetal rights

The Yale Law Journal   Vol. 95: 599, 1986

and interrelatedness with the body of the woman, virtually every act of the pregnant woman has some effect on the fetus. A woman could be held civilly or criminally liable for fetal injuries caused by accidents resulting from maternal negligence, such as automobile or household accidents. She could also be held liable for any behavior during her pregnancy having potentially adverse effects on her fetus,[28] including failing to eat properly,[29] using prescription, nonprescription and illegal drugs,[30] smoking,[31] drinking alcohol,[32] exposing herself to infectious disease[33] or to workplace

without paying adequate attention to the potential infringements on women's liberty. *See, e.g.*, King, *The Juridical Status of the Fetus: A Proposal for Legal Protection of the Unborn*, 77 MICH. L. REV. 1647, 1687 (1979) ("There are no serious legal problems to recognizing legal protection of viable fetuses equal to that already afforded newborns."); Parness & Pritchard, *To Be or Not to Be: Protecting the Unborn's Potentiality of Life*, 51 U. CIN. L. REV. 257 (1982) (advocating more extensive legal protection of the fetus, including legal rights assertable against woman bearing the fetus); Walker & Puzder, *State Protection of the Unborn After* Roe v. Wade: *A Legislative Proposal*, 13 STETSON L. REV. 237, 240-41 (1984) (advocating passage of legislation granting "to unborn children, from the moment of conception, the basic rights, immunities, and protections available to all other persons, subject only to such limitations as are mandated by the Constitution of the United States"); Note, *Parental Liability for Prenatal Injury*, 14 COLUM. J.L. & SOC. PROBS. 47, 90 (1978) ("The parents' rights to autonomy should be limited when they conflict with the right of the child to be born whole."). Several of the relatively few commentators who have acknowledged that extensive, unprecedented restrictions on women's autonomy would result have nevertheless advocated expanded fetal rights. *See, e.g.*, Shaw, *Conditional Prospective Rights of the Fetus*, 5 J. LEGAL MED. 63, 67-69 (1984) ("It will take courage to reverse the well-established legal presumption that the mother's rights transcend those of the fetus."); Robertson, *Procreative Liberty and the Control of Conception, Pregnancy, and Childbirth*, 69 VA. L. REV. 405, 437 (1983) ("Once she decides to forgo abortion and the state chooses to protect the fetus, the woman loses the liberty to act in ways that would adversely affect the fetus."). Members of the medical community have advocated similar proposals. *See infra* note 46 and accompanying text.

In contrast, however, several commentators have written convincingly of the dangers of an unthinking expansion of fetal rights. *See* Westfall, *supra*; Parness, *Social Commentary: Values and Legal Personhood*, 83 W. VA. L. REV. 487 (1981); *see also infra* note 97.

28. The following examples, cited in notes 29-38 and accompanying text, were offered by commentators advocating the imposition of liability or state regulation on pregnant women.

29. Substandard nutrition during pregnancy may result in low birth weight, which causes higher incidence of defects, such as impairment of fetal brain development, and mortality. *See* Note, *supra* note 27, at 73 ("Nutrition is the single most important exogenous influence in the life of the fetus.").

30. For example, cough medicines may cause congenital goiter or skeletal, liver or brain damage; antacids and laxatives may cause kidney and brain damage; quinine and its derivatives may cause deafness; aspirin may cause damage to the nervous system, kidneys and liver; heroin may cause prematurity, deformity or death. *See id.* at 73-74.

31. Smoking reduces the fetus's oxygen supply, which is correlated with low birth weight, prematurity and perinatal mortality. "Indeed, a single cigarette smoked by a pregnant woman can disrupt the fetus' heartbeat." *See id.* at 74.

32. Heavy alcohol use may result in fetal alcohol syndrome, which "consists of growth retardation, facial anomalies, mental retardation, and assorted congenital defects affecting other organs." *See* Shaw, *supra* note 27, at 73. There is some evidence that the fetus may be adversely affected by even very small amounts of alcohol, *see id.* at 73, and by heavy alcohol use that occurred even prior to pregnancy, *see* Beal, *"Can I Sue Mommy?" An Analysis of a Woman's Tort Liability for Prenatal Injuries to her Child Born Alive*, 21 SAN DIEGO L. REV. 325, 360-61 (1984).

33. For example, diabetes in the mother may cause cerebral palsy with mental retardation; congenital syphilis may cause blindness, retardation, and birth defects; and genital herpes may cause brain damage. All may cause fetal death. *See* Shaw, *supra* note 27, at 67-69. In addition, maternal mumps, scarlet fever, malaria, small pox, chickenpox, measles and rubella all have potential adverse effects on fetal development. *See* Note, *supra* note 27, at 74 n.227.

Women's Rights/Fetal Rights

hazards,[34] engaging in immoderate exercise or sexual intercourse,[35] residing at high altitudes for prolonged periods,[36] or using a general anesthetic or drugs to induce rapid labor during delivery.[37] If the current trend in fetal rights continues, pregnant women would live in constant fear that any accident or "error" in judgment could be deemed "unacceptable" and become the basis for a criminal prosecution by the state or a civil suit by a disenchanted husband or relative.[38]

34. Exposure of the pregnant woman to teratogenic substances may result in harm to the fetus, including brain damage, behavioral disturbances, growth retardation, and gross birth defects. According to Dr. Shaw, "Exposure to organic or inorganic compounds in the chemical industry, dry-cleaning establishments, and gasoline stations are particularly suspect." *See* Shaw, *supra* note 27, at 70. Employers are excluding fertile women from working near teratogenic chemicals, claiming concern for their own financial or moral liability for causing birth defects. Some women have been faced with the "choice" of losing their jobs or undergoing sterilization. *See* Westfall, *supra* note 27, at 121. For an intelligent discussion of the problem of fetal hazards in the workplace as they affect women's employment rights, see Note, *Getting Beyond Discrimination: A Regulatory Solution to the Problem of Fetal Hazards in the Workplace*, 95 YALE L.J. 577 (1986).

35. Late in a pregnancy, exercise or sexual intercourse may cause premature labor due to trauma. *See* Note, *supra* note 27, at 75 & n.234. Furthermore, a study by Dr. Richard Naeye, Chairperson of the Department of Pathology at Pennsylvania State University found that "[a] pregnant woman's engaging in sexual intercourse is more dangerous to the fetus than the combined effects of her use of alcohol and cigarets [sic] . . . due to a bacterial infection known as chorioamnionitis which is apparently transmitted to the womb by semen." Chicago Trib., June 13, 1981, at 22, col. 1.

36. *See* Note, *supra* note 27, at 75.

37. These activities reduce the fetus's oxygen supply, and thus may cause cerebral palsy, epilepsy, lowered intelligence or mental illness. *See id.* at 75 & n.236.

38. Were prenatal tort claims against the mother widely recognized, courts would probably hold pregnant women to the standard of a "reasonable pregnant woman." *See* Grodin v. Grodin, 102 Mich. App. 396, 400–02, 301 N.W.2d 869, 870–71 (1980). The woman would be required to have knowledge of the potential risks of her behavior at least equal to the typical person in the community. If she had superior knowledge, she would have a duty to act according to that higher standard. The converse, however, would not be true: Courts would apply the community standard if she had inferior knowledge. *See* Beal, *supra* note 32, at 353–58.

A number of commentators have written approvingly of this development and have encouraged courts to allow such suits. *See* Note, *supra* note 27, at 84 ("Given that the child's right to sue his parents in negligence has already been established in many jurisdictions, no purpose would be served by singling out and denying the proposed cause of action [of a child prenatally injured by parental negligence].") (footnote omitted); Note, *Recovery for Prenatal Injuries: The Right of a Child Against Its Mother*, 10 SUFFOLK U.L. REV. 582, 609 (1976) (pregnant woman should be held to standard of gross negligence).

In the course of advocating greatly expanded legal restrictions on the actions of pregnant women, Dr. Shaw describes what might be expected of a "reasonable pregnant woman." Her "prenatal duties" would include "regular prenatal checkups, a balanced diet with vitamin, iron, and calcium supplementation, weight control, and judicious use of medications, tobacco, and caffeine. Alcohol and narcotic use in pregnancy should be avoided entirely." Shaw, *supra* note 27, at 83. In addition, "[n]egligent exposure to noxious chemicals and drugs, refusal to accept genetic counseling and prenatal diagnosis, refusal to obtain prenatal therapy, or failure to provide a modified diet, could give rise to a cause of action." *Id.* at 95. In some high-risk cases, Dr. Shaw would find women negligent for not taking affirmative actions to minimize risks to the fetus even before they could possibly have known that they were pregnant. *Id.* at 83–84. Finally, if a woman gave birth at home using a midwife after a physician strongly recommended hospital delivery, "she could be liable for fetal neglect." *Id.* at 89.

In the criminal context Dr. Shaw has stated that "health care professionals and others could be required, by properly drawn statutes, to report both *potential* and *actual* fetal abuse." Shaw, *supra* note 27, at 100 (emphasis in original). In Massachusetts, given the holding in *Commonwealth v. Cass* that a viable fetus is a person for purposes of the state's vehicular homicide statute, a woman whose reckless driving results in the loss of her late pregnancy may be subject to prosecution for homicide.

The Yale Law Journal   Vol. 95: 599, 1986

In addition to advocating expansion of criminal penalties and tort recovery, commentators have advocated a wide range of new forms of state regulation of pregnant women's behavior. One such suggestion is that public benefits be withheld from pregnant women who refuse to submit to physical examinations or to abstain from drugs or alcohol.[39] "High risk" parents could be required to undergo genetic or post-conception screening.[40] Pregnant women could be prohibited from drinking alcohol and required to submit to breathalyzer tests to ensure compliance.[41] One commentator has even proposed allowing punitive damages against women who intentionally harm their fetuses.[42]

Perhaps the most foreboding aspect of allowing increased state involvement in pregnant women's lives in the name of the fetus is that the state may impose direct injunctive regulation of women's actions. When expanded to cover fetuses, child custody provisions may be used as a basis for seizing custody of the fetus to control the woman's behavior. As noted by one commentator, "[t]he principal difficulty with the state taking custody of a conceived but unborn child is that the mother herself necessarily is taken into custody."[43] This fact forcefully demonstrates the threat to women's autonomy inherent in the creation of any fetal right that treats the fetus as an entity independent from the woman. Nevertheless, advocates of fetal rights have proposed that the state increasingly take custody of fetuses and, in some cases, civilly commit pregnant women to "protect" their fetuses.[44]

This threat appears particularly immediate in the area of coerced medical treatment of pregnant women. Women already have been compelled to submit to blood transfusions and cesarean sections against their will, when it was believed to be in the interest of the fetus.[45] This phenomenon, troubling in its own right, is susceptible to even more dangerous expan-

---

467 N.E.2d 1324 (1984). It would be difficult to make an exception for the pregnant woman under *Cass* given its blanket holding that the fetus is a legal person with rights completely independent from those of the woman.

39. Note, *Constitutional Limitations on State Intervention in Prenatal Care*, 67 Va. L. Rev. 1051, 1051–53 (1981).

40. *Id.*

41. Shaw, *supra* note 27, at 74, 103.

42. *Id.* at 104.

43. Parness & Pritchard, *supra* note 27, at 294.

44. For example, the commentators who observed that taking a fetus into custody would necessarily entail taking a pregnant woman into custody nevertheless strongly advocate doing just that. *Id.* ("The failure of states to use child custody provisions on a wide scale to compel conduct benefitting the conceived unborn is both perplexing and troubling."); *see also* Shaw, *supra* note 27, at 89 ("[A]n alcoholic or an addict could be institutionalized for the specific purpose of protecting the fetus."); Note, *supra* note 39, at 1051–52 ("A more effective means of preventing prenatal injury [than allowing tort suits against mother for prenatal injuries] would be for states to intervene in prenatal health care by imposing requirements or restrictions on expectant mothers.") (footnote omitted).

45. *See supra* notes 25–26 and accompanying text.

Women's Rights/Fetal Rights

sion given new procedures in fetal therapy and fetal surgery. When fully developed, these procedures, which had promised to enhance women's reproductive freedom, may be used to restrict it. Some in the medical profession advocate compulsory medical treatment, including forced surgery, where it is determined by medical professionals to be in the interest of the fetus.[46] The threat to women's autonomy is intensified by the fact that fetal therapy is still in the very early stages of development and, as one physician has noted: "Excessive enthusiasm, combined with inexperience, can be dangerous. Eager to learn and refine these procedures, physicians and surgeons may rush ahead."[47]

C. *Expansionary Forces*

1. *Careless Lawmaking*

The threat to the autonomy of pregnant women posed by the expansion of fetal rights has been largely unintentional. When making laws that involve fetuses and pregnant women, courts (as well as legislatures) have felt constrained by the existing law as developed for born persons and have considered the granting of fetal rights an all-or-nothing proposition.

---

46. *See, e.g.*, Leiberman, Mazor, Chaim & Cohen, *The Fetal Right to Live*, 53 OBSTETRICS & GYNECOLOGY 515, 517 (1979) ("If . . . the patient does not consent to undergo a given treatment directed to save the fetus, and which involves no undue risk to the patient, the doctor must be legally entitled to warn the patient that she is committing a felony."). Others argue against allowing physicians or the state to interfere with the wishes of the pregnant woman concerning medical treatment, pointing out that if such intrusion were permitted, fetal therapy might "foreclose current options, rather than create new ones." Ruddick & Wilcox, *Operating on the Fetus*, HASTINGS CENTER REP., Oct. 1982, at 10, 11. *See also* Shriner, *Maternal Versus Fetal Rights—A Clinical Dilemma*, 53 OBSTETRICS & GYNECOLOGY 518, 519 (1979) ("There is no acceptable alternative to requiring the woman's consent to surgery, and the obstetrician's role must remain one of informing, counseling, and persuading . . . ."). For further discussion of the potential conflicts created between the interests of the pregnant woman and the fetus by viewing the fetus as a separate patient, see Lenow, *The Fetus as a Patient: Emerging Rights as a Person?*, 9 AM. J.L. & MED. 1, 15–29 (1983); Ryan, *Medical Implications of Bestowing Personhood on the Unborn*, in DEFINING HUMAN LIFE, *supra* note 1, at 84.

47. Shriner, *supra* note 46, at 10. Even in cases involving well-established medical procedures, decisions about whether and how to proceed should be left to the woman. Because choices about medical treatment necessarily involve a consideration of competing concerns, the law should encourage physicians to disclose fully the potential risks and benefits of the procedure to enable the woman to make an informed choice. Despite the physician's presumed competence to inform the patient of the possible results of the medical treatment, the physician is not capable of making the required value choices for the woman. *See* Schultz, *From Informed Consent to Patient Choice: A New Protected Interest*, 95 YALE L.J. 219, 270–72 (1985). Furthermore, the physician's professional opinion is not always definitive. It is significant that in two of the very few reported cases where cesarean sections were ordered against the woman's consent (but never performed), the cesareans were later found to be unnecessary for the health of the fetuses, both of which were born through vaginal delivery without injury. Annas, *supra* note 26, at 16. Similarly, subsequent to a court ordering his client to submit to a blood transfusion, an attorney expressed his belief that the transfusion was not, in fact, medically necessary: "In point of fact an order was made against this woman when there was no serious problem at all. Two young resident doctors imagined that something might happen. A one-pint blood transfusion for an adult person is never justified. It is simply placing her in a state of risk with no correlative value." Letter from Glen How to the National Council on Crime and Delinquency (May 16, 1967), *quoted in* Lenow, *supra* note 46, at 20 n.119.

They have mistakenly viewed their options as being limited to either granting the fetus personhood status without regard to either the context or the parties involved, or denying the very existence of the fetus. It is thus not surprising that these lawmakers have extended the rights of persons to fetuses when faced with instances of clear harm and injustice, such as when an assailant negligently or willfully destroys a fetus through violence to a pregnant woman.

Courts have also employed unnecessarily simplistic reasoning when adopting the other extreme and refusing to recognize the existence of the fetus at all. For example, in denying a wrongful death action by a fetus, one court stated that it was "incongruous" to allow a woman the constitutional right to abort and yet hold a third party liable to the fetus for unintended but merely negligent acts.[48] Another court denied a child's wrongful life claim against a physician out of fear that allowing it would necessitate holding liable for wrongful life women who had knowledge of probable fetal defects yet chose not to abort.[49] Similarly, in limiting a feticide statute to the destruction of viable fetuses (where the statute on its face made no such distinction), the California Supreme Court stated: "If destruction of a nonviable fetus were susceptible to classification as the taking of human life and therefore murder, then the mother no more than the father would have the right to take human life."[50]

In thus treating the fetus, courts have glossed over crucial differences between fetuses and persons, and have lost sight of the interests that narrow legal recognition of the fetus traditionally has attempted to protect. They have ignored alternatives to equating the fetus with a person that would have more appropriately served their goals. In some cases, they have too quickly applied the legal status of the fetus in one context to entirely new contexts,[51] and in others they have unnecessarily refused to

---

48. Wallace v. Wallace, 120 N.H. 675, 679, 421 A.2d 134, 137 (1980); *see also* Toth v. Goree, 65 Mich. App. 296, 304, 237 N.W.2d 297, 301 (1975) ("There would be an inherent conflict in giving the mother the right to terminate the pregnancy yet holding that an action may be brought on behalf of the same fetus under the wrongful death act.") (footnote omitted).

49. Elliott v. Brown, 361 So.2d 546, 548 (Ala. 1978) (denying claim for wrongful life against physician reasoning that " '[i]mplicit, beyond this claim against a physician for faulty advice, is the proposition that a pregnant woman who, duly informed, does not seek an abortion, and all who urge her to see the pregnancy through, are guilty of wrongful injury to the fetus' ") (quoting Gleitman v. Cosgrove, 49 N.J. 22, 63, 227 A.2d 689, 711 (1967) (Weintraub, J., dissenting)).

50. People v. Smith, 59 Cal. App. 3d 751, 757, 129 Cal. Rptr. 498, 502 (1976).

51. In *Commonwealth v. Cass*, for example, the court relied on a prior decision that a fetus could bring a wrongful death action as the basis for holding that a fetus could be the legal victim of a homicide in the absence of a feticide statute or any evidence of legislative intent to include fetuses under the homicide statute. 467 N.E.2d 1324 (1984). Given the very different goals and effects of tort law and criminal law, and the absence of evidence of legislative intent, this is a particularly weak ground for deviating from the centuries of unwavering adherence by American courts to the born alive rule. *See supra* text accompanying notes 12–13.

In holding that a viable fetus was a person within the meaning of 42 U.S.C. § 1983 (1982) (despite the Supreme Court's holding that a fetus is not a person under the Fourteenth Amendment), a federal

Women's Rights/Fetal Rights

recognize and protect important interests.[52] Most importantly, the courts
have failed to recognize the fundamental differences between a woman
deciding to terminate her own pregnancy and a third party intruding
upon her body to end that pregnancy against her will.

To the extent that the expansion of fetal rights is the result of inadequate attention to the particular contexts in which those rights are
granted, courts and legislatures should take strict care to ensure that the
interests of pregnant women are not impaired by enhancing the legal status of the fetus. Given the physical reality of the fetus as part of the pregnant woman, there exists an inherent potential for conflict between the
autonomy of pregnant women and any "right" granted the fetus *qua* fetus. The law should continue to recognize the existence of the fetus insofar
as is necessary to protect the interests of the subsequently born child and
is consistent with the pregnant woman's interests, as, for example, in suits
by children against third parties for prenatal injuries. In their attempt to
protect pregnant women from violent criminal or tortious acts, however,
lawmakers should structure the laws so that they retain their focus on the
primary subject of protection—the pregnant woman. Attempts to deter the
destruction of fetuses by third parties against the will of pregnant women
should recognize that the actual physical injury is inflicted on and suffered
by the pregnant woman and that the fetus is affected only through her.
Courts should, in allowing a tort claim for the negligent destruction of a
fetus by third party, make clear that recovery is to compensate parents for
the loss of their expected and desired child.[53] Similarly, an assault on a
pregnant woman that causes her to lose her pregnancy could be considered a more serious crime than an assault on a nonpregnant person in
recognition of the increased harm suffered by the woman and thereby providing the desired added deterrence.[54]

2. *The anti-abortion movement*

Many anti-abortion activists strongly urge an enhanced legal status for
the fetus in nonabortion contexts.[55] Some of these activists are motivated

---

district court relied simply on what it perceived as a general expansion of legal rights to fetuses.
Douglas v. Town of Hartford, 542 F. Supp. 1267 (D. Conn. 1982). *But see* Harman v. Daniels, 525
F. Supp. 798 (W.D. Va. 1981) (on almost identical facts, viable fetus held not a person under §
1983).

52. *See supra* notes 48–50.

53. *Compare* cases cited *supra* note 15 *with* cases cited *supra* note 17.

54. New Mexico recently became the first state to enact such legislation in a manner that explicitly focuses on protection of the pregnant woman rather than the fetus. If in the course of committing
a felony, such as rape or assault, an individual causes a pregnant woman to suffer a miscarriage, that
individual is guilty of a third degree felony. The new law stipulates that voluntarily induced abortions
are not affected. N.M. Stat. Ann. §30-3-7 (Supp. 1985).

55. For two of the more explicit, but by no means unique, expressions of the anti-abortion effort,

The Yale Law Journal   Vol. 95: 599, 1986

by a sincere belief that a fetus is the moral equivalent of a born person. Others recognize that greater fetal protection serves to create a general atmosphere that is more hostile to the abortion right. Yet the fetal interests involved in the fetal rights debate differ greatly from those raised by the issue of abortion. In the nonabortion context, the woman intends no injury to the fetus; rather, she seeks to carry her pregnancy to term and is likely to act with the interests of the fetus in mind. In this context, the "state purpose" is not to preserve the life of the fetus against the pregnant woman's will, but to prescribe a woman's behavior during her *wanted* pregnancy. If the state were to deprive women of their right to choose to have an abortion, it would impose on women a duty to bear unwanted children; by creating fetal rights susceptible to use against pregnant women, the state compels women who desire to bear children to reorganize their lives in accordance with judicially-defined norms of behavior.[56]

3. *Concern for health of children*

To date the expansion of fetal rights assertable against pregnant women has been largely the product of accident and of zealous and imprecise political forces. Yet some commentators now argue that granting fetuses rights assertable against the women bearing them serves the legitimate, and even important, purpose of protecting the interests of the subsequently born child.[57] Precisely because the fetus is dependent upon the body of the woman for its continued life, these critics note, the health of the child depends in part on the conduct of the woman during pregnancy. They contend, therefore, that where the acts of a pregnant woman threaten to harm her future child, the state should intervene and dictate pregnant women's behavior.

This argument, too, misconceives the nature of the relationship between the fetus and the pregnant woman and is insensitive to the great harm

---

see President Reagan's 1985 State of the Union address, in which he stated: "Abortion is either the taking of a human life or it isn't. And if it is—and medical technology is increasingly showing that it is—it must be stopped." Nat'l NOW Times, May 1985, at 5, col. 2; and Illinois's abortion law, in which the legislature sets forth "the longstanding policy of this State, that the unborn child is a human being from the moment of conception" and states that the "longstanding policy of this State to protect the right to life of the unborn child from conception by prohibiting abortion unless necessary to preserve the life of the mother is impermissible only because of the decisions of the United States Supreme Court." ILL. ANN. STAT. ch. 38, § 81-21 (Smith-Hurd Supp. 1985).

56. The potential infringements on women's liberty could actually discourage women from becoming pregnant, and, given certain adverse precedents, could in fact create an incentive for them to abort. For example, a woman with an alcohol or drug problem might abort if faced with the possibility of civil commitment. Alternatively, in order to avoid being "caught" by the authorities, she might not seek any prenatal care, thereby endangering both her own and her future child's health. Extending personhood to fetuses in nonabortion contexts thus threatens not the abortion right, but women's freedom to bear children, and is a particularly inappropriate method for opposing *Roe*, 410 U.S 113.

57. See *supra* note 27.

Women's Rights/Fetal Rights

that would be inflicted on women by such an interventionist policy. A woman should not behave during pregnancy so as to avoid any risks to the fetus regardless of the costs to her, just as no individual should refrain from all activities that pose any threat to her or his well-being. Rather, the relevant question is what is in the interests of the woman, given that she is pregnant. Allowing the state to control women's actions in the name of fetal rights, however, reflects a view of the fetus as an entity separate from the pregnant woman, with interests that are hostile to her interests. In fact, by granting rights to the fetus assertable against the pregnant woman, and thus depriving the woman of decisionmaking autonomy, the state affirmatively acts to create an adversarial relationship between the woman and the fetus. By separating the interests of the fetus from those of the pregnant woman, and then examining, often post hoc, the effect on the fetus of isolated decisions made by the woman on a daily basis during pregnancy, the state is likely to exaggerate the potential risks to the fetus and undervalue the costs of the loss of autonomy suffered by the woman.[58]

Where the woman has chosen not to exercise her right to abort her fetus, she is likely to care deeply about the well-being of the child she will bear. It is therefore more rational to assume that women will consider potentially harmful effects to their children resulting from their actions during pregnancy than to subject all women to state regulation of their actions during pregnancy. Furthermore, because the decisions a woman makes throughout her pregnancy depend on her individual values and preferences, complicated sets of life circumstances, and uncertain probabilities of daily risk, the woman herself is best situated to make these complex evaluations.

But we should not be concerned merely with whether the state or the woman is better situated to decide how to reconcile fetal and maternal interests. Another fundamental issue is who has the right to make the value choices required to decide such questions. By substituting its judgment for that of the woman, the state deprives women of their right to control their lives during pregnancy—a right to liberty and privacy protected by the Constitution. Furthermore, by regulating women as if their lives were defined solely by their reproductive capacity, the state perpetuates a system of sex discrimination that is based on the biological difference between the sexes, thus depriving women of their constitutional right to the equal protection of the laws. Lawmakers should carefully consider the liberty and equality interests at stake, as well as the value of the state involvement, before imposing intrusive regulations on pregnant women in the name of fetal protection.

---

58. See *infra* note 68.

II. CONSTITUTIONAL LIMITATIONS ON RECOGNITION OF FETAL RIGHTS

A. *The Fetus and the Constitution*

The Supreme Court has never considered the possible deleterious effects of granting fetal rights in nonabortion contexts on women's exercise of their constitutional rights. In recognizing a woman's right to choose to have an abortion, however, the Court did make a number of relevant observations.[59] In *Roe v. Wade*, the Court acknowledged that fetuses differ from persons in very basic and legally relevant ways, and that the extension of rights to fetuses reflects an affirmative value choice by the state not compelled by biological fact.[60] The Court rejected the notion that the state could avoid the great complexities involved in determining the legal status of the fetus simply by equating the fetus with a person. In holding that the state could not adopt a concept of the fetus that conflicted with the right of women to terminate their pregnancies, the Court stated: "In view of all this, we do not agree that, by adopting one theory of life, Texas may override the rights of the pregnant woman that are at stake."[61]

B. *Infringements of Women's Liberty and Privacy*

Vesting fetuses with rights that are assertable against the women bearing them would create an unprecedented intrusion on women's bodies and personal lives. The magnitude of the intrusion on women's rights threatened by the current expansion of fetal rights implicates basic constitutional liberty and privacy interests that have been recognized by the Court in *Roe* and in other cases. The Court has long held that the Constitution protects certain aspects of personal autonomy from state interven-

---

59. Roe v. Wade, 410 U.S. 113 (1973). Yet the Court's discussion in *Roe* clearly is not determinative of the constitutionality of fetal rights in nonabortion contexts. The Court did not fully analyze the nature of the relationship between the fetus and the woman, nor did it address the equality concerns raised by restrictions on access to abortion given that only women, and not men, are subject to those restrictions. Furthermore, the factors relevant in determining the legal status of the fetus in nonabortion contexts are significantly different from those considered in *Roe*. *See supra* text accompanying notes 55–56; *infra* note 82. Neither the Supreme Court nor any lower court has fully considered the threat that legal recognition of the fetus poses to women's constitutional rights of liberty and privacy and to the equal protection of the laws.

60. These implications naturally arise from *Roe*'s holding that even a viable fetus is not a person under the Fourteenth Amendment, and are further supported by the Court's discussion of the legal status of the fetus in nonabortion contexts. 410 U.S. at 161–62. *See supra* text accompanying notes 2–4.

61. 410 U.S. at 162. In *Roe*, the Court held that the state's interest in the "potentiality for life" of the fetus becomes compelling after viability and can be used to restrict third trimester abortions that are not necessary to preserve the life or health of the woman. *Id.* at 163–64. The Court defined a viable fetus as one "potentially able to live outside the mother's womb, albeit with artificial aid." *Id.* at 160 (citing L. HELLMAN & J. PRITCHARD, WILLIAMS OBSTETRICS 493 (14th ed. 1971)). For further discussion of the viability standard, see *infra* note 82.

Women's Rights/Fetal Rights

tion. The Court has described the "right to be left alone" as "the most comprehensive of rights and the right most valued by civilized man."[62] This right is particularly important when the state intervention involves a physical intrusion on an individual's body: "No right is held more sacred, [n]or is more carefully guarded . . . than the right of every individual to the possession and control of his own person."[63] The right to be free from government control of one's physical person has been described as the right to "personal privacy and dignity,"[64] "personal security,"[65] and "bodily security and personal privacy."[66]

There have been few attempts at state intrusion of the magnitude and sweeping nature involved in state regulation of pregnant women's actions.[67] Courts have held unconstitutional even isolated instances of the type of intrusions to which pregnant women would be continually subjected.[68] For example, the Supreme Court has held that the state may not

---

62. In an often-quoted dissent in *Olmstead v. United States*, Justice Brandeis wrote: "The makers of our Constitution undertook to secure conditions favorable to the pursuit of happiness. They recognized the significance of man's spiritual nature, of his feelings and of his intellect. They knew that only a part of the pain, pleasure and satisfactions of life are to be found in material things. They sought to protect Americans in their beliefs, their thoughts, their emotions and their sensations. They conferred, as against the Government, the right to be left alone—the most comprehensive of rights and the right most valued by civilized men." 277 U.S. 438, 478 (1928) (Brandeis, J., dissenting), *quoted in* Stanley v. Georgia, 394 U.S. 557, 564 (1969) (Constitution prohibits making private possession of obscene matter a crime).

63. Union Pac. Ry. v. Botsford, 141 U.S. 250, 251 (1891) (under common law, court has no power to require plaintiff in tort action to submit to surgical examination for purpose of verifying injuries), *quoted in* Terry v. Ohio, 392 U.S. 1, 9 (1968). The Court further stated, "'The right to one's person may be said to be a right of complete immunity: to be let alone.'" *Union Pac. Ry.*, 141 U.S. at 251 (citation omitted).

In discussing the scope of the right to "personal security" as protected by the Fourth Amendment's prohibition of unreasonable search and seizure, the Court stated, "We have recently held that 'the Fourth Amendment protects people, not places,' and wherever an individual may harbor a reasonable 'expectation of privacy,' he is entitled to be free from unreasonable governmental intrusion." *Terry*, 392 U.S. at 9 (citations omitted).

64. Schmerber v. California, 384 U.S. 757, 767 (1966) ("The overriding function of the Fourth Amendment is to protect personal privacy and dignity against unwarranted intrusion by the State.").

65. Ingraham v. Wright, 430 U.S. 651, 673 (1977) ("Among the historic liberties so protected [substantively by the Fourteenth Amendment] was a right to be free from, and to obtain judicial relief for, unjustified intrusions on personal security.").

66. Winston v. Lee, 105 S.Ct. 1611 (1985), *aff'g* 717 F.2d 888 (4th Cir. 1983) (involuntary removal of bullet from suspect unconstitutional; decided on Fourth Amendment grounds, but lower court noted could be decided on Fourteenth Amendment grounds); *see also* Rochin v. California, 342 U.S. 165 (1952) (forcible pumping of criminal suspect's stomach violates substantive protection of Fourteenth Amendment); Pruneyard Shopping Center v. Robins, 447 U.S. 74, 93–94 (1980) (Marshall, J., concurring) ("The constitutional terms 'life, liberty, and property' . . . have a normative dimension as well, establishing a sphere of private autonomy which government is bound to respect. Quite serious constitutional questions might be raised if a legislature attempted to abolish certain categories of common-law rights in some general way. Indeed, our cases demonstrate that there are limits on governmental authority to abolish 'core' common-law rights . . . .") (footnotes omitted).

67. It is significant that the types of restrictions that would be imposed on pregnant women far exceed any that we as a culture would allow children to impose on parents. For example, we would not compel an individual to move to a different climate if her or his child's health required it and we would not permit a child to sue her or his parents for deciding not to relocate.

68. The privacy and autonomy cases and doctrines discussed herein deal exclusively with regula-

The Yale Law Journal   Vol. 95: 599, 1986

compel criminal suspects to undergo certain medical procedures,[69] and a
federal circuit court has recognized the right of even involuntarily committed mental patients to refuse medical treatment.[70] The fact that these pro-

---

tions that "directly" infringe on protected interests, either by making criminal certain behavior, or by
actually forcing the individual to engage in or refrain from specified behavior through the use of the
injunctive power of the state. It might be argued that privacy and autonomy rights are not as clearly
threatened by a more "indirect" regulation, namely, the threat of post-natal civil liability. This sort of
"deterrent" regulation was involved in such cases as the denial of child custody, *see supra* text accompanying note 22, and actions for damages against the mother by the child, *see supra* text accompanying notes 18–20. Though the threat to a woman's autonomy may not be as immediately apparent in
post-natal cases as in cases involving criminal sanctions or direct state appropriation of a woman's
body, the threat is, nevertheless, just as severe. Fear of liability for damages or of the denial of child
custody obviously could have an enormous impact on a woman's behavior.

The potential impact is intensified by the fact that the standards for behavior are not likely to be as
clearly delineated as in the more "direct" cases. Women would be at the mercy of an undefined and
ever-developing common law. Not only are the standards of the state common law courts constantly
changing and often incoherent, but also women would confront varying jury conceptions of "reasonable" behavior. Given common stereotypical public conceptions of the "proper" role of women, particularly pregnant women, there is very little behavior that might not be found by a jury to be "unreasonable." This is particularly a risk when juries are confronted with injuries that will otherwise go
unremedied, as is likely often to be true in such cases. It would not, in fact, be "unreasonable" for a
pregnant woman, faced with the prospect of post-natal civil liability according to community standards of propriety, to assume that the only safe course of behavior is to lie prone for nine months.
Thus, the distinction between "direct" and "indirect" sanctions in the fetal rights context is a distinction without a difference. The actual diminution of women's autonomy to make decisions is just as
severe whether the regulation is immediate or merely lurking in some vague threat of future penalties.

69.   For example, in *Rochin v. California*, the Court held that the forcible pumping of a criminal
suspect's stomach violated the individual's Fourteenth Amendment due process rights, and was "conduct that shocks the conscience." 342 U.S. 165, 172 (1952). This was true despite the fact that the
individual was a criminal suspect; police officers witnessed the suspect swallow two pills, which they
believed to be narcotics, in an attempt to hide them from the officers; the stomach pumping involved
an isolated instance of intrusion; and the Court stressed that it must review criminal convictions from
state courts "with due humility," *id.* at 168.

In *Winston v. Lee*, the Court held that to remove surgically a bullet from a suspect's body against
his will for use as evidence against him would violate his constitutional rights. 105 S. Ct. 1611 (1985).
The Court considered "[whether] the community's need for evidence outweighs the substantial privacy
interests at stake," *id.* at 1616–17 and stated "[a] compelled surgical intrusion into an individual's
body for evidence . . . implicates expectations of privacy and security of such magnitude that the
intrusion may be 'unreasonable' even if likely to produce evidence of a crime," *id.* at 1616. The Court
found the proposed surgery to be an "unreasonable" intrusion even though the risks of general anesthesia were considered "minimal" in this case, *id.* at 1618 n.7, and the Court noted, "whether the
surgery is to be characterized in medical terms as 'major' or 'minor' is not controlling," *id.* at 1618
n.8.

Although the Supreme Court in *Schmerber v. California* held that the state could compel an individual to take a blood test, the Court stated it could do so only if it could demonstrate that it was
necessary to perform the test immediately or else the evidence would be lost, thereby making it impossible to obtain a search warrant. 384 U.S. 757 (1966). The Court stressed, moreover, the very limited
application of this case:

> It bears repeating, however, that we reach this judgment only on the facts of the present
> record. The integrity of an individual's person is a cherished value of our society. That we
> today hold that the Constitution does not forbid the States minor intrusions into an individual's
> body under stringently limited conditions in no way indicates that it permits more substantial
> intrusions, or intrusions under other conditions.

Id. at 772.

70.   The Court of Appeals for the Third Circuit has held that the substantive right to refuse
medical treatment derives from the constitutional right to liberty and is not extinguished if an individual is committed involuntarily to a mental institution. Rennie v. Klein, 653 F.2d 836 (3d Cir. 1981),
vacated on other grounds, 458 U.S. 1119 (1982), *on remand*, 720 F.2d 266 (3d Cir. 1983) (reaffirm-

Women's Rights/Fetal Rights

hibited attempts at intrusions have involved those over whom the state traditionally exerts a great deal of authority—criminal defendants and mental patients—suggests the radical nature of the fetal rights trend and its incompatibility with our heritage of civil liberties.[71] One judge, concurring in an order compelling a pregnant woman to submit to a cesarean section, acknowledged this anomaly: "The power of a court to order a competent adult to submit to surgery is exceedingly limited. Indeed, until this unique case arose, I would have thought such power to be nonexistent."[72]

Although this judge suggests that protecting the life of the fetus should represent a unique exception to the state's traditional deference to adults' personal decisions, the law suggests the opposite: The protection against state intrusion afforded by the Constitution is especially strong where issues of childbearing are involved. The Supreme Court, in a long line of cases, has affirmed, as part of the constitutional "right of personal privacy,"[73] an individual's right to "independence in making certain kinds of important decisions,"[74] at "the very heart" of which lie decisions in matters of childbearing.[75] Because the Court has emphasized that the right of

ing constitutional right to refuse drugs). The court quoted a state court as follows: " '[L]iberty includes the freedom to decide about one's own health. This principle need not give way to medical judgment.' " *Id.* at 847 (quoting *In re* KKB, 609 P.2d 747, 749 (Ok. 1980)). Even when involuntarily committed, "the patient's liberty is diminished only to the extent necessary to allow for confinement by the state so as to prevent him from being a danger to himself or to others." *Id.* at 843.

71. A number of state courts have held that the right to refuse medical treatment as protected by the right to privacy extends to situations where the treatment is necessary to preserve the patient's life. As one court stated, "The constitutional right to privacy, as we conceive it, is an expression of the sanctity of individual free choice and self-determination as fundamental constituents of life. The value of life . . . is lessened . . . by the failure to allow a competent human being the right of choice." Superintendent of Belchertown State School v. Saikewicz, 373 Mass. 728, 742, 370 N.E.2d 417, 426 (1977) (footnote omitted). One court has stated that, even when an individual is mentally incompetent, because the right to refuse medical treatment is a "very personal right to control one's own life," the correct standard to be used in deciding whether to withdraw life-sustaining treatment "is not what a reasonable or average person would have chosen to do under the circumstances but what the particular patient would have done if able to choose for himself." *In re* Conroy, 98 N.J. 321, 360-61, 486 A.2d 1209, 1229 (1985). *See also In re* Quinlan, 70 N.J. 10, 355 A.2d 647, *cert. denied,* 429 U.S. 922 (1976); *In re* Yetter, 62 Pa. D. & C.2d 619 (C.P. of Northampton County 1973).

72. Jefferson v. Griffin Spalding County Hosp. Auth., 247 Ga. 86, 89, 274 S.E.2d 457, 460 (1981) (Hill, J., concurring) (per curiam).

73. Carey v. Population Servs. Int'l, 431 U.S. 678, 684 (1977) (right to use contraceptives).

74. *Id.* (quoting Whalen v. Roe, 429 U.S. 589, 599-600 (1977)).

75. *Carey,* 431 U.S. at 685. "[T]he Constitution protects individual decisions in matters of childbearing from unjustified intrusion by the State." *Id.* at 687. Significantly, the Court has characterized the right to privacy as protecting autonomy in "matters relating to marriage, procreation, contraception, family relationships, and child rearing and education. In these areas, it has been held that there are limitations on the States' power to substantively regulate conduct." Whalen v. Roe, 429 U.S. at 600 n.26 (quoting Paul v. Davis, 424 U.S. 693, 713 (1976)). *See, e.g.,* Skinner v. Oklahoma, 316 U.S. 535 (1942) (right to procreation); Griswold v. Connecticut, 381 U.S. 479 (1965) (right to use contraceptives; applied to married individuals); Loving v. Virginia, 388 U.S. 1 (1967) (right to marry); Eisenstadt v. Baird, 405 U.S. 438 (1972) (right to purchase and use contraceptives; applied to unmarried individuals); Roe v. Wade, 410 U.S. 113 (1973) (right to abortion); Carey v. Population Servs. Int'l, 431 U.S. 678 (1977) (right to purchase and use contraceptives; applied to minors under

privacy is the right to make decisions free from state intrusion, not only is the state prohibited from infringing directly on the protected right, but it also may not act in any way to interfere with the individual's decision-making autonomy. For example, although there is no "independent fundamental 'right of access to contraceptives,' "[76] state restrictions on access to contraception must be narrowly drawn to serve a compelling state interest, because they infringe on the "exercise of the constitutionally protected right of decision in matters of childbearing . . . ."[77]

Just as the state may not force a woman to bear a child against her will, it may not act to penalize her for deciding to bear a child. In *Cleveland Board of Education v. LaFleur*,[78] the Court found unconstitutional a rule that required pregnant school teachers to take unpaid maternity leave for the five months prior to an expected childbirth. Noting that "freedom of personal choice in matters of marriage and family life is one of the liberties protected by the Due Process Clause of the Fourteenth Amendment," the Court stated that "[b]y acting to penalize the pregnant teacher for deciding to bear a child, overly restrictive maternity leave regulations can constitute a heavy burden on the exercise of these protected freedoms."[79] By creating fetal rights that can be used against the woman bearing the fetus to restrict her conduct, the state appropriates a woman's right to control her actions and imposes a burden at least as great as that imposed in *LaFleur*.

In determining how great a burden a state regulation imposes on privacy interests, courts often focus on the intrusiveness of the necessary

---

sixteen years of age); Zablocki v. Redhail, 434 U.S. 374 (1978) (right to marry). The Court has further stated: "If the right of privacy means anything, it is the right of the *individual*, married or single, to be free from unwarranted governmental intrusion into matters so fundamentally affecting a person as the decision whether to bear or beget a child." Eisenstadt v. Baird, 405 U.S. 438, 453 (1972) (emphasis in original).

76. *Carey*, 431 U.S. at 688.

77. *Id.* Similarly, the Court held that a statute that placed restrictions on the right of individuals obligated to pay child support to marry was unconstitutional in that it "significantly" interfered with the right to marry, part of the "fundamental 'right of privacy' implicit in the Fourteenth Amendment's Due Process Clause." Zablocki v. Redhail, 434 U.S. 374, 383–84 (1978). In addition to holding that the state may not prohibit abortion, Roe v. Wade, 410 U.S. 113 (1973), the Court has also held unconstitutional statutes that infringe on a woman's right to choose to abort. *See, e.g.*, Doe v. Bolton, 410 U.S. 179, 195–200 (1973) (Court struck down as "unduly restrictive" statutory requirements that all abortions be performed in accredited hospitals, be approved by committee of at least three members of hospital's staff and two physicians in addition to woman's physician, and be restricted to state residents); Planned Parenthood v. Danforth, 428 U.S. 52, 67–71, 75–79 (1976) (Court held unconstitutional statutory requirement of spousal consent for abortions and statutory prohibition of saline amniocentesis as method of abortion); Akron Center for Reproductive Health v. City of Akron, 462 U.S. 416 (1983) (Court held unconstitutional various provisions of abortion statute, including mandatory twenty-four hour waiting period before performance of any abortion, requirement that post first trimester abortions be performed in hospital, "informed consent" provision, and requirement concerning disposition of remains of abortions).

78. 414 U.S. 632 (1974).

79. *Id.* at 639–40.

Women's Rights/Fetal Rights

means of enforcement. In *Griswold v. Connecticut*, for example, the Court held that a statute prohibiting the use of contraceptives violated the right to privacy in part because the state intrusions necessary for enforcement would be tremendous.[80] Similarly, in order to enforce fetal rights or state regulations dictating behavior during pregnancy, the state would necessarily intrude in the most private areas of a woman's life. The state would have to police what a woman ate and drank, the types of physical activity in which she engaged, with whom and how often she had sexual intercourse, and where she worked—to name only a few areas of regulation. The enforcement of direct state regulation of pregnant women's actions, as in cases involving court-ordered medical treatment against the pregnant woman's wishes, would require the state forcibly to take the pregnant woman into physical custody in order to impose the ordered action.

In order to withstand the strict scrutiny necessitated by the infringements on women's constitutional rights to liberty and privacy, any state recognition of fetuses that operates to the detriment of women must be necessary to protect a compelling state interest.[81] That is, not only must the law promote a compelling state interest, but it must also be narrowly tailored to do so in the manner that is least intrusive on protected rights. Laws that attempt to regulate the actions of pregnant women by creating fetal rights clearly do not survive this standard.[82] Rather, they allow pre-

---

80. The Court wrote, "Would we allow the police to search the sacred precincts of marital bedrooms for telltale signs of the use of contraceptives? The very idea is repulsive to the notions of privacy surrounding the marriage relationship." 381 U.S. 479, 485–86 (1965).

81. When a law infringes upon a fundamental constitutional right or involves a suspect classification, the courts must apply strict scrutiny in evaluating its constitutional validity. San Antonio Indep. School Dist. v. Rodriguez, 411 U.S. 1, 16 (1973). The law must be narrowly tailored so as not to infringe unduly on the protected freedom, and the means selected must be the least intrusive available:

> [S]trict scrutiny means that the State's system is not entitled to the usual presumption of validity, that the State rather than the complainants must carry a 'heavy burden of justification,' that the State must demonstrate that [the law] has been structured with 'precision,' and is 'tailored' narrowly to serve legitimate objectives and that it has selected the 'less drastic means' for effectuating its objectives.

Id. at 16–17; *see also* Shelton v. Tucker, 364 U.S. 479, 488 (1960) ("[E]ven though the governmental purpose be legitimate and substantial, that purpose cannot be pursued by means that broadly stifle fundamental personal liberties when the end can be more narrowly achieved."); Cantwell v. Connecticut, 310 U.S. 296, 304 (1940) ("In every case the power to regulate must be so exercised as not, in attaining a permissible end, unduly to infringe the protected freedom.").

82. Those advocating state regulation of pregnant women's actions might argue that the "potentiality for life" of the viable fetus qualifies as a compelling state interest that justifies giving the fetus rights that can be used against the pregnant woman in nonabortion contexts. The "logical and biological justifications" for drawing the line at viability discussed by the Court in *Roe*, however, are simply nonexistent in the fetal rights context. As discussed above, *see supra* text accompanying notes 55–56, the concerns in nonabortion contexts differ significantly from those present in the abortion context. When restricting access to abortions after viability, the state seeks to prevent the destruction of a fetus that, by definition, has the potential to live outside of the woman's womb. In the nonabortion context, the state seeks to create fetal rights out of a concern for the health of the fetus, and, where those rights are contingent upon live birth, the health of its future citizens. It seeks to further this interest by

The Yale Law Journal   Vol. 95: 599, 1986

cisely the type of unnecessarily sweeping state intrusion upon basic individual rights that the Constitution prohibits. To deprive women of their right to control their actions during pregnancy is to deprive women of their legal personhood.

C. *Fetal Rights and Sex Equality*

Existing liberty and privacy doctrine recognizes the threat to pregnant women's autonomy posed by fetal rights laws. Yet existing doctrine does not describe the full extent of the injury involved, for it does not identify the sex-specific nature of that injury. Only women can suffer the great intrusions of such laws, for only women have the ability to bear children. Fetal rights laws would not only infringe on constitutionally protected liberty and privacy rights of individual women, they would also serve to disadvantage women as women by further stigmatizing and penalizing them on the basis of the very characteristic that historically has been used to perpetuate a system of sex inequality.

The equal protection clause of the Fourteenth Amendment protects individuals from discrimination that is based on their membership in a disadvantaged group. It is now well established that the equal protection

---

substituting its judgment for that of the pregnant woman concerning how she should behave during pregnancy and by preventing her from acting in ways that it views as posing unacceptable risks to the health of the fetus. As this Note has argued, this asserted state interest fails to qualify as compelling, and, in fact, is clearly illegitimate. *See* Shapiro v. Thompson, 394 U.S. 618, 631 (1969) (invalidating restriction of constitutional right to travel, stating, "[i]f a law has 'no other purpose . . . than to chill the assertion of constitutional rights by penalizing those who choose to exercise them then it [is] patently unconstitutional' ") (quoting United States v. Jackson, 390 U.S. 570, 581 (1968)).

Furthermore, viability is a meaningless distinction in the fetal rights context because the state's interest in the health of its future citizens is equally strong throughout pregnancy. Drawing a line at the third trimester would be an ineffective means of preventing unintentional harm to the fetus resulting from the behavior of the pregnant woman. In fact, the woman's actions have the greatest impact on the development of the fetus during the first trimester of pregnancy, during most of which time she typically does not know that she is pregnant. Trying to enforce the viability distinction in cases of prenatal injury due to the woman's behavior during pregnancy also presents huge problems of proof, as it would require identifying a specific point at which a woman's actions harmed the fetus. Thus, viability is an arbitrary point at which to begin restricting the woman's actions in these contexts.

In fact, application of the viability requirement in nonabortion contexts has actually hindered the courts from protecting the ability of born children to recover damages from third parties for injuries inflicted prenatally. When recognizing fetal rights contingent upon live birth and against third parties, courts sometimes feel constrained by the viability distinction drawn in *Roe* and by potential conceptual conflicts with the abortion right. *See, e.g., supra* notes 48–50 and accompanying text. Continuing to view this legal recognition as protecting the interests of born children and their parents would eliminate those constraints. For example, allowing recovery for prenatal injuries against third parties as compensation for real harm that the born child presently suffers reveals that the injury is identical whether it was inflicted before or after the attainment of viability, thus permitting more complete protection. Recognizing this, many courts have abandoned the viability distinction in cases involving prenatal injuries, see PROSSER & KEETON, *supra* note 8, at 369, and one court has allowed a child to sue a pharmaceutical company for personal injuries resulting from damage to its mother's chromosomes that occured prior to conception. Jorgensen v. Meade-Johnson Labs., 483 F.2d 237 (10th Cir. 1973).

Women's Rights/Fetal Rights

clause protects women from discrimination on the basis of sex.[83] Current doctrine, however, offers women no protection against discrimination that is based on real biological differences between women and men, and in fact denies that such discrimination is sex-based. Women are granted equal protection of the laws only to the extent that they are "similarly situated" to men. In the contexts of both equal protection and Title VII challenges, the Court has stated that discrimination on the basis of pregnancy does not discriminate against women, but rationally discriminates between pregnant people and nonpregnant people.[84] Through its passage of the Pregnancy Discrimination Act, Congress immediately rejected the Court's position for purposes of employment discrimination under Title VII.[85] This Act amended Title VII's definition of sex discrimination to include pregnancy-related discrimination. Yet the Court has not to date reevaluated its holding that pregnancy discrimination is not sex discrimination for purposes of equal protection analysis. Unless the Court reverses itself, it is likely to uphold, without even employing heightened scrutiny, any unequal treatment of the sexes that is predicated on the reproductive difference, regardless of the magnitude of the harm imposed on women.

By blindly applying a requirement that the groups being compared be similarly situated, and by viewing reproductive differences as a permissible basis for differential treatment, the Court has substituted misguided formalism for what should be the true goal of equal protection analysis in cases of alleged discrimination—that is, to prevent the state from systematically disadvantaging on the basis of an immutable characteristic a class of people who historically have been disadvantaged on the basis of that

---

83. Laws that discriminate on the basis of sex are currently subject to "intermediate scrutiny," a standard that requires that "classifications by gender must serve important governmental objectives and must be substantially related to the achievement of those objectives." Craig v. Boren, 429 U.S. 190, 197 (1976). The Court has never articulated clearly why "strict scrutiny," the more stringent standard used for race, should not also apply for sex. In fact, in an earlier decision, four Justices had ruled that sex should be regarded as a suspect class and strict scrutiny applied. Frontiero v. Richardson, 411 U.S. 677, 682–88 (1973) (plurality opinion). In a recent decision, the Court invalidated a sex-based classification as not surviving intermediate scrutiny, and stated "we need not decide whether classifications based upon gender are inherently suspect." Mississippi Univ. for Women v. Hogan, 458 U.S. 718, 724 n.9 (1982).

84. Geduldig v. Aiello, 417 U.S. 484 (1974) (equal protection); General Elec. v. Gilbert, 429 U.S. 125 (1976) (Title VII).

85. Pub. L. No. 95-555, § 1, 92 Stat. 2076 (codified at 42 U.S.C. § 2000e(k) (1982)). The Pregnancy Discrimination Act reads in relevant part:

The terms 'because of sex' or 'on the basis of sex' include, but are not limited to, because of or on the basis of pregnancy, childbirth, or related medical conditions; and women affected by pregnancy, childbirth, or related medical conditions shall be treated the same for all employment-related purposes, including receipt of benefits under fringe benefit programs, as other persons not so affected but similar in their ability or inability to work . . . .

While *Gilbert* was effectively overruled by the Pregnancy Discrimination Act, *Geduldig* remains controlling for purposes of equal protection analysis.

characteristic.[86] In the race context, the standard for equal protection analysis that requires that similarly situated people be treated the same generally functions well as a proxy for the goal of avoiding the real harm of detrimental discriminatory treatment under the law. In most cases, skin color is irrelevant and attempts to classify according to race are properly suspect.[87]

The ability to bear children is to sex discrimination what dark skin is to race discrimination. It is the immutable characteristic that distinguishes the disadvantaged from the advantaged and which historically has been used to justify the subordination of the disadvantaged. Yet the similarly situated model designed for race is simply inappropriate in cases of sex discrimination.[88] In the case of sex, it is a *dis*similar situation[89] that has been used to erect and justify a system of male dominance. By dismissing claims of sex discrimination on the grounds that the sexes are differently situated in matters of reproduction, the Court rationalizes differential treatment of the sexes as legitimate and as merely "reflecting" the fact of biological difference. In fact, it is society's *disvaluing* of that difference, and not its mere existence, that has created the existing inequalities between the sexes.[90]

---

86. Several leading scholars have written persuasively in support of such an anti-caste approach. *See* Black, *The Lawfulness of the Segregation Decisions*, 69 YALE L.J. 421 (1960); Dimond, *The Anti-Cast Principle—Toward a Constitutional Standard for Review of Race Cases*, 30 WAYNE L. REV. 1 (1983); Fiss, *Groups and the Equal Protection Clause*, 5 PHIL. & PUB. AFF. 107 (1976).

87. There may be some relatively rare instances where blacks and whites are not similarly situated in some sense, as, for example, when there exist statistical differences between the races that might be useful for determining insurance rates. Race remains an impermissible basis for classification in these cases, despite its relevance, as a result of our larger commitment to securing equality. In cases of affirmative action, on the other hand, differential treatment on the basis of an otherwise forbidden classification is permitted because its object is to reduce the targeted harm.

88. For insightful discussions of the shortcomings of current equal protection analysis as applied to sex, see Law, *Rethinking Sex and the Constitution*, 132 U. PA. L. REV. 955 (1984); C. MACKIN-NON, THE SEXUAL HARASSMENT OF WORKING WOMEN: A CASE OF SEX DISCRIMINATION 101–41 (1979).

89. The reproductive difference between the sexes is occasionally of great relevance and legitimately legally cognizable. Women's ability to bear children is essential to the survival of humankind and should be accomodated and rewarded. It is only when that ability is used to disadvantage women that it is an impermissible basis for legal action. *See* Law, *supra* note 88, at 1007–40; Note, *Employment Equality Under the Pregnancy Discrimination Act of 1978*, 94 YALE L.J. 929, 929–30 (1985) (arguing Title VII as amended by Pregnancy Discrimination Act requires "not only comparable treatment [for female employees], but that measure of institutional accomodation necessary to bear children without forfeiture of employment opportunites").

90. Although the reproductive difference is the one significant biological difference between the sexes, as is frequently observed, "women's reproductive situation is never the result of biology alone, but of biology mediated by social and cultural organization." R. PETCHESKY, ABORTION AND WO-MAN'S CHOICE 5 (1984). *See also* S. DE BEAUVOIR, THE SECOND SEX 3–41 (1974).

Not only does the Court refuse to recognize equality claims based on reproductive difference, it also continues to confuse socially-created, sex-based stereotypes with natural, biological differences between the sexes. *See, e.g.*, Michael M. v. Superior Court, 450 U.S. 464 (1981) (upholding California's statutory rape law making it criminal for any man, regardless of age, to have sex with minor woman, but imposing no penalties on women for having sex with minor men); Parham v. Hughes, 441 U.S. 347 (1979) (upholding statute that permitted unmarried mothers to bring tort claims for wrong-

Women's Rights/Fetal Rights

State and social regulations concerning reproductive differences have served to create and reinforce separate and unequal sex-segregated spheres in the United States. Women's ability to bear children has been used to systematically disadvantage women by defining their "proper" role in terms of that ability. Social determinations concerning the reproductive difference underlie our present patriarchal society in which men and male norms have dominated the "public" sphere, the locus of political and economic power, while women have been relegated to the "private" sphere, where they provide the socially-necessary but socially-unrewarded work of care for children and home.[91] Conformity to prescribed sex roles has been accomplished through the imposition of economic, social and legal constraints, such as protectionist legislation. For example, in the past the Court has upheld restrictions placed on the hours women could work, citing a "public interest" in protecting the well-being of the fetus.[92] The Court has also upheld the exclusion of women from the legal profession, citing the "wide difference in the respective spheres and destinies of men

---

ful death of their children but denied unmarried fathers the right to bring such claims); *see also* Law, *supra* note 88, at 987-1002. Law writes that these "cases illustrate more than the Court's consistent confusion of biology with the social consequences of biology. They also demonstate the breakdown in current sex equality doctrine that occurs when the Court reviews a classification that, in its view, is based upon biological differences." *Id.* at 1001.

The Court also trivializes the impact on women's lives of laws that use women's biology in ways that disadvantage them. In failing to recognize the equality interests raised by the social treatment of the reproductive difference, the Court acts as if "women need only be treated as persons when they are not engaged in their childbearing function." Scales, *Towards a Feminist Jurisprudence*, 56 INDIANA L.J. 375, 398 (1981).

> By so doing, the Court ignores the effects of centuries of such disadvantaging. Women cannot be separated thus from their reproductive capacity, and laws that disadvantage women on the basis of that difference inevitably will affect all aspects of their lives. Because pregnancies occur in women's bodies, the continued possibility of an 'unwanted' pregnancy affects women in a very specific sense, not only as potential bearers of fetuses but also in their capacity to enjoy sexuality and maintain health. A woman's right to decide on abortion, and, it follows, on childbearing issues when her health and sexual self-determination are at stake is 'nearly allied to her right to be.' Reproduction affects women as women; it transcends class divisions and penetrates everything: work, political and community involvements, sexuality, creativity, and dreams.

R. PETCHESKY, *supra* at 5.

91. *See generally* Z. EISENSTEIN, FEMINISM AND SEXUAL EQUALITY: CRISIS IN LIBERAL AMERICA 87-113 (1984).

92. In *Muller v. Oregon*, the Court upheld a statute that restricted the hours women could work but did not place similar restrictions on men. The Court used as a rationale for this differential and clearly disadvantageous treatment a "public interest" in protecting the well-being of the fetus through preserving the health of women:

> That woman's physical structure and the performance of maternal functions place her at a disadvantage in the struggle for subsistence is obvious. This is especially true when the burdens of motherhood are upon her. Even when they are not, by abundant testimony of the medical fraternity continuance for a long time on her feet at work, repeating this from day to day, tends to injurious effects upon the body, and as healthy mothers are essential to vigorous offspring, the physical well- being of woman becomes an object of public interest and care in order to preserve the strength and vigor of the race.

208 U.S. 412, 421 (1908).

The Yale Law Journal   Vol. 95: 599, 1986

and women."[93] The "burdens necessarily borne by women for the preservation of the race" were even used as an excuse to justify exempting women from paying poll taxes if they "chose" not to vote, thus discouraging women from participating in the political process.[94] More recently, the Court upheld a statute exempting all women from compulsory jury duty in recognition of women's "special responsibilities" in the home.[95]

The social and legal treatment accorded women's reproductive capacity will inevitably shape the status of women in the United States. Despite the Court's pronouncements to the contrary, laws that disadvantage people on the basis of pregnancy disadvantage only women. Given that women's ability to bear children historically has served as the primary justification for denying women equality, courts should scrutinize with particular care laws that deal with matters of reproduction to ensure that they do not operate to the detriment of women. Equal protection doctrine should incorporate the approach advocated by Professor Sylvia Law. Law proposes that "laws governing reproductive biology be scrutinized by courts to ensure that (1) the law has no significant impact in perpetuating either the oppression of women or culturally imposed sex-role constraints on individual freedom or (2) if the law has this impact, it is justified as the best means of serving a compelling state purpose."[96]

Granting rights to fetuses in a manner that conflicts with women's autonomy reinforces the tradition of disadvantaging women on the basis of their reproductive capability. By subjecting women's decisions and actions during pregnancy to judicial review, the state simultaneously questions women's abilities and seizes women's rights to make decisions essential to

---

93. In *Bradwell v. Illinois*, the Court upheld a decision by the Supreme Court of Illinois to prohibit women from practicing law, relying on the "natural" differences between the sexes:
> [T]he civil law, as well as nature herself, has always recognized a wide difference in the respective spheres and destinies of man and woman . . . . The constitution of the family organization, which is founded in the divine ordinance, as well as in the nature of things, indicates the domestic sphere as that which properly belongs to the domain and functions of womanhood . . . . [T]he paramount destiny and mission of women are to fulfill the noble and benign offices of wife and mother. This is the law of the Creator. And the rules of civil society must be adapted to the general constitution of things.

83 U.S. 130, 141–42 (1873) (Bradley, J., concurring).

94. "In view of burdens necessarily borne by them for the preservation of the race, the State reasonably may exempt [women] from poll taxes." Breedlove v. Suttles, 302 U.S. 277, 282 (1937).

95. Hoyt v. Florida, 368 U.S 57, 62 (1961). The Florida statute in question exempted all women from jury duty unless they registered with the clerk a desire to be placed on the jury list. This exclusion resulted in only 220 women volunteering for jury duty in a county with approximately 46,000 registered female voters in the year 1957. *Id.* at 64. Despite this great discrepancy, the Court, noting that "woman is still regarded as the center of home and family life," held that the state constitutionally could permit women to determine if jury duty was consistent with their own "special responsibilities." *Id.* at 62.

96. Law, *supra* note 88, at 1008–09. Law says further: "Given how central state regulation of biology has been to the subjugation of women, the normal presumption of constitutionality is inappropriate and the state should bear the burden of justifying its rule in relation to either proposition." *Id.* at 1009.

Women's Rights/Fetal Rights

their very personhood. The rationale behind using fetal rights laws to control the actions of women during pregnancy is strikingly similar to that used in the past to exclude women from the paid labor force and to confine them to the "private" sphere. Fetal rights could be used to restrict pregnant women's autonomy in both their personal and professional lives, in decisions ranging from nutrition to employment, in ways far surpassing any regulation of the actions of competent adult men. The state would thus define women in terms of their childbearing capacity, valuing the reproductive difference between women and men in such a way as to render it impossible for women to participate as full members of society.[97] In light of the great threat to women's right to equality posed by legal recognition of the fetus, the state should bear the burden of ensuring that any law granting fetal rights does not disadvantage women or in any way infringe on the autonomy of pregnant women.

---

97. In discussing the potential effects of an amendment to the U.S. Constitution that would label the fetus a legal person under the Constitution, one commentator has noted:

[Women] might be required to lead less active life-styles in order to preserve the life of a conceptus (or possible conceptus). The interests of the conceptus will often diverge from those of the woman in such matters. From the standpoint of the conceptus, a passive carrier who exposes it to the minimum risk of miscarriage or prenatal injury is preferred. She should not smoke, drink, or use any drugs with possible adverse effects on the conceptus. Skiing, working in hazardous environments, flying, and riding in automobiles might be prohibited for such women in order to minimize possible adverse effects on the conceptus. Indeed, the Victorian regime for upper-class pregnant women that minimizes activities either inside or outside the home might be ideal.

Westfall, *supra* note 27, at 111. Another commentator noted that, in addition to the above, "maternal discretion to . . . engage in immoderate exercise or sexual intercourse . . . or reside at high altitudes for a prolonged period might be limited." Parness, *supra* note 27, at 500. Such restrictions might not be limited to pregnant women, but might be extended to all women as "potentially pregnant": "Restricting the activities of potentially pregnant women might similarly be justified on the ground that such classification is necessary to protect the conceptus during the period between conception and proof of pregnancy." Westfall, *supra* note 27, at 111.

[11]

Hastings Center Report, February/March 1988

Angela C was a twenty-eight-year old married woman who was approximately twenty-six weeks pregnant. She had suffered from cancer since she was thirteen years old, but had been in remission for approximately two years before she became pregnant. The pregnancy was planned, and she very much looked forward to the birth. Her health seemed reasonably good until about the twenty-fifth week of pregnancy, when she was admitted to George Washington University Hospital, and a tumor was found in her lung.

Within a few days the physicians determined that her condition was terminal and she would die within weeks. At approximately 4:00 p.m. on June 15, 1987, she was told that she might die much sooner. Because her fetus would have a much better chance to be born healthy at twenty-eight weeks or more gestation, she agreed to treatment that might help her survive longer, but insisted that her own care and comfort be primary.

Ms. C's husband, her mother, and her physicians agreed that keeping her comfortable while she died was what she wanted and that her wishes should be honored. The next morning this information was communicated to hospital administration. Legal counsel was consulted, who decided to consult the university's outside counsel. Outside counsel asked a judge to come to the hospital to decide what to do.

The Hearing

Judge Emmett Sullivan of the District of Columbia Superior Court summoned volunteer lawyers, and with a police escort rushed to the hospital where he set up "court." Legal counsel was, of course, present for the hospital. In addition, lawyers were appointed to represent Ms. C, and her fetus, and the judge invited the District of Columbia Corporation Counsel to participate as well. The

George J. Annas is Utley Professor of Health Law and Chief, Health Law Section, Boston University Schools of Medicine and Public Health.

She's Going to Die: The Case of Angela C

by George J. Annas

lawyer for the hospital opened the proceeding:

[T]he apparent desire of the patient and her family is that if the patient is to die, that no intervention be done on behalf of the fetus.... The hospital is seeking declaratory relief from the court to direct the hospital as to what it should do in terms of the fetus, whether to intervene and save its life.

The lawyer for the fetus expressed the view that the fetus was "a probably viable fetus, presumptively viable fetus, age twenty-six weeks," and that the court's task was to "balance" the interests of the fetus "with whatever life is left for the fetus's mother...." Ms. C's lawyer argued simply that she opposed surgical intervention to remove the fetus.

Her attending physician, Louis Hamner, testified that Ms. C had agreed to have the child at twenty-eight weeks, but that because the odds of a major handicap were much higher at twenty-six weeks gestation, she did not want the fetus delivered earlier. He said Ms. C was heavily sedated, and would likely die within twenty-four hours.

A neonatologist testified hypothetically, having "had no direct involvement with the mother or the family." She strongly supported intervention on the basis that for any individual fetus, survival and morbidity are "very difficult to predict." When pressed she put the likelihood of fetal viability at 50 to 60 percent and the risk of serious handicap at less than 20 percent.

The patient's mother testified that the previous day, after her daughter had been informed that her condition was terminal, she said, "I only want to die, just give me something to get me out of this pain."

Hospital counsel then asked the court to decide "what medical care, if any, should be performed for the benefit of the fetus of [Ms. C]." The lawyers' arguments focused not on what Ms. C wanted or even on her best interests, but on the best interests of the fetus and on Ms. C's terminal condition. The lawyer for the fetus, for example, urged that a cesarean be performed because, "sadly, the life of the mother is lost to us no matter what decision is made at this point." Ms. C's lawyer, on the other hand, argued the case on the basis of Ms. C's wishes, noting (correctly) that "we can't order abortions even to protect the post-viability and potentiality of life if a woman objects." The lawyer for the District of Columbia argued that Ms. C's interests need not concern the court because of the "sad fact" that "the mother will die regardless of what we do...." A subsequent exchange between Ms. C's lawyer and Judge Sullivan captures the essence of the hearing:

Mr. Sylvester: As I see this, as I understand the medical testimony, if we were to do a C-section on this woman in a very weakened medical state, we would in effect be terminating her life, and I can't—

The Court: She's going to die, Mr. Sylvester.

Hastings Center Report, February/March 1988

The lawyer for the fetus concluded: "All we are arguing is the state's obligation to rescue a potential life from a dying mother." The judge took a short recess and then issued his opinion orally. The decisive consideration was Ms. C's terminal condition: "The uncontroverted medical testimony is that Angela will probably die within the next twenty-four to forty-eight hours." He did "not clearly know what Angela's present views are" respecting the cesarean section, but found that the fetus had a 50 to 60 percent chance to survive and a less than 20 percent chance for serious handicap. The judge concluded: "It's not an easy decision to make, but given the choices, the court is of the view the fetus should be given an opportunity to live." He cited only one case, an unreported 1986 opinion from the District of Columbia Court of Appeals (the only case anyone present had a copy of). That case was based in large part on dicta from a New Jersey case that had previously been largely overruled and was, in any event, easily distinguishable.

After the Hearing

Shortly after the court recessed at 4:15 p.m., Hamner informed Ms. C of the decision. Ms. C was on a ventilator, but was able to mouth agreement. The court reconvened upon learning that Ms. C was awake and communicating.

The chief of obstetrics, Alan Weingold, reported a more recent discussion with the patient in which she "clearly communicated" and after being informed that Hamner would only do the cesarean section if she consented to it, "very clearly mouthed words several times, I don't want it done. I don't want it done." Hamner confirmed this exchange. Weingold concluded:

I think she's in contact with reality, clearly understood who Dr. Hamner was. Because of her attachment to him wanted him to perform the surgery. Understood he would not unless she consented and did not consent. This is, in my mind, very clear evidence that she is responding, understanding, and is capable of making such decisions.

The judge indicated that he was still not sure what her intent was. Counsel for the District of Columbia then suggested that her current refusal did not change anything because the entire proceeding had been premised on the belief that she was refusing to consent. In his words, "I don't think we would be here if she had said she wants it." The judge concurred, and reaffirmed his original order.

The Appeal

Less than an hour later three judges heard by telephone a request for stay of at least fifteen minutes so that arguments could be heard. Ms. C's lawyer told the judges that the cesarean section had been scheduled for 6:30 p.m., which gave them approximately sixteen minutes to hear arguments and make a decision. He argued that the cesarean section would likely end Ms. C's life, and that it was unconstitutional to favor the life of the fetus over that of the mother without the mother's consent. The lawyer for the fetus argued that Ms. C had no important interests in this decision because she was dying; "unintended consequences on the mother" are "insignificant in respect to the mother's very short life expectancy." The state's interest, she said, "overrides any interest in the mother's continued very short life, which is under heavy medication and very short duration."

A discussion ensued about the possibility of the fetus surviving, which the chief judge cut short by asking: "Let me ask you this, if it's relevant at all. Obviously the fetus has a better chance than the mother?" The lawyer for the fetus responded, "Obviously. Right." A few minutes later, the court denied the request for a stay, reserving the right to file an opinion at a later date. The proceeding was concluded at 6:40 p.m.

What Went Wrong?

The cesarean section was performed and the nonviable fetus died approximately two hours later. Ms. C, now confronted with both recovery from major surgery and the knowledge of her child's death, died approximately two days later. Five months later the Court of Appeals issued its written opinion (*In re A.C.,* D.C. Ct. Appeals, No. 87-609, Nov. 10, 1987). The opinion reads more like a Hallmark sympathy card. Its first paragraph, for example, concludes: "Condolences are extended to those who lost the mother and child." The court acknowledged that its opinion might "reasonably" be seen as "self-justifying" and then went on to rationalize the denial of the stay.

The opinion rests on a number of false assumptions. The most serious error is the statement that "as a matter of law, the right of a woman to an abortion is different and distinct from her obligations to the fetus once she has decided not to timely terminate her pregnancy." This is incorrect as both a factual and legal matter. Ms. C never "decided not to timely terminate her pregnancy," and because of her fetus's effect on her health, under *Roe v. Wade* she could have authorized her pregnancy to be terminated (to protect her health) at any time prior to her death. In essence, the court forced Ms. C to have an abortion prior to her death, doing so on the false premise that a terminal diagnosis strips a pregnant woman of her constitutional rights.

The second basis for the opinion is that a parent cannot refuse treatment necessary to save the life of a child (true) and therefore a pregnant woman cannot refuse treatment necessary to save the life of her fetus (false). The child must be treated because parents have obligations to act in the "best interests" of their children (as defined by child neglect laws), and treatment in no way compromises the bodily integrity of the parents. Fetuses, however, are not independent persons, and cannot be treated without invading the mother's body. There are no "fetal neglect" statutes, and it is unlikely that any could withstand constitutional scrutiny. Treating the fetus against the will of the mother degrades and dehumanizes the mother and treats her as an inert container. This *is* acceptable once the mother is dead, but is never acceptable when the mother is alive. The court seems to understand this, at least at the instinctive level, and thus ultimately justified its opinion on the basis that Ms. C was as good as dead and had no "good health" to be "sacrificed." "The cesarean section would not significantly affect A.C.'s condition because she had, at best, two days of sedated life...." But this reasoning will not do. It would, for example, permit the involuntary removal of vital organs prior to death when they were needed to "save a life." But if the child had already been born, no court (not even this one) would require its mother to undergo major surgery for its sake (for example, a kidney "donation") no matter how dire the potential consequences of refusal to the child. And certainly no court would ever require the father of a child to undergo surgery, even to save the child's life. The ultimate rationale for the decision may be purely sexist: this situation could never apply to males like these judges; they are unable to identify with the pregnant woman and thus need not concern themselves about the future application of their decision to themselves.

This is a cavalierly lawless and unprincipled opinion that merits condemnation and reversal. The proper question the opinion poses is not whether the patient was competent, but whether the lawyers and judges were competent. What went wrong with the judicial process? At least three things: (1) the emergency nature of the hearing and the question asked of the judge; (2) the refusal to recognize the patient as a person with rights; and (3) the self-justifying nature of the appeals court's opinion.

This case illustrates the general rule that judges should never go to the hospital to make emergency treatment decisions. First, judges know nothing about treatment decisions. Judges can render an opinion about the lawfulness of a proposed course of treatment or nontreatment (although even this is seldom needed). But to ask judges to make the treatment decision to protect the hospital from some speculative potential liability simply invites them to play doctor; something they might enjoy, but something about which judges possess no more competence than the average person on the street. Rushed to an unfamiliar environment, asked to make a decision under great stress, and having no time either for reflection or to study existing law and precedents, a judge cannot act

judiciously. Facts cannot be properly developed and the law cannot be accurately determined or fairly applied to the facts. The "emergency hearing" scenario invites arbitrariness.

[The judges] treated a live woman as though she were already dead, forced her to undergo an abortion, and then justified their brutal and unprincipled opinion on the basis that she was almost dead and her fetus's interests in life outweighed any interest she might have in her own life or health.

The only reason a judge should ever go to a hospital is to determine the competence of a patient. This *is* a proper judicial task. Thus it is astonishing that the judge never even bothered to go the short distance to her hospital room to talk directly with Ms. C. The reason, of course, is that he viewed her simply as an inanimate container and so didn't care what the container's wishes were; this is what makes the decision so offensive. Angela C was legally presumed competent, did not consent to the surgical intervention, and surgery was ultimately performed over her express objection. She was totally dehumanized, her wishes and best interests ignored.

Finally, the appeals court did not act like an appeals court. It initially heard brief arguments over the phone and made a snap decision. It did not wait for the "trial" judge to write a more formal opinion before issuing its own; did not hear or invite arguments from the parties; and ultimately wrote a "self-justifying" opinion instead of a neutral and fair rendering of the law.

When asked how he would make decisions on the U.S. Supreme Court in his confirmation hearings, Judge Anthony Kennedy replied that he

would carefully consider all of the facts, listen to the legal arguments, review all of the legal precedents, and then reflect long and hard about the case and how to apply the law to the facts properly to arrive at a fair and just opinion. Many commentators were disappointed in this response, noting that it was just a summary of what judges do. In fact, it is a summary of what judges *should do*, but unfortunately does not in any way reflect what the judges involved in Ms. C's case did. They treated a live woman as though she were already dead, forced her to undergo an abortion, and then justified their brutal and unprincipled opinion on the basis that she was almost dead and her fetus's interests in life outweighed any interest she might have in her own life or health. This is what happens when judges (and hospital lawyers that call them) forget what judging is all about and combine rescue fantasy with dehumanization of the dying.

This was *not* a hard case. The patient's wishes should have been honored. If there really were facts in dispute, a case conference involving the patient, family, and all attending health care personnel could have been held to assess them. Direct communication with the patient is almost always the most useful and constructive response to "problems" like those presented by this case. Calling a judge was a counterproductive panic reaction.

[12]

J. K. Mason

Unwanted Pregnancy: A Case of Retroversion?

Perhaps the main reason why the judgment of the House of Lords in *McFarlane* v *Tayside Health Board*[1] has provoked such interest lies in the wonder that it ever happened. The great majority of those engaged in the study of medical jurisprudence would have regarded the decision of the Lord Ordinary in the Outer House[2] as a unique exception to the established precedents which would be reversed on appeal.[3] The action in delict, which was one based on the unwanted birth of a child as a result of alleged negligence on the part of the defenders, developed according to that script until, with an unexpected twist, it transpired that the case was to be heard in the House of Lords.

An unexpected twist? Possibly but, at the same time, understandable. As Lord Slynn was to say later:

> Although these judgments refer to the law of Scotland . . . it is as I understand it accepted that the law of England and that of Scotland should be the same in respect of the matters which arise on this appeal. It would be strange, even absurd, if they were not.[4]

No comparable English cases had been referred to the highest legal tribunal. Here, then, was an opportunity to establish the law in such a way that it was not only clarified but was, at the same time, harmonised throughout Great Britain.

But, as in any good drama, peripety is reserved for the third act. In the event, the House agreed that the movement in England and Scotland has been towards allowing damages not only for the pain and distress of an unplanned pregnancy and birth but also for the cost of rearing the resultant child. Yet, when it came to the point, the latter was rejected unanimously as a tenable principle. The purpose of this note is to examine the reasons for what is, at first glance, a remarkable *volte face*.

A. THE PRECEDENTS

All five Law Lords considered the early precedents derived from litigation in the United States and the Commonwealth. None found them particularly helpful and, in any event, "the discipline of comparative law does not aim at a poll of the solutions adopted in different countries".[5] The present writer believes that, by a process of

---

1 2000 SLT 154; [1999] 4 All ER 96.
2 *McFarlane* v *Tayside Health Board* 1997 SLT 211. It is only fair to add that Lord Gill had powerful support: e.g. P S Atiyah, *The Damages Lottery* (1997), 54.
3 *McFarlane* v *Tayside Health Board* 1998 SLT 307.
4 2000 SLT 154 at 158.
5 Per Lord Steyn, 2000 SLT 154 at 164. Admittedly, some opinions referred to the "overwhelming majority of US jurisdictions" as rejecting claims for the cost of bringing up the child, but few of the appellate decisions have been unanimous, and many of them contain powerful and persuasive dissenting judgments (per Lord Millett at 179).

judicious selection of decisions, almost any "solution" to the problems posed can be derived from overseas jurisdictions and, particularly, from the United States. By contrast, the House recognised the clarity of the trend in the United Kingdom towards allowing damages for births associated with negligent contraceptive surgery. As a result, it is proposed, here, to limit a constructed analysis of the precedents to those of the British jurisdictions.[6]

Udale v *Bloomsbury Area Health Authority* is not, chronologically speaking, the first relevant British case. But, in outlining the circumstances of the case, Jupp J said:

> Fortunately or unfortunately, she gave birth to a normal healthy boy. . . . The phrase "fortunately or unfortunately" encapsulates the most part of the legal argument which has surrounded the plaintiff's claim for damages.[7]

Udale, thus, grasped the nettle firmly at a very early stage in the development of the law in this area and can be looked upon as the index case. The circumstances were relatively simple. Mrs Udale underwent a sterilising operation but, nonetheless, conceived a fifth child. After a stormy start, she came to terms with her pregnancy and was delivered of a healthy boy who was received into the family with love and affection. In due course, she sued the Area Health Authority under what have now come to be seen as relatively standard headings—for the pain and suffering associated with pregnancy and childbirth, for associated loss of earnings and, of major importance in the current context, for the upkeep of the child until its majority.

In the event, Jupp J rejected all these—and on grounds which have, again, become standard bases for argument. These included the disadvantage to the child who later found that he had been rejected; the fact that to offset the joys of parenthood against the economic damage sustained would mean that virtue went unrewarded, while the "unnatural rejection of womanhood and motherhood would be generously compensated"; that doctors would be under pressure to arrange abortions; and, finally, having directed us to the Gospel of St John,[8] that:

> It has been the assumption of our culture from time immemorial that a child coming into the world, even if, as some say, "the world is a vale of tears", is a blessing and a reason for rejoicing.[9]

Jupp J's decision was avowedly based on public policy and depended very much on the reasoning in the barely relevant "wrongful life" case of *McKay* v *Essex Area Health Authority*.[10] In the instant case, he concluded that: "on the grounds of public policy, the plaintiff's claims . . . insofar as they are based on negligence which allowed David Udale to come into this world alive, should not be allowed".[11] Even so, damages in respect of pain and suffering and of the necessary extensions to the plaintiffs' house were allowed—this being largely because doing so did not imply rejection of the child.

---

6 The court in *McFarlane* derived particular benefit from A Stewart, "Damages for the birth of a child" (1995) 40 *Journal of the Law Society of Scotland* 298, which should be consulted.
7 [1983] 2 All ER 522 at 523.
8 John 16.21.
9 At 531.
10 *McKay* v *Essex Area Health Authority* [1982] QB 1166.
11 At 531.

However, Peter Pain J who, in his own words, firmly put sentiment on one side, was unable to see the logic of this in the closely following case of *Thake v Maurice*.[12] The award of damages was, to him, an all or nothing reaction—and he chose the all. He used the powerful words:

> [E]very baby has a belly to be filled and a body to be clothed. The law relating to damages is concerned with reparation in money terms and this is what is needed for the maintenance of a baby.[13]

Thus he proposed an award of damages not only for the pain and suffering attending an unexpected pregnancy and birth but also for the child's support. He would not, however, go the whole way and conceded that there must be some offset as measured by the joy of having a healthy child. In order to circumvent the injustice anticipated by Jupp J, he balanced this against the sorrows of pregnancy and childbirth, rather than against the economic costs of rearing the child. This solution was, however, rejected on appeal,[14] with the result that damages under both these heads could be awarded without offset.

Meantime, however, the other major English case, *Emeh v Kensington and Chelsea and Westminster Area Health Authority*,[15] was weaving its way through the courts in the manner of a double helix. Here, however, the issues were rather different and arose, primarily, from the fact that the trial judge regarded the refusal to abort a physically abnormal child as a *novus actus interveniens*—a problem that is discussed below. Even so, the Court of Appeal specifically rejected the concept of there being a public policy objection to the award of damages for the negligent conception and birth of a healthy, as opposed to a congenitally abnormal, child.[16]

As Slade LJ put it:

> In these circumstances [a negligent operation], it seems to me clear that the loss suffered by the plaintiff as a result of the defendant's negligence would be any reasonably foreseeable financial loss directly caused by the unexpected pregnancy, and the subsequent birth of her child.

Or:

> If a woman wants to be sterilised, I can see no reason why, under public policy, she should not recover such financial damage as she can prove she has sustained by the surgeon's negligent failure to perform the operation properly whether or not the child is healthy.[17]

Emeh has been generally regarded as representing the English law in this area,[18] but it is only fair to point out that the House of Lords in *McFarlane* accepted this analysis with more than a little scepticism. *Emeh* was, for example, concerned with

---

12 [1986] QB 644.
13 At 666.
14 Per Kerr LJ, [1986] QB 644 at 683.
15 *The Times*, 3 Jan 1983 (QBD), [1985] QB 1012 (CA).
16 Per Waller LJ at 1022.
17 Per Slade LJ at 1025. The court also rejected the variation on "offset" that, in the event of the child being handicapped, the damages awarded should be those for rearing that child less the costs of bringing up a normal child.
18 "It is the critical decision in the line of authority in England" per Lord Steyn, 2000 SLT 154 at 163. See also E J Russell, "Is parenthood always an 'unblemished blessing' in every case?" 1998 SLT (News) 191.

the birth of a congenitally disabled child and it was suggested that the arguments presented in the case were, perhaps, less than ideal. Moreover, Lord Hope considered that the authorities relied on in *Emeh* were of doubtful status.[19] Even so, *Emeh* has founded Scottish decisions in the Outer House,[20] and there is nothing in the several later cases cited in the House of Lords to suggest that it had been displaced—at least in a *de facto* sense.

As Butler-Sloss LJ intimated in one such case,[21] these issues are often difficult to evaluate entirely unemotionally. For this reason, the present writer attaches considerable importance to the unusual case of *Walkin* v *South Manchester Health Authority*.[22] Here the question was couched simply in terms of the application of the English Limitation Act 1980, s 11—did the expenses and tribulations of rearing the child form part of the personal injury[23] resulting from negligence giving rise to an unwanted pregnancy or did they not? Auld LJ was in no doubt:

> In my view, it clearly did. It is true . . . that the claim depended on the birth of the child, but the birth was not an intervening act; it was caused by the personal injury, namely the unwanted pregnancy.[24]

Neill LJ summarised thus: "There is one cause of action which arises at the moment of conception."[25]

It is concluded that, until *McFarlane* had run its course, an award of damages for the upkeep of an unexpected—albeit not, eventually, unwanted—child was acceptable under both English and Scots law.

B. THE PRESENT CASE

The present case arose from a vasectomy performed on Mr McFarlane in October 1989. In March 1990, having undergone the necessary tests, he was informed that his sperm count was negative and that he could safely resume sexual intercourse without contraceptive measures. Mrs McFarlane, who already had four children, became pregnant in September 1991 and was delivered of a healthy female child in May 1992. The child was subsequently admitted as a loved and integral member of the family.

An action in negligence was raised against the Health Board. The claim was in two parts. The first, later described by Lord Hope as the "mother's" claim, was in respect

---

19 While the present writer fully agrees that the importance attached to *Sherlock* v *Stillwater Clinic* (1977) 260 NW 2d 169 by several courts in the United Kingdom is disproportionate, it is to be noted that Purchas LJ quoted the case only "to identify the problem, not to solve it". The same criticism might be levelled at the frequent reference to the "purely personal" opinion of Ognall J in *Jones* v *Berkshire Health Authority* QBD, unreported, 2 July 1986.

20 *Allan* v *Greater Glasgow Health Board* 1998 SLT 580; *Anderson* v *Forth Valley Health Board* 1998 SLT 588, a case which post-dated the Outer House decision in *McFarlane* (see note 2 above).

21 *Salih and another* v *Enfield Health Authority* (1991) 7 BMLR 1 at 4.

22 (1995) 25 BMLR 108.

23 Assuming, as this writer does, that a normal *unwanted* pregnancy can be regarded as an injury—a question which particularly concerned the Lord Ordinary in *McFarlane*.

24 At 116.

25 At 120.

of pain and suffering due to pregnancy and childbirth. The second, or "parents'",
claim was for the upkeep of the child until the age of majority.

The Lord Ordinary, Lord Gill, rejected both claims, concluding:

> In my view, a pregnancy occurring in the circumstances of this case cannot be equiparated
> with a physical injury. Pregnancy and labour are natural processes resulting in a happy
> outcome. . . . Even if otherwise, I do not consider that it is an injury for which damages are
> recoverable. I cannot see how [the happiness Mrs McFarlane has and will have] can either
> be disregarded altogether or be held not to outweigh the natural pain and discomfort in
> the creation of life. I am of the opinion that this case should be decided on the principle
> that the privilege of being a parent is immeasurable in money terms; that the benefits of
> parenthood transcend patrimonial loss . . . ; and that the parents in a case such as this
> cannot be said to be in a position of loss.[26]

The Inner House of the Court of Session then unanimously allowed a reclaiming
motion.[27] The reasons given by Lord Justice-Clerk Cullen can be summarised: the
defenders' contention that the costs of maintaining the child could not be due to
their negligence was unsustainable; it was unwarrantable to assume that the birth of
a child was a blessing in every case; the principle that the value of a child outweighed
its costs was not one that was recognised in Scots law; and there were no overriding
considerations of public policy that would be contravened by awarding damages to
the pursuers.

All three judges, as particularly carefully explained by Lord McCluskey,[28] agreed
that the concurrence of *iniuria* (in this case the provision of incorrect information)
and *damnum* (prejudice to the McFarlanes' legitimate interests in not having any
more children) derived from conception and pregnancy and provided grounds for an
action for reparation—and the costs of rearing the child flowed directly from her
conception. It may be noted that, as Lord McCluskey demonstrated, there is no
satisfactory English equivalent of the Scots concept of *damnum*; thus, while it is
clearly correct to invoke *damnum* in the Scots law of delict, it does, at the same time,
neatly sidestep the English difficulty of equating a natural process such as pregnancy
with a "personal injury".[29]

The Health Authority then appealed to the House of Lords, the bench consisting
of Lords Slynn, Steyn, Hope, Clyde and Millett. In the event, the appeal was allowed
unanimously in respect of the parents' claim for costs of the child's upbringing but
was dismissed as to the mother's *solatium* by a majority—Lord Millett dissenting.[30]

As described above, the McFarlanes' action in delict was in two parts. Even so, as
Lord Clyde put it, if the action was to any extent relevant, there was only one right of
action for the pursuers—a right which arose, if it did, at conception. Few people, if

---

26 1997 SLT 211 at 214 and 216.

27 Thus, negligence has, so far, never been admitted or proved. The defender's duty of care to the
pursuers was, however, admitted.

28 1998 SLT 307 at 313.

29 *Damnum*, as described by Lord McCluskey, means a loss in the sense of a material prejudice to an
interest that the law recognises as a legal interest (at 313).

30 It is somewhat ironic that the report on *McFarlane* in *The Times* of 26 Nov 1999 was juxtaposed
with the very similar case of *Nunnerley v Warrington Health Authority*. In that case the costs awarded
for the upkeep of a disabled child were not confined to those arising from the care which the
parents were under a legal duty to provide; the case may, however, be one involving wrongful birth.

any, can have qualms as to the mother's claim *per se* once negligence has been demonstrated.[31] Its validity will only be questioned when the two claims are taken as dependent upon each other. It is then possible to argue that it is illogical to accept the one without the other and that, accordingly, both should be denied if one is unacceptable—and this was the route taken by the Lord Ordinary and Lord Millett in the House of Lords in *McFarlane*.

The present writer finds it hard to understand why, given the same circumstances, it is not equally logical to hold that both claims should be upheld if one is found acceptable—and it will be seen that this form of argument arises at several points in the assessment of the case. Beyond this somewhat esoteric point, however, the mother's claim is regarded as unexceptional and the reader should understand that the remainder of this article is devoted solely to the joint claim for recovery of the costs involved in maintaining an unexpected, albeit healthy, child during its minority.

C. ASPECTS OF THE CASE

(1) The nature of the case

Before embarking on a discussion of the House of Lords' decision in *McFarlane*, it is important to clarify the nature of the action—which Lord Steyn, giving the second speech, describes as one for "wrongful birth".[32] With the greatest respect, I do not believe that this is how the majority of commentators would regard it.

Certainly it is an action brought by the parents for harm that is done to them, but such actions can be divided into two types.[33] The classic "wrongful birth" action results from a failure to advise a termination of pregnancy in the face of fetal abnormality which should have been discovered but which was not diagnosed until birth by reason of negligent ante-natal care. *Anderson* v *Forth Valley Health Board*[34] is a recent Scottish example. However, cases of the present type, which derive from failure of the sterilisation process, are often described, particularly in the American jurisdictions, as actions for "wrongful conception",[35] and this was Lord Clyde's definition of the action.[36] Lord Clyde's assessment is to be preferred to that of Lord Steyn, although this writer prefers the term "wrongful pregnancy" to that of "wrongful conception", largely on the ground that "harm" results only following implantation; the woman may, indeed, be quite unaware, and never become aware, of a conception— that is, the union of male and female gametes—*per se*.[37]

The distinction between "wrongful birth" and "wrongful pregnancy" is important for several reasons. Firstly, the defender may well differ in the two cases. Thus, in a

---

31 The exception seems to have been Peter Pain J in *Thake*, note 12 above.

32 2000 SLT 154 at 162.

33 See J K Mason, "Wrongful pregnancy" in *The Laws of Scotland: Stair Memorial Encyclopaedia*, vol 15 (1996), para 305.

34 1998 SLT 588.

35 See, for example, *Sherlock* v *Stillwater Clinic*, note 19 above, as quoted by Lord Hope at 170.

36 2000 SLT 154 at 174.

37 Some commentators go further and distinguish a "wrongful conception" from a "wrongful pregnancy" when the former has been negatived by lawful termination. See B Dickens, "Wrongful birth and life, wrongful death before birth and wrongful law" in S A M McLean (ed), *Legal Issues in Human Reproduction* (1989), ch 4.

wrongful pregnancy case, action will be brought against the surgeon who performs the sterilisation operation, whether this be by way of doubtful expertise or of inadequate provision of information; the manager of the pregnancy, or even the laboratory technician, is far more likely to be found negligent in an action for wrongful birth. Secondly, the distinction may lie at the heart of—and go some way to explaining—the anomaly that results when damages for an unwanted birth are or are not awarded according to whether the neonate is handicapped or normal. Whereas *McFarlane* now tells us that no damages are to be awarded for maintenance of the latter child, Lord Steyn conceded that the rule might have to be different in the case of a child who was born seriously disabled.[38] The issue did not, however, arise in *McFarlane*, and the House declined to follow up the proposition. The widespread agreement that damages for upkeep are available in the former case, thus, remains undisturbed—yet the reasons for this are seldom convincing or, indeed, argued.

In seeking an explanation, it is important to appreciate that there are two ways in which the birth of a defective child can occur within the present context. In the first scenario, the woman is unexpectedly pregnant following contraceptive surgery; she goes through the modern ante-natal regime, is told that her fetus is healthy and resigns herself to a normal pregnancy. A defective child is born, and she claims that, but for the negligent advice as to the condition of the fetus, she would have sought a termination. It is now perfectly logical to award costs to cover the child's upkeep, despite the fact that they might not have been available had the neonate been healthy, for the action has become one for wrongful birth rather than one for wrongful pregnancy.[39] However, no such absolute distinction can be discerned if, in what may well be the more likely scenario, the child is born defective despite exemplary ante-natal management and because of the in-built hazards of fetal development. The only action then available is for wrongful pregnancy, within which normality and abnormality can be seen as variations within a continuum rather than as distinct entities: arguably, only the quantum of damages should be in doubt.[40] This, however, is an aspect of major significance to the discussion on "setting off" which follows below.

(2) Their Lordships' misgivings

It is easy to read too much into a written opinion. Yet, throughout the opinions, one senses a conflict within the minds of each member of the House, the probable reason for which lies in the interweave between the legal and the moral issues involved and the near impossibility of disentangling these. It is important to emphasise this crucial difficulty before embarking on a discussion of the case. We can do this by repeating some of the legal observations made by their Lordships which they were, in the end, unable to follow—presumably because of their moral misgivings.

38 2000 SLT 154 at 166.
39 There is, of course, no reason why, in such circumstances, actions for wrongful pregnancy and wrongful birth should not be raised in parallel, although the same Health Board would probably be responsible for both surgery and pregnancy management.
40 See Watkins J in *Sciuriaga* v *Powell* (1979) 123 Sol Jo 406; also *Salih* v *Enfield Health Authority*, note 21 above.

Thus, we have Lord Slynn, first, allowing without qualm the mother's claim for damages in respect of the pregnancy and birth itself. Turning, however, to the question of recovery of costs for the child's maintenance, he said:

> Logically, the position may seem to be the same. If she had not conceived because of the Board's negligence there would not have been a baby and then a child and then a young person to house, to feed and to educate.[41]

This is an observation which few would dispute. Yet, we will see that he was unable to pursue this logic to its logical conclusion.

In the same vein, we have Lord Steyn:

> It is possible to view the case simply from the perspective of corrective justice. It requires somebody who has harmed another without justification to indemnify the other. On this approach the parents' claim for the bringing up of Catherine must succeed.[42]

But he was, then, forced to an opposite conclusion on largely moral grounds.

And we have Lord Millett:

> The defenders do not admit that they were negligent . . . but they rightly concede that [the pregnancy and birth] were the direct and foreseeable consequences of the information [as to sterility] being wrong. Causation is not in issue.[43]

All this must leave us anxiously seeking their Lordships' reasons for refusing the recovery of the resultant costs.

D. THEIR LORDSHIPS' REASONS

Before discussing these, it will be convenient to dispose of some matters which the House rejected as being significant to their conclusions.

(1) *Novus actus interveniens*

Since the action for the upkeep of the unexpected child depends upon there being a child for which the parents are responsible,[44] it must be open to the defenders to hold that the parents could have solved the problem, either by lawful termination of pregnancy or by arranging for the neonate's adoption. This was accepted at first instance in *Emeh* where, as we have seen, Park J was of the opinion that the plaintiff's refusal to terminate the pregnancy was so unreasonable as to constitute a *novus actus interveniens*.[45]

This was forcefully rejected on appeal where Slade LJ considered that:

> The judge . . . was, I think, really saying that the defendants had the right to expect that, if they had not performed the operation properly, she would procure an abortion . . . I do not, for my part, think that the defendants had the right to expect any such thing.[46]

41 2000 SLT 154 at 161.
42 2000 SLT 154 at 165.
43 2000 SLT 154 at 178.
44 Children (Scotland) Act 1995, s 1; Family Law (Scotland) Act 1985, s 1(1)(c).
45 *The Times*, 3 Jan 1983. As a consequence, damages were awarded only for the discomfort associated with the first four months of pregnancy.
46 [1985] QB at 1024.

Slade LJ's approach has been followed almost universally—not least in the House of Lords in *McFarlane* where Lord Steyn, for example, was unable to conceive of any circumstances in which the decision of the parents not to resort even to a lawful abortion could be questioned.[47] Yet their Lordships, as a whole, gave little reason for their unanimity on the question. Lord Hope, while clearly wishing to play down the significance of the parental decision, was content to accept that they had no other choice.[48] Lord Clyde stated only that: "the decision to keep the child, to accept into the family a baby who was originally unwanted, cannot rank as an acting on the part of the pursuers sufficient to break the causal chain".[49] Lord Millett regarded the proposition that it is unreasonable for parents not to have an abortion or place a child for adoption as far more repugnant than the characterisation of the birth of a healthy and normal child as a detriment,[50] and the vast majority would agree with those sentiments.

But one has to ask whether it is so unreasonable to deny the concept of a *novus actus* to the defendants. The House of Lords quoted widely from the Australian case *CES v Superclinics (Australia) Pty Ltd* in which Priestly JA said:

> The point in the present case is that the plaintiff chose to keep her child. The anguish of having to make the choice is part of the damage caused by the negligent breach of duty, but the fact remains, however compelling the psychological pressure on the plaintiff may have been to keep the child, the opportunity of choice was in my opinion real and the choice made was voluntary. It was this choice which was the cause, in my opinion, of the subsequent cost of rearing a child . . . The plaintiff having chosen to keep the child in the human way that . . . I think most people in the community would approve of, is not entitled to damages for the financial consequences of having made that difficult but ordinary human choice.[51]

Lords Steyn and Millett were, in fact, the only Law Lords to discuss this aspect of causation in depth, and the latter even offered grudging support for this view. We are, however, effectively left to fend for ourselves in establishing why it is unacceptable. The primary reason, it is suggested, is that to hold otherwise would be to imply that abortion is available on demand in the United Kingdom and, while I have argued that this is the situation *de facto*,[52] it certainly cannot be seen as that *de jure*.[53] Secondly, the moral implications in electing for abortion are of such intensity and variety that it could scarcely be right to lay down a rule as to the legal implications of the decision reached. Thirdly, the circumstances are such that neither consent to nor refusal of abortion could be said to be unfettered and, therefore, truly valid. And, finally—and,

47 2000 SLT 154 at 164. This discussion of an aspect of "wrongful pregnancy" which particularly troubles the writer is, here, really of academic interest only as *novus actus* was not seriously argued in *McFarlane*.

48 2000 SLT 154 at 173.

49 2000 SLT 154 at 177.

50 2000 SLT 154 at 181.

51 (1995) 38 NSWLR 47 at 84–85. *CES* is certainly not on all fours with *McFarlane*. In the first place, it was an action for wrongful birth rather than wrongful pregnancy, and, secondly, New South Wales has no statute comparable to the Abortion Act 1967, the law being currently based on *R v Bourne* [1939] 1 KB 687. The case turned largely on whether an abortion would have been legal.

52 See, for example, J K Mason, *Medico-legal Aspects of Reproduction and Parenthood*, 2nd edn (1998), 116–117.

53 This may be the reason for Lord Hope saying that the parents had no other choice.

perhaps, most importantly—one must agree with Lord Steyn that the law does and must respect these decisions of parents which are so closely tied to their basic freedoms and rights of personal autonomy.[54]

Perhaps the last word may be left to Lord Millett:

> Catherine's conception and birth, and the restoration of the *status quo* by abortion or adoption, were the very things that the defenders were engaged to prevent. . . . The costs of bringing her up are no more remote than the costs of an abortion or adoption would have been. In each case the causal connection is strong, direct and foreseeable.[55]

(2) Public policy

Much of the reasoning in *McFarlane* is devoted to considerations of public policy. It might be assumed that for public policy reasons damages should not be awarded for the birth of a healthy child—albeit one conceived as a result of another's negligence. But, as Lord Clyde indicated, it is difficult to find any policy ground supporting one course of action without unearthing a countervailing consideration that points to the opposite conclusion. In the event, all five Law Lords were at pains to exclude public policy from their reasoning—the issue was to be settled by recourse to principle. The frequent difficulty is, however, to distinguish the two. If, for example, as Lord Slynn proposed, the question of whether reparation for the expenses incurred in the upbringing of a loved child is resolved by way of legal principle, it is not easy to distinguish the result from a formulated policy. Or where lies the difference between applying the principle of distributive justice and accepting that principle as a matter of policy—a distinction which Lord Steyn manages to make with ease?

(3) The principles accepted

Each of the five judges involved gave individual reasons in principle for allowing the defenders' appeal.[56]

Lord Slynn, pointing to the fact that the issue was one of the extent of liability, considered it neither fair, just nor reasonable to impose on the doctor "liability for the consequential responsibilities, imposed on or accepted by the parents to bring up a child".[57] A line is to be drawn before such losses are recoverable—but how fair, just or reasonable is it from the parents' point of view to do so? Lord Slynn did not comment on the question. He was, however, strongly supported by Lord Hope who, in addition, stressed that, in the absence of a threshold, liability could be stretched almost indefinitely so as to include, for example, the costs of a private education for the resultant child.[58] Lord Hope's reasons for rejecting *any* restitution are, however, less easy to accommodate:

---

54 It could be held that only the last two considerations apply to adoption. Nevertheless, they carry their own powerful reasoning.

55 2000 SLT 154 at 182.

56 It is interesting to note in another recent case that much the same arguments can be used, based upon Roman-Dutch law, to reach a different conclusion. See *Mukheiber* v *Raath and Raath* (Supreme Court of Appeal of South Africa, 1999, reported online at http://www.uovs.ac.za/law/appeals/).

57 2000 SLT 154 at 162, relying on *Caparo Industries plc* v *Dickman* [1990] 2 AC 605.

58 The case of *Benarr* v *Kettering Health Authority* [1988] NLJR 179, which was the first to allow such costs, has much to answer for as to its influence in *McFarlane*.

It cannot be established that, overall and in the long run, these costs [of meeting the obligations to the child during her childhood] will exceed the value of the benefits. This is economic loss of a kind which must be held to fall outside the ambit of the duty of care which was owed . . . by the persons who carried out the procedures in the hospital and the laboratory.[59]

One wonders why this constitutes a *sequitur*—and Lord Hope's analysis is considered again below.

Reasonableness as to the extent of liability was also considered by Lord Clyde, who believed that it includes an element of proportionality between the wrongdoing and the resulting loss suffered. Lord Clyde found it difficult to accept that, in a case such as *McFarlane*, there would be any reasonable relationship between the fault and the claim such as would "accord with the idea of restitution",[60] and he accepted that the expense of child rearing could be wholly disproportionate to the doctor's culpability—a reason for limiting liability which was, incidentally, specifically rejected by Lord Millett. Once again, it is possible to argue from the other side—that the costs to the McFarlanes were wholly disproportionate to those anticipated when they acted on advice to resume non-contraceptive sexual intercourse.

Lord Millett's analysis of the principles involved was, possibly, the most comprehensive but is also the most difficult to interpret.[61] The impression gained is that this is because he was the most anxious of the judges that the McFarlanes should "not go away empty handed". In the end, it was almost by a process of elimination that he finally concluded that the reason why the costs of bringing up the child should not be recoverable lay in the fact that the law must take the birth of a normal, healthy baby to be a blessing, not a detriment—in other words, he joined hands with Jupp J in *Udale* and Lord Gill in the Outer House in *McFarlane* in making what can only be seen, *pace* Lord Gill, as a policy decision. Lord Millett concluded:

It would be repugnant to [society's] own sense of values to do otherwise. It is morally offensive to regard a normal, healthy baby as more trouble and expense than it is worth.[62]

Lord Steyn almost hoed a row of his own in a direct appeal to distributive justice and, thereby, to the common man. It may, he said, become relevant to ask commuters on the Underground the following question:

Should the parents of an unwanted but healthy child be able to sue the doctor or the hospital for compensation equivalent to the cost of bringing up the child for the years of his or her minority—i.e. until about eighteen years?[63]

His view was that an overwhelming number of ordinary men and women would answer the question with an emphatic "no". Well—maybe; but very few of the commuters on the Underground are already striving to bring up four demanding children—and we will return to the commuter later on.

---

59 2000 SLT 154 at 173.
60 2000 SLT 154 at 177.
61 Lord Millett's distinction between the recovery of costs for, on the one hand, acquiring and, on the other, replacing a high chair is an interesting detail.
62 2000 SLT 154 at 182.
63 2000 SLT 154 at 165.

There are a number of other difficulties in Lord Steyn's approach. In the first place, he did not explain how justice was to be distributed in the present case. If pressed, he said, he would say that the claim did not satisfy the requirement of being fair, just and reasonable—but this is no explanation and, as we have seen, fairness depends very much on the viewpoint; it is not difficult to visualise the *McFarlane* decision as an example of distributive *in*justice. Secondly, he relied on the twin cases of *Alcock* v *Chief Constable of South Yorkshire Police*[64] and *Frost* v *Chief Constable of South Yorkshire Police*.[65] Both these cases can be seen as unsatisfying. One may have little sympathy for police officers who claim damages for carrying out duties for which they have been trained and paid; but the fact that others were ineligible does not constitute an adequate reason to deny them compensation. Thirdly, in a search for coherence, Lord Steyn quoted the case, and deprecated the result, of *McKay* v *Essex Area Health Authority*,[66] in which an action for damages by a child born handicapped was rejected while the parallel action by her mother was allowed to proceed[67]—and this was regarded as incoherent. However, these two actions are distinct entities. The former—for "wrongful life"—implies, *inter alia*, that the defective fetus has a right to be killed, a proposition which has been rejected in the vast majority of jurisdictions.[68] The latter—for "wrongful birth"—is one seeking compensation for the costs and anguish resulting from negligently depriving a woman of a choice available to her under the Abortion Act 1967, s 1(1)(d). The one is not dependent on the other. Even if it were otherwise, to disallow the parental action simply because of the inadmissibility of the neonate's would be another example of equating two wrongs with a right. It is hard to realise any major explanatory gain from applying the moral doctrine of distributive justice to the solution of the present case.

(4) The uncertainties of "offset"

McFarlane, thus, contains something of a hidden agenda. We have seen that all five Law Lords were prepared to see a good case for rejecting the appeal. The foregoing analysis suggests that their reasons for allowing it are not immediately attractive and are, at least, open to reasoned counter-argument. What, then, lies behind their salmon-leap against the current of opinion?

The more one reads the judgments, the more one is convinced that the main stumbling block on the road to restitution of the McFarlanes' costs lies in the problem of "offset". Every principle of damage assessment dictated that there should be *some* offset for the advantages to the parents of a new child, albeit one that was originally unwanted. But the problem became, firstly, one of comparing the emotional advantages with the pecuniary disadvantages and, at least equally, of putting a monetary value on the life of a child. The combined difficulty was expressed by Lord Millett:

64 [1992] 1 AC 310.
65 [1998] QB 254.
66 [1982] QB 1166.
67 Inferred from Stephenson LJ at 1175.
68 See A Shapira, "'Wrongful life' lawsuits for faulty genetic counselling: should the impaired newborn be entitled to sue?" (1998) 24 *Journal of Medical Ethics* 369.

There is something distasteful, if not morally offensive, in treating the birth of a normal, healthy child as a matter for compensation. I cannot accept that the solution lies in requiring the costs of maintaining the child to be offset by the benefits derived from the child's existence. . . . The placing of a monetary value on the birth of a normal and healthy child . . . provides no solution to the moral problem. The exercise must either be superfluous or produce the very result which is said to be morally repugnant.[69]

In this he was fully supported by Lords Slynn and Steyn. Lord Hope expressed the sentiments of the House in saying that:

[T]he value which is to be attached to these benefits [of rearing a child] is incalculable. The costs can be calculated but the benefits, which in fairness must be set against them, cannot. The logical conclusion, as a matter of law, is that the costs to the pursuers of meeting their obligations to the child . . . are not recoverable as damages.[70]

One must, of course, bow to his Lordship on a matter of law but it is difficult to see where the logic lies as a matter of common sense. The net costs to the parents of rearing the child are the gross costs less the beneficial "offsets". The fact that the extent of the last cannot be assessed with accuracy provides a less than satisfactory logical basis for holding, in effect, that the first has been wished out of existence. Still less does it explain the reason why the economic loss sustained by the parents must, as a result, be held to fall outside the ambit of the duty of care which was owed to the parents by the health carers.

Lord Slynn found himself in the same difficulty. He, at least, refused to assume that the benefits of having a child always outweighed the cost, but he then described the many difficulties in estimating the values to be put on either of them over the period of childhood and adolescence. As a result, he concluded that the problems were of such gravity as to discourage the acceptance of the "benefits" approach. But, on his own admission, it *could* be done, and the fact that a process is difficult seems a lame reason for discarding it absolutely—and, then, in favour of one which appears less fair to an aggrieved person.

The *moral* problems which so beset their Lordships are, at least, minimised if one accepts that the McFarlanes' action is not about the resultant child but is simply a matter of *the costs of* the resultant child. This is not a wholly novel conclusion— Kirby A C-J was widely quoted, from a judgment in the Supreme Court of New South Wales, to the effect:

In most cases, it was not the child as revealed that was unwanted. Nor is the child's existence the *damage* in the action. . . . It is the economic damage which is the principal unwanted element, rather than the birth or existence of the child as such.[71]

Once this is accepted, the moral opprobrium associated with apparent commodification of an infant is avoided. True, several difficulties remain but, at least, the consequences of whether the child is loved or unloved are eliminated. However, given that the unsought child *is* loved, it can still be argued that the parents who are compensated are, so to speak, "getting something for nothing". But this is nothing new—Lord McCluskey's quoted example of the miner who is compensated for injury

---

69 2000 SLT 154 at 180.

70 2000 SLT 154 at 173.

71 *CES*, note 51 above, at 75.

sustained in the pits but who is not disadvantaged if he subsequently enjoys life in the open air[72] is a compelling analogy. The problem remains that the costs of rearing a child will vary with the family circumstances and this brings one to the concept of a conventional child as a possible way of reconciling the opposing philosophies on the issue.

Surely the damage may be assessed not on the basis of the actual circumstances but, rather, on the basis of the cost involved in the upkeep of the average child born to the average family. Not only would the "odious" task of assessing the attitudes of and the resources available to the injured parents be avoided, but the professionals involved would know the extent of their liabilities should negligence be proved. This again is not a novel idea. To quote Lord Cameron:

> [A]ccount [can] be taken of the parents' means in the sense that it will be unreasonable to compensate the well-to-do parents to any substantially greater level than the parents of more modest means. To take an example, the amount of the layette of which an allowance would be made should be set at a reasonable and not an extravagant level, albeit that the well-to-do may well have exceeded that level because they have the means to enable them to express their love and care for the child in a more expensive fashion. Equally the same principle of reasonableness should apply in relation to items as divergent as necessary accommodation and fees for schooling.[73]

(5) The defective neonate

The question of the defective neonate remains for consideration. This is more than a matter of completeness—it is an integral aspect of the "offset" debate. We have seen that it has been generally agreed that damages can be awarded for the unsought birth of a defective child, but the reasons for this have not been analysed. Moreover, any comments are pre-*McFarlane* and it is to be noted that, in that case, the most that could be conceded was that the rule may have to be different in such a case.[74] One way round this could be, as we have discussed, to look upon the actions in the two eventualities as being of different types—but we have also seen that this manoeuvre may not always be available. The case then falls into what can be regarded as a sub-category of wrongful pregnancy terminating in a handicapped neonate.

The action is the same, however, irrespective of the outcome, and to allow full damages in the event of handicap is to do no more than assess the "offset" in terms of parental benefit as nil. On the face of things, this supports the case for "offset" in that the degree of handicap can be assessed and the associated costs of maintenance can be adjusted accordingly. What it does not do, however, is to look in the mirror and explain why expenses associated with the birth of a healthy child should be assessed as being 100% offset by the resulting advantages. Neither the joys of parenthood nor the heartbreak associated with caring for children with a varied degree of handicap can be accurately quantified in monetary terms. The logic of the *McFarlane* decision must, then, be that damages should be denied in either case. But, given an all-or-nothing rule, the alternative—and better—view is that, if damages *ought to be* and

---

72 1998 SLT 307 at 316.

73 *Allan*, 1998 SLT 580 at 585.

74 2000 SLT 154 per Lord Steyn at 166.

are available in the case of handicap, they must also be awarded in the case of normality. Returning, again, to Lord Cameron:

> The question must be asked whether there is any reason why the law . . . should not recognise as elements sounding in damages, circumstances such as the additional financial hardships imposed on the parent or parents who require to take into the family the unexpected and unplanned child after birth, in accommodating and caring for that child thereafter and, particularly in the case of a handicapped child, in meeting the additional burdens arising from the distress occasioned by its handicap and the extra payments which they require to make to enable the child to live as near to a normal life as possible. Why, in the case of a handicapped child, for instance, should not a parent who requires to give up employment or the like to care for the child, sue for the loss so occasioned? I see nothing in principle to prevent this. If that be so, why should a healthy child be dealt with differently in regard to a similar loss?[75]

Neither solution is incompatible with the majority reasoning in *McFarlane*; in this writer's opinion, the latter at least goes to show that two rights do not make a wrong.

E. CONCLUSION

A fellow commentator has written of the House of Lords stage of *McFarlane*: "I can think of few decisions that are . . . as odious, unsound and unsafe as this one."[76] This, of course, carries a ring of hyperbole. Nevertheless, it is well nigh impossible to read the case without experiencing a feeling of dissatisfaction. Try as one may, it is difficult to see the House of Lords' judgments in *McFarlane* as other than a scholarly and thoughtful elaboration of a single word—distaste—and it could be argued that we are entitled to disclosure of better grounds on which to reverse an established line of decisions.

I have every sympathy with their Lordships. They may have been in an impossible situation. Despite their protestations, they were, effectively, being forced into the field of public policy and, as Lord Hope agreed, the legislature is the proper forum in which competing social philosophies should be considered in establishing the law.[77] We have already noted how close Lord Steyn and others were to acknowledging the validity of the parents' claim. But it was really left to Lord Millett to distinguish between Mr and Mrs McFarlane on the one hand and the public at large on the other. Lord Millett conceded and, indeed, elaborated on the real damage that had been done to them. They were, he reasoned, at least entitled to general damages[78]— and I suspect strongly that the public would follow Lord Millett and, indeed, go further.

Lord Steyn's commuter on the Underground is a tough person, inured to the slings and arrows of outrageous conditions; he might well come to the simple pragmatic conclusion attributed to him. I fancy, however, that the traveller on Strathtay Scottish Omnibuses has more time and space in which to consider the problem put to him— or more appropriately, her. He or she is, in my view, far more likely to say: "these people find themselves in a position which they sought to avoid. The reason they are

---

75 *Allan v Greater Glasgow Health Board* 1998 SLT 580, at 584.

76 E Cameron-Perry, "Return of the burden of the 'blessing'" (1999) 149 NLJ 1887. See also the remarkably prescient article: A Mullis, "*Wrongful conception unravelled*" (1993) 1 Med L Rev 320.

77 Quoting from *Johnson v University Hospitals of Cleveland* (1989) 540 NE 2d 1370.

78 But, even then, damages which would amount only to a conventional sum.

there is, in the end, the result of a failure of professional duty. True, there is some good in their new condition but, so far as they are concerned, there is also a lot of bad. True, also, that it may be difficult to set one off against the other. Nevertheless, justice tells me that the effort should be made and that they should be compensated for their financial loss". And, in so saying, he or she would be emphasising that there is no implied denigration of a newborn child and no underlying attack on family values; it is simply a matter of common observation that an outside agency has diverted the family resources in a way that the family neither intended nor desired.

Ultimately one might ask whether it is fair, just and reasonable to *deny* restitution to those whose lives have been impaired. *McFarlane* was, at base, a matter between two individual parties—can it be said that justice was seen to be done? At the end of the day, might not even the commuter on the Underground admit to a sense of unease not only as to the result but also as to how that result was achieved?

J K Mason
Professor (Emeritus) of Forensic Medicine
University of Edinburgh

(The author has invited a number of legal colleagues to review his paper and is particularly indebted to Dr G T Laurie and Ms E Sutherland. It is, however, entirely his own responsibility.)

Part III
Human Experimentation and Research

[13]

ETHICS AND CLINICAL RESEARCH*

HENRY K. BEECHER, M.D.†

BOSTON

HUMAN experimentation since World War II has created some difficult problems with the increasing employment of patients as experimental subjects when it must be apparent that they would not have been available if they had been truly aware of the uses that would be made of them. Evidence is at hand that many of the patients in the examples to follow never had the risk satisfactorily explained to them, and it seems obvious that further hundreds have not known that they were the subjects of an experiment although grave consequences have been suffered as a direct result of experiments described here. There is a belief prevalent in some sophisticated circles that attention to these matters would "block progress." But, according to Pope Pius XII,[1] ". . . science is not the highest value to which all other orders of values . . . should be subordinated."

I am aware that these are troubling charges. They have grown out of troubling practices. They can be documented, as I propose to do, by examples from leading medical schools, university hospitals, private military departments (the Army, the Navy and the Air Force), governmental institutes (the National Institutes of Health), Vet-

erans Administration hospitals and industry. The basis for the charges is broad.‡

I should like to affirm that American medicine is sound, and most progress in it soundly attained. There is, however, a reason for concern in certain areas, and I believe the type of activities to be mentioned will do great harm to medicine unless soon corrected. It will certainly be charged that any mention of these matters does a disservice to medicine, but not one so great, I believe, as a continuation of the practices to be cited.

Experimentation in man takes place in several areas: in self-experimentation; in patient volunteers and normal subjects; in therapy; and in the different areas of *experimentation on a patient not for his benefit but for that, at least in theory, of patients in general*. The present study is limited to this last category.

REASONS FOR URGENCY OF STUDY

Ethical errors are increasing not only in numbers but in variety — for example, in the recently added problems arising in transplantation of organs.

---

*From the Anaesthesia Laboratory of the Harvard Medical School at the Massachusetts General Hospital.

†Dorr Professor of Research in Anaesthesia, Harvard Medical School.

‡At the Brook Lodge Conference on "Problems and Complexities of Clinical Research" I commented that "what seem to be breaches of ethical conduct in experimentation are by no means rare, but are almost, one fears, universal." I thought it was obvious that I was by "universal" referring to the fact that examples could easily be found in all categories where research in man takes place to any significant extent. Judging by press comments, that was not obvious: hence, this note.

There are a number of reasons why serious attention to the general problem is urgent.

Of transcendent importance is the enormous and continuing increase in available funds, as shown below.

MONEY AVAILABLE FOR RESEARCH EACH YEAR

	MASSACHUSETTS GENERAL HOSPITAL	NATIONAL INSTITUTES OF HEALTH*
1945	$ 500,000†	$ 701,800
1955	2,222,816	36,063,200
1965	8,384,342	436,600,000

*National Institutes of Health figures based upon decade averages, excluding funds for construction, kindly supplied by Dr. John Sherman, of National Institutes of Health.

†Approximation, supplied by Mr. David C. Crockett, of Massachusetts General Hospital.

Since World War II the annual expenditure for research (in large part in man) in the Massachusetts General Hospital has increased a remarkable 17-fold. At the National Institutes of Health, the increase has been a gigantic 624-fold. This "national" rate of increase is over 36 times that of the Massachusetts General Hospital. These data, rough as they are, illustrate vast opportunities and concomitantly expanded responsibilities.

Taking into account the sound and increasing emphasis of recent years that experimentation in man must precede general application of new procedures in therapy, plus the great sums of money available, there is reason to fear that these requirements and these resources may be greater than the supply of responsible investigators. All this heightens the problems under discussion.

Medical schools and university hospitals are increasingly dominated by investigators. Every young man knows that he will never be promoted to a tenure post, to a professorship in a major medical school, unless he has proved himself as an investigator. If the ready availability of money for conducting research is added to this fact, one can see how great the pressures are on ambitious young physicians.

Implementation of the recommendations of the President's Commission on Heart Disease, Cancer and Stroke means that further astronomical sums of money will become available for research in man.

In addition to the foregoing three practical points there are others that Sir Robert Platt[2] has pointed out: a general awakening of social conscience; greater power for good or harm in new remedies, new operations and new investigative procedures than was formerly the case; new methods of preventive treatment with their advantages and dangers that are now applied to communities as a whole as well as to individuals, with multiplication of the possibilities for injury; medical science has shown how valuable human experimentation can be in solving problems of disease and its treatment; one can therefore anticipate an increase in experimentation; and the newly developed concept of clinical research as a profession (for example, clinical pharmacology) — and this, of course, can lead to unfortunate separation between the interests of science and the interests of the patient.

FREQUENCY OF UNETHICAL OR QUESTIONABLY ETHICAL PROCEDURES

Nearly everyone agrees that ethical violations do occur. The practical question is, how often? A preliminary examination of the matter was based on 17 examples, which were easily increased to 50. These 50 studies contained references to 186 further likely examples, on the average 3.7 leads per study; they at times overlapped from paper to paper, but this figure indicates how conveniently one can proceed in a search for such material. The data are suggestive of widespread problems, but there is need for another kind of information, which was obtained by examination of 100 consecutive human studies published in 1964, in an excellent journal; 12 of these seemed to be unethical. If only one quarter of them is truly unethical, this still indicates the existence of a serious situation. Pappworth,[3] in England, has collected, he says, more than 500 papers based upon unethical experimentation. It is evident from such observations that unethical or questionably ethical procedures are not uncommon.

THE PROBLEM OF CONSENT

All so-called codes are based on the bland assumption that meaningful or informed consent is readily available for the asking. As pointed out elsewhere,[4] this is very often not the case. Consent in any fully informed sense may not be obtainable. Nevertheless, except, possibly, in the most trivial situations, it remains a goal toward which one must strive for sociologic, ethical and clear-cut legal reasons. There is no choice in the matter.

If suitably approached, patients will accede, on the basis of trust, to about any request their physician may make. At the same time, every experienced clinician investigator knows that patients will often submit to inconvenience and some discomfort, if they do not last very long, but the usual patient will never agree to jeopardize seriously his health or his life for the sake of "science."

In only 2 of the 50* examples originally compiled for this study was consent mentioned. Actually, it should be emphasized in all cases for obvious moral and legal reasons, but it would be unrealistic to place much dependence on it. In any precise sense statements regarding consent are meaningless unless one knows how fully the patient was informed of all risks, and if these are not known, that fact should also be made clear. A far more dependable safeguard than consent is the presence of a truly *responsible* investigator.

EXAMPLES OF UNETHICAL OR QUESTIONABLY ETHICAL STUDIES

These examples are not cited for the condemna-

*Reduced here to 22 for reasons of space.

tion of individuals; they are recorded to call attention to a variety of ethical problems found in experimental medicine, for it is hoped that calling attention to them will help to correct abuses present. During ten years of study of these matters it has become apparent that thoughtlessness and carelessness, not a willful disregard of the patient's rights, account for most of the cases encountered. Nonetheless, it is evident that in many of the examples presented, the investigators have risked the health or the life of their subjects. No attempt has been made to present the "worst" possible examples; rather, the aim has been to show the variety of problems encountered.

References to the examples presented are not given, for there is no intention of pointing to individuals, but rather, a wish to call attention to widespread practices. All, however, are documented to the satisfaction of the editors of the *Journal*.

Known Effective Treatment Withheld

Example 1. It is known that rheumatic fever can usually be prevented by adequate treatment of streptococcal respiratory infections by the parenteral administration of penicillin. Nevertheless, definitive treatment was withheld, and placebos were given to a group of 109 men in service, while benzathine penicillin G. was given to others.

The therapy that each patient received was determined automatically by his military serial number arranged so that more men received penicillin than received placebo. In the small group of patients studied 2 cases of acute rheumatic fever and 1 of acute nephritis developed in the control patients, whereas these complications did not occur among those who received the benzathine penicillin G.

Example 2. The sulfonamides were for many years the only antibacterial drugs effective in shortening the duration of acute streptococcal pharyngitis and in reducing its suppurative complications. The investigators in this study undertook to determine if the occurrence of the serious nonsuppurative complications, rheumatic fever and acute glomerulonephritis, would be reduced by this treatment. This study was made despite the general experience that certain antibiotics, including penicillin, will prevent the development of rheumatic fever.

The subjects were a large group of hospital patients; a control group of approximately the same size, also with exudative Group A streptococcus, was included. The latter group received only nonspecific therapy (no sulfadiazine). The total group denied the effective penicillin comprised over 500 men.

Rheumatic fever was diagnosed in 5.4 per cent of those treated with sulfadiazine. In the control group rheumatic fever developed in 4.2 per cent.

In reference to this study a medical officer stated in writing that the subjects were not informed, did not consent and were not aware that they had been involved in an experiment, and yet admittedly 25 acquired rheumatic fever. According to this same medical officer *more than 70* who had had known definitive treatment withheld were on the wards with rheumatic fever when he was there.

Example 3. This involved a study of the relapse rate· in typhoid fever treated in two ways. In an earlier study by the present investigators chloramphenicol had been recognized as an effective treatment for typhoid fever, being attended by half the mortality that was experienced when this agent was not used. Others had made the same observations, indicating that to withhold this effective remedy can be a life-or-death decision. The present study was carried out to determine the relapse rate under the two methods of treatment; of 408 charity patients 251 were treated with chloramphenicol, of whom 20, or 7.97 per cent, died. Symptomatic treatment was given, but chloramphenicol was withheld in 157, of whom 36, or 22.9 per cent, died. According to the data presented, 23 patients died in the course of this study who would not have been expected to succumb if they had received specific therapy.

Study of Therapy

Example 4. TriA (triacetyloleandomycin) was originally introduced for the treatment of infection with gram-positive organisms. Spotty evidence of hepatic dysfunction emerged, especially in children, and so the present study was undertaken on 50 patients, including mental defectives or juvenile delinquents who were inmates of a children's center. No disease other than acne was present; the drug was given for treatment of this. The ages of the subjects ranged from thirteen to thirty-nine years. "By the time half the patients had received the drug for four weeks, the high incidence of significant hepatic dysfunction . . . led to the discontinuation of administration to the remainder of the group at three weeks." (However, only two weeks after the start of the administration of the drug, 54 per cent of the patients showed abnormal excretion of bromsulfalein.) Eight patients with marked hepatic dysfunction were transferred to the hospital "for more intensive study." Liver biopsy was carried out in these 8 patients and repeated in 4 of them. Liver damage was evident. Four of these hospitalized patients, after their liver-function tests returned to normal limits, received a "challenge" dose of the drug. Within two days hepatic dysfunction was evident in 3 of the 4 patients. In 1 patient a second challenge dose was given after the first challenge and again led to evidence of abnormal liver function. Flocculation tests remained abnormal in some patients as long as five weeks after discontinuance of the drug.

Physiologic Studies

Example 5. In this controlled, double-blind study of the hematologic toxicity of chloramphenicol, it was recognized that chloramphenicol is "well known as a cause of aplastic anemia" and that there is a "prolonged morbidity and high mortality of aplastic anemia" and that ". . . chloramphenicol-induced aplastic anemia can be related to dose . . ." The aim of the study was "further definition of the toxicology of the drug. . . ."

Forty-one randomly chosen patients were given either 2 or 6 gm. of chloramphenicol per day; 12 control patients were used. "Toxic bone-marrow depression, predominantly affecting erythropoiesis, developed in 2 of 20 patients given 2.0 gm. and in 18 of 21 given 6 gm. of chloramphenicol daily." The smaller dose is recommended for routine use.

Example 6. In a study of the effect of thymectomy on the survival of skin homografts 18 children, three and a half months to eighteen years of age, about to undergo surgery for congenital heart disease, were selected. Eleven were to have total thymectomy as part of the operation, and 7 were to serve as controls. As part of the experiment, full-thickness skin homografts from an unrelated adult donor were sutured to the chest wall in each case. (Total thymectomy is occasionally, although not usually part of the primary cardiovascular surgery involved, and whereas it may not greatly add to the hazards of the necessary operation, its eventual effects in children are not known.) This work was proposed as part of a long-range study of "the growth and development of these children over the years." No difference in the survival of the skin homograft was observed in the 2 groups.

Example 7. This study of cyclopropane anesthesia and cardiac arrhythmias consisted of 31 patients. The average duration of the study was three hours, ranging from two to four and a half hours. "Minor surgical procedures" were carried out in all but 1 subject. Moderate to deep anesthesia, with endotracheal intubation and controlled respiration, was used. Carbon dioxide was injected into the closed respiratory system until cardiac arrhythmias appeared. Toxic levels of carbon dioxide were achieved and maintained for considerable periods. During the cyclopropane anesthesia a variety of pathologic cardiac arrhythmias occurred. When the carbon dioxide tension was elevated above normal, ventricular extrasystoles were more numerous than when the carbon dioxide tension was normal, ventricular arrhythmias being continuous in 1 subject for ninety minutes. (This can lead to fatal fibrillation.)

Example 8. Since the minimum blood-flow requirements of the cerebral circulation are not accurately known, this study was carried out to determine "cerebral hemodynamic and metabolic changes . . . before and during acute reductions in arterial pressure induced by drug administration and/or postural adjustments." Forty-four patients whose ages varied from the second to the tenth decade were involved. They included normotensive subjects, those with essential hypertension and finally a group with malignant hypertension. Fifteen

had abnormal electrocardiograms. Few details about the reasons for hospitalization are given.

Signs of cerebral circulatory insufficiency, which were easily recognized, included confusion and in some cases a nonresponsive state. By alteration in the tilt of the patient "the clinical state of the subject could be changed in a matter of seconds from one of alertness to confusion, and for the remainder of the flow, the subject was maintained in the latter state." The femoral arteries were cannulated in all subjects, and the internal jugular veins in 14.

The mean arterial pressure fell in 37 subjects from 109 to 48 mm. of mercury, with signs of cerebral ischemia. "With the onset of collapse, cardiac output and right ventricular pressures decreased sharply."

Since signs of cerebral insufficiency developed without evidence of coronary insufficiency the authors concluded that "the brain may be more sensitive to acute hypotension than is the heart."

Example 9. This is a study of the adverse circulatory responses elicited by intra-abdominal maneuvers:

> When the peritoneal cavity was entered, a deliberate series of maneuvers was carried out [in 68 patients] to ascertain the effective stimuli and the areas responsible for development of the expected circulatory changes. Accordingly, the surgeon rubbed localized areas of the parietal and visceral peritoneum with a small ball sponge as discretely as possible. Traction on the mesenteries, pressure in the area of the celiac plexus, traction on the gallbladder and stomach, and occlusion of the portal and caval veins were the other stimuli applied.

Thirty-four of the patients were sixty years of age or older; 11 were seventy or older. In 44 patients the hypotension produced by the deliberate stimulation was "moderate to marked." The maximum fall produced by manipulation was from 200 systolic, 105 diastolic, to 42 systolic, 20 diastolic; the average fall in mean pressure in 26 patients was 53 mm. of mercury.

Of the 50 patients studied, 17 showed either atrioventricular dissociation with nodal rhythm or nodal rhythm alone. A decrease in the amplitude of the T wave and elevation or depression of the ST segment were noted in 25 cases in association with manipulation and hypotension or, at other times, in the course of anesthesia and operation. In only 1 case was the change pronounced enough to suggest myocardial ischemia. No case of myocardial infarction was noted in the group studied although routine electrocardiograms were not taken after operation to detect silent infarcts. Two cases in which electrocardiograms were taken after operation showed T-wave and ST-segment changes that had not been present before.

These authors refer to a similar study in which more alarming electrocardiographic changes were observed. Four patients in the series sustained silent myocardial infarctions; most of their patients were undergoing gallbladder surgery because of

1358 THE NEW ENGLAND JOURNAL OF MEDICINE June 16, 1966

associated heart disease. It can be added further that in the 34 patients referred to above as being sixty years of age or older, some doubtless had heart disease that could have made risky the maneuvers carried out. In any event, this possibility might have been a deterrent.

Example 10. Starling's law — "that the heart output per beat is directly proportional to the diastolic filling" — was studied in 30 adult patients with atrial fibrillation and mitral stenosis sufficiently severe to require valvulotomy. "Continuous alterations of the length of a segment of left ventricular muscle were recorded simultaneously in 13 of these patients by means of a mercury-filled resistance gauge sutured to the surface of the left ventricle." Pressures in the left ventricle were determined by direct puncture simultaneously with the segment length in 13 patients and without the segment length in an additional 13 patients. Four similar unanesthetized patients were studied through catheterization of the left side of the heart transeptally. In all 30 patients arterial pressure was measured through the catheterized brachial artery.

Example 11. To study the sequence of ventricular contraction in human bundle-branch block, simultaneous catheterization of both ventricles was performed in 22 subjects; catheterization of the right side of the heart was carried out in the usual manner; the left side was catheterized transbronchially. Extrasystoles were produced by tapping on the epicardium in subjects with normal myocardium while they were undergoing thoracotomy. Simultaneous pressures were measured in both ventricles through needle puncture in this group.

The purpose of this study was to gain increased insight into the physiology involved.

Example 12. This investigation was carried out to examine the possible effect of vagal stimulation on cardiac arrest. The authors had in recent years transected the homolateral vagus nerve immediately below the origin of the recurrent laryngeal nerve as palliation against cough and pain in bronchogenic carcinoma. Having been impressed with the number of reports of cardiac arrest that seemed to follow vagal stimulation, they tested the effects of intrathoracic vagal stimulation during 30 of their surgical procedures, concluding, from these observations in patients under satisfactory anesthesia, that cardiac irregularities and cardiac arrest due to vagovagal reflex were less common than had previously been supposed.

Example 13. This study presented a technic for determining portal circulation time and hepatic blood flow. It involved the transcutaneous injection of the spleen and catheterization of the hepatic vein. This was carried out in 43 subjects, of whom 14 were normal; 16 had cirrhosis (varying degrees), 9 acute hepatitis, and 4 hemolytic anemia.

No mention is made of what information was divulged to the subjects, some of whom were seriously ill. This study consisted in the development of a technic, not of therapy, in the 14 normal subjects.

Studies to Improve the Understanding of Disease

Example 14. In this study of the syndrome of impending hepatic coma in patients with cirrhosis of the liver certain nitrogenous substances were administered to 9 patients with chronic alcoholism and advanced cirrhosis: ammonium chloride, di-ammonium citrate, urea or dietary protein. In all patients a reaction that included mental disturbances, a "flapping tremor" and electroencephalographic changes developed. Similar signs had occurred in only 1 of the patients before these substances were administered:

> The first sign noted was usually clouding of the consciousness. Three patients had a second or a third course of administration of a nitrogenous substance with the same results. It was concluded that marked resemblance between this reaction and impending hepatic coma, implied that the administration of these [nitrogenous] substances to patients with cirrhosis may be hazardous.

Example 15. The relation of the effects of ingested ammonia to liver disease was investigated in 11 normal subjects, 6 with acute virus hepatitis, 26 with cirrhosis, and 8 miscellaneous patients. Ten of these patients had neurologic changes associated with either hepatitis or cirrhosis.

The hepatic and renal veins were cannulated. Ammonium chloride was administered by mouth. After this, a tremor that lasted for three days developed in 1 patient. When ammonium chloride was ingested by 4 cirrhotic patients with tremor and mental confusion the symptoms were exaggerated during the test. The same thing was true of a fifth patient in another group.

Example 16. This study was directed toward determining the period of infectivity of infectious hepatitis. Artificial induction of hepatitis was carried out in an institution for mentally defective children in which a mild form of hepatitis was endemic. The parents gave consent for the intramuscular injection or oral administration of the virus, but nothing is said regarding what was told them concerning the appreciable hazards involved.

A resolution adopted by the World Medical Association states explicitly: "Under no circumstances is a doctor permitted to do anything which would weaken the physical or mental resistance of a human being except from strictly therapeutic or prophylactic indications imposed in the interest of the patient." There is no right to risk an injury to 1 person for the benefit of others.

Example 17. Live cancer cells were injected into 22 human subjects as part of a study of immunity to cancer. According to a recent review, the subjects (hospitalized patients) were "merely told they would be receiving 'some cells'" — ". . . the word cancer was entirely omitted. . . ."

Example 18. Melanoma was transplanted from a

daughter to her volunteering and informed mother, "in the hope of gaining a little better understanding of cancer immunity and in the hope that the production of tumor antibodies might be helpful in the treatment of the cancer patient." Since the daughter died on the day after the transplantation of the tumor into her mother, the hope expressed seems to have been more theoretical than practical, and the daughter's condition was described as "terminal" at the time the mother volunteered to be a recipient. The primary implant was widely excised on the twenty-fourth day after it had been placed in the mother. She died from metastatic melanoma on the four hundred and fifty-first day after transplantation. The evidence that this patient died of diffuse melanoma that metastasized from a small piece of transplanted tumor was considered conclusive.

Technical Study of Disease

Example 19. During bronchoscopy a special needle was inserted through a bronchus into the left atrium of the heart. This was done in an unspecified number of subjects, both with cardiac disease and with normal hearts.

The technic was a new approach whose hazards were at the beginning quite unknown. The subjects with normal hearts were used, not for their possible benefit but for that of patients in general.

Example 20. The percutaneous method of catheterization of the left side of the heart has, it is reported, led to 8 deaths (1.09 per cent death rate) and other serious accidents in 732 cases. There was, therefore, need for another method, the transbronchial approach, which was carried out in the present study in more than 500 cases, with no deaths.

Granted that a delicate problem arises regarding how much should be discussed with the patients involved in the use of a new method, nevertheless where the method is employed in a given patient for *his* benefit, the ethical problems are far less than when this potentially extremely dangerous method is used "in 15 patients with normal hearts, undergoing bronchoscopy for other reasons." Nothing was said about what was told any of the subjects, and nothing was said about the granting of permission, which was certainly indicated in the 15 normal subjects used.

Example 21. This was a study of the effect of exercise on cardiac output and pulmonary-artery pressure in 8 "normal" persons (that is, patients whose diseases were not related to the cardiovascular system), in 8 with congestive heart failure severe enough to have recently required complete bed rest, in 6 with hypertension, in 2 with aortic insufficiency, in 7 with mitral stenosis and in 5 with pulmonary emphysema.

Intracardiac catheterization was carried out, and the catheter then inserted into the right or left main branch of the pulmonary artery. The brachial artery was usually catheterized; sometimes, the radial or femoral arteries were catheterized. The subjects exercised in a supine position by pushing their feet against weighted pedals. "The ability of these patients to carry on sustained work was severely limited by weakness and dyspnea." Several were in severe failure. This was not a therapeutic attempt but rather a physiologic study.

Bizarre Study

Example 22. There is a question whether ureteral reflux can occur in the normal bladder. With this in mind, vesicourethrography was carried out on 26 normal babies less than forty-eight hours old. The infants were exposed to x-rays while the bladder was filling and during voiding. Multiple spot films were made to record the presence or absence of ureteral reflux. None was found in this group, and fortunately no infection followed the catheterization. What the results of the extensive x-ray exposure may be, no one can yet say.

COMMENT ON DEATH RATES

In the foregoing examples a number of procedures, some with their own demonstrated death rates, were carried out. The following data were provided by 3 distinguished investigators in the field and represent widely held views.

Cardiac catheterization: right side of the heart, about 1 death per 1000 cases; left side, 5 deaths per 1000 cases. "Probably considerably higher in some places, depending on the portal of entry." (One investigator had 15 deaths in his first 150 cases.) It is possible that catheterization of a hepatic vein or the renal vein would have a lower death rate than that of catheterization of the right side of the heart, for if it is properly carried out, only the atrium is entered en route to the liver or the kidney, not the right ventricle, which can lead to serious cardiac irregularities. There is always the possibility, however, that the ventricle will be entered inadvertently. This occurs in at least half the cases, according to 1 expert — "but if properly done is too transient to be of importance."

Liver biopsy: the death rate here is estimated at 2 to 3 per 1000, depending in considerable part on the condition of the subject.

Anesthesia: the anesthesia death rate can be placed in general at about 1 death per 2000 cases. The hazard is doubtless higher when certain practices such as deliberate evocation of ventricular extrasystoles under cyclopropane are involved.

PUBLICATION

In the view of the British Medical Research Council[5] it is not enough to ensure that all investigation is carried out in an ethical manner: it must be made unmistakably clear in the publications that the proprieties have been observed. This implies editorial responsibility in addition to the investiga-

1360 THE NEW ENGLAND JOURNAL OF MEDICINE June 16, 1966

tor's. The question rises, then, about valuable data that have been improperly obtained.* It is my view that such material should not be published.[5] There is a practical aspect to the matter: failure to obtain publication would discourage unethical experimentation. How many would carry out such experimentation if they *knew* its results would never be published? Even though suppression of such data (by not publishing it) would constitute a loss to medicine, in a specific localized sense, this loss, it seems, would be less important than the far reaching moral loss to medicine if the data thus obtained were to be published. Admittedly, there is room for debate. Others believe that such data, because of their intrinsic value, obtained at a cost of great risk or damage to the subjects, should not be wasted but should be published with stern editorial comment. This would have to be done with exceptional skill, to avoid an odor of hypocrisy.

SUMMARY AND CONCLUSIONS

The ethical approach to experimentation in man has several components; two are more important than the others, the first being informed consent. The difficulty of obtaining this is discussed in detail. But it is absolutely essential to *strive* for it for moral, sociologic and legal reasons. The statement that consent has been obtained has little meaning unless the subject or his guardian is capable of understanding what is to be undertaken and unless all

*As far as principle goes, a parallel can be seen in the recent Mapp decision by the United States Supreme Court. It was stated there that evidence unconstitutionally obtained cannot be used in any judicial decision, no matter how important the evidence is to the ends of justice.

hazards are made clear. If these are not known this, too, should be stated. In such a situation the subject at least knows that he is to be a participant in an experiment. Secondly, there is the more reliable safeguard provided by the presence of an intelligent, informed, conscientious, compassionate, responsible investigator.

Ordinary patients will not knowingly risk their health or their life for the sake of "science." Every experienced clinician investigator knows this. When such risks are taken and a considerable number of patients are involved, it may be assumed that informed consent has not been obtained in all cases.

The gain anticipated from an experiment must be commensurate with the risk involved.

An experiment is ethical or not at its inception; it does not become ethical *post hoc* — ends do not justify means. There is no ethical distinction between ends and means.

In the publication of experimental results it must be made unmistakably clear that the proprieties have been observed. It is debatable whether data obtained unethically should be published even with stern editorial comment.

REFERENCES

1. Pope Pius XII. Address. Presented at First International Congress on Histopathology of Nervous System, Rome, Italy, September 14, 1952.
2. Platt (Sir Robert). 1st bart. *Doctor and Patient: Ethics, morals, government.* 87 pp. London: Nuffield provincial hospitals trust, 1963. Pp. 62 and 63.
3. Pappworth, M. H. Personal communication.
4. Beecher, H. K. Consent in clinical experimentation: myth and reality. *J.A.M.A.* **195**:34, 1966.
5. Great Britain, Medical Research Council. *Memorandum*, 1953.

[14]

A REPORT FROM NEW ZEALAND: AN "UNFORTUNATE EXPERIMENT"

ALASTAIR V. CAMPBELL

At the beginning of June 1987 the Auckland monthly magazine, *Metro*, published as its cover story a 16 page article entitled, 'An "Unfortunate Experiment" At National Women's'. Written by Sandra Coney, a freelance journalist and Phillida Bunkle, a Wellington academic specialising in Women's Studies, the article described a policy for treating cervical cancer adopted by Associate Professor Herbert Green, an obstetrician and gynae-cologist at National Women's Hospital, Auckland. Professor Green was described as 'a man with a mission' who wanted to save women from mutilating surgery and 'so he had to prove . . . that CIS [carcinoma in situ] was a harmless disease which hardly, if ever, progressed to invasive cancer.'

The authors were at pains to explain fully what was a somewhat complex medical debate. Basing their assertions on papers in medical journals, on interviews with various medical authorities and on the story of one particular patient, 'Ruth', they pointed out that before Professor Green started his 'conservative' treatment policy in 1966 there was an established view that CIS (a symptomless condition detected by observation and by cervical smear) should be eradicated, normally by the technique of cone biopsy.. The effectiveness of this procedure would then be checked by negative cervical smears taken at regular intervals. Contesting this established view, Green believed that most of the area affected by CIS should be left undisturbed and that observation over the years would demonstrate that there was no spread of cancer, even with continuing positive smears. On the basis of this view—the authors alleged—Professor Green conducted an experi-ment without the patients' knowledge or consent over a period of 15 to 20 years, which entailed not fully treating some women who had continuing abnormal cervical smear results in order to establish the hypothesis of non-progression. This required frequent visits to the hospital, with the women believing that they were

60 ALASTAIR V. CAMPBELL

receiving standard treatment and diagnostic checks. In a highlighted paragraph the article stated:

> Some women with evidence of disease were to be left. They would be followed—that is, brought back for regular smears and possibly more biopsies—but there was no intention to cure them.

The response to the *Metro* article was dramatic and virtually instantaneous—in marked contrast with the virtual absence of any reaction from the medical profession to the technical articles upon which it was based. On 8 June 1987 the Superintendent-in-Chief of the Auckland Hospital Board wrote a memo to the Minister of Health recommending an official inquiry. Two days later the Minister appointed District Judge Silvia Cartwright to conduct a full investigation and report to him. The Minister said that he favoured a 'short, sharp' inquiry and set a date for reporting of 31 August 1987. This highly optimistic deadline was subsequently revised on three occasions, and the Inquiry Report was finally submitted to the Minister on 29th July 1988.

Judge Cartwright was given nine terms of reference, ranging from establishng whether there had been failures in treatment of patients (and whether there had been an experiment conducted without the knowledge and consent of the subjects) to wider questions concerned with the oversight of treatment and research in the hospital, the protection for patients' rights and the policies governing detection and treatment of cervical cancer in New Zealand. She was assisted by three medical advisers (Professor E. V. Mackay, Professor of Obstetrics and Gynaecology at the University of Queensland, Dr. Charlotte Paul, an epidemiologist from Otago Medical School and Dr. Linda Holloway, a pathologist from Wellington Medical School) and by two counsel, Lowell Goddard QC and Philippa Cunningham. The judge called evidence from 64 parties and in addition interviewed or held informal meetings with several other groups, including 81 patients or relatives of patients, nurses and social workers from the hospital, a group of Samoan women and Te Whare Tangate, a group of Maori women interested in the Inquiry. Another important aspect of the Inquiry's work was the reviewing by the medical advisers of more than 1200 patient files and the subsequent submission to the Minister of the names of 123 patients requiring tracing and follow-up treatment.

It would be unrealistic to attempt to do justice to all the issues contained in the 288 closely printed pages of the Report and Appendices (see *The Report of the Cervical Cancer Enquiry*, Government Printing Office, Auckland, New Zealand, July 1988.) Instead, I must concentrate on those aspects which raise wider issues for bioethics internationally as well as in New Zealand. This emerges naturally from my own involvement in the Inquiry, when, as a Visiting Professor in Biomedical Ethics to the Otago Medical School, I was called to give evidence on the ethical guidelines relevant to the policy adopted at National Women's Hospital from 1960 to the present.

However, it is not sensible to discuss the emergent ethical issues without first summarising the main findings of the Inquiry regarding the alleged failures to treat, and experimentation without consent. Unravelling the complexities of these matters took much of the judge's attention since it was claimed in defence that Professor Green's policies were within the parameters of the normal 'clinical freedom' due to any medical consultant. After obtaining evidence from international experts on cervical cancer treatment, studying Professor Green's own publications, and hearing detailed evidence of the discussions over the years with colleagues in personal conversations and in the relevant hospital committees, the judge reached some decisive judgements. As regards failures to treat, she described the outcome of treatment for the majority of women as 'adequate', but went on to state that 'for a minority of women, their management resulted in persisting disease, the development of invasive cancer and, in some cases, death.' (*Report*, p. 210). She also found that there had indeed been a major research trial commencing in 1966, which, although reviewed by the Hospital Medical Committee in 1975, had never been formally ended and that the great majority of patients did not know, except intuitively, that they were participants and had clearly not given consent. The judge did not mince her words when she came to assess the seriousness of these failures by all those responsible:

> The fact that the women did not know they were in a trial, were not informed that their treatment was not conventional and received little detail of the nature of their condition were grave omissions. The responsibilty for these omissions extends to all those who, having approved the trial, knew or ought to have known of its mounting consequences and design faults and allowed it to continue. (*Report*, p. 69).

A further quotation from the Report will illustrate how strongly the judge felt about the failure of the medical profession to deal on its own initiative with the mounting expressions of concern:

For 20 years there was criticism, yet no special effort was made to ensure that patients' health did not suffer as a result of Dr Green's attempt to prove his hypothesis. Until the Auckland Hospital Board recommended the current Inquiry, no person or body with the power or responsibility to intervene took steps to deal decisively with its consequences. The medical profession failed in its basic duty to its patients. (*Report*, p. 70).

What then of the ethical issues involved? They may seem so obvious to students of bioethics that they hardly need restating, yet it is clear that they were by no means obvious to all who held clinical and administrative responsibility at the time. The issue which emerges again and again from the Report is the basic ethical requirement for valid consent, not only to participation in research (including the right to refuse to participate without any sense of duress), but also to the *specific details* of proposed treatments. Gone are the days when vague assurances that all is well or that 'just a few tests' are needed, can be seen as professional medical advice and care. We do not know the details of the consultations conducted by Dr. Green and his colleagues during the period in question—and we do know that his care was much appreciated by many patients. However, the practical effect of the policy was that patients were not party to the unusual treatment regimen being pursued and were often falsely assured that there was no cause for concern. Such things are now labelled as 'paternalistic' and are rightly seen as serious affronts to the dignity and autonomy of patients. In this context it is certainly not irrelevant that failures to inform and consult were found in gynaecology—an area of medical care in which women can feel particularly vulnerable, disabled and subject to humiliating treatment by male doctors (however well intentioned they are). Cultural factors are also of great importance in this field of medicine. These issues were treated with particular care by the Inquiry and attention was drawn to the special shame felt by Maori women when undergoing gynaecological examinations.

Why do even the most well-meaning health care professionals still have such difficulty in treating these patients or clients as self-determining adults? Perhaps it is partly the fault of the ethos of professionalism, which affects students from an early stage in their training. What may be loosely termed the 'Hippocratic Tradition' puts all the stress on the dedication, good judgment and benevolent disposition of the doctor, whose first concern is to do what is best for 'his' patient. If we add to this the difficulties entailed in explaining the complexities and uncertainties of modern diagnosis and treatment to patients (especially when their anxiety is raised by the presence of a 'dread disease' like cancer), it is possible to understand how easily paternalistic approaches can be adopted. Yet, whatever the emphasis of the traditional Codes, respect for the individual patient and an awareness of her essential humanity has also been a contantly repeated ideal of medical practice. The so-called Prayer of Maimonides reminds us of a venerable tradition: 'May I never see in the patient anything else but a fellow creature in pain'.

But noble sentiments, however ancient, are unlikely to be sufficient to safeguard the rights of patients, especially in these times of ever-increasing demands on professions, matched by a rationing of resources. Perhaps wisely, the Inquiry came forward with a *legislative* solution as part of the answer to the problem, proposing an amendment to the NZ Human Rights Commission Act 1977 to include a statement of patients' rights and to provide for the appointment of a Heath Commissioner, who would heighten professionals' understanding of these rights and mediate and negotiate in cases of grievance. Should the NZ government act on this recommendation, the outcome will be of paramount interest to bioethics, for, it will make professionals in health care (and not only doctors) answerable in a new way to their patients, and so could bring the ideal of patient autonomy closer to the reality of day to day practice.

In a further effort to protect patients in the hospital under review the Report proposed the appointment of a patient advocate who would be responsible directly to the Director-General of Health. Her task would be to ensure that there was adequate information given to patients, that their complaints were properly attended to and that their rights were protected, especially if they were to be included in research projects. This is a genuinely innovative proposal, seeking to bring about a real change in the balance of power within the hospital. The Report recognises that the task will be a very difficult one, and only experience can show whether such a person can be both effective and respected by all the parties concerned. Whatever the practical outcome, however, the point of principle remains vital: patients' rights to information and adequate consultation cannot be left to the vagaries of professional benevolence. The analogy with a court of law is telling—due process is required, not just good intentions.

Related quite closely to the proposal to appoint a patient advocate is the judge's disenchantment with 'peer review' as it operated in the period under scrutiny. Commenting on the failure of the relevant committees to take note of the expressions of

64   ALASTAIR V. CAMPBELL

concern about the policy followed by Dr. Green, she states:

> I reserve particular disquiet not only for the fate of the . . .
> patients . . . but also for the future of peer review within the
> medical profession, if it cannot confront issues squarely and
> resolve them after such sustained, detailed and well documented
> statements of concern . . . (*Report* p. 101).

The issue at stake here is the claim to 'clinical freedom' which has
long been the shibboleth of professional status. The Report quotes
with approval from a celebrated leader in the *BMJ* by Professor
Hampton of Nottingham Medical School, which states

> Clinical freedom is dead, and no-one need regret its passing.
> Clinical freedom was the right—some seemed to believe the
> divine right—of doctors to do whatever in their opinion was
> best for their patients. (*BMJ* 1983, vol. 287, 1237.)

Of course this death is only a *theoretical* one. It can become a
reality only if peer review and interprofessional consultation are
made standard features of all hospital practice. The judge was not
sanguine about the effectiveness of such controls, at least in the
current climate in Auckland Women's. The *Report* describes a
general air of 'institutionalism', in which nurses must protect
patients' interest 'by stealth' and where 'The patient, her needs,
her pain, her views and her . . . family responsibilities sometimes
take second place.' (*Report*, p. 173).

Thus, in addition to the more effective communication with
patients to be ensured by the patient advocate, the Report called
for formal treatment protocols which would be regularly revised
by all medical staff, for both scientific and ethical assessments of
any significant shifts in treatment and for in-hospital and possibly
external audit for the quality of treatment being provided. In
short, the scope of the traditional autonomy of the individual
practitioner and of the medical professional group as a whole
would be circumscribed for the sake of the enhanced autonomy
and health prospects of patients. The Report makes this explicit:

> Now the patient must be involved in decisions concerning her
> management and colleagues must intervene if there is risk to
> the patient for any reason. The doctor is no longer wholly
> autonomous. (*Report*, p. 129).

Such views are very much in line with the contractual models
which have been gaining currency in recent theoretical accounts
of bioethics (see, for example, the 'triple contract' theory in R.
Veatch's *A Theory of Medical Ethics*). The crucial question, which

will be answered only when such measures are genuinely tried, is whether institutional change will achieve the desired ethical goal. Some may fear that without the requisite 'covenantal' spirit, external control will achieve little (see for example W. F. May, *Physician's Covenant*).

What, finally, are the ethical lessons to be learned from the 'unfortunate experiment'? The authors borrowed the phrase from a letter written to the *NE Medical Journal* by Dr. David Skegg, Professor of Preventive and Social Medicine in the University of Otago and Director of the Hugh Adam Cancer Epidemiology Unit. Professor Skegg was responding to an earlier letter from Dr. Green which had criticised the recommendations of a working group on the introduction of routine cervical screening in New Zealand. In his reply Skegg argues that 'the unfortunate experiment' at the National Women's Hospital had no bearing on the case for cervical screening, because those cases with continuing abnormal cytology which progressed to invasive cancer were dismissed by Green as being due to either inadequate exclusion of invasion at the outset or over-diagnosis of invasion later. Skegg's comments are worth quoting in full, since they neatly summarise two of the most fundamental issues in the ethics of clinical research:

> ... the whole argument betrays circular thinking. If the experiment was incapable of falsifying Green's hypothesis why was it carried out? Moreover, if invasion could not be excluded at the outset, were the patients warned of the risk that was being taken? (*NZ Med J*, Jan 1986, p. 26).

Fundamental to codes governing the ethics of experimentation (from the time of the Nuremberg trials onwards) are the requirements that there should be no undue risk to subjects, that the research should be scientifically sound, and that wherever possible the consent of subjects should be obtained. Yet the Inquiry found that a research proposal first considered by a meeting of the senior medical staff in 1956 (two years after the Declaration of Helsinki was adopted by the WMA and nearly four years after the first draft of the code was published in the *BMJ*) was 'an attempt to prove a theory that lacked scientific validity' (*Report*, p. 69), that failed to gain consent of patients and failed to take adequate account of predictable risks.

Perhaps this is the issue which must give the profession and the general public in New Zealand the greatest cause for concern. It could well be the tip of a singularly dangerous iceberg. The system of ethics committees in New Zealand has, to date, been very similar to that adopted in the UK, depending on guidelines issued by the MRC or the Royal Colleges rather than on government directives. There has been little or no monitoring of the extent to which the guidelines have been followed in individual centres of research. Scientists and clinical doctors naturally dislike what they regard as 'bureaucratic interference' and much prefer a voluntary system to control by a government department. But, as the Book of Judges observes, when there is no king in Israel, each man tends to do merely what is right in his own eyes! There is evidence to suggest that, as a result of the Inquiry, approaches taken by the NHMRC in Australia and by the Department of Health in the USA are being seriously considered by the NZ Director General of Health. An especially important issue will be the constitution and membership of committees and the extent to which lay participation in them is more than mere tokenism. The time is long past for 'gentleman's honour' in the control of research, especially when the majority of the 'gentlemen' are themselves researchers and very many of their patients or subjects are women.

Yet, although the Cervical Cancer Report reveals some disquieting things about the control of clinical research and of clinical practice in the particular hospital under review, it is by no means a totally bleak picture, nor can we suppose that it is only in New Zealand that medicine is prone to the dangers uncovered by the Inquiry. On the contrary, a Report which gives such detailed and well researched attention to ethical issues offers to all those professionally involved in the delivery of health care much to think about. One should especially note the care taken by the Inquiry to redress injustices done to women patients and its attention to the influence of professional education on the attitudes of future practitioners. All in all, it is a powerful endorsement of the centrality of ethical issues both in professional education and in the public debate about the quality of health care. If the Report gets the attention it deserves from the NZ government and from the professions worldwide, then the news from New Zealand is good news, manifesting two striking national qualities—openness and honesty about past mistakes and a real willingness to create a new future out of the lessons learned from such honest self appraisal.

Department of Christian Ethics and Practical Theology,
University of Edinburgh

[15]

Ian Kennedy

RESEARCH AND EXPERIMENTATION

A. Introduction

13.01 This Chapter is concerned with biomedical research on human subjects.[1] Research here principally refers to any intervention by touching or more, whereby the law as it relates to the inviolability of the person is engaged. This approach highlights the perspective of human rights which has been the central focus of discussion and analysis, particularly since the end of the Second World War. It also offers a way of understanding the underlying principles which inform and condition the law. To qualify as research, an intervention must form part of a programme of enquiry based on a scientifically plausible hypothesis, must follow a scientifically valid methodology, and be intended to produce data of a generalisable nature. The principal focus in this Chapter is on the doctor as medical researcher.[2] Research which

---

[1] For discussion of research on embryos and foetuses, see Chapters 10 and 15.

[2] Thus, this Chapter will not be concerned with such matters as the regulatory systems under which medicinal products or devices are licensed, once tested satisfactorily.

Introduction

does not involve touching, for example, observational or epidemiological research, will also be briefly discussed. In such research, the legal interests engaged are those of privacy and confidentiality.

Research on human subjects is most commonly associated with the development and testing of pharmaceutical products. Of course, research is conducted in all areas of medicine, but it should be noted that the case of surgery is somewhat exceptional. Developments in surgery are often described and reported as 'innovative therapy'.[3] This may not reflect any desire to avoid or finesse the regulatory mechanisms surrounding research. It may merely mean that surgeons oftentimes do not see themselves as engaged in research when they test out new procedures or techniques. The response of the law is that any innovation which departs from standard practice(s) will be regarded as research if it can be shown that the ordinary principles defining research (see para 13.01) apply. In such a case, the researcher will be expected to have observed the regulatory procedures, (see para 13.65). If the innovation does not qualify as research, the ordinary rules of the common law apply.

13.02

The focus in this Chapter is on the law. Much has been and, increasingly, is being written on the ethics of research.[4] There also exist a growing number of Codes of Ethics relating to research, both nationally—emanating from the medical profession, through, for example, the Royal Colleges and their Faculties, from industry, and from public bodies—and internationally from international agencies.[5] Clearly, the law takes account of and seeks to reflect what is thought to be ethically appropriate. Codes of Research Ethics may indeed set the standards which the law will seek to adopt.[6] Despite the very considerable growth in the number of Codes and the range of activities they address, however, the law, by contrast or maybe because of the increased availability of Codes, remains singularly underdeveloped. Remarkably, perhaps, there is no specific regime of law regulating research on humans. This is in contrast to the comprehensive legislative framework regulating the conduct of research on non-human animals.[7] Furthermore, there are no cases in English law directly related to the conduct of research, (and few in the

13.03

---

[3] See Kennedy and Grubb, *Medical Law: Text with Materials* (2nd edn, Butterworths, 1994), 1073 *et seq*.

[4] See eg, *Manual For Research Ethics Committees* (4th edn, Centre of Medical Law and Ethics, King's College London, 1996).

[5] ibid. And see Council of Europe's Convention on Human Rights and Biomedicine, 1997, Arts 16 and 17 and the Explanatory Report thereto from the Directorate of Legal Affairs, DIR/JUR(97)1. A detailed Protocol on Research is under consideration by the Council of Europe.

[6] See, for example, the detailed ethical requirements relating to consent set out in the European Guidelines on Good Clinical Practice, *Manual* (n 4 above).

[7] Consolidated currently in the Animals (Scientific Procedures) Act 1986.

13: Research and Experimentation

Commonwealth), on which to draw. Thus, the exposition of the law which follows is fundamentally a matter of applying the relevant common law principles—particularly the law relating to consent and to the torts of battery and negligence—and the relevant European law.[8]

13.04 At the most general level, there are two major areas which need to be examined:

(a) the lawfulness of any proposed research procedure; and

(b) the relevant regulatory/supervisory mechanisms.

B. Lawfulness

13.05 It will be recalled that the principal concern here is with research which involves touching the research subject. For the purposes of analysis, the common classification of research as being either **therapeutic** or **non-therapeutic** will be adopted. These two types of research are distinguished from each other by reference to the intention of the researcher. In the case of therapeutic research, there is a dual intention, both to seek to benefit the patient who is the research subject *and* to gather data of a generalisable nature. In non-therapeutic research, there is only a *single* intention: to gather data. Whether any proposed intervention qualifies as research (see para 13.01) is measured, prima facie, by reference to the views of peers. This means that, as regards any claim for damages brought by someone harmed as a consequence of alleged research, the complainant must show that the procedure should not have been carried out because it had no scientific plausibility or the methodology was flawed. The cause of action would be in negligence. The court would largely rely on expert evidence such that *Bolam*[9] would apply, as modified by *Bolitho*.[10]

13.06 There are certain general legal themes which are common to the consideration of all forms of research. The most important is the theme of **consent**. As regards medical *treatment*, the general law provides that consent is required before a patient may lawfully be touched, (save in the special circumstances of

---

[8] See further, Kennedy and Grubb (n 3 above), ch 14. Curiously, one of the very, very few examples of legislation concerned with research on human subjects can be found in the rather obscure statutory instrument, SI 1992/3146, Sch 3 implementing 90/385/EEC, The Active Implantable Medical Devices Regulations 1992. By Sch 3, clinical investigations must be carried out in accordance with the Declaration of Helsinki, as amended (on which, see *Manual*, n 4 above).

[9] *Bolam v Friern Hospital Management Committee* [1957] 1 WLR 582.

[10] *Bolitho v City and Hackney Health Authority* [1997] 4 All ER 771, and see discussion in Chapter 7.

Lawfulness

an emergency). The consent must come from the patient, if competent, or, in the case of an incompetent child, from someone with parental responsibility. Failure to obtain consent will result in liability for battery or negligence. The current law contemplates circumstances in which a doctor would not be liable in negligence for failing, in the process of obtaining consent to treatment, to pass on certain information to a patient, if, in the opinion of fellow professionals, it would not be in the patient's interests to do so. This approach, (not without its critics[11]), will be examined later as to its application to research, (see paras. 13.23–13.25). However, the law allows no exception to the requirement that, at the very least, that degree of consent necessary to defeat a claim in battery must be obtained from a patient prior to treatment. By the same token, the law is clear that a patient who refuses consent may not thereafter be treated.[12] *A fortiori*, therefore, the general law applies in the case of therapeutic *research*. *Consent*, at least sufficient to counter any claim in battery, *is required*.

13.07 Participation in research entails an act of altruism. Thus, the law's concern for the need to obtain legally valid and effective consent to any proposed research comes as no surprise. As will be seen later, however, this concern for consent is not free of difficulties. In particular, it creates problems for those who wish to conduct certain forms of research, for example on young children and on incompetent adults.

13.08 The examination of consent which follows will concentrate on the various, interrelated legal issues which arise from the law's concern for consent. The first is concerned with **competence** to consent to research. The second relates to **who** may consent: whether the law recognises the authority to consent of anyone other than the research subject. The third issue is how the **validity** of any apparent consent is established. The fourth issue is what may be consented to: the **limits** of consent.

13.09 As a matter of everyday practice, the various legal issues considered here, in so far as they are also matters of ethics, are scrutinised by Research Ethics Committees (RECs)[13] to which research proposals are ordinarily submitted. The role and status of these Committees will be considered later (see para 13.70 *et seq*). Suffice it to say here that they have developed working practices which require researchers to give their minds to, and set out their responses to, the legal issues arising from the conduct of research.

---

[11] See eg Kennedy, I, *Treat Me Right* (Clarendon Press, 1992), ch 9; and Chalmers and Schwartz, '*Rogers v Whitaker* and Informed Consent in Australia' (1993) 1 Med L Rev 139.   [12] *Re MB* [1997] 8 Med LR 217.
[13] On which see *Manual* (n 4 above).

C. Therapeutic Research

Research Subjects

13.10 For the purposes of analysing the legal issues referred to (para 13.08 above), it is helpful to consider research on **children** (ie persons under 18 years of age) and on **adults** (ie persons over 18 years of age) separately.

1. Children

(i) *Consent: Competence*

13.11 If it is the word *'therapeutic'*, in the term therapeutic research, which is dominant, then the ordinary common law should apply. This would mean that a child over sixteen years of age would appear, by virtue of section 8(1) of the Family Law Reform Act, 1969,[14] to have the capacity to consent to therapeutic research. As regards a child under sixteen, the law as laid down in *Gillick v West Norfolk and Wisbech AHA* [15] would apply, namely that such a child's consent would be valid in law if the child had sufficient maturity and understanding. Of course, since something more than treatment alone is involved, the degree of understanding required would be commensurately high. On this view, however, there would be no general rule that therapeutic research on children under the age of sixteen may not be carried out solely on the basis of the child's consent, despite the child's apparent competence. The decision would rest on the facts of each case. Alternatively, and this is the more cautious view adopted by a number of bodies concerned with the ethics of research, it may be that the law would take a paternalistic position and decide that as regards any procedure other than the very simple and risk-free, there would be the strongest presumption against competence.[16] By contrast, should a competent child refuse permission rather than consent to take part in a therapeutic research project, current law could have it that the child's refusal may be ignored if the parents give consent. This is the case as regards medical treatment *simpliciter*.[17] The criticism to which this view has been

---

[14] See Kennedy and Grubb (n 3 above), 108–9.
[15] [1986] AC 112, and see Kennedy and Grubb (n 3 above), 109 *et seq*.
[16] See eg, *Research Involving Patients* (Royal College of Physicians, 1990), para 7.32. The Department of Health's guidance goes further and states that 'it would . . . be unacceptable not to have the consent of the parent or guardian where the child is under 16', Local Research Ethics Committees, HSG (91) 5 para 4.2.
[17] *Re W* (*A Minor*) (*Medical Treatment*) [1992] 4 All ER 627, but cf the view taken in HSG (91) 15, written before the decision in *Re W.*

subjected,[18] however, would suggest that it would be unwise to ignore the refusal of a competent child. Certainly, the prevailing view in medical ethics is that the refusal of a competent child, or even the dissent of a child not deemed competent, should be honoured.

If the word 'research' is dominant, then section 8(1) may not apply. Lord **13.12** Donaldson MR and Nolan LJ in *Re W (A Minor) (Medical Treatment)*[19] made it clear that the wording of the section was limited to 'surgical, medical or dental *treatment*' (emphasis added), and did not apply to non-therapeutic research. It could well be that this reasoning could be extended to therapeutic research. In this case, the common law would govern until the child reached adulthood. The question then becomes whether the different emphasis, whereby the word research is stressed, would lead to a different view of the common law from that just stated (para 13.11). The probable answer is that it would reinforce the more cautious view of the law. Thus, save in those cases involving the most trivial intervention, carrying minimal risk or inconvenience, a child would be deemed—by virtue of being a child and thus presumed to be lacking maturity and the ability to weigh risks against benefits—as a matter of law to be incompetent to consent to therapeutic research.

Where a child is judged incompetent to give a valid consent, a researcher **13.13** must seek consent elsewhere. Although not strictly required in law, it is deemed proper to seek the assent of the child before proceeding. Equally, while, in principle, the refusal of an incompetent child to participate lacks any legal effect, it is deemed good ethical practice at the very least to take seriously any refusal or expression of dissent by the child.[20]

(ii) *Consent: Who*

Where a child is competent and the proposed intervention is deemed to be **13.14** one to which the child can consent, the child's consent will be valid. In this regard, the child is in no different a position in law than the competent adult, such that references hereafter to a competent child can be read as referring equally to a competent adult. Where the child is not competent, consent must be obtained from a parent, or person with parental responsibility, (including, where relevant, the court).

---

[18] See eg, Kennedy and Grubb (n 3 above), 392–6.   [19] N 17 above.
[20] *Research Involving Patients* (n 16 above), para 7.34.

(iii) *Consent: Validity*

13.15 Does the law stipulate the *form* in which consent to participate in therapeutic research must be expressed? The general common law rule relating to medical treatment is, of course, that there are no requirements as to form. This is so despite the elevation of the 'consent form' to the status of an icon in medical practice (at least in hospitals though, oddly, not in general practice). It is trite law that the consent form may be evidence of consent, but the law's real concern is with real consent, as established by all the evidence and not just a consent form. The law relating to therapeutic research may not be different, even though superficially it may appear to be. It is standard practice for RECs to require that they be informed about the procedures to be adopted by the researcher in order to obtain consent. This will normally involve the submission of a draft consent form to the REC for approval. It does not follow that any failure to use the approved form would render legally invalid any consent obtained which is otherwise valid. It may well be that the researcher would be guilty of unethical conduct, but, provided the law was satisfied that real consent was, in fact obtained, the precise form would be of no concern.

13.16 Consent, to be valid, must be both *voluntary*, that is freely given, and properly *informed*. The ordinary principles of the common law apply, but given that research is involved, observance of them is subject to particular scrutiny. Both of the requirements pose problems in the case of children.

13.17 As regards *voluntariness*, in the, perhaps rare, case in which a child may be judged prima facie competent, the law's concern is to be vigilant to ensure that no pressure or persuasion has been brought to bear which could have overborne the child's capacity to refuse participation. Clearly, there is an interaction here with the law on competence, since in both cases a high level of maturity would be insisted upon. Where a child is incompetent to consent, it may be thought that the problem of voluntariness would be less serious, since the parents would be involved and have to consent. However, parents caring both for and about sick children are vulnerable to pressure. The law would again be vigilant to ensure that they have freely agreed that their child should participate in the proposed research. In other words, there must be no indication of pressure, however subtle, by, for example, being told that their child must be part of the research project as a condition of receiving any treatment, (save in the rare case where this is so). In practice, the relevant REC will have explored this issue, if it is doing its job properly. As has been said, it is standard practice for RECs to require consent forms to be submitted by researchers as part of the research proposal. These must then be approved,

Children

as must any accompanying information sheet. In the relatively rare case where research is conducted without prior submission to an REC, the law would probably treat evidence of what RECs regard as reasonable practice as its guide.

As regards *information*, again, in the case of a child who is prima facie **13.18** competent, there is an obvious interaction between competence and being properly informed. The relative complexity of the information which it is intended to pass on to the child and the child's ability both to comprehend it and deal with it emotionally will necessarily condition any view as to the child's competence. That said, there is clearly a duty properly to inform the competent child. The general law on the doctor's duty to inform a patient about proposed treatment is currently that laid down in *Sidaway v Governors of Bethlem Hospital*.[21] In the context of research, however, there must be added to the somewhat minimalist approach of *Sidaway*, the law's proper recognition of the fact that the patient is acting in the public interest. Consequently, any discretion not to disclose information which may be enjoyed by doctors under the general law is limited, in the context of research, by the law's desire to ensure that the patient's interests are appropriately secured. Thus, at the very least, the doctor is under a duty to inform the competent child of the fact that the treatment being proposed is part of a research project, and also of the implications and consequences of this fact. The former means that the patient is entitled to be told how involvement in research will affect the proposed therapeutic procedure and future health status. It also involves being told, for example, if the proposed research is, as is usual in the case of pharmaceutical research, a Randomised Controlled Trial (RCT) and what this means.[22] The latter involves such questions as whether there will be more than the usual number of interventions (for example, more blood samples taken), or more visits to the hospital or doctor than would be normal, or whether a lengthier than usual stay in hospital will be required, or more follow-up examinations called for. It also requires that the patient must be told of such matters as the foreseeable risks (both present and longer term), what provision exists for after care in the event that matters do not proceed as intended, and what alternatives exist to the therapeutic research being proposed. It may also involve, if the circumstances warrant it, informing the patient of any arrangements for compensation should things go wrong. Critically, patients must be told that they can withdraw from the research at any time without incurring any disadvantage in treatment, or

---

[21] [1985] AC 871.
[22] For an explanation and discussion of RCTs, see *Research Involving Patients* (n 16 above), para 7.93 *et seq*.

13: Research and Experimentation

generally (save in the unusual circumstances in which treatment is only available under a research protocol).[23]

13.19 The REC, in carrying out its responsibility to approve the proposed consent form and information sheet, is concerned to insist on what is judged to be ethically appropriate. It is unlikely that the ethical and the legal will diverge. To the extent that they do, the requirements of the law must be observed, if otherwise that which is judged ethically appropriate detracts in any significant way from that required by law. To the extent that the REC requires more of the researcher than the current law demands, the point may arrive at which such requirements themselves become incorporated into the law. Such a view is a consequence of the reasoning in the *Bolam/Sidaway* approach, namely that the views of the REC reflect a responsible body of informed and expert opinion, including that of doctors. In this way, the law will develop a framework of regulation which meets proper ethical standards, drawing *inter alia* on such principles as those laid down in the various International Conventions post-Nuremberg, as well as more recent European developments.[24]

13.20 It is important here to notice a development in Europe, the precise legal effect of which remains unclear. The Committee for Proprietary Medicinal Products (CPMP) of the European Community in 1991 issued its *Guidelines on Good Clinical Practice for Trials on Medicinal Products in the European Community*.[25] As the name indicates, the *Guidelines on GCP* do not themselves have the force of law although they were intended to be, and have since become, the basis for the conduct of the relevant research. The *Guidelines on GCP* have extensive provisions relating to 'informed consent' which could be thought to go beyond the requirements of the common law, in detailing the extent of the researcher's duty to disclose.[26] Subsequently, as part of the process of the harmonisation of European law relating to the testing and licensing of medicinal products, Directive 91/507/EEC was issued. This was incorporated into English law by the Medicines (Applications for Grant of Product Licences—Products for Human Use) Regulations 1993.[27] The

---

[23] The matters referred to are among the many addressed in such guides as *Research Involving Patients* (n 16 above) and form part of the legal duty to inform to the extent that, in the circumstances, the patient reasonably needs to know them so as to make a considered decision.

[24] For instance, the European Convention on Human Rights and Biomedicine.

[25] See *Manual* (n 4 above). These *Guidelines* have been superseded by International Guidelines, ICH Good Clinical Practice, Step 4 Consolidated Guideline i.5.96 (CPMP/ICH/135/95) but there is no reference to them in any law which could justify the argument that *they* have been incorporated by reference into European and hence English law.

[26] See the text and dicussion in Kennedy and Grubb (n 3 above), 1047–8.

[27] SI 1993/2538.

Children

Directive, (and thus the Regulations), provides that, '[a]ll phases of clinical investigation . . . shall be designed, implemented and reported in accordance with *good clinical practice*' (emphasis added).[28] On one view, this reference to 'good clinical practice' incorporates by reference the 1991 *Guidelines on GCP* into English law, at least as regards research leading to an application for a product licence for a medicinal product. Thus, the consent requirements generally, and specifically those relating to the researcher's duty to inform, must be read in the light of the *Guidelines on GCP.* Alternatively, and perhaps this is the better view with regard to the researcher's *legal* duty, the *Guidelines on GCP* were not incorporated into English law by the Regulations. Thus, their legal significance lies not in the fact that they are embodied in delegated legislation, but rather that they represent what a reasonable REC should require and take account of. As such, of course, they begin to mark out the boundaries of the researcher's legal duty.

13.21 The fact that the child, though competent, is, by definition, ill (in that the concern here is with therapeutic research), may appear to serve as a ground for arguing that, notwithstanding the general principles discussed above (para 13.18), *Sidaway* (discredited as it may be) allows the doctor engaged in the research a wide discretion as to what to tell the child. The response is that the law would not permit a researcher to use the fact of illness as a ground for not properly informing the patient. It has been argued, for example, that a patient suffering from cancer should not be told that she is involved in a research project, since that would inevitably involve telling her that she had cancer, something which the attending doctors had decided not to do. However, this is to turn on its head the respect for the person which underlies the law. It is to suggest that if consent to participate in research may be difficult to obtain, it should be dispensed with. The law's response is that if informing a competent patient of the fact that she is participating in a research project would not be in the patient's interests, the patient should not participate. To argue that it is in the interests of the patient, who is otherwise competent, to be protected from information, is either to say that the patient (here a child), in fact is not competent, or that the pursuit of research has a greater priority under the law than the protection of a patient's rights, a proposition which the law would emphatically reject.

13.22 Where a child is incompetent to give a valid consent, it is the person with parental authority who must be informed. Here there is no room at all for arguments in favour of allowing doctors a discretion as to what parents (or others) should be told. The duty placed on them by the law to act in the

---

[28] Para 1.1, Part 4B, Annex to Directive 91/507/1991.

13: Research and Experimentation

child's best interests[29] means that as regards treatment *simpliciter*, a doctor has a duty to inform the parents as fully as possible. Only thus will a parent be able to fulfil the role which the law imposes. Consequently, a doctor has no discretion to withhold any information necessary for making a considered decision about treatment. *A fortiori*, no such discretion exists when there is the added dimension that the parent is being asked to involve a child in research, at least in part for the common good. It follows that parents must be given all that information which will allow them properly to weigh the risks and benefits and thus determine the interests of the child.

(iv) *Consent: Limits*

13.23 As was discussed above, the competent child can, theoretically at least, consent to anything which is otherwise permissable under the general law. In practice, however, the better view is that the law will be slow to find a child competent, save in those cases in which the proposed intervention is trivial. Thus, to the question, to what may a competent child consent, the answer is, not very much: only that which is readily comprehensible and does not pose any but the remotest risk, in the form of short or long-term physical or psychological harm.

13.24 As regards the incompetent child, the law is obviously keen to set limits to what the child may be volunteered for by the parent or other. As will be seen, these limits differ depending on whether the proposed research is therapeutic or non-therapeutic. As regards therapeutic research, given the therapeutic element, the relevant legal criterion as regards the limits of consent is the same as that which the law uses in the case of treatment *simpliciter*, namely, the best interests of the child. The parent must weigh up the risks and benefits to the child of participating in the research project. Clearly, the more ill the child, the more potentially beneficial the consequences if the child is exposed to what is proposed, and the more dire the consequences if the child is not, the greater the risks to which the parent may expose the child. This is no more than an application of the more general proportionality test, which must be satisfied so as to honour the law's commitment to the paramountcy of the child's welfare.[30]

13.25 The European *Guidelines on Good Clinical Practice*, referred to above (para 13.20) specifically address the issue of research on those unable to consent. As

---

[29] See, Kennedy and Grubb (n 3 above), 255 *et seq.*   [30] ibid.
[31] Para 1.13, Guidelines on GCP, *Manual* (n 4 above).

Adults

regards therapeutic research on children, they contemplate that this is both ethical and lawful, provided there is approval from the REC and from those with parental authority, on the basis that the research will promote the interests and welfare of the child.[31]

2. Adults

(i) *Consent: Competence*

The criteria of competence to consent to participate in therapeutic research **13.26** mirror those laid down by Thorpe J in *Re C*[32] as regards consent to treatment; namely, that the patient first, comprehends and retains treatment information, secondly, believes it and thirdly weighs it in the balance to arrive at a choice.[33] The only question which arises is whether the fact that the patient is consenting to something in addition to treatment means that the criteria for consent are more demanding. The answer must be that the comprehension referred to in *Re C* must extend to participation in the research project. Thus, the criteria are not different, they must merely be applied to the facts of involvement in research.

(ii) *Consent: Who*

Obviously, in the case of the *competent* adult, it is the adult and no one else **13.27** whose consent must be sought and given.

As regards the *incompetent* adult, the picture is less clear. It is settled law that, **13.28** unlike a child, no one can consent to treatment on behalf of an adult in English law.[34] This cannot mean, however, as the House of Lords in *Re F* made clear, that the inability to consent makes it always unlawful to treat an incompetent adult. Such a result would be grotesque. Rather, the law is that consent, in the case of the incompetent adult, is no longer the relevant legal consideration. Instead, the doctor stands as a proxy and is entitled in law to treat if such treatment is in the patient's best interests. Where what is contemplated is therapeutic research, the therapeutic element would suggest that the same rule applies. By this reasoning, the doctor may involve the incompetent adult in therapeutic research if what is to be undertaken is in the

---

[31] *Re C (Refusal of Medical Treatment)* [1994] 1 FLR 31 as explained in *Re MB* (n 12 above).
[33] ibid, 36. See also the similar approach adopted by the Law Commission in *Mental Incapacity*, Law Com No 231 (1995).
[34] *Re F (A Mental Patient: Sterilisation)* [1990] 2 AC 1.

patient's best interests. Clearly, if the treatment holds out a prospect of benefit and is not available other than in a research project, or if the prospects of benefit outweigh both any risks that may be involved and the consequences of not being exposed to the procedure, the involvement of the incompetent adult would seem to be prima facie lawful.[35]

13.29   Much depends, however, on what is chosen as the appropriate legal basis for determining best interests. One approach is that *Bolam* governs;[36] that a patient's best interests are determined by reference to what an informed body of medical opinion would decide. This approach, however, could weight the scales in favour of a view that being involved in research is, ipso facto, in a patient's best interests, not least because most doctors are persuaded of the benefits of carrying out therapeutic research and can rationalise their decision by referring, for example, to the heightened quality of care often associated with involvement in research. An alternative, and arguably more defensible position, is that *Bolam* is not relevant and that any determination of best interests must be made by reference to more explicit and objective criteria. The question remains where the onus should be. If research, even therapeutic research, is seen as raising human rights issues, (which are, of course, always lurking in medical law), then the onus ought to be on those proposing the research to justify it and to do so by means of evidence which addresses specific questions, rather than allowing research to go through on the nod of interested parties, for example, doctors. This would entail the development of a conceptual shortlist of the sort of matters relating to best interests which are raised by research.

(iii)   *Consent: Validity*

13.30   As regards the *form* which consent must take, the law relating to research on the competent adult is *mutatis mutandis* the same as that set out above (para 13.15). In the case of the incompetent adult, as has been made clear, consent, strictly speaking, has no place. Rather, the doctor must make a judgment of the patient's best interests. The intention to involve incompetent adults in a research project will have been made clear to the REC, which will have insisted on being satisfied that the proposed research was, in fact, in the patient's best interests. The recording of the REC's approval and the doctor's judgment in the patient's notes will, if the involvement of the patient is thereafter challenged, serve as evidence that consideration was given by the

---

[35] See further, the discussion in Kennedy and Grubb (n 3 above), 1052–4.

[36] See *Re F* (n 34 above), *per* Lord Goff, and discussion in Kennedy and Grubb (n 3 above), 321 *et seq*.

Adults

doctor to the relevant issues. It would, of course, only be evidence of form. It would still be open to a court to conclude that the research was not, in fact, in the patient's best interests.

What was said previously (paras 13.16–13.20) concerning the need for **13.31** consent to be both *voluntary* and *informed* applies *mutatis mutandis* to therapeutic research on the competent adult. These requirements cannot, of course, apply in the case of the adult who is incapable of giving consent. That said, the law will regard it as part of the doctor's obligation, in reaching the conclusion that involvement in a research project is in the patient's best interests, to have taken account of and weighed appropriately all relevant information before reaching this conclusion.

(iv) *Consent: Limits*

As noted above (para 13.23) the law limits the extent to which a competent **13.32** child may consent to therapeutic research by the device of adopting a demanding set of criteria for establishing competence. The law's concern to protect the vulnerable is less pronounced in the case of such research on competent adults. The assumption, intrinsic to the notion of competence, applies that people should be left to make their own decisions. Thus, the law places no limit on what the competent adult may consent to by way of therapeutic research, subject to any overarching prohibitions contained in the general law.[37] The prior scrutiny of an REC will, of course, serve to ensure that the patient is not invited to consent to that which it would be unethical to carry out.

When the adult patient is incompetent, the limits to what therapeutic **13.33** research may be carried out are contained within the concept of best interests. This being so, it is clearly desirable, as was suggested above (para 13.29), that, from the point of view of safeguarding the patient, some flesh, by way of explicit criteria, should be put on the bones of the otherwise unsatisfactorily vague concept of best interests. The Law Commission made some efforts in this direction in its Report on Mental Incapacity.[38] These do not have the force of law but they do suggest and, it is argued, reflect the kind of factors a

---

[37] See eg, *R v Brown* [1993] 2 All ER 65.
[38] N 33 above, Part III, para 3.26 *et seq*. A 'checklist of factors' is proposed in para 3.28. In its Consultation Paper, 'Who Decides?' (Cm 3803) (1997), which reviews the Law Commission's Report, the Government 'endorses the need for guidance as to the criteria that must be taken into account when a decision-maker is considering what is in a person without capacity's best interests' but seeks views on whether the proposed checklist 'would prove workable, and useful, in practice', at 14.

court should take into account. Thus, they and other similar considerations are what should guide the REC, in its prior evaluation of a research proposal, and the doctor, in deciding whether to involve an incompetent adult patient. Above all, in therapeutic research, where there is an intention to benefit the particular patient as well as to produce generalisable data, the principle of proportionality applies. If the patient is severely ill, greater risks may be taken if the possibility of benefit is medically plausible and the alternative is otherwise bleak. Clearly, if the research involves extra interventions, or greater inconvenience or pain, the justification, that it is in the patient's best interests, must be that much stronger. As has been said, these would be matters that the REC would be expected to examine.

13.34   The question then arises whether, if the researcher has complied with the criteria of best interests stipulated by the REC, this would serve as a defence to any action subsequently brought by a patient or his representative, alleging that the research project was not in his best interests? The answer must be that compliance would be good evidence of the reasonableness of the doctor's judgment as to the patient's best interests, such that an action, whether in battery or negligence, would be unlikely to succeed.

D. Non-Therapeutic Research

Introduction

13.35   Non-therapeutic research, it will be recalled, is research carried out to produce generalisable scientific data but with no intention to benefit the research subject. It is ordinarily conducted on healthy volunteers, although it may, rarely, be carried out also on patients if it is concerned with matters other than the patient's specific illness and does not expose the patient to any additional risk of harm. Clearly, because of the altruism of the volunteer and of the fact that no benefit is intended, since no procedure can be free of risk, the law is, arguably, particularly vigilant to ensure that the volunteer is protected from harm or exploitation. This is, however, an assertion of general principle, since, as was pointed out at the outset, there is, surprisingly, no specific regime of law governing medical research, not even non-therapeutic research.

13.36   In the paragraphs which follow, the issues considered earlier in the context of therapeutic research will again be analysed as they affect non-therapeutic research. As before, the principal focus of the law is on **consent**. The same distinctions will be drawn between the child under eighteen years of age and the adult, and between the competent and the incompetent.

1. Consent: Competence

The criteria governing competence to consent are the same for non-thera-   **13.37**
peutic as for therapeutic research. While the application of these criteria is
relatively unproblematic in the case of *adult* volunteers, the legal position
regarding a *child* volunteer is not without difficulty. The law's concern to
protect the vulnerable even from themselves could, on one view, suggest that a
child should always be regarded, as a matter of law, as incompetent to
consent. Such a view is hard to support. It would involve the adoption of a
status approach to competence, (that competence depends on the fact of
minority), rejected by the House of Lords in *Gillick*[39] in favour of an
approach based on comprehension. As a matter of law, therefore, there is
no room for a blanket assumption of incompetence. Furthermore, as a matter
of logic, it is perfectly plausible to contend that, in certain circumstances, a
particular child may be competent to consent to a particular non-therapeutic
research procedure. Such a view, of course, reflects the pragmatism of the
common law and its commitment to the supremacy of the particular facts. It
is, however, a view which causes concern lest it go too far.[40] The best view,
therefore, may be as follows. A sweeping prohibition on all non-therapeutic
research on children relying solely on the child's consent, on the basis of an
irrebuttable presumption of incompetence to consent, cannot be justified. A
strong presumption exists, however, against the use of a child volunteer,
without the involvement of parents, such that very clear evidence of competence to consent will be required before non-therapeutic research may legitimately be carried out on the child.

2. Consent: Who

In the case of a competent adult, it is the adult whose consent must be sought   **13.38**
and given. In those, albeit very limited, circumstances in which a child is
deemed competent, it is the child who must consent.

In the case of an incompetent child, the general law provides that it is the   **13.39**
person with parental responsibility who may consent on behalf of the child.
The criterion governing this power to consent is, as before, the best interests
of the child. Here a difficulty arises. It can be argued that non-therapeutic
research, because it is not intended to benefit the child and is never entirely
free of risk when some form of intervention is to be carried out, can never, as

---

[39] N 15 above.
[40] See eg, the view taken in the Department of Health's guidance (n 16 above), para 4.3.

a consequence, be said to be in the child's *best* interests. On the other hand, it can be objected that some non-therapeutic research on incompetetent children ought to be permissable. It is clear that children suffer from children's diseases. Thus, data on healthy children are essential, for example, so as to identify what deviations from a norm are pathological. Data generated from research on adults may not be relevant. In such circumstances, it would be at least unfortunate, the argument goes, if such data could not be collected because of an overall ban on non-therapeutic research on incompetent children.

13.40 A compromise which is probably acceptable to the law is as follows. The criterion for consent to non-therapeutic research by those with parental responsibility should be the more relaxed test of whether the proposed research is *not against* the child's interests, rather than the need to show it is in the child's best interests.[41] The law should only follow this approach, however, subject to two crucial provisos. The first is that the research be approved independently by an REC. The second is that there should be strict limits to that for which the parent may volunteer the child. These all important limits are considered below (paras 13.55–13.56). Translated into legal analysis, therefore, the law would be that it would serve as an answer to an action, whether in battery or negligence, for the researcher to point to the fact that the child's interests had been carefully considered and a decision had been taken that what was proposed was not against the child's interests, viewed objectively and provided the proper limits were observed.

13.41 It is important to note that this view appears to be at odds with that expressed in the European *Guidelines on GCP.* By paragraph 1.15, '[c]onsent must always be given by the signature of the subject in a non-therapeutic study,[42] ie when there is no direct clinical benefit to the subject'.[43] If a subject is incompetent to consent, *ex hypothesi* no valid signature can be given. Thus, non-therapeutic research on such a subject is prohibited. A parent, consequently, may not authorise non-therapeutic research on a child. As has been seen, there is some doubt as to whether the *Guidelines on GCP* form part of English law even in that area to which they are addressed, namely research leading to an application for a product licence for a medicinal product. If they do, the view taken above (para 13.40) on the conduct of non-therapeutic research on incompetent children may to that extent need to be revised. Such

---

[41] For discussion of this test, see Kennedy and Grubb (n 3 above), 256–8, 1061–5 and *S v S, W v Official Solicitor* (or *W*) [1972] AC 24, *per* Lord Reid.

[42] It should be noted that the ICH Guidelines (n 25 above) appear to be somewhat less restrictive as regards research on the incompetent (para 4.8.14), but the wording is by no means unequivocal. [43] See *Manual* (n 4 above).

a consequence, however, may well be regarded as unfortunate, and would provide an argument for a court's holding that the Regulations translating European Directive 91/507/EEC into English law do not, in fact, incorporate the *Guidelines on GCP.*

Non-therapeutic research on an incompetent *adult* poses even greater pro-   **13.42**
blems. As has been seen, no one has authority to consent on behalf of an adult. Moreover, a proxy decision-maker must act in the best interests of the adult. Given the nature of non-therapeutic research (that it confers no benefit but carries some risk), it would appear to follow that a proxy decision-maker, who unlike the person with parental responsibility is not consenting on behalf of the adult, has no authority to volunteer an incompetent adult for involvement in such research. From this would follow the inevitable conclusion that non-therapeutic research on an incompetent adult is unlawful.

Furthermore, the interaction of the European *Guidelines on GCP,* Directive   **13.43**
91/507/EEC, and the 1993 Regulations, which was examined above (paras 13.20 and 13.41), adds further force to this view. The apparent prohibition on non-therapeutic research on the incompetent, at least in the context of research leading to an application for a product licence for a medicinal product, would clearly apply to the incompetent adult. It is no surprise, therefore, that the Law Commission in its Report on Mental Incapacity also concluded that non-therapeutic research on adults incompetent to consent for themselves is currently unlawful.[44]

It is important, therefore, to identify what, if any, legal counter-arguments   **13.44**
may exist to justify some, albeit very limited, research on the incompetent adult. First, the same sort of arguments set out in para 13.39 above can be advanced here. Research into certain diseases which result in incompetence may be impeded if, for example, tests on the incompetent themselves, so as to discover possible variations from the norm, were outlawed. On the other hand, concern to protect the vulnerable from exploitation is particularly keen in this context. The law cannot be seen to condone circumstances in which the incompetent are converted into guinea pigs for the benefit of the more fortunate. The central question is as follows. The law may, as was suggested above (para 13.40), accept a less demanding test of when non-therapeutic research may be carried out on incompetent children, namely that the proposed research is not against the child's interests, provided certain safeguards are observed. Even if this is the law as regards children, does it apply to incompetent adults, (whether generally, or, in the event that they are part of

---

[44] N 33 above, paras 6.28 *et seq.*

English law, where the *Guidelines on GCP* do not apply)? Clearly, there is no definitive answer to this question. Equally clearly, any view expressed by the Law Commission, that non-therapeutic research on incompetent adults is currently unlawful, would not lightly be disregarded by a court. Nonetheless, the view taken here is that such non-therapeutic research on incompetent adults may be lawful, subject to the strictest safeguards, as set out below (paras 13.55–13.56). The basis of its lawfulness rests on the reasoning and the test advanced above (paras 13.39–13.40), that the research is *not against* the interests of the incompetent person and is subject to strict limits, supervised by the REC.[45] The position of the Law Commission can, perhaps be explained by its desire to expose the uncertainties of current law with a view, then, to proposing a comprehensive legislative solution. This case is better made if the current law is viewed abstractly in the least favourable light rather than pragmatically as being the only law there currently is.

13.45 Indeed, the Law Commission recommended that non-therapeutic research *should* be lawful if, besides involving no more than minimal risk and invasiveness, the research was into the condition which the patient suffered from and provided that certain procedures were satisfied. (The recommended procedures are in Clause 11(i) of the Draft Bill). The insistence that the research be limited to the condition which a patient has seems difficult to justify. Apart from the hope that the patient may one day benefit, which, by definition is not the intended reason for doing the research, the patient's incompetence presumably relates as much to his own condition as to others. It seems, therefore, that what is being offered is an apparent ethical life-line to those seeking to justify the otherwise unjustifiable, in particular so as to allow research on such conditions as Alzheimer's Disease to be conducted on those suffering from it. The Government's response in its Consultation Paper is suitably cautious about contemplating even this limited degree of non-therapeutic research on the incompetent. Baldly it asks, 'Should procedures not intended to benefit the patient be allowed?'[46]

3. Consent: Validity

13.46 *Competent* volunteers, as a matter of law, may consent to non-therapeutic research without observing any particular *form*, providing they have in fact given consent. Ordinarily, of course, the relevant REC will have insisted on written consent, in an approved form, as a requirement of the ethical accept-

---

[45] Support for this approach, from an ethical point of view, can be found, for example, in guidance from the Medical Research Council, *The Ethical Conduct of Research on the Mentally Incapacitated*, 1991.   [46] See 'Who Decides?' (n 38 above), 41.

ability of the research proposal. To the extent that the *Guidelines on GCP* are part of English law, (as discussed in para 13.20 above), they stipulate, in Para 1.14, that consent must 'always be given by the signature of the subject', that is to say, in writing.

As regards non-therapeutic research on an *incompetent child*, to the extent, **13.47** argued above, that such research can be lawful, the law does not specify any particular form which consent must take. If consent may be given, it must be given by the person with parental responsibility, and, as a matter of proper caution, it would be wise for it to be set down in writing. Ordinarily, of course, the REC, in deciding whether to approve the research proposal, will have insisted on written consent.

In the case of research involving the *incompetent adult*, strictly speaking, the **13.48** form of consent does not arise, since consent does not. However, if the view expressed above (para 13.44) represents the law and non-therapeutic research, generally or subject to the application of the *Guidelines on GCP,* may lawfully be carried out within limits, some formal recording of the process leading to the decision would appear to be at least desirable. The decision-maker would wish to record the factors taken into account in reaching the view that the proposed non-therapeutic research was not against the adult's interests, and the fact that the relevant REC had been consulted and given its approval. This record, although not formally required as a prerequisite for undertaking the research, would serve as evidence that the researcher's mind was directed to the factors deemed relevant by the law, (assuming that the view of the law being advanced is valid), should the involvement of the adult be challenged.

As has been seen earlier, consent to be valid must be given voluntarily and **13.49** must be properly informed. The requirement of *voluntariness*, which, of course, only applies to the competent volunteer, is of particular importance in the case of non-therapeutic research. More generally, the fact that no benefit is intended to accrue to the volunteer causes the law to be vigilant to ensure that participation results from genuine agreement rather than from duress or coercion. Mention of duress is not intended to suggest that strong-arm tactics might be employed by medical researchers. Rather, it is to draw attention to the many pressures, subtle and otherwise, which may operate on the mind of the person asked to volunteer.

Two particular areas of difficulty warrant mention here. The first relates to **13.50** *payment*. There are those who argue that the payment of research subjects puts at risk the voluntariness of their participation. Certainly, concern has been expressed, for example, at the recruitment of participants for drug trials in areas of high unemployment, where involvement in such research could take on the quality of alternative employment. The argument is that financial exigencies cause people to expose themselves to risks they would otherwise choose to avoid. This is a complex subject, not free from an element of paternalism. Suffice it to say that it has caused considerable concern to RECs and has resulted in an uneasy compromise in which payment (in addition to reasonable expenses) is tolerated, provided it is not inappropriate or disproportionately large.[47] The law's position would tend to be rather more robust. Payment is unlikely to be regarded as vitiating consent unless, applying the principle of proportionality, it is so obviously out of proportion to that which was asked of the volunteer, that the ability of a reasonable person, in the volunteer's shoes, to refuse would have been overborne.

13.51 The second area of difficulty relates to those who, by virtue of their status or *relationship* with the researcher, may find it difficult to refuse consent, though they might wish to do so. What these groups have in common is their vulnerability to exploitation. Examples include: students asked to participate by teachers who also are responsible for grading their examinations; armed forces personnel asked by their superiors in rank; employees recruited by employers, explicitly on terms that no reward, by way of promotion or preferment will follow, but where the employee believes some reward will in fact follow; prisoners, again in circumstances where they hope for advantage despite explicit disclaimers; and mentally disordered persons, who, by virtue of their condition may be particularly vulnerable. One ethical response is that such relationships are so affected by the inevitable imbalance of power that research involving these and similar categories of persons should not be permitted. An alternative approach is that prohibition is too extreme and unnecessary. Instead, wherever the consent of someone in such a relationship is involved, extra vigilance is called for to ensure that the apparent consent is in fact real. Whatever view is taken on the ethics, the law probably reflects this latter position. Perhaps before moving on, it is worthwhile noticing here another group as regards whom extra vigilance is urged before they be involved in non-therapeutic research. The group is women. The argument advanced is that all women of child-bearing age should, on the precautionary principle, be regarded as potentially pregnant (subject to obvious exceptions). This being so, the research could put at risk the life of the embryo/foetus and, thus, cannot be justified. This approach, not suprisingly, has been strongly criticised as discriminating against women by distorting the data generated by

---

[47] The Department of Health's guidance (n 16 above), states, for example, in para 3.16 that '[p]ayment in cash or kind . . . should only be for expense, time and inconvenience reasonably incurred. It should not be at the level of an inducement which would encourage people to take part in studies against their better judgement.'

research. Data become, in fact, data on men not on people. Given the differences between men and women, this distortion can only act to the detriment of women.[48] Whatever the merits of the arguments, it will be obvious that the origin of the exclusionary principle lies with lawyers. It is an eminently sensible piece of preventive lawyering to counsel against the recruitment of women in circumstances where liability might flow if the woman were pregnant and damage were done to the unborn child. It is a matter for speculation whether an explicit waiver of responsibility, excusing the researcher of any liability, by the woman on her own and any unborn child's behalf would be legally valid or ethically acceptable.

13.52 The issue of voluntariness obviously does not arise in the case of those incompetent to consent. This does not mean that factors such as money or other possible inducements—which might cause the decision-maker to decide in favour of volunteering someone for non-therapeutic research—cease to be important. They remain relevant and, to the extent that the law allows, form part of the assessment of whether a particular procedure is or is not against the interests of the person involved.

13.53 As regards the *information* which must be supplied to the volunteer, the starting point for the law is that, since no therapeutic benefit is intended, there can be no case for withholding any information necessary to allow the volunteer to make a reasoned decision. The researcher's duty, as has been said, is not confined to what was set out by the House of Lords in *Sidaway*.[49] Rather, it is a much more extensive duty, namely, to bring to the attention of the volunteer all that information which, from what the volunteer has said and the researcher knows and reasonably ought to know, the volunteer would wish to know. What is known to the researcher about such matters as risks, inconvenience, or side-effects of the proposed procedure must be passed on to the volunteer in a manner and form which is comprehensible. Furthermore, the comprehensibility should be tested and checked to ensure, to the extent that is reasonably possible, that in the particular case the volunteer has, in fact, understood. As has been said before, the REC will ordinarily have called for and seen both an information sheet and a consent form, thereby providing a mechanism for translating the legal duty into practice.

13.54 In those circumstances, if any, in which the law permits non-therapeutic research on those incompetent to consent, the issue of information translates, if the legal analysis offered above is valid, into the duty of the decision-maker not to act against the incompetent person's interests. Thus, not only is it the

---

[48] See eg, Institute of Medicine, *Women and Health Research* (National Academic Press, 1994).   [49] N 21 above.

duty of the researcher to impart all relevant (as defined in para 13.53 above) information, but it is also the duty of the decision-maker, (whether parent or otherwise) to seek out this information, weigh it and reach a view on how it affects the incompetent person's interests. Again, the REC's involvement will tend to ensure that these duties are complied with.

4. Consent: Limits

13.55 The law's concern here is to set proper limits to that which volunteers may be exposed to, so as to protect the more eager from themselves and the more vulnerable from others. The question of limits, therefore, is of the greatest importance. The focus of attention clearly must be on the level or degree of *risk* involved in any particular procedure. The prevailing ethical standpoint is that volunteers in non-therapeutic research should never be exposed to a risk greater than that which can be described as *minimal*.[50] This limit also reflects the position in law. Thus, to expose a healthy volunteer or, in those circumstances in which it may be permissable, an incompetent child or adult, to risks other than those which objectively can be categorised as minimal (and, clearly, the test must be objective), is to behave unlawfully. The consent, real or apparent, of the research subject would be no defence to possible criminal liability.[51] Equally, it would probably not be admissable as a defence of consent or voluntary assumption of risk in any civil suit, whether in battery or negligence, for reasons of public policy.

13.56 In addition to setting the limit to non-therapeutic research at minimal risk, two further limits are recognised as ethically appropriate in the case of research on those incompetent to consent, where such research is permissable. The first is that the case for carrying out the research on the incompetent should be compelling. It is not enough merely to wish to know. What is required is strong evidence that the information which is sought will be gained and that, once gained, it is likely to have significant practical consequences. The second additional limitation is that the researcher must clearly demonstrate that the research must be carried out on the incompetent, or, put another way, no other group of research subjects would be suitable to generate

---

[50] See eg, Department of Health's guidance (n 16 above) para 4.3 and see the definition offered in *Research on Healthy Volunteers*, Royal College of Physicians 1986, *Manual* (n 4 above): 'We . . . use the term "minimal risk" to cover two types of situation. The first is where there is a small chance of a recognised reaction which is itself trivial, eg a headache or feeling of lethargy. The second is where there is a very remote chance of a serious disability or death. We regard this second risk to the healthy volunteer as comparable, for example, to that of flying as a passenger in a scheduled aircraft.' For further discussion, see Kennedy and Grubb (n 3 above), 1060.   [51] See eg, *R v Brown* (n 37 above).

the desired data. There is no doubt that these two ethical concerns would be recognised as a legally relevant part of the process of determining whether the proposed research is or is not against the interests of the incompetent child or adult.

5. Research not Involving Intervention

Not all medical research involves intervention by way of touching so as to **13.57** bring into play the law of battery and negligence. Psychologists and psychiatrists, for example, may conduct research through observation and recording of patients and volunteers.[52] Epidemiologists carry out research which usually will not even bring them into contact with the research subject. Their concern is with aggregates of patients or healthy volunteers, rather than individuals. Such research attracts its own ethical guidance.[53] The task here is to identify areas of legal concern. The approach adopted will be to identify possible harm or grounds for complaint which might flow from these forms of research and analyse the law's response.

The first area of concern is that *psychiatric or psychological research* could **13.58** expose the research subject to *psychological damage* actionable in negligence.[54] Such damage may occur as a consequence of therapeutic research on a patient or non-therapeutic research on a volunteer. The law's response is that the researcher in either set of circumstances is under a duty of care owed to the subject, which must not be breached. A breach may occur because the research was ill-conceived or improperly conducted, or because the subject was not properly informed as to what might transpire. How will the law define the standard of care? The situation in which it is alleged that the research was ill-conceived, in that it lacked scientific plausibility, is different from the others. The court would rely there on expert evidence. In the other cases, the standard of care to which the researcher will be held will not be determined simply by reference to *Bolam*.[55] The views and practice of other researchers (*per Bolam*) would be regarded by the court as relevant but by no means determinative of the degree of care required by law. The fact that research was involved and, thus, that someone was acting altruistically, would persuade the court to impose its own standard. In the context of *therapeutic* research, if the complaint was as to the conduct of the research, the court would weigh the risks against the alleged benefits, in the light of

---

[52] See Guidelines issued by the Royal College of Psychiatrists and the British Psychological Society in *Manual* (n 4 above).
[53] See eg, British Sociological Association, Statement of Ethical Practice, in *Manual* (n 4 above).   [54] On which see *Alcock v Chief Constable of South Yorkshire* [1992] 1 AC 310.
[55] N 9 above.

13: Research and Experimentation

the circumstances, not least the subject's mental state. If the complaint rested on breach of the duty to inform, it is equally unlikely that *Sidaway*[56] *simpliciter*, derived as it is from *Bolam*, would be relied on. Instead, the court in all probability would opt for a test based on the reasonable patient in the particular patient's position.[57] In the context of *non-therapeutic* research, the fact that no benefit is intended to accrue to the subject would, *a fortiori*, result in the court going beyond *Bolam*. Researchers would be held to a standard of care which, though it took account of, was not determined by evidence of professional standards or practice.

13.59 The second area of concern relates to *privacy* and *confidentiality*. There are a number of circumstances in which a research subject might complain of an invasion of privacy or a breach of confidence.

13.60 The first relates to research involving *observation* of the subject. By its nature this would ordinarily be non-therapeutic research. Obviously, if the subject has given effective consent beforehand, no problems arise. This is what an REC would insist on. But, what of the situation in which, whatever the REC may have stipulated, the research is conducted surreptitiously, without consent? The question arises whether the subject, once aware of what has taken place, can bring any legal action if upset thereby. There is no doubt that, as a matter of ethics, the subject has been wronged. Recourse to the relevant Professional Codes of Conduct[58] would, therefore, be an option open to the subject. It is doubtful, however, that any legal redress would be available. The English law of privacy is extremely undeveloped.[59]

13.61 The following question then arises: what if it were proposed to carry out such research on someone incompetent to consent? The limitations on carrying out non-therapeutic research on the incompetent have been set out in detail above. It could be argued, however, that these limitations do not apply here. It could be said that they apply only to those circumstances in which the incompetent person is touched and thereby put at risk. Whatever the validity of this view, it is likely that, from an ethical perspective, in the case of research on an incompetent child, the consent of the person with parental responsibility will be required. Furthermore, the parent will be constrained in what may be consented to, whether by reference to the child's best interests or that the research is not against the child's interests. It is most likely, moreover, that

---

[56] N 21 above.
[57] Following, eg, the reasoning in *Reibl v Hughes* (1980) 114 DLR (3rd) 1.
[58] See eg, nn 52 and 53 above.
[59] See eg, Salmond and Heuston, *Law of Torts*, 21st edn (Sweet and Maxwell, 1996), 32–4. It is a separate question whether an action would be sustainable under Article VIII of the European Convention on Human Rights, once all domestic remedies were exhausted.

this also represents the legal position, bearing in mind the law's paramount concern for the welfare of the child. Thus, any research carried out without the parent's consent or which, despite consent, violates the child's interests, will be unlawful.[60] In the case of an incompetent adult, it may similarly be argued that the limits or prohibitions on non-therapeutic research discussed above (para 13.44) do not, or should not, apply to research which does not involve touching. The answer would be that the primary ethical concern would be to safeguard the interests of the incompetent adult, at the very least so as to ensure that nothing is done which is against those interests. Whether the incompetent adult would have any legal redress if those interests were violated is by no means clear. As has been said, the law of privacy is wholly undeveloped. Clearly, if some harm were suffered as a consequence of negligence, an action would lie. Equally, a remedy may exist if harm were caused intentionally. Beyond these, the subject's protection lies with those who police the relevant Ethical Codes.

The second situation which could give rise to legal complaint is where *access*   **13.62**
to personal medical details relating to a current or former patient is granted to a researcher, ordinarily in the context of non-therapeutic research. Again, no complaint can be made if the patient has given effective consent, whether at the time of treatment or subsequently. If the patient is an incompetent child, arguably the person with parental authority could authorise access. It may well be, however, that the test against which any decision would be judged would be the traditional test of the child's best interests. There does not seem to be a strong argument in favour of the more relaxed test of 'not against the child's interests' in this context, bearing in mind the possible damaging effect to a child of the release of personal medical details. What if the patient is an adult, incompetent to give, or have given, consent? As has been seen, the general law makes it clear that no one else has authority to consent *to treatment* on behalf of an adult. Does this prohibition apply equally where what is at issue is not treatment but access to personal medical details, usually in the form of records? It could be said that those who have the responsibility of managing the affairs of the incompetent person could give consent, all other things being equal, namely that the adult's interests are not violated. This may not be the law, however, since medical records are not the property of the patient.[61] Thus, if the authority to manage affairs is limited to property, it would not extend to authorising access to medical details. If

---

[60] It is a separate question, and one not easy to resolve, whether the conduct described as unlawful would give rise to a civil cause of action at the suit of the child. Negligence suggests itself as one candidate, if the child suffered harm. Clearly, family law remedies would also be available to seek to protect the child for the future.

[61] See Kennedy and Grubb (n 3 above), 610 *et seq.*

the authority goes further—and Ungoed-Thomas J's judgment in *Re W* (*EEM*)[62] is somewhat equivocal, since it draws the line at treatment decisions and what is being considered here is somewhere in-between—access could be granted. Perhaps the better view is that the authority does not, in fact, extend this far. Thus, prima facie, access is impermissable. If such a conclusion were judged to be too restrictive in circumstances where very good reasons could be advanced for access, the law could adopt a more permissive position. This could be that access is lawful, provided that it is not against the interests of the incompetent adult and is deemed acceptable by a reasonable body of informed people, by being approved, after proper deliberation, by an REC.

13.63 In the absence of lawful authority, the person granting access, usually the doctor, has committed a breach of confidence. This would be actionable at the suit of the patient.[63] The legal position in the case of those incompetent to consent, however, is less clear. While any release of personal medical details to persons other than those who need them for the purposes of rendering medical care would provoke ethical disapproval and, perhaps, sanction, it is by no means clear that any legal action would lie in the case of an incompetent child or adult.[64] If such an action were to lie, the only possible defence would be to argue that the public interest in pursuing the particular research outweighed the public interest in maintaining the law's commitment to confidentiality. It is difficult to envisage circumstances in which such a defence would succeed.

13.64 The third situation warranting attention here is where *information is published* as part of a research project which allows a research subject, usually a patient, to be identified. The publication can take such diverse forms as personal details in a learned paper, a photograph in an article or book illustrating a particular condition, or a video shown at a research conference. Once again, if effective consent has been given, no problem arises. By contrast, it would be hard to justify publication in any other case, whether of those who are incompetent to consent or those whose consent has not been sought. The reasons are twofold. First, it would appear to be a significant intrusion into

---

[62] [1971] Ch 123.

[63] It should be noticed that the NHS executive in HSG (96) 48, *The Protection and Use of Patient Information*, takes a different view. Broadly speaking, it contemplates that NHS records are available to any NHS employee for NHS purposes. This somewhat self-serving view, by which a number of managerial tasks can be more readily accomplished, flies in the face of long-standing medical tradition and the law. In the context of research and access to personal medical details, it advises that NHS staff may have access to patients' notes for the purpose of research without the consent of the patients. With all due respect, this is not the law and the NHS Executive does itself no favours by taking the position that by saying something frequently enough it will become true.   [64] Kennedy and Grubb (n 3 above), 640 *et seq.*

the privacy of the research subject. Secondly, publication of identifying details is rarely, if ever, necessary. Data can be anonymised. Photographs and other pictorial representations can be so disguised as to prevent identification. Professional bodies regard the anonymisation of data, wherever possible, and consent, if feasible, when anonymisation is not possible, as required from an ethical perspective.[65] The legal position, however, is less clear. Once again, what is being complained of is, in essence, an invasion of privacy. As was said above in (para 13.60) the existence of any legal remedy is, at best, problematical.

E. Regulatory/Supervisory Mechanism

1. Introduction

As was said at the outset, there is no overarching statutory framework **13.65** regulating the conduct of biomedical research on humans. With the limited exception of the Regulations referred to above (para 13.20), those conducting research must, therefore, look to the common law for guidance. As the foregoing exposition has made clear, it is no easy task to state the law with any degree of certainty. This is because, until very recently, medical research has been conducted out of the public limelight, in an atmosphere of trust (or at least tolerance) and responsibility, and, apparently, with very few cases of harm ensuing. For these among many reasons, remarkably, no cases involving research have been brought to the English courts from which guidance could be obtained.

2. HSG *(91) 5—Department of Health Guidelines*

In the absence of any specific regulatory system, various institutional bodies, in **13.66** particular the Royal College of Physicians and the Association of the British Pharmaceutical Industry, began to develop frameworks for guidance during the early 1980s.[66] Eventually, the Department of Health, having taken advice, issued Guidelines in 1991 through the NHS Management Executive (HSG (91) 5). Perhaps the principal factor which persuaded government to act, albeit in a non-statutory manner, was a concern at the lack of legal protection available to research subjects. The Guidelines which emerged, entitled *Local Research Ethics Committees*, are the closest the United Kingdom government has come to regulating the conduct of research on human subjects.

---

[65] See eg, *Duties of a Doctor: Confidentiality* (General Medical Council, 1995), paras 15 and 16.   [66] See, *Manual* (n 4 above).

13.67   The Guidelines lay certain duties on various bodies within the NHS under the auspices of which research is conducted. Ultimately, the duties fall upon the relevant District Health Authority (DHA). Principal among these duties is the creation of a local REC and consultation of it in matters relating to the ethics of any proposed research project. These duties form part of the contractual obligations of the manager of the DHA. In turn, through its contractual relationship with NHS employees, management then ensures that the procedures and safeguards set out in the Circular are observed. In this way, the provisions of the Guidelines, at least as they affect those employed within the NHS, operate as if they had the force of law.

13.68   The Guidelines only apply, of course, to activities undertaken within the ambit of the NHS. To that extent, those who conduct research outside the NHS are under no duty to comply with them. Given the status of the Guidelines, in practice if not in law, as some form of quasi-legislation, this limitation on their reach might seem to represent a significant hiatus. In practice, however, this limitation may be more apparent than real. First, the Circular extends to any research involving the use of NHS patients or premises. To the extent that non-NHS researchers, (that is, researchers who are not employed within the NHS), might wish to conduct research, it is difficult to do so without using NHS patients or premises. Secondly, companies sponsoring research will ordinarily wish to ensure that the Guidelines are followed, both because they represent considered public policy but also because it is clearly in their commercial interests to be seen to behave responsibly. Thirdly, the Guidelines' most significant regulatory mechanism, the REC, is now a standard feature of biomedical research, whether conducted within or outside the NHS. Indeed, bodies which provide financial support for research and editors of journals which publish research results both tend to insist on evidence that research has received approval from an REC.

13.69   Nonetheless, whatever the situation may be in practice, it remains odd, and some would say unfortunate, that there is no formal law regulating research. It means, among other things, that, as a matter of law, there is no requirement that a research proposal even be submitted to, let alone be approved by, an REC. Thus, in principle at least, the safeguards referred to earlier whereby, for example, RECs will have had to be satisfied as to the scientific plausibility of a research proposal and have called for and approved consent forms or information sheets, may not always apply. To this extent, the law's protection of the interests and welfare of research subjects is less than satisfactory. Of course, the common law remains. However, the extent and prevalence of biomedical research suggest that something better than relying on the common law is called for, not least something which is prescriptive, setting out in a pro-active manner what ought to be done, rather than a system which only provides for complaint after the event, when damage may already have been done.

As will have become clear, the REC is seen as the single most important and, **13.70**
ex hypothesi, most effective mechanism to ensure that research proceeds in a way which meets the twin public policy objectives widely recognised as justifying biomedical research: that it should proceed without unnecessary impediment; and that the welfare and safety of research subjects should at all times be the primary consideration in deciding whether to proceed. There-fore, given the significance of the REC, it is important, first, to notice the membership. The Guidelines make certain recommendations but, in practice, the size and composition vary considerably.[67] It is equally important to determine its precise legal status. The short answer is that the REC, in law, is no more than a group of individuals. It has no separate legal personality, distinct from its members.[68] Thus, any action complaining of an REC's conduct must be brought either against the individual members or the Health Authority, as the appointing body and, as regards some at least of the members, the employer. That said, in the case of *R v Ethical Committee of St Mary's Hospital (Manchester), ex p H*,[69] the court, by admitting the suit, appeared to accept that RECs are amenable to judicial review in the exercise of their functions. This must be right since they are a quasi-public body, chosen by government to perform an important public role.

Although there is no legal requirement that RECs should exist, and although, **13.71**
once established, they have no legal personality, the members, once appointed, take on a number of legal duties. As has been seen, the REC is amenable to judicial review in the exercise of these duties and members are also individually responsible. Principal among these duties is the duty of each member to act with due care. The role of each member is to review proposals for research and make recommendations as to the ethical propriety, or otherwise, of them. In carying out this role, members must take account of the twin aims, referred to above (para 13.70), of fostering research while safeguarding the welfare of research subjects. Members must, therefore, seek to understand, so as to take an ethical view about, complex issues of, *inter alia*, biomedical science, statistics and moral philosophy. The members' duty, expressed in this way, may seem somewhat daunting. The standard of care demanded by the law, however, is that of reasonableness. The REC member

---

[67] See eg, Neuberger, *Ethics and Healthcare: The Role of Research Ethics Committees in the UK*, King's Fund Research Report No 13, 1992.
[68] See Brazier, 'Liability of Ethics Committees and Their Members', (1990) PN 186.
[69] [1988] 1 FLR 512.

must behave as a reasonable REC member. While this does not mean that the quantum of care demanded of a member may be intentionally kept at a low point through the expedient of appointing members whose experience and expertise is limited, it does mean that the law recognises that it will be a rare member who is at home in all areas of concern to the REC. The upshot is that the member will not be held to too high a standard, but at the same time will be expected to recognise the limits of his own expertise. Where such limits exist, the law would expect that the member would not take a view until information and reassurance had been sought from others. A member, and the Health Authority, would also be expected to take advantage of whatever training opportunities may exist. Equally, a member has a duty to ensure that the decision-making process which the REC operates is one which, for example, ensures that expertise is drawn upon and shared, that decisions are only taken after proper consultation and that the REC follows appropriate standing procedures.[70]

13.72 It is fair to say that not all RECs function in as appropriate a manner as the law would expect.[71] Standing operating procedures may not exist or may not be observed. The expertise available within the REC may be too limited. The REC may be dominated by one section of the local community, whether medical, nursing or anti-medical. These deficiencies are unfortunate when it is recalled that RECs are the bodies with which the pharmaceutical industry, with its huge investment in research, must deal. Arguably, the industry should be entitled to a rather more professional and, it would follow, better resourced system than the somewhat amateurish and overworked RECs which currently exist in some parts of the country. Moreover, it will be clear from what has been said that the industry, among others, is limited as regards any redress it may have in the face of adverse decisions by the REC. An action in theory exists against any member who has failed to behave reasonably, for example, by reaching a perverse decision or simply failing to read the papers before making a decision. Not only would it be difficult to prove breach but it would also be extremely difficult to demonstrate any actionable harm or a causal link between the conduct complained of and the harm suffered. Furthermore, only those members of the REC who were employees of the Health Authority would have any insurance cover to meet any claim, such that the existence of a cause of action against members is more theoretical than real. That said, the threat exists that a test case, whether by judicial review or common law action, may be brought by researchers

---

[70] See eg, Bendall, 'Standard Operating Procedures for Local RECs', *Manual* (n 4 above).
[71] See Neuberger (n 67 above).

frustrated by the conduct of an REC which has very considerable power and very little accountability.

The alternative to ensuring greater professionalism and accountability of **13.73** RECs through litigation is though political action. The development of a new system for dealing with *multi-centre trials* illustrates this latter approach. Multi-centre trials, as their name makes clear, are trials, usually of a medicinal product, conducted simultaneously at a number of places, often in a number of countries. Conflict has arisen over the years because RECs at different research centres, in considering a proposal for multi-centre research, have reached different decisions as to the acceptability of the research or have imposed different terms as the condition for acceptability. Those in charge of multi-centre trials have complained about the variability of approach, its unpredictability and, hence, its cost. RECs have responded that they exist to make independent judgments. Local circumstances may well affect the ethical acceptability of a proposal, such as, for instance, the ethnic composition of a particular area. Furthermore, they have urged that on issues of ethical acceptability, it should not be assumed, nor may it be desirable for every REC to take the same view. In the event, after considerable consultation between industry, RECs and the Department of Health, a compromise position was agreed. HSG (97) 23 was issued. It is concerned with the ethical review of multi-centre research. Eleven new MRECs, (multi-centre RECs) were established, one each in Scotland, Northern Ireland, and Wales and the remainder in England. They will consider all multi-centre research proposals involving the use of human subjects. RECs at local level will still be involved in review but their powers have been limited. They may insist on changes to the patient information sheet, but only if local reasons justify them. They are not, however, permitted to change the scientific basis of the research proposal.[72]

The final matter which warrants mention is *compensation* for research subjects **13.74** who may be injured as a result of their participation in research. Of course, it is open to any research subject to pursue an action at common law. The difficulties of doing so and the uncertainty of success, coupled with the argument that, as public-spirited volunteers, research subjects deserved some special treatment, led to the emergence of proposals that compensation be available without the need for litigation. The Association of the British Pharmaceutical Industry (ABPI) proposed a scheme whereby compensation based on no-fault would be paid to the subject.[73] The subject still had to

---

[72] See, for the full text, HSG (97) 23.

[73] For a discussion of this and other schemes, see Hodges, 'Harmonisation of European Controls over Research: Ethics Committees, Consent, Compensation and Indemnity', in Goldberg, (ed) *Pharmaceutical Medicine and the Law* (1991). and Kennedy and Grubb (n 3 above), 1067–73.

prove that it was the research which caused the harm complained of. The Royal College of Physicians, in its 1986 guidance, made a number of proposals designed to ensure that a research subject who was harmed through taking part in research would obtain compensation with a minimum of legal obstacles and delay.[74] The Department of Health's Guidelines, however, are somewhat guarded on the issue, not least because of the Treasury convention that open-ended financial commitments are not made by government. It cannot be said, therefore, that arrangements for compensation outside the framework of litigation, regarded by most as eminently desirable, are currently satisfactory.

---

[74] *Research on Healthy Volunteers* (n 50 above).

Part IV
Death and Dying

[16]

Helga Kuhse

Some Reflections on the Problem of Advance Directives, Personhood, and Personal Identity[*]

ABSTRACT. In this paper, I consider objections to advance directives based on the claim that there is a discontinuity of interests, and of personal identity, between the time a person executes an advance directive and the time when the patient has become severely demented. Focusing narrowly on refusals of life-sustaining treatment for severely demented patients, I argue that acceptance of the psychological view of personal identity does not entail that treatment refusals should be overridden. Although severely demented patients are morally considerable beings, and must be kept comfortable whilst alive, they no longer have an interest in receiving life-sustaining treatment.

F OLLOWING U.S. JUSTICE Benjamin Cardozo's declaration in 1914 that "Every human being of adult years and sound mind has a right to determine what shall be done with his own body" (*Schloendorff v. Society of New York Hospital*, 211 N.Y. 125, 105 N.E. 92 (1914), "Dissenting Opinion"), societies have, in their institutions and laws, increasingly recognized that there is no absolute obligation to preserve and prolong life. Rather, there is now widespread agreement that competent and informed patients have a moral and legal right to refuse unwanted medical treatment, including life-sustaining treatment, for themselves. It is also widely assumed that this right can be extended into the future by way of advance directives, such as living wills and proxy directives. A living will allows a competent person to specify that she does not, when incompetent, wish to receive certain medical treatments, and a proxy directive

---

[*]This paper is a revised and expanded version of a paper published in a collection of articles presented at the Tagung der Österreichischen Sektion der IVR in Graz, 29-30 November 1996: Peter Strasser and Edgar Starz, eds. *Personsein aus bioethischer Sicht*, pp. 81-89. Stuttgart: Franz Steiner Verlag, 1997.

Kennedy Institute of Ethics Journal Vol. 9, No. 4, 347–364 © 1999 by The Johns Hopkins University Press

KENNEDY INSTITUTE OF ETHICS JOURNAL • DECEMBER 1999

allows her to appoint an agent or proxy who will be able to make treatment decisions for her should accident or illness render her incompetent.

It is easy to see why advance directives enjoy great initial appeal. Medicine is continually increasing its capacity to prolong life, without, however, always being able to restore function and well-being. Many people regard such diminished lives as undesirable. Moreover, given that death is often preceded by a period of mental incapacity, advance directives seem to offer a relatively simple and morally defensible way of guiding medical decision making in accordance with the formerly competent person's values and beliefs. They can give those who execute them a sense of control over their lives and provide guidance to health care professionals and family members, alleviating them of some of the burdens of making difficult and contested quality-of-life judgments for incompetent patients (Robertson 1991).

Despite the seeming advantages of advance directives and an impressive ethical and legal agreement on their use, it has been claimed that such directives are problematic and should be treated with considerable caution. Some writers argue that treatment decisions or preferences expressed in these instruments rarely are specific enough to prevent unwanted treatment, and may in fact create opportunities for abuse (Stone 1994). Others point out that advance directives are not necessarily expressions of the patient's autonomy because the person executing the advance directive is likely to have an inadequate understanding of future options and may lack the imagination necessary to adequately consider the particular circumstances in which the actual medical decision must be made (Buchanan and Brock 1989, pp. 101-7; Savulescu 1994).

Although these practical difficulties cannot be ignored and may raise questions about the validity of individual instruments, they do not undermine the validity of advance directives as such. A more serious threat is posed by the charge—put forward by writers, such as John Robertson (1991) and Rebecca Dresser (1986; 1989; 1995)—that advance directives are conceptually confused because they rely on inapplicable notions of self-determination and personal identity. Given this conceptual confusion, these writers hold that advance directives should, in some circumstances, be overridden. If it is in an incompetent patient's interests to live, he or she should not be made to die, simply because the formerly competent person executed an advance directive that refused readily available treatment.

KUHSE • ADVANCE DIRECTIVES, PERSONHOOD, AND PERSONAL IDENTITY

The focus of the present paper is a narrow one. Setting empirical questions relating to the validity of particular directives to one side, I shall address myself exclusively to the above conceptual issues and their ethical ramifications. Moreover, although similar issues would be raised in other health care contexts, such as psychiatry (Radden 1996) and dementia research (Berghmans 1998), I shall limit my discussion for the most part to refusals of life-sustaining treatment. Only toward the end of the paper will I touch briefly on questions relating to the refusal of palliative measures. Given certain assumptions, to be explained below, I shall argue that *even if* writers such as Robertson and Dresser are correct in holding that advance directives are conceptually confused in the relevant sense, it does not follow that refusals of life-sustaining treatment should be overridden in the kind of cases they have in mind. Matters are, however, different when it comes to the advance refusal of pain relief. There are good ethical reasons, I shall suggest, for not honoring such directives.

SETTING THE SCENE: ALZHEIMER'S DISEASE

The charge that advance directives are conceptually confused is often raised in the context of dementia. Alzheimer's disease is the most common and probably best known form of dementia, and I shall largely focus on this disease. Although the risk of suffering from Alzheimer's disease before age 65 is relatively small, the incidence may increase to about 50 percent in those aged 85 or more (Whitehouse 1992, p. 23). The symptoms of early Alzheimer's disease can be subtle. A person may feel somewhat disorganized at times and experience some mild loss of memory, without realizing that she is suffering from a progressive medical condition. As the disease progresses, symptoms will increase, accompanied by cognitive decline. Patients will eventually lose many of the characteristics that defined them as particular persons—their memories, their skills, the ability to sustain even simple projects or desires. They may be unable to recognize, and respond to, others and speech may be limited to a word or two. There is often incontinence, the patient may be unable to walk and to feed herself and will ultimately need total care (Office of Technology Assessment 1987; Whitehouse 1992). One care giver describes Alzheimer's disease as "a funeral that never ends" (Smith 1992, p. 49), and many others lament the fact that the patient they care for "is no longer the same person" he or she once was (Smith 1992, p. 46).

Many people regard incurable severe dementia as a fate worse than death—not, or not only, because of any suffering, pain, or distress that may be associated with the condition, but because it depersonalizes the sufferer and robs her of her very character and personality. One commentator expresses his horror of the condition in the following way:

> [A]lthough cancer kills you . . . it doesn't remove your very humanity. . . . It doesn't turn you into a vegetable. . . . All diseases are depersonalizing to some extent. But you're still human. But a person with a serious dementia is no longer human. He's a vegetable. That's devastating. Fearsome. Terrifying, to anyone who's ever seen it—the thought that it could happen to you. (Smith 1992, p. 51)

Those who wish to protect themselves against this fate may execute advance directives, stipulating that they refuse all life-sustaining treatment should this "saddest of the tragedies" (Dworkin 1993, p. 218) befall them.

THE CASE OF MARGO

There are many situations, particularly in the case of permanent unconsciousness or end-stage terminal illness, where the advance refusal of life-sustaining treatment raises little concern. In the case of permanent unconsciousness, continued treatment would not benefit the patient and, in the case of end-stage terminal illness, an extension of life would more often harm, rather than benefit, the dying patient. The same is true in many cases of advanced Alzheimer's disease. Patients will often display signs of agitation and distress, and it is plausible to think that the formerly competent person's non-treatment decision, particularly if it involves the refusal of burdensome treatment, is at least not contrary to the best interests of the now incompetent patient.

However, Alzheimer's disease does not render all patients seriously distressed. Rather, some patients are "pleasantly demented" (Rhoden 1990). Such a case is described by a medical student, Andrew Firlik (1991), in the *Journal of the American Medical Association* (see also, Dworkin 1993, pp. 226ff; Dresser 1995). As part of his gerontology elective, Firlik paid daily visits to "Margo," who was suffering from Alzheimer's disease and who, Firlik observed, seemed to be extraordinarily happy.

Margo lived at home, being cared for by an attendant. On his visits, Firlik often found Margo reading. She told him she was particularly fond of mysteries, but, Firlik noticed, "her place in the book jump[ed] randomly from day to day." Although Margo did not seem to remember his name, she always seemed pleased to see him. In her art therapy class,

Margo enjoyed painting—the same soft-hued circles, day after day. She also enjoyed listening to music. Indeed, she seemed happy to listen to the same song again and again, as if she were hearing it for the first time.

Firlik described Margo as "undeniably one of the happiest people" he had known. The degeneration of her mind, he mused, seemed to leave her carefree and always cheerful. "Do her problems, whatever she may perceive them to be, simply fail to make it to the worry centers of her brain? How does Margo maintain a sense of self? When a person can no longer accumulate new memories as the old rapidly fade, what remains? Who is Margo?"

Let us suppose that years ago, Margo was a philosophy professor who relished complex mental activities. Let us also suppose that Margo, while fully competent, executed an advance directive. Adequately informed, she knows that dementia affects different people differently, leaving some happy and some distressed. She makes it quite clear that even if she were to be experiencing no visible distress and were seemingly "pleasantly demented," she would wish to be allowed to die if and when the opportunity were to present itself. Margo, now demented, contracts pneumonia. This is likely to be fatal, unless Margo were prescribed a course of antibiotics. Should Margo be treated or not?

THE PHILOSOPHICAL CRITIQUE OF ADVANCE DIRECTIVES

As noted above, it is widely assumed that the moral force of advance directives derives from a competent patient's right to refuse unwanted medical treatment for herself. This right is commonly grounded in one of two further assumptions: first, that a competent persons is best-placed to decide what is in her future interests and, second, that the competent person's interest in controlling her life takes precedence over any interests the future incompetent individual might have.

Critics of advance directives, such as Robertson (1991) and Dresser (1986; 1995) argue that these justifications are problematic. They hold that there is insufficient continuity of interests between the competent person who executes the advance directive and the later incompetent patient to justify the implementation of the directive. This, they say, makes it far from self-evident that a person's right to self-determination at time t_1 can justify the withholding of life- sustaining treatment from an incompetent patient at time t_2. Robertson's argument rests on the relatively straightforward claim that the competent and the incompetent individual— while the same person—have different interests; Dresser sharpens and radicalizes this interests-based critique by also challenging the common assumption that the incompetent patient is the same person as the author of the advance directive.

Discontinuity of Interests

John Robertson (1991, p.7) advances a convincing argument for the view that there is a radical break between the value-based interests or preferences possessed by competent persons and the simple interests that remain in seriously cognitively impaired patients. As he puts it:

> The values and interests of the competent person no longer are relevant to someone who has lost the rational structure on which those values and interests rested. Unless we are to view competently held values and interests as extending even into situations in which, because of incompetency, they can no longer have meaning, it matters not that as a competent person the individual would not wish to be maintained in a debilitated or disabled state. If the person is no longer competent enough to appreciate the degree of divergence from her previous activity that produced the choice against treatment, the prior directive does not represent her current interests merely because a competent directive was issued. (See also Dresser 1986.)

Robertson (1991, p. 7) does not deny that competent individuals have an interest in controlling their future, but, he holds, this is not the same as showing that the directive will reflect the future incompetent patient's best interests. Rather, in some situations there is "conflict between past competent interests and current incompetent interests—between the need of the competent patient for control and certainty and the need of the incompetent patient for treatment." If that conflict is resolved in favor of past competent interests, then we are implicitly favoring one interest over another. This, then, is the problem with advance directives, as Robertson sees it:

> Because [advance directives] either confuse the present interests of an incompetent patient with interests she had when competent, or forthrightly privilege the competent person's interests in control and certainty over the incompetent patient's current interests, they pose a threat to incompetent patients.

One of the practical conclusions Robertson (1991, p. 8) draws from this is that advance directives should not always be enforced. Rather, in situations where the incompetent patient "has an interest in further life," those caring for the patient should be able to question the directive. Although Robertson does not provide any concrete examples of when a patient might be said to have an interest in further life, the thrust of his argument suggests that it is cases such as Margo's that would be among those he has in mind.

If Robertson's arguments are correct, he would seem to have undermined the first justification of advance directives which, it will be recalled, was based on the assumption that a competent person is best-placed to decide what is in her future interests. Cases such as Margo's, he would argue, suggest otherwise. To the extent that the life of an incompetent patient is free from pain and suffering and seemingly cheerful and happy, she has, according to Robertson, an "interest in further life" and this interest should, other things being equal, determine treatment decisions.

Later, I will question the assumption that the ability to experience pleasant states of consciousness is sufficient to establish an "interest in further life." For the moment, I want to set that issue aside and deal with a possible objection to Robertson's argument. Following Dworkin (1993, p. 226), I shall call this "the precedent autonomy view." Those who subscribe to this type of view do not generally deny that incompetent patients can have interests, including an interest in further life; rather they hold that a competent person's interest in controlling her life takes *precedence* over any interests the future incompetent individual might have. But this argument can be challenged on the grounds that the incompetent patient is not the same person as the competent executor of the advance directive.

Precedent Autonomy and the Other Person View

To illustrate the precedent autonomy view, Dworkin (1993, pp. 226 ff) discusses the case of Margo. He accepts that "[p]eople are not the best judges of what their own interests would be under circumstances they have never encountered and in which their preferences and desires may have drastically changed," but, he argues, this does not provide us with a sufficient reason to override a properly executed advance directive. Rather, after drawing a distinction between merely experiential interests or preferences and more significant critical interests or commitments, he argues that we should honor the critical interests of a person at t_1, even if—as in Margo's case—our doing so may seemingly not be in the best interests of the demented patient at t_2. We should do this, Dworkin holds, because our critical interests (the values and projects we consciously adopt) are more morally significant than our merely experiential interests, such as eating an ice-cream, watching television, experiencing states of well-being rather than states of pain, and so on. The reason is that our values and projects give coherence to our lives, and provide them with an ongoing narrative structure that marks them as our very own (see also Dresser 1995).

Those who, like Dworkin, take this kind of approach may thus readily admit that there can be cases of a perceived conflict between a person's prior instructions, based on what Dworkin calls her critical interests, and her current experiential interests, and yet hold that it is appropriate to give priority to the person's critical interests. As Dworkin (1993, p. 204) sees it, the competent Margo's critical interest in living her life in accordance with her deeply held values and beliefs includes an interest in how, and whether, her life as an incompetent patient continues.

But the precedent autonomy view is open to the radical philosophical challenge posed by the psychological view of personal identity (Parfit 1986, pp. 204ff). Put most simply, on this view, psychological continuity is a *necessary* condition for personal identity. This presupposes that for Margo at t_1 to be the same person as Margo at t_2, there must be sufficient psychological continuity and connectedness (exemplified by memories, intentions, beliefs, desires, and so on) between the former competent person and the now incompetent patient. If these psychological links become very weak or are absent, as often will be the case in advanced Alzheimer's disease, there are conceptual grounds for claiming that the severely demented patient is not the same person as the author of the directive. Based on the psychological view of personal identity, critics of advance directives have argued that a person's earlier choice at t_1 lacks moral authority to control what happens to the demented patient (a different person) at t_2. Although I, Helga Kuhse, may have the moral authority to decide that *I* want to die because I regard life in a certain state as undignified and not worthwhile, it does not follow that I have the moral authority to make that decision for someone else.

PSYCHOLOGICAL CONTINUITY, PERSONHOOD, AND THE INTEREST IN FURTHER LIFE

Objections based on the psychological view of personal identity pose a profound threat to advance directives. After all, as Allen Buchanan (1988, p. 280) has noted, they assert no less than "that the very process that renders the individual incompetent and brings the advance directive into play, can—and indeed often does—destroy the conditions necessary for his or her personal identity and thereby undercut entirely the moral authority of the directive."

For the purposes of my argument, I shall accept the now widely held view that psychological continuity is at least a necessary condition for personal identity, but shall deny that this is a sufficient reason for overriding advance directives in cases such as Margo's.

Psychological Continuity

Given that the continuity between mental states admits of degrees, the issue of when one person has been replaced by another remains somewhat vague (Buchanan 1988). As long as strong psychological connections continue to exist, there is little reason to doubt that the executor of the advance directive and the patient are the same person. Similarly, there is little reason to doubt that a patient who has slipped into a persistent vegetative state and has irreversibly lost the capacity to experience states of consciousness is not the same person as the executor of the advance directive. The reason is not that the patient is a *different* person, but rather that with the permanent loss of the ability to experience *any* psychological states, the patient is, on the view we are discussing, no longer a person.

Matters become more difficult when psychological continuity and connectedness are neither very strong nor totally absent, as would be the case once Alzheimer's disease has progressed beyond the initial stages of relatively mild memory loss, feelings of disorganization, and so on, but has not resulted in the obliteration of all consciousness. Patients in this broad category would have suffered varying degrees of permanent neurological damage, they would experience moderate to severe memory loss, deficits in cognition, and their ability to sustain even simple projects and desires would be much reduced and, in some cases, nearly obliterated. Provided, however, that at least some psychological continuity persists, is such a patient the same person as the individual who executed the advance directive?

Although I believe that the precise level of psychological continuity regarded as sufficient for personal identity will involve a societal choice and that there are good reasons for setting the threshold required for the persistence of psychological continuity for personal identity very low (Buchanan 1988), I do not want to pursue these complex and contentious issues here. For our limited focus on the refusal of life-sustaining treatment in the context of advanced Alzheimer's disease, a more straightforward approach is available, which distinguishes the question of whether personal identity has been destroyed from the question of whether personhood has been destroyed. Even if some psychological continuity continues to exist between the person at t_1 and the incompetent patient at t_2, it does not follow that the incompetent patient at t_2 is a *person*.

Personhood

The question of personhood is, of course, an extremely complex one, and I cannot adequately discuss, let alone settle, all the relevant issues here. Like Buchanan's (1988, pp. 283-84) personhood approach, my view falls broadly in the Lockean tradition according to which persons are conscious beings, who have the capacity for rationality, self-consciousness, and purposive agency; they have the ability to see themselves as existing over time, that is, they are not only living in the present, but have the mental capacity to span time (Kuhse and Singer 1985; Kuhse 1987; see also, e.g., Warren 1973; Tooley 1983; Singer 1993; Brock 1988; Hoerster 1995).

Where would this conception of personhood leave patients severely affected by Alzheimer's disease? Although the notion of personhood, like that of psychological continuity, is somewhat vague at the margins, it seems clear that as long as we understand the term "person" in the above psychological sense (rather than as, say, describing all members of the species *homo sapiens*, or all those said to possess immortal souls), we must also accept that there are some human individuals who, short of being in a persistent vegetative state, are not persons. For the remainder of this paper, I shall—whenever I speak of patients suffering from advanced Alzheimer's disease or from severe dementia—assume that these individuals no longer have the cognitive abilities thought necessary for personhood. I shall, as before, be concerned with "pleasantly demented" patients only, that is, with patients who, like Margo at t_2, continue to be able to experience states of consciousness and whose lives contain a balance of pleasant experiences over unpleasant or painful ones.

Now, if a severely demented patient is not a person, it follows that she, like a patient in a persistent vegetative state, cannot be the same person as the author of the advance directive. There is, however, an important morally relevant difference that distinguishes these two groups of patients. Severely demented patients, but not patients in a persistent vegetative state, are capable of experiencing states of consciousness and have interests. This is why the problem raised by advance directives is so poignantly posed in the context of these patients: if a patient such as Margo at t_2 is not the same person as the author of the advance directive at t_1, and can seemingly derive some benefit from life-sustaining treatment, what possible justification could there be for allowing her to die?

Can the moral authority of advance directives be upheld? Before I give my own affirmative answer, I want to show why the approach taken by Buchanan (1988) is at best inconclusive. Although Buchanan accepts both the psychological continuity view, and agrees that patients affected by severe dementia[1] are not persons, his substantive conclusion—that the moral authority of advance directives is not seriously threatened by cases of this kind—is not, or is only inadequately, supported by the arguments advanced in its favor.

Buchanan (1988, p. 286ff) argues that advance directives can be seen as tools to protect interests other than merely experiential interests. To the extent that these interests survive the author of the directive, they have a much greater moral weight than the experiential interests of the nonperson that "succeeds" the author of the directive. Although the person's successor is clearly still a morally considerable being, she or he has only limited interests. The interests of such nonpersons would "consist solely in the interest in avoiding pain and the interest in having whatever fleeting, fragmentary, and unanticipated experiences of simple physical pleasures his or her damaged nervous system still allows." These interests, Buchanan holds, would be easily overridden by the "surviving interests" of the author of the advance directive. Such surviving interests might be the financial and emotional well-being of our loved ones, or concern about how our mortal remains are treated after our death. And just as a person's interest in what happens to her corpse once she is dead is legitimate, so, Buchanan holds, is her interest in what happens to her living remains: "We would be justified in thwarting the latter interest only if satisfying it required the thwarting of other, morally weightier interests." Given that a patient suffering from advanced Alzheimer's disease would only have the severely truncated interests already referred to above, the overriding of the incompetent patient's interests is, Buchanan concludes, easily justified.

As it stands, this defense is problematical. The fundamental question Buchanan fails to answer is this: How do interests—in dignity or the well-being of one's loved ones, for example—survive the profound changes the patient has undergone? (On this and the following points, see also Kuczewski 1994, p. 34ff.) Buchanan does not seem to subscribe to the view that a person such as Margo at t_1 would have been harmed directly

KENNEDY INSTITUTE OF ETHICS JOURNAL • DECEMBER 1999

if her wishes were not implemented at t_2. Moreover, to the extent that on the psychological view of personal identity (which Buchanan endorses), "surviving interests" have their source in, and are tied to, our continued psychological existence, it is not clear how, or where, these interests can survive once the person has ceased to exist. In fact, it is this very question that provokes and underpins the challenge posed by the psychological view of personal identity: the assumption that a person's interests at t_1 continue to have any force to determine what happens to a different individual at t_2. After all, critics of advance directives have pointed out, the latter individual may be *harmed* by that decision. As Dresser (1995, p. 36) puts it when reflecting on the case of Margo: "Happy and contented Margo will experience clear harm from the decision that purports to advance the critical interests she no longer cares about."

Interests

Although Buchanan's account is thus question begging, a stronger defense of advance directives is available. Rather than appeal to the, in this context, dubious notion of "surviving interests," those who accept the psychological continuity view, would be standing on much firmer ground if they were to look for a justification of advance directives in the value they have for their authors. Persons care about events that happen after their death and in that sense have an interest in controlling (what they see as) their future. In other words, the value of advance directives lies, as Robertson (1991, p. 7) has noted, in the comfort and assurance those of us who are persons derive from the knowledge that our wishes will be honored after we have ceased to exist.

To say that advance directives serve the interests of persons is not, of course, sufficient to justify their use. Other interests, foremost among them the interests of the surviving incompetent patient, must also be taken into account. As noted before, Dresser (1995, p. 36) holds that a patient such as Margo "will experience clear harm" from a nontreatment decision, and Robertson (1991, p. 8) appears to express a similar view when he writes of such patients having an "interest in further life." If the moral authority of advance directive is to be upheld, it is necessary to question these assumptions. Buchanan fails to do this directly. Although he takes pains to point out that patients suffering from advanced Alzheimer's disease have only very truncated interests and mental capacities that "are much less sophisticated than those of a small child or a nonhuman animal such as a dog" (Buchanan 1988, p. 285), he does not tackle the problem head-on. On the contrary, his remark that the interests of a nonpersons would include not only an interest in avoiding pain but also an interest "in having ... experiences of simple physical pleasures" might be read to imply agreement with those views.

Buchanan's comparison of severely demented human individuals with nonhuman animals is, however, instructive. It would be widely agreed, I think, that most animals are not persons. They are not persons because they, like severely demented human individuals, lack the capacity for self-consciousness, rationality, and purposive agency, and have no conception of themselves as existing over time. Although such beings are sentient, that is, they are capable of experiencing states of pleasure and pain, they· lack the capacity to sustain hopes and fears and, more generally, a vision of their lives as extending into the future.

As has been noted (Tooley 1983; Singer 1993; see also Kuhse and Singer 1985; Brock 1988), the fact that most animals seem to lack a conception of themselves as existing as a single being through time may explain the widely shared view that it is, on the one hand, seriously morally wrong to inflict gratuitous suffering on animals, but that it is not wrong to kill them painlessly. On the other hand, it is also widely believed that the killing of a person, against her will, is probably the most serious wrong we can do to that person—and a much more serious wrong than the infliction of pain and suffering. What explains the difference in our attitude to the treatment of animals and persons in these two respects? The answer lies, I believe, in the differences that distinguish persons from those animals that lack the capacities widely believed to be necessary for personhood. Although persons and all sentient animals can experience pain, only persons can anticipate, and have desires about, their own future. These desires can be thwarted by a person being killed.

Michael Tooley (1983) has developed this position more thoroughly than anybody else. He argues, convincingly in my view, that the ability to see oneself as existing over time is a necessary condition for being a person and for having what he calls a "right to life." What Tooley suggests is that the wrongness of an action is related to the extent to which the action prevents some interests, desires, or preferences from being fulfilled. This basic principle explains both why it is wrong, other things being equal, to inflict pain, and why it is wrong, other things being equal, to kill a being with a desire to go on living. Any being capable of feeling pain can have a desire that the pain stop, but only a being capable of understanding that it has a prospect of future existence can have a desire to go on living, and only a continuing self—or "person"—can have an interest in continued life.

In seeing the capacity to be conscious of oneself as existing over time as a necessary condition for personhood, Tooley does not stand alone. Rather there is considerable philosophical agreement that this ability is a necessary condition for being considered a person. (In addition to Buchanan 1988, see also, for example, Singer 1993; Kuhse 1987; Hoerster 1995; Engelhardt 1986; Warren 1973; Brock 1988; Rachels 1987.) On this view, it would thus not be *directly* wrong to allow a human individual who is not a person to die painlessly, and would permit one to accept both the psychological view of personal identity and to argue that the advance refusal of life-sustaining treatment by a person should be honored if the individual that succeeds her is not a person, that is, does not have an interest in her own continued existence.

Two points need emphasizing: First, to say that an individual lacks an interest in future life and hence in life-sustaining treatments is not the same as saying that she has also lost an interest in the kinds of experience she will have while alive. All patients capable of experiencing states of consciousness have an interest in avoiding pain and discomfort, and hence in receiving pain and symptom control, and in receiving care that ensures comfort and provides simple pleasures. Second, to affirm that severely demented patients retain an interest in experiencing simple pleasures while alive is quite different from saying that these patients retain an interest in being kept alive, so as to experience whatever pleasures are available to them (Brock 1988, p. 90).

The preceding analysis suggests that the psychological view of personal identity does not pose a serious challenge to advance refusals of life-sustaining treatments. Matters are, however, different when it comes to the refusal of palliative care. Some modes of dying are excruciatingly painful, and even though severely demented patients no longer have an interest in their own continued existence, they retain a strong interest in not experiencing pain and discomfort. In other words, although these patients cannot be harmed by being allowed to die painlessly, they are being harmed if pain and discomfort are allowed to persist. Given, then, that severely demented patients retain a strong interest in receiving pain and symptom control, it is far from clear that this basic interest should be trumped by the interests persons might have in knowing that the values and beliefs they hold dear (for example, a belief in the redemptive value of suffering) will find expression after their lives as persons have ceased.

CONCLUSION

I have argued that it would not be *directly* wrong to allow a severely demented patient to die painlessly, in accordance with the wishes laid down in a competently executed advance directive. Contrary to what is widely assumed, this conclusion can, however, not—given the truth of the psychological continuity view—be justified by traditional appeals to self-determination. Rather, a different justification is required. I have argued that such a justification can be found in the different interests possessed by persons on the one hand, and severely demented patients who are no longer persons on the other. The advance refusal of life-sustaining treatment will satisfy the interests or preferences of the author of the directive to control what she sees as her future, without thereby thwarting any of the severely demented patient's interests. The reason is that severely demented patients, in distinction from persons, no longer have an interest in their own continued existence.

This conclusion challenges the traditional sanctity-of-life view (Kuhse 1987), that is, the view that all innocent human lives are equally valuable and inviolable and that one human individual has no authority to make life and death decisions for another. Any theory of personhood that wedges the concept of human life apart and suggests that some human beings do not have a "right to life" is thus highly controversial. This may explain why the present moral defense of advance directives is so rarely articulated in the literature, and why attempts to establish their moral authority rely so heavily on the widely accepted belief in the value of self-determination. But, as we have seen, there are good reasons for thinking that self-determination provides only a conceptually confused justificatory basis for advance directives.

In summary, I have suggested that those who argue that advance directives rest on a confused understanding of personal identity may well be correct, but acceptance of that position does not by itself provide sound reasons for overriding refusals of life-sustaining treatment. Rather, an examination of plausible understandings of the concepts of "person," "human individual," and "interests" may lead one to conclude that the implementation of advance directives will, other things being equal, be justified, even when the now incompetent patient is not experiencing suffering and distress, and seemingly is capable of experiencing some simple but psychologically disjointed pleasures.

KENNEDY INSTITUTE OF ETHICS JOURNAL • DECEMBER 1999

One important set of concerns I have not discussed is whether, and if so how, this conclusion ought to be translated into health care policy. Although Margo at t_2 is severely demented, she is capable of experiencing pleasurable states of consciousness, and is not suffering great pain or distress. It may be emotionally difficult for health care professionals, who do not generally draw philosophical distinctions between persons and nonpersons, to withhold a simple life-sustaining treatment from a patient who clearly is deriving some pleasures from her existence. Would we really want health care professionals who are prepared to end the lives of people such as Margo at t_2? Our answer might, for a number of symbolic and practical reasons, well be "no" (see also Dworkin 1993, pp. 228-32; Dresser 1995, p. 34). But if that is the answer we will want to give, it would require articulation and defense, and much more public discussion than it has until now received.

NOTE

1. Buchanan (1988) does not specifically address the issue of "pleasantly demented" nonpersons. Rather, he limits his discussion to the arguably much easier case of a severely demented patient who is close to death and "typically suffers a number of serious and often painful ailments as well" (see, e.g., pp. 285, 299). Although this kind of scenario makes nontreatment decisions intuitively more acceptable, his conceptual framework should support nontreatment decisions for pleasantly demented patients as well.

REFERENCES

Berghmans, R. L. P. 1998. Advance Directives for Non-Therapeutic Dementia Research: Some Ethical and Policy Considerations. *Journal of Medical Ethics* 24: 32-37.

Brock, Daniel. 1988. Justice and the Severely Demented Elderly. *Journal of Medicine and Philosophy* 13: 73-99.

Buchanan, Allen. 1988. Advance Directives and the Personal Identity Problem. *Philosophy and Public Affairs* 17: 277-302.

———, and Brock, Dan. 1989. *Deciding for Others: The Ethics of Surrogate Decision Making*. New York: Cambridge University Press.

Dresser, Rebecca. 1986. Life, Death, and Incompetent Patients: Conceptual Infirmities and Hidden Values in the Law. *Arizona Law Review* 28: 373-405.

———. 1989. Advance Directives, Self-Determination, and Personal Identity. In *Advance Directives in Medicine*, ed. Chris Hackler, Ray Moseley, and Dorothy E. Vawter, pp. 155-70. New York: Praeger.

————. 1995. Dworkin on Dementia—Elegant Theory, Questionable Policy. *Hastings Center Report* 25 (6): 32-38.

Dworkin, Ronald. 1993. *Life's Dominion: An Argument about Abortion and Euthanasia*. Hammersmith, London: Harper Collins.

Engelhardt, H. Tristram, Jr.. 1986. *The Foundations of Bioethics*. New York: Oxford University Press.

Firlik, Andrew D. 1991. Margo's Logo. *Journal of the American Medical Association* 9: 201.

Hoerster, Norbert. 1995. Neugeborene und das Recht auf Leben. Frankfurt: Suhrkamp.

Kuczewski, Mark G. 1994. Whose Will is it, Anyway? A Discussion of Advance Directives, Personal Identity and Consensus in Medical Ethics. *Bioethics* 8: 27-48.

Kuhse, Helga 1987. *The Sanctity-of-Life Doctrine in Medicine: A Critique*. Oxford: Clarendon Press.

————, and Singer, Peter. 1985. *Should the Baby Live: The Problem of Handicapped Infants*. Oxford: Oxford University Press.

Office of Technology Assessment, U.S. Congress. 1987. *Losing a Million Minds: Confronting the Tragedy of Alzheimer's Disease and Other Dementias*. Washington, DC: U.S. Government Printing Office.

Parfit, Derek. 1984. *Reasons and Persons*. Oxford: Oxford University Press.

Rachels, James. 1987. *The End of Life*. New York: Oxford.

Rhoden, Nancy K. 1990. The Limits of Legal Objectivity. *North Carolina Law Review* 68: 845- 65.

Radden, Jennifer. 1996. *Divided Minds and Successive Selves: Ethical Issues in Disorders of Identity and Personality*. Cambridge, MA: MIT Press.

Robertson, John A. 1991. Second Thoughts on Living Wills. *Hastings Center Report* 21 (6): 6-9.

Savulescu, Julian. 1994. Rational Desires and the Limitation of Life-Sustaining Treatment. *Bioethics* 8: 191-222.

Singer, Peter. 1993. *Practical Ethics*. Cambridge and New York: Cambridge University Press.

Smith, David H. 1992. Seeing and Knowing Dementia. In *Dementia and Aging: Ethics, Values, and Policy Choices*, ed. Robert H. Binstock, Stephen G. Post, and Peter J. Whitehouse, pp. 44- 54. Baltimore: Johns Hopkins University Press.

Stone, Jim. 1994. Advance Directives, Autonomy and Unintended Death. *Bioethics* 8: 223-46.

Tooley, Michael. 1983. *Abortion and Infanticide*. Oxford: Clarendon Press.

KENNEDY INSTITUTE OF ETHICS JOURNAL • DECEMBER 1999

Warren, Mary Anne. 1973. On the Moral and Legal Status of Abortion. *The Monist* 57 (1): 43- 61.

Whitehouse, Peter J. 1992. Dementia: The Medical Perspective. In *Dementia and Aging: Ethics, Values, and Policy Choices*. ed. Robert H. Binstock, Stephen, G. Post, and Peter J. Whitehouse, pp. 21-29. Baltimore: Johns Hopkins University Press.

[17]

dvance directives in their many variations continue to be the preferred solution to treatment decisions for incompetent patients.[1] Recommended by most medical ethicists and advisory bodies, they have achieved judicial or legislative recognition in more than forty states. The *Cruzan* decision came close to granting them constitutional status. And through the Patient Self-Determination Act federal law now encourages their use by requiring hospitals to inform patients of their right to make such directives.

Given the rising tide in favor of living wills it might seem surprising—and surely politically incorrect—to call their use into question. Yet living wills strike me as an initially appealing but inadequate solution to decisionmaking for incompetent patients.[2] Despite their allure and short-term benefits, they are full of contradictions that threaten the welfare of incompetent patients. Before discussing my objections, however, let me forthrightly acknowledge two benefits of living wills that explain much of their appeal.

One is that advance directives do give competent persons a sense of control over future decisions if they become incompetent. The living will thus empowers people, by extending the scope of personal autonomy to situations in which autonomy cannot be directly exercised. The individual when competent determines the course of her life

John A. Robertson is Thomas Watt Gregory Professor, School of Law, University of Texas, Austin, Tex.

Second Thoughts on Living Wills

by John A. Robertson

Advance directives such as living wills are attractive in that they give us a sense of control over our futures. But they also tend to obscure conflicts between a patient's competent wishes and later, incompetent interests. They allow caregivers to avoid evaluating quality of life in assessing the best interests of incompetent patients.

when incompetent, thus gaining the assurance that she will later be viewed in light of previously expressed preferences. In addition, the certainty that excessive treatment will not be imposed at a later time reassures those fearful of a debilitated future.

The second advantage is that living wills, if specific enough, provide a workable rule for nontreatment decisions that *appears* to respect autonomy without compromising respect for incompetent patients. Rather than wrestle with difficult questions about the quality or worth of an incompetent patient's life, treatment can be withheld if the prior directive so specifies. Thus living wills have played an important role in achieving the now widely accepted recognition that treatment can be withheld, in appropriate circumstances, from both competent and incompetent patients.

Yet despite these advantages, it is noteworthy that in practice advance directives have not been so warmly embraced by those they are intended to help. Polls show that only a few people actually make them out.[3] Even when they do, physicians sometimes are very reluctant to follow them. Moreover, living will laws have traditionally been limited to narrowly defined "terminal conditions," leaving other debilitating conditions outside of their purview.[4]

While federal law will increase the use of advance directives by notifying hospital patients of their availability, existing statutory restrictions and the limited use of living wills even where available suggest that ordinary people and policy makers alike distrust—or are am-

6

Hastings Center Report, November-December 1991

bivalent about—their use in many circumstances. (Indeed, they are accepted most readily only in those circumstances where they are least needed.) Interestingly, this distrust stems from the same source as their advantages. Both grow out of the conceptual confusions and contradictions that inhere in the use of an advance directive to control a future situation.

Confusions and Inconsistencies

A main problem with living wills is that the assumptions underlying their use are confused or not clearly distinguished. It is usually assumed that the justification for giving the competent person power over decisions when she is incompetent is that the competent person is best situated to identify what those future interests are. That is, the prior directive is taken to be the most accurate indicator of the person's interests once she becomes incompetent.

The problem, however, is that the patient's interests when incompetent—viewed from her current perspective—are no longer informed by the interests and values she had when competent. The values and interests of the competent person no longer are relevant to someone who has lost the rational structure on which those values and interests rested. Unless we are to view competently held values and interests as extending even to situations in which, because of incompetency, they can no longer have meaning, it matters not that as a competent person the individual would not wish to be maintained in a debilitated or disabled state. If the person is no longer competent enough to appreciate the degree of divergence from her previous activity that produced the choice against treatment, the prior directive does not represent her current interests merely because a competent directive was issued.[5] Although still the same person, the patient's interests have changed radically once she becomes incompetent. Yet the premise of the prior directive is that patient interests and values remain significantly the same, so that those interests are best served by following the directive issued when competent.

The point stated here will be rejected by persons who believe that the self should be viewed as a whole that exists over one's entire life.[6] In their view,

focussing on the situation of the incompetent patient without taking account of his or her previously held interests and values misdescribes patients by treating them too narrowly. Since previously competent persons have a history of values and preferences, they should be treated as having the same values and interests even when they become incompetent.

In my view, this position overlooks the important fact that at different stages and times of life we have different interests. When our situations change drastically, our interests and preferences also change. The difference between competent and incompetent interests is so great that if we are to respect incompetent persons, we should focus on their needs and interests as they now exist, and not view them as retaining interests and values which, because of their incompetency, no longer apply.

The confusion between past competent and present incompetent interests risks harming incompetent patients in situations in which competent and incompetent interests diverge. Advance directives, which reflect competent values and interests, may inaccurately reflect the interests of the incompetent patient who is in a radically different situation, in which values and interests dependent on a rational structure no longer apply. Yet the situation of the incompetent patient is viewed through the lens of her prior competent self rather than how she now is, which tends to devalue the more limited interests of a patient no longer moved by the concerns that once animated her when competent.

A more accurate justification for living wills would focus on their value to competent patients in controlling their future. Although advance directives do not always accurately reflect incompetent patients' interests, they do reflect the interests of competent persons in determining their future. Indeed, the clearest and most honest justification for the living will is that it gives competent persons certainty and assurance about how they will be treated when incompetent, thus serving the interests of competent patients in controlling their future.

But this rationale makes all the clearer the possibility of conflict between past competent and current incompetent interests—between the

need of the competent patient for control and certainty and the need of the incompetent patient for treatment. Except when both sets of interests coincide, the competent person's advance certainty is bought at the possible cost of denying needed treatment to the incompetent person he or she has become. Under either rationale, the possibility of conflict with the incompetent patient's interests arises, yet is not acknowledged. This tradeoff may be an acceptable policy choice, but it cannot always be justified either as protection for the incompetent patient or as a necessary or desirable implication of personal autonomy.

To determine whether this conflict has practical rather than merely theoretic significance, we need to know how often incompetent persons have interests in being treated that are denied on the basis of prior directives. It is impossible to gauge the frequency of conflict at the present time because so little attention has been given to this problem. Still, anecdotes abound of cases in which patients treated despite a directive recover and are grateful. We also often hear of situations in which doctors are reluctant to follow living wills because they think the patient should be treated.[7] In any event, it is plausible to think that there will be many cases in which conscious incompetent patients clearly have interests in treatment that a prior directive would deny. As the use of living wills expands, there are likely to be many more such conflicts. Of course, in many situations—particularly of terminal illness—there will be no conflict, because the incompetent patient will have no current interest in treatment. But in those circumstances it should not be necessary to rely on an advance directive to have treatment withheld.

This then is the nub of the problem that I see with living wills. Because they either confuse the present interests of an incompetent patient with interests she had when competent, or forthrightly privilege the competent person's interest in control and certainty over the incompetent patient's current interests, they pose a threat to incompetent patients. If this threat arises in many cases, it is a serious problem for an ethical-legal position that purports to be patient-centered. Of course, a patient-centered policy may not be morally required in all circumstances, and perhaps should be modified. However, when respect for the incompetent patient purports to be the central value animating ethical and legal norms for nontreatment, deviations from this standard should not be hidden by the legerdemain of prior directives.

At the very least the possibility of such conflicts should be recognized, and some attempt made to assess their frequency. Yet medical ethicists and policy makers have hardly noted, much less addressed this risk (though it is reflected in the ambivalence and distrust that surrounds living wills in practice).[8] Moreover, doubts arise about whether those who execute advance directives are exercising autonomy in an informed way if they are not even aware of the conflict. Rarely are they told that the directive they make reflects their current interests and may not be a good indicator of their interests as an incompetent patient. If this conflict were forthrightly acknowledged, living wills would at least be made in an informed manner, and thus more clearly deserve respect as an indicator of the competent person's autonomy.

Finally, the implications of the autonomy principle for other kinds of prior directives should be noted. If prior directives are to control, even when patient interests conflict, would not this same principle apply to other directives or contracts that regulate the future, including directives that take effect when the person is later competent, such as surrogate mother contracts or agreements for the disposition of frozen embryos? Persons who oppose enforcing such contracts will say that the individual's competent change of mind distinguishes these situations from that of the living will, but autonomy in controlling the future by advance directive nonetheless appears to be involved in both cases.[9]

Once acknowledged, the possibility of conflict between competent wishes and incompetent interests will direct attention away from the question of what the incompetent patient wanted when competent, to the central issue of whether treatment or nontreatment best serves the interests of the now incompetent patient. If this question were faced squarely there would be no need to rely on the prior directive (unless in cases of conflict we want to privilege the competent person's certainty over the incompetent patient's need). The needs of the incompetent patient would be directly addressed, and treatment given or withheld on the basis of her current interests, as the appropriate proxy or other decisionmakers decide.

In fact, we can usefully understand the living will as a device that functions to avoid assessing incompetent patient interests (though avoiding the question directly is itself a value judgment about the worth of incompetent lives). Introduced at a time of great uncertainty about the legitimacy of nontreatment of incompetent patients, the living will purported to allow nontreatment to occur without assessing quality of life. In fact, however, a quality of life assessment was hidden in the narrow definitions of "terminal condition" for which the living will was most easily accepted. With more than fifteen years of debate over nontreatment of incompetent patients behind us, it is now time to address quality of life directly, and not cloak it with diversionary investigations into prior wishes. Indeed, a direct assessment of patient interests, now undertaken when the patient never was competent and in many jurisdictions when no prior directive was made, focuses directly on the incompetent patient's welfare, and thus is most respectful of the now incompetent patient.

Looking to the Future

Where does this leave us with regard to advance directives and public policy? It would seem useless at this point—the equivalent of tilting at bioethical windmills—to try to stave off or reverse the living will juggernaut. So let me suggest the following steps to alleviate the worst problems that an unblinking faith in prior directives brings.

First, assure at the very least that makers of living wills are informed of the potential conflict between their future interests when incompetent and their current interests in achieving certainty about how they will be treated when incompetent. There is a tradeoff here that should be recognized so that the exercise of present autonomy is truly informed.

Second, prepare for the more frequent emergence of conflicts over whether advance directives should be enforced when they conflict with the incompetent patient's current interests. The theory of the living will does not even acknowledge such a conflict, yet many situations will arise in which the incompetent patient appears to have an interest in treatment that conflicts with a prior directive. Rather than simply enforce all prior directives, doctors, family, and others involved in the care of incompetent patients should be able to question whether the patient's interests would best be served by actions contrary to the living will, in situations in which the incompetent patient appears to have an interest in further life. A procedure that avoids an overly rigid vitalism will have to be devised to resolve these conflicts.

Third, begin direct, explicit assessments of the quality of life and best interests of incompetent patients. Distinguishing those situations of incompetent existence that have value for incompetent patients will be difficult in many cases. But this is the basic value question that treatment decisions for incompetent patients necessarily raise, and it should be forthrightly addressed. States deemed to have sufficient value for such patients to warrant treatment should be identified and guidelines formulated to prevent manipulation and abuse of a best interests approach.

Advance directives at present neatly evade these messy questions, but they inexorably arise. They are unavoidable with regard to patients who have never been competent, or who when competent never issued a prior directive. Rather than always treat, most courts and commentators recognize some room for a best interests test in these circumstances. It is time to bring such assessments out of the closet and apply them to all situations involving incompetent patients. Indeed, such assessments will help determine whether living wills are actually hurting patient interests. Ironically, if they are not, there is no need to rely on them, because treatment may be withheld when patients have no further interests in treatment regardless of a prior directive. On the other hand, if enforcing living wills harms incompetent patients, the rationale for enforcing them is questionable.

Fourth, do not constitutionalize ad-

Hastings Center Report, November-December 1991

vance directives. The opinions in *Cruzan* suggest that a majority of the Supreme Court may be ready to protect health care directives as part of Fourteenth Amendment liberty.[10] Such a move would be unwise and constitutionally unjustified. Constitutionalizing prior directives will limit state efforts to protect the welfare of incompetent patients when their interests conflict with a prior directive. Moreover, the autonomy interest in avoiding bodily intrusions, which deserves constitutional status under the Fourteenth Amendment when those intrusions are imposed on a competent patient, is not implicated in a person's interest in controlling future situations of incompetency. At the very least, states should be free to balance competent and incompetent patient interests as they see fit, free of constitutional constraints that enshrine living wills as beyond challenge.

Living wills have played an important role in the ethical and policy debate over treatment decisions for incompetent patients, but it is time to move beyond them to the central issues of what quality of life for incompetent patients is worth protecting. Although not explicitly acknowledged, such assessments are now occurring with patients who were never competent or who never issued a health care directive. They are also figuring in the growing debate over allocation of medical resources at the end of life.

Directly assessing quality of life, however, is difficult and threatening, and may be too politically divisive to be done openly. If so, these questions will continue to be framed in terms of prior directives and substituted judgment when directives are lacking. As a second best solution, this approach is preferable to a vitalist rule of always treat. But the living will's conceptual frailties limit its usefulness, and it is of little help where prior directives or wishes cannot be ascertained.

Ironically, just as advance directives gain wide acceptance, their inherent problems emerge. Unless we want to privilege competent choice over incompetent interests, the living will focuses on the wrong issue. It can no longer save us from the difficult task of determining which incompetent states of existence are worth protecting.

References

1. I include here living wills, durable powers of attorney, appointment of health care proxies, advance directives for or against treatment, and other devices that allow a competent person to give directions concerning her medical treatment if she becomes incompetent, although there are important differences among them.

2. See Rebecca Dresser and John A. Robertson, "Quality of Life and Nontreatment Decisions for Incompetent Patients: A Critique of the Orthodox Approach," *Law, Medicine & Health Care* 17 (1989): 234-44.

3. Linda Emanuel and Ezekiel Emanuel, "The Medical Directive: A New Comprehensive Care Document," *JAMA* 261 (1989): 3288-93.

4. John A. Robertson, "*Cruzan* and the Constitutional Status of Nontreatment Decisions for Incompetent Patients," *Georgia Law Review* 25 (1991): 1139-1202. See also Gregory Gelfand, "Living Wills: The First Decade," *Wisconsin Law Review* (1987): 737-822.

5. Rebecca Dresser, "Life, Death and Incompetent Patients: Conceptual Infirmities and Hidden Values in the Law," *Arizona Law Review* 28 (1986): 373-405; Rebecca Dresser, "Relitigating Life and Death," *Ohio State Journal* 51 (1990): 425-37.

6. Nancy Rhoden, "Litigating Life and Death," *Harvard Law Review* 102 (1988): 375-446.

7. See for example "*Evans v. Bellevue Hospital*," *New York Law Journal* 28 (July 1987): 11.

8. See for example Emanuel and Emanuel, "The Medical Directive."

9. Robertson, "*Cruzan* and the Constitutional Status of Nontreatment Decisions."

10. See especially Justice O'Connor's concurring opinion at 110 S.Ct. 2857 (1990).

9

[18]

I n the past decade, formal advance directives have come to be viewed by nearly all parties as having the potential to be a very important component of medical decisionmaking. For the past year, they have been the main object of a federal initiative under the Patient Self-Determination Act, intended to encourage patients to claim their rights in regard to decisionmaking. The PSDA requires that notice of the possibility of formulating advance directives be given to nearly all patients in the health care system; it also carries substantial requirements for documentation, transfer, clarification of the law, and public education.

While theoretical justifications for use of advance directives are easy to marshall,[1] to date little empirical research has been done to assess the merits of advance directives in practice.[2] For all we know, advance directives could be costly, irrelevant, or harmful. If so, encouraging their use would not be good policy. Here we will outline the issues needing to be addressed about formal advance directives and give an overview of what is now known. We will not assess what we could and should know about informal advance directives

Joanne Lynn is professor of medicine and of community & family medicine, Center for Evaluative Clinical Sciences, Dartmouth Medical School, Hanover, N.H.; Joan M. Teno is assistant professor of community & family medicine, Center for the Evaluative Clinical Sciences, Dartmouth Medical School.

Joanne Lynn and Joan M. Teno, "After the Patient Self-Determination Act: The Need for Empirical Research on Formal Advance Directives," *Hastings Center Report* 23, no. 1 (1993): 20-24.

After the Patient Self-Determination Act
The Need for Empirical Research on Formal Advance Directives
by Joanne Lynn and Joan M. Teno

(oral communications, letters, medical records, etc.). They are both more difficult to measure and have been even less often studied. Nonetheless, we would note that these informal advance directives are probably more important to clinical practice than are formal advance directives.

The Rationale for Advance Directives

The fundamental claim of mainstream American medical ethics today is, roughly, this: the decisions made in the care of a patient should be those that are expected to deliver the best possible outcome for that patient, as judged by the patient.[3] Although beyond the scope of this article, the merits of this decisionmaking model also could be studied empirically, although virtually no such research has been done.

However, when the patient cannot make his or her own assessment of alternative outcomes it is very difficult to make decisions that reflect patient preferences. Especially since illness is now so commonly chronic

and incompetence is so often the result of long-term illness in old age, clinicians can anticipate incompetence and enable patients to direct in advance the kinds of treatments and/or outcomes they would prefer. This provides a way to have the patient's nearly absolute authority endure into a period of incompetence and thereby greatly simplifies decisionmaking, both by making it more expeditious and by making it more likely to comport with the patient's own preferences. Having the patient make decisions in advance of incompetence allows others to avoid the often quite difficult and uncertain task of making the choices and provides a way for the patient to continue to bear the responsibility for decisions. Thus, various formal measures have been implemented to effectuate this endeavor. The most common are "living wills" and "durable powers of attorney."

These fundamental claims were at the heart of the Patient Self-Determination Act. However, good policy must depend upon effective implementation at least as much as

Hastings Center Report, January-February 1993

sound argument. How effective has the implementation of advance directives been?

Prevalence: Awareness and Completion of Advance Directives

Most people now seem to have at least a passing acquaintance with formal advance directives.[4] Support groups for persons with AIDS appear to have been singularly effective in assuring that this population is well informed.

Descriptive research to date has shown that advance directives enjoy widespread approval but that the rate at which they are actually written is much lower and varies with the population. In 1988, a public opinion survey conducted by the American Medical Association found that 56 percent of the general population had discussed with family their treatment preferences if they were in a coma. However, only 15 percent had a living will.[5] Emanuel and colleagues found that greater than 90 percent of respondents had a positive attitude toward advance directives but fewer than one in ten had completed one.[6] In contrast, about two in ten persons with AIDS treated in established community settings have a written directive.[7] In SUPPORT (The Study to Understand Prognoses and Preferences for Outcomes and Risks of Treatments), 21 percent of a population of very seriously ill hospitalized patients has been reported to have advance directives, with 7 percent living wills only, 9 percent durable powers of attorney only, and 5 percent having both.[8]

Characteristics associated with completing advance directives are known only for select populations with limited generalizability. Among persons with AIDS, white or well-educated respondents were more likely to have written a directive.[9] An association of ethnicity and intent to complete an advance directive has been reported in a population admitted to one Veteran's Administration hospital, with 91 percent of whites and 66 percent of blacks expressing an intent to complete an advance directive.[10]

One persistent concern about use of advance directives has been

whether their meaning and usefulness might be linked to a rational, "middle-class" approach to health care. The very meaning of offering an advance directive might be ineluctably altered when the patient is too poor to demand health care at all.

Few studies have examined whether the rate of advance directive use in practice can be improved. Among ambulatory patients in a residency program at a tertiary care hospital, an intervention consisting of an educational booklet and physician-initiated discussion resulted in only eight of fifty-two patients writing an advance directive.[11] In a randomized controlled trial of an educational intervention, Greg Sachs and colleagues found that a majority of patients (85%) did not implement a living will.[12] In contrast, Lawrence Markson and Knight Steel reported that forty-eight out of seventy-four homebound patients who were counseled about a durable power of attorney completed one.[13] The potential for increasing the rate of use of directives through an educational intervention is, therefore, uncertain.

Patients' Intent

We do not know the intent of patients who chose to complete a formal directive, or, for that matter, why some do not. Clearly, at least prior to the PSDA, advance directives have not figured centrally in patients' and physicians' interactions. The directives that have been reported to exist in the community at present do not seem to be based on discussion with a physician. In the AIDS population reported above, only one-half of persons with an advance directive discussed it with a physician, even after surviving a year of treatment.[14] Much anecdotal evidence favors the claim that physician involvement is uncommon.

In SUPPORT, we found that of the 735 patients who were reported (by self or surrogate) to have an advance directive, its existence was mentioned in the physician or nurse progress notes in only 45 cases. In this study, patient and surrogate preferences against resuscitation did not have a substantial association with having a living will. This suggests that patients

may intend more to avoid loss of control while dying and incompetent, rather than to shape a palliative plan of care throughout the course of their terminal illness.

Since treatment directives are commonly vague and difficult to interpret, it is important to know what the patient understood and what he or she was hoping to accomplish by completing the directive. However, no study yet reported has asked patients what they thought they were doing and how confident they were that they had succeeded. Likewise, no study yet has examined a full range of possible incentives, including the obvious possibility that the patient is heavily motivated by a fear of loss of control, or by a concern for the well-being of family.

Patients might execute advance directives to keep decisionmaking out of the courts—avoiding certain kinds of judicial involvement seems likely with some advance directives. However, once there is a legal document, the opportunities for legal wrangling may escalate rather than decline. No study has yet addressed the actual effects. This may be especially important for instruction directives, which are often too vague for ready application or are clouded by uncertainty about patient understanding at the time the directive was constructed.

A flurry of articles has documented that surrogates (next of kin, usually) err substantially in predicting patient preferences.[15] This is often taken to be a strong argument for encouraging advance directives, especially treatment directives, since the major alternative strategy of relying on a (family) surrogate seems so flawed. Not only is this problematic in that patients might have a stronger interest in who makes decisions than in having a particular choice made,[16] but the finding of discordance is also inconclusive since no one has yet studied the efficacy of advance directives in evading this problem.

Do the preferences articulated during a time of health and prior to a pressing need for a decision endure into a period marked by serious illness and imminence of the impact of the choice? The few research endeavors that have examined the stability of preferences have shown only moderate agreement over time, with a clinically significant number of people changing their stated preferences (in both directions).[17] To date, this research has examined patient responses to a standardized interview, which is a limited method but still leads to the important question, What are we to do if competent patients often disagree later with what they said earlier in a formal advance directive?

Impact of Advance Directives on Medical Decisionmaking

Formal advance directives are not worth much unless they can be shown to improve decisionmaking. To date, only a few research projects have generated relevant insights, and none have done so definitively. Physicians who had used written directives felt that they were helpful.[18] However, in-depth interviews with fifty-seven physicians from California and Vermont yielded little indication that advance directives were helpful in medical decisionmaking.[19] Marion Danis and colleagues noted that one in four directives were not honored by the attending physicians.[20] This study did not address whether these failures to follow a directive were justifiable or not.

Only two studies have addressed the fundamental question of whether care differs between patients with and without advance directives. An abstract from the SUPPORT project indicates that seriously ill persons with and without advance directives tend to get about the same care patterns, even if the advance directives are treatment directives.[21] In a randomized trial, Lawrence Schneiderman and colleagues assigned subjects to be offered the opportunity to complete written directives or to receive routine care.[22] This intervention did not affect subsequent resource utilization prior to death. Nor did it have an impact upon DNR rates, CPR, survival, or well-being. However, the patients were not very ill (although they had long-term, life-threatening illnesses) and did not often have cognitive deficits as they died, and the sample was small (183 patients with 100 deaths during at least thirty-four months of follow-up).

In both of these studies, subjects had a treatment and/or a proxy directive. It will take some focused attention on the matter to discern whether advance directives that designate proxies are followed and whether the same proxy would have been identified without the directive. Likewise, the impact of instruction directives will have to be elucidated much more clearly. If they turn out to have little or no effect, then one is obliged to examine whether that is because very good decisionmaking practices apply in the case of the patients without formal advance directives, so that the differences are slight, or whether the formal advance directives are too easily ignored, even though they would have stipulated substantial differences in care. Of course, for the latter to be the case, there must be a substantial rate of incompetence near death.

In doing such research, certain methodological issues are recurrent and need careful consideration. For example, it turns out to be quite difficult to define the necessary components of a formal advance directive. Must it have met the witnessing and registration requirements of the state? Must it have been shared with some health care provider? If it is a surrogate designation, must it name someone who is actually available and appropriate? If an instruction directive, is it enough to state general sentiments about the appropriateness of dying, or must it also say something more directly applicable, such as addressing the acceptance of particular treatments or outcomes? Should an advance directive have substantial force if it is likely to be based on serious misunderstandings by the patient about his or her situation and its likely outcomes? Probably most

important, is a written document ever as important as comprehensive communication about preferences and likely outcomes among patient, providers, and potential surrogates? These last policy issues would be decided much more wisely if there were more understanding of the effects of enforcing even directives that are acknowledged to be deficient as compared with the effects of alternative strategies for decisionmaking.

Whatever was the practice before the Patient Self-Determination Act may well have changed substantially since, and those changes will need to be described. In addition, other initiatives might well have promise in encouraging optimization of decisionmaking through more extensive use of advance directives. The burgeoning array of efforts to enhance use of advance directives includes values history forms,[23] better formal advance directive forms, consumer education material (including the descriptions of patients' rights under state law that are required by the PSDA), videos, interactive videodiscs, and skilled legal counseling (mostly during estate planning). The merits of these are unknown without careful assessment. Some are probably helpful. Some are probably unreasonably costly or actually misleading. Program evaluation and demonstration projects are urgently needed.

One must eventually define the outcomes of interest in assessing the merits of advance directives. It

---

> Making decisions in advance of incompetence seems to reconstitute the competent decisionmaker and to evade the obvious ambiguities and compromises inherent in allowing decisions to be made by physicians and families. What is not clear is that the solution works.

---

cannot be adequate to document the frequency of directives, or to show that an intervention can increase the rate of completion. One must show that decisionmaking is improved by the presence of formal advance directives, or that patient outcomes are improved. Specifying the measures for either of these is quite difficult. Patient outcomes might include survival, function, symptoms, satisfaction, and global quality of life.[24] Perhaps it is also an "outcome" to have had the treatment course that one preferred. How to measure each dimension and how to combine them is largely unresolved. Nevertheless, patient outcomes do matter, and we must develop a serviceable metric and accomplish the research necessary to assess whether advance directives improve outcomes and, if so, in which forms and which populations.

Asking the Right Questions

Patients face decisions among potential courses of care; for reasons as diverse as caregivers' desire to leave the patient responsible for the outcome and society's investment in the moral value of letting people make their own decisions, we want to have the patient's preferences dictate the choice. When the patient is adult but incompetent, our community value of honoring self-determination becomes hard to implement, as there is no process that ensures decisions are made so as to honor the patient's preferences. Making decisions in advance of incompetence seems to reconstitute the competent decisionmaker and to evade the obvious ambiguities and compromises inherent in allowing decisions to be made by physicians and families. What is not clear is that the solution works or, more precisely, that it works better than alternative strategies. Nor is it clear that we have a common conception of what it would mean to "work"; that is, What is the standard to which one would compare any policy choice?

There are a few fundamental issues about advance directives in practice that must be researched if we are to be at all confident about the appropriate role for them. First, research must elucidate the degree to which patients' preferences are stable and represent important beliefs. If patients' preferences are quite unstable, then carrying them forward into incompetence is unjustified. Likewise, some preferences might be strongly held, so that thwarting them wrongs the patient, while others are lightly

held, and thwarting them is barely perceived by the patient. Such considerations must be incorporated into the implementation and evaluation of advance directives. Second, the effects of advance directives under various conditions need to be compared with various alternative strategies to guide decisionmaking for adults with incompetence. Otherwise, we will not be able to assess whether the policy of encouraging advance directives is, on the whole, an improvement over alternatives. Third, we need to understand why people do and do not write advance directives, especially the barriers to writing one when the concept is understood and is relevant to the patient. If many people do not write advance directives, for example because they do not want to have responsibility for these choices, that rationale should reshape the policy and practice.

In sum, advance directives have been proposed as the answer to the problem of how to empower patients so that they maintain control of their care even when incompetent. We have not yet shown that directives will answer that need. Indeed, the question may well be better articulated as one of defining and implementing an optimal procedure to make care decisions on behalf of incompetent adults. We certainly do not know how well advance directives answer that need, especially in comparison to alternative strategies. We may have the wrong answer; in fact, we may have answered the wrong question. We must seek to do the research on these issues before substantial social resources are committed to any particular strategy.

References

1. Allen E. Buchanan and Dan Brock, *Deciding for Others: The Ethics of Surrogate Decision Making* (Cambridge: Cambridge University Press, 1989); The Hastings Center, *Guidelines on the Termination of Life-Sustaining Treatment and the Care of the Dying* (Bloomington: Indiana University Press, 1987); The Appleton International Conference, "Developing Guidelines for Decisions to Forgo Life-Prolonging Medical Treatment," supplement, *Journal of Medical Ethics* 18 (September 1992): 1-23.

2. Kent W. Davidson, Chris Hackler, Debra R. Caradine, and Ronald S. Mc-

Cord, "Physicians' Attitudes on Advance Directives," *JAMA* 262 (1989): 2415-19; Marion Danis, Leslie I. Southerland, Joanne M. Garret, et al., "A Prospective Study of Advance Directives for Life-Sustaining Care," *NEJM* 324 (1991): 882-87; Joel M. Zimberg,"Decisions for the Dying: An Empirical Study of Physicians' Responses to Advance Directives," *Vermont Law Review* 13 (1989): 445-49; Joan M. Teno, Joanne Lynn, Donald J. Murphy, et al., "Impact of Advance Directives on Decisionmaking," *Gerontologist* 31 (1991): 41; Lawrence J. Schneiderman, Richard Kronick, Robert M. Kaplan, et al., "Effects of Offering Advance Directives on Medical Treatments and Costs," *Annals of Internal Medicine* 117 (1992): 599-606.

3. Buchanan and Brock, *Deciding for Others;* President's Commission for the Study of Ethical Problems in Medicine and Biomedical and Behavioral Research, *Deciding to Forego Life-Sustaining Treatment* (Washington, D.C.: U.S. Government Printing Office, 1983); Joanne Lynn and David DeGrazia, "An Outcomes Model of Medical Decision-Making," *Theoretical Medicine* 12 (1991): 325-43; *Cruzan v. Director, Missouri Department of Health,* 110 S. Ct. 2841 (1990).

4. American Medical Association, "Physician and Public Attitudes on Health Care Issues"; Linda L. Emanuel, Michelle Barry, John D. Stoeckle, et al., "Advance Directives for Medical Care: A Case for Greater Use," *NEJM* 324 (1991): 889-95; Joan M. Teno, John Fleishman, Dan Brock, and Vincent Mor, "The Use of Formal Prior Directives among Patients with HIV-Related Diseases," *Journal of General Medicine* 5 (1990): 490-94; Elizabeth R. Gamble, Penelope J. McDonald, and Peter R. Lichstein, "Knowledge, Attitudes and Behavior of Elderly Persons Regarding Living Wills," *Archives of Internal Medicine* 151 (1991): 277-80; Jiska Cohen-Mansfield, Beth A. Rabinovich, Steven Lipson, et al., "The Decision to Execute a Durable Power of Attorney for Health Care and Preferences Regarding Utilization of Life Sustaining Treatments in Nursing Home Residents," *Archives of Internal Medicine* 151 (1991): 289-94; Robert Steinbrock, Bernard Lo, Jeffrey Moulton, et al., "Preferences of Homosexual Men with AIDS for Life-Sustaining Treatment," *NEJM* 314 (1986): 457-60.

5. American Medical Association, "Physician and Public Attitudes."

6. Emanuel et al., "Advance Directives for Health Care."

7. Teno et al., "The Use of Formal Prior Directives."

8. Teno et al., "Impact of Advance Directives."

9. Teno et al., "The Use of Formal Prior Directives."

Hastings Center Report, January-February 1993

10. Jeremy Sugarman, Morris Weinberger, and Greg Samsa, "Factors Associated with Veterans' Decisions about Living Wills," *Archives of Internal Medicine* 152 (1992): 343-47.

11. Jan Hare and Carrie Nelson, "Will Outpatients Complete Living Wills? A Comparison of the Two Interventions," *Journal of General Internal Medicine* 64 (1991): 41-46.

12. Greg A. Sachs, Carol E. Stocking, and Steven H. Miles, "Failure of an Intervention to Promote Discussion of Advance Directives," *Journal of the American Geriatrics Society* 40, no. 3 (1992): 269-73, at 269.

13. Lawrence Markson and Knight Steel, "Using Advance Directives in the Home-Care Setting: A Pilot Project," supplement, *Generations* 14 (1990): 25-29.

14. Joan M. Teno, Vincent Mor and John Fleishman, "Communications Regarding Formal Advance Directives," *Clinical Research* 39, no. 2 (1991): 532a.

15. Jan Hare, Clara Pratt, and Carrie Nelson, "Agreement between Patients and Their Self-Selected Surrogates on Difficult Medical Decisions," *Archives of Internal Medicine* 152 (1992): 1049-54; N. Zweibel and Christine Cassel, "Treatment Choices at the End of Life: A Comparison of Decisions by Older Patients and Their Physician-Selected Proxies," *Gerontologist* 29 (1989): 622-26; Joseph G. Outslander, Alexander J. Tymchuk, and Biba Rahbar, "Health Care Decisions among Elderly Long-Term Care Residents and Their Potential Proxies," *Archives of Internal Medicine* 149 (1989): 1367-72; Richard F. Uhlman, Robert A. Pearlman, and Kevin C. Cain, "Physicians' and Spouses' Predictions of Elderly Patients' Resuscitation Preferences," *Journal of Gerontology* 43 (1988): 115-21; Allison Seckler, Diana Meir, Michael Mulvihill, and Barbara Cammer, "Substituted Judgment: How Accurate Are Proxy Predictions?" *Annals of Internal Medicine* 115 (1991): 92-98.

16. Joanne Lynn, "Why I Don't Have a Living Will," *Law, Medicine & Health Care* 19 (1992): 101-4.

17. Maria A. Everhart and Robert A. Pearlman, "Stability of Patient Preferences Regarding Life-Sustaining Treatments," *Chest* 97 (1990): 159-64; Mark D. Silverstein, Carol B. Stocking, Jack P. Antel, et al., "Amyotrophic Lateral Sclerosis and Life-Sustaining Therapy: Patients' Desires for Information, Participation in Decision Making, and Life-Sustaining Therapy," *Mayo Clinic Proceedings* 66 (1991): 906-13; Joan M. Teno, John Fleishman, Dan W. Brock, and Vincent Mor, "Stability of Preferences among Patients with HIV-Related Illnesses," unpublished.

18. Davidson et al., "Physicians' Attitudes."

19. Zimberg, "Decisions for the Dying."

20. Danis et al., "A Prospective Study of Advance Directives on Decision-Making."

21. Teno et al., "Impact of Advance Directives on Decision-Making."

22. Schneiderman et al., "Effects of Offering Advance Directives on Medical Treatments and Costs."

23. Joan Gibson, "National Values History Project," supplement, *Generations* (1990): 51-64.

24. Joanne Lynn and William A. Knaus, "Background for Support," supplement, *Journal of Clinical Epidemiology* 43 (1990): 1S-5S.

24

[19]

A dvance care directives, whether these consist of written instructions or proxy designation, are justified on the grounds that they allow patients to exercise their autonomy.[1] The primary purpose for using advance directives has been to give patients the opportunity to control their medical care even if they become incapable of making contemporaneous decisions. As Sissela Bok noted in 1976, living wills (or, more generally, instructional directives) "represent an effort to retain some control on what happens at the end of one's life, even if one is then no longer competent to make personal choices, or to see that they are carried out."[2] Because instructional directives may only imperfectly convey patients' wishes, another modality in advance directives, proxy designation, has been developed. This modality is similarly justified as, in George Annas's words, the best way to ensure "that the patient's wishes will be followed."[3] However, the inability of proxies to know and predict patients' wishes has stimulated a different round of discussions, this time about the legitimate interests of patients' family and community. As one set of commentators noted recently, "Some values—in this case, the importance of family, and of decisions reached through struggle by our loved ones—are at least as important as a rigid devotion to the goal of patient autonomy."[4] Nevertheless, awareness that incompetent patients are vulnerable to harm when their families act on inappropriate motives has limited the appeal of arguments of this sort and refocused the discussion on patient autonomy.[5]

Using currently available data we will try to quantify how well instructional directives and proxy decision-

Decisions at the End of Life
Guided by Communities
of Patients

by Linda L. Emanuel and Ezekiel J. Emanuel

To guide treatment decisions for incompetent patients who have no advance directives, health care institutions should look to the preferences of their own communities of patients. That is the best way to ensure that incompetent patients' wishes will be followed.

making realize the ideal of patient autonomy. We will then consider alternative policies for decisionmaking for incompetent patients who have no advance directives. We will propose that life-sustaining treatment decisions for these patients be made according to default guidelines that follow the preferences of the local community of patients. These default decisions can: (1) realize the ideal of patient autonomy for this group of people better than other alternatives; (2) simultaneously honor some of the interests of patients' families; and (3) realize other important values.

Limitations of Living Wills and Other Instructional Directives

At first glance, prior written directives seem to be an unproblematic way of ensuring desired care when it is not possible to speak for oneself. However, two distinct types of limitations have become evident. First, there are intrinsic limitations to giving prior instructions. Patients may find it difficult to understand all the relevant medical issues, or they may change their decisions. Moreover, the clinical circumstances may be different from what the patient anticipated, making it necessary to adapt the patient's explicitly stated preferences to the ac-

tual situation. Second, there are procedural limitations, including the fact that few people ever use advance directives, and even when they do, physicians do not always honor them. In addition, the documents may be unavailable when relevant.

Empirical studies have quantified some of the intrinsic limitations. First, there is the fact that lay people are often not medically well informed. While measuring the frequency with which patients and members of the public make mistakes based on lack of clinical understanding is difficult, we know that patients make clinically inapplicable treatment-specific decisions about 1 percent of the time.[6]

Second, not surprisingly, people do change their minds about what medical treatments they want. Studies on the topic show a wide range of estimates;[7] those showing moderately good stability indicate that 70 to 85 percent of patient preferences regarding life-sustaining treatments are stable over periods of time up to two years.[8] These figures include decisions made by people facing hospitalization, but not specifically life-threatening illness. Interestingly, 3 to 7 percent of decisions to decline treatment in poor prognoses are unstable, which is similar to the propor-

Linda L. Emanuel is an internist and the assistant director of the Division of Medical Ethics at Harvard Medical School, Boston, Mass.; **Ezekiel J. Emanuel** is an oncologist and a medical ethicist at Harvard Medical School.

Linda L. Emanuel and Ezekiel J. Emanuel, "Decisions at the End of Life: Guided by Communities of Patients," *Hastings Center Report* 23, no. 5 (1993): 6-14.

Hastings Center Report, September-October 1993

tion of decisions to marry that are reversed (4.7% of marriages end in divorce within two years).[9]

The third intrinsic limitation is that a patient's previously stated preferences may need to be applied to unanticipated circumstances. When the instructions are simply general statements, such as to avoid "artificial means, or heroic measures,"[10] it is not possible to quantify the accuracy of application because of lack of specificity. However, we know that scenario and treatment-specific decisions, such as those in The Medical Directive, can be quite accurately extrapolated to alternative circumstances and decisions in 67 to 100 percent of studied cases.[11]

The procedural hurdles involved in use of instructional directives are more serious. The failure of patients to complete living wills or other instructional directives is perhaps the largest impediment. Even after the well-publicized *Cruzan* decision and the implementation of the Patient Self-Determination Act, it appears that only about 20 percent of patients make use of these directives.[12] It is difficult to know whether additional time, publicity, and directed educational efforts will increase the number of people who will complete living will forms. We can estimate that

at a maximum there might be as many as the number of people who have wills covering their property and estate—approximately 50 percent of adult patients.[13]

As for the other procedural impediments, evidence indicates that of all the advance directives that were completed, only 31 percent were available when life-sustaining treatment decisions were being made, and 22.8 percent were ignored or overridden even when they were available.[14] The Patient Self-Determination Act may improve the availability of advance directives, but the reluctance of physicians to follow them may represent a more serious barrier.

Overall, when we combine data we can conclude that living wills and other written instructional directives can be relied on to represent a patient's wishes accurately, under good circumstances, in 46 to 84 percent of decisions. The more serious limitations are that only about 20 percent of the population use them, and the directions of even fewer will be honored.

Limits of Proxies' Ability to Match the Patient's Wishes

For a proxy to carry out the patient's wishes, several things must

happen. First, patients must designate a proxy. Then they must discuss their treatment preferences with the proxy. Next, the proxy must understand the patient's preferences, and finally, the proxy must make the same choices as the patient would have.

The existing research suggests that these events are not taking place very well.[15] Currently available data indicate that few patients formally designate a proxy decisionmaker. Only 20.6 percent of patients had a formal proxy even after *Cruzan* and the implementation of the Patient Self-Determination Act. (Many of these people also had instructional directives, so that only 25% of the population has some formal advance care planning.) Extrapolating again from the rate at which estate wills are made, the proportion of patients who might eventually formally designate a proxy could go as high as 50 percent. The numbers of those who designate a proxy informally, by word of mouth, could conceivably reach a higher level but will doubtless never embrace the entire population.

Second, many studies have shown that only between 16 percent and 55 percent of patients have had discussions of their preferences for life-sustaining treatment with their family or proxy.[16] A family member is the designated proxy in about 80 percent of cases, but the discussions tend to be vague and do not provide specific information on end-of-life treatment preferences.[17] This is true especially among those who designate their proxy only by word of mouth. Only half of the patients who designated a proxy in a written document have discussed with that person their preferences regarding specific interventions, such as mechanical breathing or artificial feeding and fluids.

Third, many studies have indicated that concordance between patient and proxy is far from perfect. The patient's prior wishes and proxy predictions of the patient's prior wishes in circumstances other than the patient's current health overlap only from 33 to 68 percent of the time.[18] It is possible that proxies will become more accurate if the incidence of specific discussions rises, but there are currently no available data to support this hypothesis.

Limitations of Instructional Directives

Limitation	Accuracy Rate
Clinically applicable decisions*	99%
Durable decisions*	70-85%
Extrapolation to new clinical circumstances*	67-100%
Cumulative accuracy rate†	46-84%

Limitations of Proxy Designation

Limitation	Accuracy Rate
Patient-proxy concordance on treatment decision involving situations of incompetence*	33-68%
Willingness to act on presumed wishes of a loved one to withdraw support*	60%
Cumulative accuracy rate†	20-41%

Based on data from references. †Product of above accuracy rates.

Use of Advance Care Documents

	Living Wills and Other Instructional Directives*	Formal (Written) Proxies **
Current use	18.1%	20.6%
Potential maximal use	50.0%	50.0%

*Includes those patients who have completed living will forms or other instructional directives and may have a formal proxy designation, but excludes those patients who have only completed formal proxy designation without an instructional directive.

**Includes those patients who have completed formal proxy designation forms and may have also completed an instructional directive, but excludes those patients who have only completed a living will or other instructional directive but no proxy form.

Fourth, it appears that potential proxies are more hesitant to withdraw or terminate life-sustaining treatment than patients are. The burden of decisionmaking is heavy, and produces much greater reluctance to withhold care from a loved one than from oneself. Whereas 77 percent of people wanted life-sustaining treatment removed for themselves if in a permanent coma, less than two-thirds of that number would be prepared to withdraw support from a loved one in the same situation.[19]

When we combine these data, it appears that at best, proxies will accurately reflect the wishes regarding life-sustaining treatment of about 68 percent of the patients who have appointed them, but such patients represent only 20.6 percent of the population. Moreover, of the proxies who do manage accurately to judge patients' wishes, less than two-thirds will be emotionally capable of carrying them out.

Supplemental Policies for Incompetent Patients

As this summary of studies shows, self-determination for incompetent patients cannot be ensured completely with current policies using either instructional directives or proxy decisions. Some other policy will be needed to determine what care to provide incompetent patients. One possibility is to combine instructional directives with proxy designation so that proxies have patients' prior written advice to guide them.[20] Many states have statutes to protect both living wills and proxy designation, and more are currently considering such combinations. The primary merit of this double approach is that, on the one hand, proxies have the benefit of advisory documents, and on the other, the patient's written instructions are accompanied by an advocate to implement them. While this may represent an ideal, it is not a complete solution to the problem of desuetude; there will always be a significant proportion of people who have neither an instructional directive nor a formal proxy.

Default Proxies

Another approach is to endorse proxy decisionmaking even if the proxy cannot accurately determine what the patient would have wanted, and to give authority to proxies even if they are not formally designated by patients.[21] This policy of default proxy decisionmaking in the absence of any advance directive is justified not because it honors the patient's autonomy in treatment choices, but for other reasons. First, it is argued, it is better to have an imperfect, default system for making decisions for incompetent patients than for patients to be kept alive because they did not execute an advance directive. Second, using families to make decisions is efficient, usually better than going to court to obtain a legally appointed guardian.

Third, while a default system that empowers the family to make decisions for the incompetent patient may do little to promote patient autonomy, it does stress other values, especially "the importance of family." Finally, the power to choose who decides is, it is argued, the next best level of self-determination for incompetent patients if the choices themselves cannot be directed.

Although default proxy decisionmaking has merit, its advocates minimize the burdens proxies must bear. Making a life or death decision for a family member is especially stressful if the person has not left clear indications of his or her wishes. As noted, there is evidence to suggest that the anxiety caused by this uncertainty makes family members hesitant to withdraw life-sustaining medical treatment. We have no evidence that the incidence of prolonged and unwanted vegetative life will drop merely because a proxy is empowered to stop it. The case of Helga Wanglie can serve to remind us of this.[22] Although Mr. Wanglie apparently believed he was acting as his wife would have wanted when he demanded that life-support be continued, we also know that spouses can often be wrong about one another's supposed wishes.[23]

Furthermore, especially without a specific proxy designation, there may be family controversy over who really speaks for the patient. In a society with a changing family structure, default proxies may cause problems the patient is no longer in a position to help resolve. Without a patient-appointed proxy, the physician must be especially careful to ensure that there are no conflicts of interest.[24] Finally, family members may not be available at the relevant moment when decisions must be made. In general, default proxies give legal endorsement to the rather troubled traditional system that was used before advance directives.

Default Guidelines Defined by Communities of Patients

We propose another supplement to instructional directives and formal proxy designation that can help realize patient autonomy for those at risk of losing it, namely, have default

Hastings Center Report, September-October 1993

guidelines based on a "local patient community medical directive" for incompetent patients with no advance directives.

A community of patients bears only a mild resemblance to more commonly accepted notions of community. Nevertheless, we suggest that it is a potentially meaningful community, necessitated by the *de facto* existence of groups of underrepresented people who end up having issues in common.[25] Patient communities, in contrast to other communities, take on meaning only in the realm of health care. They do so in the following ways.

First, patients are the group of people with the greatest authority to define the local medical directive, as patient preferences take ethical precedence over healthy people's preferences. We would allow for limited participation by the family or proxy of the enrolled patients. A view of the community that includes these participants provides for contributions by patients' immediate circle of supporting people, but permits the community to retain its primary focus on the importance of patient self-determination.

Second, this defining community derives special authority from the fact that patients and their supporters constitute a population with special and relevant experience. They can be considered a "valuable advise" community because all its members have personal experience with some kind of health care needs. Many of these patients will have experienced significant illness and the associated phenomena of emotional, social, and financial stress. It is naturally not possible for competent people to know fully what incompetent patients would want, even if the incompetent patients are their own future selves,[26] but this community does have an enrichment of experience relevant to those judgments.

Third, we suggest that the health care organization be considered the unit of this community, for the practical reason that it is the organizational unit for other aspects of patients' health care. It is reasonable to expect that most members of this group will eventually seek health care from the organization in which they are en-

rolled, and reasonable to expect that many of the incompetent patients served by the organization will come from this group. Furthermore, when life-sustaining treatment decisions are made, a natural source of guidance to the team of providers and family or proxy is the population of patients served by the organization. A similar conception of community has also been used in the Patient Self-Determination Act, in which health care facilities are charged with the obligation of educating their community about the right to refuse life-sustaining treatment.

Fourth, patients do have some freedom to select a facility whose policies reflect values they can affirm as their own. In the real world the choices for many may be limited. The extent of actual choice will become clear as health care reform takes its course.

Indeed, until health care delivery systems are stable it is difficult to suggest precisely which organizations devoted to health care would be best suited for defining the communities of patients involved in creating the local medical directive. But the inability to address such organizational questions, important though they may be, does not affect the underlying argument in favor of patient-directed default guidelines, and some preliminary general points can be made. As managed care becomes more prominent in the United States, many group health care plans will have contractual relationships with health care facilities and vice versa. Group plans may also provide an organizational structure for defining the community of patients, combining patient populations for the pur-

pose of defining the community medical directive and making provisions for respecting the group's guidelines within the health care facilities they use, even if those facilities have different guidelines. Alternatively, group health care plans may

---

> We propose another supplement to instructional directives and formal proxy designation that can help realize patient autonomy for those at risk of losing it, namely, have default guidelines based on a "local patient community medical directive" for incompetent patients with no advance directives.

---

choose simply to advise patients to be aware of differences among the facilities they choose, enabling patients to complete personal advance directives if they desire.

Fifth, members of health care plans are the people who are ultimately paying for the health care—including life-sustaining care. While we do not suggest that financial responsibility constitutes a prime claim to authority over life-sustaining treatment decisions, we do note that cost is one among the competing issues in such decisions. We suggest that patient communities have intrinsic authority to participate in decisions about where their financial resources should be concentrated.

For those who cannot affirm the community choices, it is very important to note that the individual remains free to designate a proxy and complete instructional directives according to existing methods. The individual's choices may differ from and would supersede the default community directive. Such traditional directives could reflect the patient's more permanent community as desired; the directives could be personal in origin or they could reflect the values of a group to which the patient belonged, such as a religious group, chosen interest group, or household. Thus, the notion of a community of patients whose base is a health care organization is not in

Hastings Center Report, September-October 1993

conflict with other notions of ethnic, political, or other morally meaningful communities.

Procedures for Defining Community Default Guidelines

Within these communities of patients, guidelines for care of patients without prior directives can be constructed in a four-step process. First, using rigorous and validated survey methodology, a random selection of patients enrolled in the health care facility would be surveyed to document their specific preferences for care in a full range of illness scenarios involving incompetence. Patients would select treatment goals and options as if they were completing their actual instructional directives. The scenarios would be designed to allow patients to identify states that they believe to be worse than death.[27] This approach has been used in several studies, all of which show a generally positive response by survey participants.[28] While most early studies were conducted on outpatients, high mortality patients and intensive care unit patients have been included in recent studies, still with negligible adverse response.[29] We would encourage health care facilities to sample a numerically representative set of adult in-patients and out-patients, with decisionmaking competence as the sole inclusion criterion.

Second, an institutional committee representing physicians, nurses, social workers, the chaplaincy, administration, and the lay community would be convened to use the survey results to develop guidelines on life-sustaining treatments. This committee would be defined by the institution; while it might have much in common with either ethics committees or an institutional review board, it would have the distinct and specific function of setting default guidelines in accordance with patients' surveyed preferences. The guidelines would be directed by the most common patient preferences in any scenario, in order that community standards guiding end-of-life care for incompetent patients have the highest chance of matching an individual patient's unvoiced preference.

Third, emulating processes used by the Oregon Health Decisions and Group Health Cooperative of Puget Sound, this committee would convene a variety of open community meetings to present and discuss the proposed policies.[30] These meetings, which would be held at the health care facility or in nearby community locations, would be announced to patients but open to all, and suggestions would be welcomed from anyone, including proxies and patients' families. These meetings would not be expected to constitute a thorough deliberative discussion; rather, they would provide an opportunity for voicing perspectives and considerations not captured by the patient survey process. The committee would assemble and analyze the comments and revise the policy proposal, always bearing in mind that patient preferences are the central focus, with family or proxy considerations having an important secondary role. Where considerations raised by family members and proxies appear to conflict with the wishes of the patients, the tendency should be to err on the side of the patients' preferences. Considerations that suit the institution but conflict with patient preferences would have to be dealt with carefully, favoring the moral authority of the community of patients over the much greater power of the institution.

Fourth, the resulting guidelines would be publicized, along with the results of the empirical survey. The guidelines must be periodically revised by resurveying the patients and holding open meetings. Such a process would ensure that the community of patients would have the opportunity for ongoing deliberation and revision of the policies based on technological advances and evolution of the community's wishes. A brochure summarizing the policies would be provided to all patients and their accompanying family members or proxies at the time of enrollment in and admission to a health care facility.

Importantly, the process should be understood as a democratic process in which the institution is accountable to its patients and their families. Each organization must establish its committee representatively, although

elections need not occur. The committees might be constituted by procedures similar to those used to establish institutional review boards for the protection of human research subjects. Essential democratic values could be realized if the committee's work is a public, open, and ongoing process. Moreover, such a process ensures that patients are informed and that the discussion of end-of-life care issues can adapt itself to changes in technology or community outlook.

A crucial reason for defining the community as a relatively small local patient population is that individuals must be able to make a difference. Defining the community using larger geographic regions such as the city or state would reduce the individual's sense of participation and might reduce the chance that the patient with no advance directive would have his or her preferences honored. While it is possible that variations among communities defined in the way we propose could be small, we believe they may be morally significant. We also note that for practical reasons, instituting large-scale processes for patient-directed default guidelines is unrealistic.

Implementing the Guidelines

Local patient community guidelines would come into play only for incompetent patients without prior advance directives of their own. Prior directives would supersede local guidelines in all cases, provided the directives are valid in other ways. However, it is worth noting that specifically designated proxies who have been provided with no guidance by the patient may be greatly aided by reviewing the local patient community decisions.

When an incompetent patient lacks an advance directive, the health care team would interpret the default directive to apply to the patient's situation in the same way it currently interprets personal instructional directives. Default proxy designation would be unnecessary in most cases. Family participation in discussions, albeit without formal proxy designation or action in that role, would be entirely possible and is usually desirable. Family members who were

Hastings Center Report, September-October 1993

not designated but who wished to act as proxies could be offered the guidelines and provided with explanations for decisionmaking based on the default directive. Family members in agreement with the default directive would not pose a problem, and decisionmaking by the medical team should not be hindered by this kind of involvement.

Family members or loved ones may occasionally claim that they should have been the designated proxy and ask for treatment that differs from the default guidelines. So, for example, a Christian Science patient from a family that permits some medical interventions but not others may correctly claim that the patient omitted to make an advance directive but would have had predictable preferences quite different from those of the rest of the local patient community. Procedures for deciding the merits of such claims would be needed. At the level of the health care facility the suitable body would be an ethics committee. Disagreement that could not be resolved by standard approaches of the ethics committee and that required the courts to adjudicate it would be rare.

Accuracy of Community Default Guidelines

How well could such community standards match patient preferences and realize the ideal of patient autonomy? Obviously, the entire process of surveying patients, formulating policies, having open discussions of the policies, and resurveying patients has never occurred. There are no estimates of the intrinsic accuracy of the default guidelines (regarding, for example, misunderstandings by

patients completing the survey or the difficulty of limiting the population to those who will not make their own advance directive). Nevertheless, we can estimate the accuracy of such community standards, using existing

data on patient preferences. For instance, data gathered from patients at one hospital indicate that in the case of the persistent vegetative state 80 percent of patients want neither mechanical respirators nor artificial nutrition. Similarly, in the case of dementia 75 percent of patients did not want a mechanical respirator and 76 percent did not want artificial nutrition. In the scenario with the most uncertainty, coma with a chance for recovery, 55 percent of patients did not want a mechanical respirator and 60 percent did not want artificial nutrition. Among the forty-six different decisions studied, the refusal of treatment rate ranged from 48 to 85 percent. In the two decisions showing less than 50 percent refusal of treatment, the remaining preferences were distributed among acceptance of treatment, uncertainty, and requests to try treatment.[31] Therefore, if the health care organization instituted policies that reflected the patients' most common preferences, among the patients to whom the

policy applied 48 to 85 percent would be treated according to their preferences, depending on the treatment and the illness scenario. Importantly, unlike the use of personal advance directives, community standards

> By having the opportunity to participate in community deliberations regarding policies affecting their lives, people can realize a deeper aspect of autonomy, namely, participation in deliberative dialogue.

could apply to every incompetent patient without an advance directive in the United States.

We can compare the three different methods of making decisions for incompetent patients—instructional directives, proxy decisionmaking, and community standards—by how well they realize the value of patient autonomy, that is, of enacting a patient's own preferences regarding life-sustaining treatment. Default guidelines may provide patients who have no advance directives with the treatments they prefer at least as often as advance directives would. Thus, from the empirical data that are available it is reasonable to think that community standards are probably very similar to instructional directives and proxy decisionmaking in their ability to match patients' preferences.

Additional Advantages of Default Guidelines

Local, patient-directed default guidelines are not only likely to promote patient autonomy by implementing a patient's wishes, they also offer other means of achieving autonomy. Patients who dissent from the prevailing standards of their community are free to complete their own advance directive, thus exercising the freedom to differ. Further, by having the opportunity to participate in community deliberations regarding policies affecting their lives, people can realize a deeper aspect of autonomy, namely, participation in deliber-

Comparative Accuracy of Instructional Directives, Proxies, and Community Standards			
Clinical Situation and Intervention	Living Will or Other Instructional Device	Proxy Designation	Community Standards
PVS and mechanical ventilation	79%	67%	80%
Dementia and CPR	71%	68%	72%

ative dialogue. A deliberative democratic process engages people in an educational process. People have the opportunity to formulate their own views, articulate them, and attempt to persuade the community of their viewpoints. In this way people examine and ally themselves with the local patient community's standards or, realizing they have a different vision of end-of-life care, make out their own advance directives. Even those patients who have no advance directive and are not personally involved in the procedures for community guidelines but who do have a proxy will benefit, as the proxy will have a useful outline, in the form of the guidelines, of the community's thinking, and this can be used to guide or counterdefine decisions for the patient.

In addition to their usefulness in achieving patient autonomy, community-based default guidelines have other distinct advantages. They are an efficient mechanism for ensuring the reasonableness of decisions made for incompetent patients with no prior directives. Every acute care hospital, rehabilitation facility, and nursing home would have a relatively simple procedure for determining what care to give their incompetent patients. No legal proceedings would have to be initiated, no hospital lawyer or ethics committee consulted in case after case. It would no longer be necessary to try to educate the family about the patient's circumstances for the purpose of getting a decision from them, nor would there be any need to negotiate family conflicts for the purposes of decisionmaking or to anticipate families' potential conflicts of interest. Although efficiency in decisionmaking is not necessarily the primary value, it is nonetheless worth noting that local patient community standards would be more efficient than default proxy decisionmaking by family members.

Further, local patient community standards can revive and nourish the value of communal solidarity. Many of the institutions of modern society, including modern health care delivery, have undermined individuals' identification with the community. Yet we can devise institutions and policies that reinforce community

and at the same time actually enrich individual rights. The policy we are advocating is of this kind.

Moreover, a policy of local patient community standards could relieve much of the uncertainty and anxiety now associated with end-of-life decisionmaking for incompetent patients. With clear guidelines for treating incompetent patients, physicians would know what to do and whom to consult for these patients. The uncertainty and anxiety that physicians experience in calling together the family, educating them about the situation, delineating the treatment options, and adjudicating any family conflicts would be alleviated.[32] Similarly, the anxiety many family members feel when forced to make a life and death decision for a patient would be reduced, as families would no longer have the responsibility of making a choice uninformed by the patient's wishes. Importantly, having local patient community standards publicly known would relieve the anxiety many patients have about their care at the end of life. They would no longer have to worry so much that they would be kept in limbo, between life and death, or that they might have life support terminated too soon.

Default Guidelines and Best Interests

Various courts and commentators have recognized that cases involving incompetent patients cannot often be resolved by guidance from an advance directive.[33] They have suggested that these mechanisms would have to be supplemented by some form of the "best interests" standard. And yet the best interests standard has its own conceptual difficulties, especially the difficulty of giving substantive content to an objective standard of what is good for particular patients. Justice Handler of the New Jersey Supreme Court summarized the attractions and problems of the "best interests" standard in his concurring opinion in the *Jobes* case:

> [No matter] how well the guardian knows the patient, and how well-intentioned that patient's guardian, family and physician

may be, there will always be some residual doubt that the decision expresses or effectuates the patient's right of self-determination. In less optimal circumstances, the doubt is greater. . . . Indeed, because doubt seems inherent in self-determination for an incompetent, objective factors may become conditions for any treatment decision. . . . [Yet] the problem with [objective factors and] the "best interests" analysis are straightforward. In our society persons have different ideas about how the value of life is affected by the loss of brain function, the loss of cognitive abilities, bodily deterioration, or unrelievable extreme pain. A "best interests" [or objective] standard assumes a consensus that is not there regarding when discontinuation of treatment is in the patient's best interest.[34]

The four-step procedure to delineate default guidelines outlined here could address the problems of the "best interests" standard. Default guidelines based on empirical evidence of patient's wishes can provide an objective means of defining the "best interests" standard for life-sustaining care.

Objections to Patient-Based Default Guidelines

There are potential objections to guidelines based on local patient community standards that must be addressed as well. Critics might contend that they diminish the responsibility and input of patients and patients' families. But in fact they can facilitate the positive while minimizing the negative aspects of having patients and their families participate in end-of-life decisions. Nothing in this proposal precludes patients from formally designating a family member to make decisions for them. Also, even family members who are not proxies can participate in the policy formulation by commenting at the open meetings. But our proposal recognizes that family decisions for patients are not always accurate reflections of the patient's wishes and that relatives who are not intimately

Hastings Center Report, September-October 1993

acquainted with the patient's views are not well situated to make decisions for the patient. Our proposal also recognizes that proxy decision-making imposes psychological burdens on the family that can be relieved by alternative policies. Clearly there will be cases where a suitable family decision will differ from the local patient community standard, and where the patient failed to execute a formal proxy designation. As noted, it is reasonable for the state to allow relatives to petition the courts for presumed proxy designation, but such cases would be rare. Such exceptional cases should not detract from a policy that can benefit the vast majority of people.

Critics also might contend that there is no precedent for adopting local patient community standards and that there will be significant resistance to them. There are, however, precedents for community guidelines. In the 1970s hospitals had to establish institutional review boards to oversee research on human subjects—boards that must include community representatives. Further, hospitals have maintained DNR policies that differ from institution to institution, including recent efforts to establish "DNR not indicated" policies.[35] While these have not always been adopted democratically, they present a precedent for establishing guidelines for each individual health care institution. Community meetings of Oregon Health Decisions can serve as a reasonable paradigm for making such procedures more democratic.

Further precedent has been set by health care facilities that have created a structure for community dialogue in implementing the Patient Self-Determination Act and in meeting standards of the Joint Commission on Accreditation of Healthcare Organizations, which recommends that patients receive assistance in creating their own advance directives. And precedent for community standards regarding other health-related decisions, such as organ donation, has also surfaced in recent proposals.[36] Such proposals testify to the merits of the idea and the readiness of the population for such approaches. Finally, compliance by health care facilities

could easily be secured if the four-step process for creating community default guidelines were made mandatory for accreditation and Medicare and Medicaid reimbursement.

While there will always be resistance to adopting new policies, especially policies that invite lay people to partake in health care policy development and formulation, such conservatism should not prevent us from exploring new approaches to problems—even if, like the establishment of institutional review boards, they involve significant institutional changes. If President Clinton's Economic Summit and town meetings are any indication, the tendency of the new administration may be to adopt procedures that promote a more democratic method of formulating policy. Local patient community standards can aptly adapt this view of governance to health care.

While the American public, courts, and medical profession now accept the use of both instructional directives and proxy decisionmaking, we are becoming aware of their limitations. The well-researched intrinsic problems of these mechanisms of advance planning, combined with the logistical problems related to their limited use, make it clear that they will never fully realize the ideal of extending patient autonomy to times of incompetence. The advantages of a supplemental policy of local patient community standards for the treatment of incompetent patients are many. Most significantly, it can help realize the ideal of patient autonomy in life-sustaining treatment decisions for the underrepresented group of patients who have no advance directive.

Acknowledgments

We thank the following colleagues for their insightful comments: Douglas Adams, Norman Daniels, Rebecca Dresser, James Ferrara, Alexandra Flather-Morgan, Robert Truog, Lynn Peterson, Jim Sabin, Benjamin Seigel, and Susan M. Wolf.

References

1. President's Commission for the Study of Ethical Problems in Medicine and Biomedical and Behavioral Research, *Deciding to Forego Life-Sustaining Treatment* (Washington, D.C.: U.S. Government Printing Office, 1983), chapter 4.

2. Sissela Bok, "Personal Directions for Care at the End of Life," *NEJM* 295 (12 August 1976): 367-69.

3. George J. Annas, "The Health Care Proxy and the Living Will," *NEJM* 324 (25 April 1991): 1210-13.

4. Jerry A. Menikoff, Greg A. Sachs, and Mark Siegler, "Beyond Advance Directives: Health Care Surrogate Laws," *NEJM* 327 (15 October 1992): 1165-69.

5. Thomas G. Gutheil and Paul S. Appelbaum, "Substituted Judgment: Best Interests in Disguise," *Hastings Center Report* 13, no. 3 (1983): 8-11.

6. Linda L. Emanuel et al., "Advance Directives for Medical Care: A Case for Greater Use," *NEJM* 324 (28 March 1991): 889-95.

7. Marc Silverstein et al., "Amyotrophic Lateral Sclerosis and Life-Sustaining Therapy: Patients' Desires for Information, Participation in Decision Making and Life-Sustaining Therapy," *Mayo Clinic Proceedings* 66 (1991): 906-13.

8. Linda L. Emanuel et al., "Advance Directives: How Do Scenario Based Treatment Choices Change Over Time?" *Archives of Internal Medicine* (in press); see also Marion A. Everhart and Robert A. Pearlman, "Stability of Patient Preferences Regarding Life-Sustaining Treatments," *Chest* 97 (1990): 159-64.

9. James A. Weed, "National Estimates of Marriage Dissolution and Survivorship: United States," U.S. Dept. of Health and Human Services Publication No. (PHS) 81-1403. Vital and Health Statistics: Series 3, Analytic Studies; #19, Table 6, 1980.

10. Concern for Dying, *A Living Will* (New York: Concern for Dying, 1984).

11. Linda L. Emanuel et al., "Advance Directives: Do Scenario Based Treatment Choices Extrapolate to Different Decisions?" *Clinical Research* 40, no. 2 (1992): 611A.

12. Ezekiel J. Emanuel et al., "How Well Is the Patient Self-Determination Act Working? An Early Assessment," *American Journal of Medicine* (in press).

13. Concern for Dying, *A Living Will.*

14. Marion Danis et al., "A Prospective Study of Advance Directives for Life-Sustaining Care," *NEJM* 324 (28 March 1991): 882-88.

15. Ezekiel J. Emanuel and Linda L. Emanuel, "Proxy Decision-Making for Incompetent Patients: An Ethical and Empirical Analysis," *JAMA* 267 (15 April 1992): 2067-71.

16. Richard F. Uhlmann, Robert A. Pearlman, and Kevin C. Cain, "Physicians' and Spouses' Predictions of Elderly Patients' Resuscitation Preferences," *Journal of Gerontology* 43 (1988): M115-21; Allison Seckler et al., "Substituted Judgment: How Accurate Are Proxy Predictions?" *Annals of Internal Medicine* 115 (1991): 92-

Hastings Center Report, September-October 1993

98; Bernard Lo, Gary A. McLeod, and Glenn Saika, "Patient Attitudes to Discussing Life-Sustaining Treatment," *Archives of Internal Medicine* 146 (1986): 1613-15; Jisha Cohen-Mansfield et al., "The Decision to Execute a Durable Power of Attorney for Health Care and Preferences Regarding the Utilization of Life-Sustaining Treatments in Nursing Home Residents," *Archives of Internal Medicine* 151 (1991): 289-94; Elizabeth R. Gamble, Penelope J. McDonald, and Peter R. Lichstein, "Knowledge, Attitudes, and Behavior of Elderly Persons Regarding Living Wills," *Archives of Internal Medicine* 151 (1991): 277-80.

17. E. Emanuel, "How Well Is the Patient Self-Determination Act Working?"; Dallas M. High, "All in the Family: Extended Autonomy and Expectations in Surrogate Health Care Decision-Making," *Gerontologist* 28 (1988): S46-S51.

18. Nancy R. Zweibel and Christine K. Cassel, "Treatment Choices at the End of Life: A Comparison of Decisions by Older Patients and Their Physician-Selected Proxies," *Gerontologist* 29 (1989): 615-21.

19. Menikoff et al. "Beyond Advance Directives"; Steven A. Steiber, "Right to Die: Public Balks at Deciding for Others," *Hospitals* 61 (1987): 72.

20. Linda L. Emanuel and Ezekiel J. Emanuel, "The Medical Directive: A New Comprehensive Advance Care Document," *JAMA* 261 (9 June 1989): 3288-93.

21. Steven A. Newman, "Treatment Refusals for the Critically and Terminally Ill: Proposed Rules for the Family, the Physician, and the State," *New York Law School Human Rights Annual* 3 (1985): 35-89; Joanne Lynn, "Why I Don't Have a Living Will," *Law, Medicine & Health Care* 19 (1991): 101-4.

22. Steven H. Miles, "Informed Demand for 'Non-Beneficial' Medical Treatment," *NEJM* 325 (15 August 1991): 512-15.

23. Emanuel and Emanuel, "Proxy Decisionmaking for Incompetent Patients"; In re Spring, 380 Mass. 629 (1980); Lane v. Candura, 376 NE 2d. 1232 (1978); John LaPuma et al., "The Standard of Care: A Case Report and Ethical Analysis," *Annals of Internal Medicine* 108 (1988): 121-24; Melinda A. Lee and Karen Berry, "Abuse of Durable Power of Attorney for Health Care: Case Report," *Journal of the American Geriatric Society* 39 (1991): 806-9.

24. Gutheil and Appelbaum, "Substituted Judgment."

25. Ezekiel J. Emanuel, *The Ends of Human Life: Medical Ethics in a Liberal Polity* (Cambridge, Mass.: Harvard University Press, 1991), chapters 5 and 6; see also his "A Communal Vision of Care for Incompetent Patients," *Hastings Center Report* 17, no. 5 (1987): 15-20.

26. Rebecca S. Dresser, "Advance Directives, Self-Determination, and Personal Identity," in *Advance Directives in Medicine*, ed. Chris Hackler et al. (New York: Praeger Publishers, 1989), pp. 155-70.

27. Robert Pearlman et al., "Insights Pertaining to Patient Assessments of States Worse than Death," *Journal of Clinical Ethics* 4, no. 1 (1993): 33-40.

28. Suzanne E. Bedell and Thomas L. Delbanco, "Choices about Cardiopulmonary Resuscitation in the Hospital: When Do Physicians Talk with Patients?" *NEJM* 310 (26 April 1984): 1089-93; Robert R. Shmerling et al., "Discussing Cardiopulmonary Resuscitation: A Study of Elderly Outpatients," *Journal of General Internal Medicine* 3 (1988): 317-21; Lo, McLeod, and Saika, "Patient Attitudes to Discussing Life-Sustaining Treatment," pp. 1613-15.

29. Thomas E. Finucane et al., "Establishing Advance Directives with Demented Patients," *Journal of Clinical Ethics* 4, no. 1 (1993): 51-54; Everhart and Pearlman, "Stability of Patient Preferences," pp. 159-64.

30. Ralph Crawshaw et al., "Oregon Health Decisions: An Experiment with Informed Community Consent," *JAMA* 254 (13 December 1985): 3213-16; Brian Hines, *Oregon and American Health Decisions: A Guide for Community Action on Bioethical Issues* (Washington, D.C.: Department of Health and Human Services, 1985).

31. L. Emanuel et al., "Advance Directives for Medical Care," pp. 889-95.

32. David Hilfiker, "Allowing the Debilitated to Die: Facing Our Ethical Choices," *NEJM* 308 (24 March 1983): 716-19; Mildred Solomon et al., "Decisions Near the End of Life: Professional Views on Life-Sustaining Treatments," *American Journal of Public Health* 83 (1993): 14-23.

33. Martha Minow, "Beyond State Intervention in the Family: For Baby Jane Doe," *University of Michigan Health Law Reform* 18 (1985): 972; Alan E. Buchanan and Dan W. Brock, *Deciding for Others* (New York: Cambridge University Press, 1989); President's Commission, *Deciding to Forego Life-Sustaining Treatment*, chapter 4.

34. In re Jobes, 108 N.J. 394 (1987) (J. Handler concurring opinion).

35. Joint Commission on Accreditation of Healthcare Organizations, *Accreditation Manual for Hospitals* (Oak Brook Terrace, Ill., 1992), p. 104.

36. James Lindemann Nelson, *The Rights and Responsibilities of Potential Organ Donors: A Communitarian Approach* (Washington, D.C.: Communitarian Network, 1992).

14

[20]

Are Advance Directives Really the Answer? And What was the Question?

ANN SOMMERVILLE
Adviser to the BMA on Medical Ethics

The extensive legal and moral debate triggered in 1991 and 1992 by the case of Anthony Bland[1] fuelled an existing clamour for the re-examination of some of society's basic preconceptions. Those preconceptions included the notion that life is always preferable to death and that life-prolonging medical treatment is necessarily a benefit to the person who receives it. The case even raised questions about what it means to be 'alive' and how to define a 'person'.

It excited disquiet and the questioning of boundaries not only on such high-flown philosophical matters as being and non-being but also on public policy issues such as the role of declaratory statements in the criminal justice system and the difference between allowing death to occur slowly by doing nothing and actively intervening to cause a quick end. There was debate about how an individual's interest in preventing the indignity of a non-consensual invasion of his or her body could be weighed against the state's interest in preserving life. Questions were raised about whether a severely mentally incapacitated person could have such interests or, indeed, any interests at all. The perceived integrity of the medical profession was seen to be potentially in doubt, and many predicted that the *Bland* case would ultimately lead to a devaluation of life and an acceptance of euthanasia. None of this debate was new, however. Courts in the USA had already thrashed out all the same arguments through a series of similar cases.[2]

In the UK, the case led some people who had never previously heard the term 'persistent vegetative state' to consider how they would want to be treated were they to lose the ability to think or communicate. Advance directives – a concept borrowed from the

USA – seemed to provide one answer, but there was widespread confusion about their status and scope. Eventually, the *Bland* case went to the ultimate appeal court, the House of Lords, whose judgement reflected much heart-searching and included a recommendation for the parliamentary review of the whole gamut of issues raised, including advance directives. Accordingly, a Select Committee of the House of Lords was set up to examine the evidence. Part of its remit was 'to consider the ethical, legal and clinical implications of a person's right to withhold consent to life-prolonging treatment, and the position of persons who are no longer able to give or withhold consent.[3] This involved clarifying the status of anticipatory decision-making and deciding whether there should be a statute on the subject. In early 1994 the Select Committee concluded that such a statute would be superfluous.

A central premise of this chapter, however, is that factors other than the House of Lords' report will ultimately decide how advance directives develop and whether or not they work well. An important factor is the common law, which by the end of 1994 had upheld the advance refusal of the first English litigant.[4] Other factors include the degree to which the public and consumer groups are really committed to advance directives, the attitudes of health care purchasers, health professionals and such bodies as the British Medical Association and Royal College of Nursing, and the extent to which all of these are prepared to take steps to make patient choice a reality. Although included in the list of factors considered, the BMA's views are not synonymous with the opinions and conclusions given in this chapter.

Why Advance Directives?

As society has attempted to protect itself from the realities of mental degeneration and death, responsibility for care of the mentally incapacitated, the elderly and the dying has been increasingly confined to institutions, hospitals and health professionals. This is what Illich in the mid-1970s called the 'medicalization' of death.[5] Although many other aspects of life – conception, childbirth, the process of ageing, manifestations of unhappiness or stress – can also be said to have been medicalized, these other facets of ordinary human experience have not been marginalized in our society as have the processes of degeneration and death. Even though, as Benjamin Franklin said, the only certainties in life are death and taxes, it seems that we put thought into avoiding the latter but not considering the former.

Advance directives or 'living wills' attempt to deal with medicalization and marginalization. They aim to permit individuals to have a voice in situations where they are otherwise unable to control what is done to them. Their purpose is to empower the individual to make future choices using present mental capacity and knowledge. The degree to which they achieve this aim depends on factors which need further examination, and this chapter attempts to place some of the rhetoric about autonomy into a practical context. The effectiveness of the advance directive depends ultimately upon wide recognition that individual views, rather than clinical opinion alone, must dictate treatment.

Part of the stimulus for advance directives derives from an increasingly misplaced fear of overtreatment at the end of life, mistrust in medical technology or lack of confidence that health professionals recognize when 'enough is enough'. But although bad practice in the form of futile prolongation of life or inappropriate resuscitation exists and should not be underemphasized, there is a growing consensus among health professionals and the courts about its unacceptability. *Patients* are being transformed into *clients* or *health-care consumers* with bargaining powers. Advance directives are both a symptom and an effect of changing practice. At the same time, lessons are being learned from the hospice movement about communication and caring for the whole person rather than responding to a set of symptoms. In practical terms, however, it must also be said that such lessons cannot be fully integrated into settings where staff–patient ratios are severely dissonant with those in the hospice context, and advance directives can do nothing to address this.

What is the Scope of an Advance Directive?

There have been many suggestions concerning the potential scope of advance directives. One useful starting-point may be the English Law Commission's description in its 1991 discussion document:

> The purpose of an advance directive is to enable a competent person to give instructions about what he wishes to be done, or who he wishes to make decisions for him, if he should subsequently lose the capacity to decide for himself. Advance directives are usually discussed in the context of medical treatment and relate mainly to the patient's right to refuse or change treatment in a disabling chronic or terminal illness.[6]

Although this definition fits into an evolving pattern of thinking about the legitimate scope of advance directives, close examination also shows it to be unsatisfactory for the current stage of debate in the UK.

The first part of the definition, for example, combines what many people see as two functions: making an anticipatory choice for oneself about specific matters and appointing another person to make proxy choices as appropriate when the need arises. Deciding in advance for oneself demands a degree of certainty about the decisions to be made and a certain clairvoyance about future options. Choosing a proxy decision-maker simply requires the individual to have confidence that the person appointed will remain alive and sane longer than himself and will indeed carry out what the appointer would like to happen. Various potential problems arise in connection with appointing a proxy, some of which are touched on later.

The second part of the definition firmly places advance directives in the category of 'end of life' medical decisions (which is the only role envisaged for them by the House of Lords too), although the Law Commission encompasses directives which change treatment rather than just refuse it. This might be seen as a variation on the common view of advance directives as only being appropriate to refuse procedures. From a legal viewpoint, however, patients can only *direct* non-treatment. If they aim to request a procedure or choose between options, then their document has to be called something other than a directive since it will not have the legal power to direct anyone. The scope of the English common law until now has only covered refusal and courts are unlikely to see health professionals as bound by statements which limit the exercise of clinical judgement by selecting between treatment options, although they might require doctors to take them into account.[7]

Comparison can be made between the manner in which the scope of advance directives has been defined in the UK and how advance directives originally developed in the USA. They were invented by Luis Kutner, a Chicago lawyer, as a means by which competent individuals could provide, in advance, evidence to rebut the legal presumption that life-prolonging treatment could be given to them when they were unable to decide for themselves.[8] The same presumption holds in the UK. Erin and Harris[9] argue that the assumption that people always want their lives sustained is frankly erroneous since evidence suggests 'that the vast majority of people would wish life-sustaining treatment withdrawn in certain situations.[10] They overturn the notion of presumed consent and propose 'as the default position that, under circumstances of irreversible loss of competence, life-sustaining treatment be withheld from all patients in the absence of an advance directive to the contrary'.[11] That is, only statements positively requesting life-prolonging treatment would have any value and health professionals should automatically allow all incompetent patients without one to die. Although Erin and Harris go on to identify some important practical disadvantages to such a system, their proposal may unfortunately have more current relevance than they suppose, as will be discussed later.

Table 3.1 The three stages in the evolution of advance directives in the USA

	Date	Legislation	Scope
Stage 1	1976	California National Death Act	• Allows withdrawal of treatment • Directive must be in a particular format • Patient must be terminally ill and death imminent
Stage 2	mid-1980s	Launch of Uniform Rights of the Terminally Ill Act	• Allows withdrawal of treatment and tube feeding • No mandatory form. Beginning of individualized form • 'Terminal' illness covers coma, PVS, dementia
Stage 3	1985	Indiana Living Wills and Life-prolonging Procedures, Declaration	• Allows for requests for, as well as refusal of, treatment

33

34   *Death, Dying and the Law*

It is possible to trace the evolution of advance directives both in the USA and the UK through three principal stages of development.[12] Table 3.1 summarizes the development of advance directives in the USA. The first generation of US laws established a model directive which could only be triggered if the patient was dying and the directive conformed to the established format. A decade later, the second generation dispensed with the mandatory form and allowed a much broader definition of terminal illness as the triggering factor. The third generation, whose prototype is seen in the Indiana legislation, incorporates the looser definition of the second generation model and permits requests for, as well as refusal of, treatment.

Discussion in the UK follows some aspects of the same pattern even though we have no statute to match US law. Initially, in the UK, advance directive forms were only available from organizations supporting voluntary euthanasia and were generally viewed as being applicable to terminal illness. A second phase witnessed arguments for the application of advance directives to non-terminal conditions, such as persistent vegetative state. The House of Lords in the *Bland* decision[13] endorsed this development. Bodies, such as the BMA, also maintained that advance statements of treatment preferences should be able to cover any condition the patient wants to provide for, but that positive requests could only be honoured if they were clinically appropriate and not detrimental to other patients.

The King's College and Terrence Higgins Trust model directive can be seen as fitting into the third generation of formats. It provides not only for refusal of treatment but for the option of asking 'to be kept alive for as long as reasonably possible using whatever forms of treatment are available'. It also permits personal requests such as the preservation of life until a particular nominated person can be called to the bedside to say goodbye. One of the important points about this type of directive is that it shows that the discussion concerns a *right to choose* rather than a *right to die*. Given the anxiety about access to medical services of some patient groups, such as smokers or the elderly, this third generation of advance directive requesting treatment may well deserve attention. For the patient, the obvious drawbacks are that it leaves open the definition of 'reasonable' and 'available'. Also some variations of this type of directive are discouragingly complex both for their drafters and interpreters: a document which is not easily understood risks being ignored or misinterpreted.

Since every modern textbook and declaration of health-care ethics calls for partnership with patients and listening skills, there seems no compelling reason for limiting the potential application of anticipatory statements or directives to chronic illness or, indeed, any illness at all. They could be accommodated as a regular part of the dialogue and continuous negotiation which is supposed to exist between patients and health professionals. Pregnant women with birth plans for the management of labour exercise a form of anticipatory decision-making, although, in most cases, women in labour do not lack capacity and can review their options according to circumstances. The point to be made here is, if advance statements really can be useful, why not adapt them to suit the myriad requirements of people facing any form of reduced capacity, whether temporary or permanent? People with Alzheimer's disease, for example, know with certainty that if they live long enough they will experience dementia. There may be a wide range of matters they would want to decide for themselves in advance rather than simply appointing an attorney with enduring powers to act for them. Arguably also, an anticipatory decision that an individual wanted her money used to maintain herself in a specific nursing home rather than other alternatives could be the basis of an advance directive. Fears are sometimes raised by doctors that relatives, anxious to get their hands on a demented patient's savings, may attempt to override the patient's strongly expressed wish to remain in the nursing home she had chosen. A witnessed statement of her intentions when competent could provide protection.

The BMA has argued that an authorizing statement would be useful – perhaps even more useful than a refusing directive – but this is partly based on the premise that the most clear and explicit refusing directives will probably apply to futile treatments which good professional practice would disallow. Authorizing statements accommodate decisions which are so personal that only the individual undertaking them could decide. For example, a person facing incapacity might wish to agree in advance to genetic testing which she does not need herself but which would benefit her children or grandchildren. She might agree to elective ventilation for organ donation if she already intends to offer to be an organ donor. At present a schizophrenic can only be sectioned for treatment under the Mental Health Act when he or she becomes dangerous but, without prior agreement, might miss out on help at a much earlier stage of illness. In lucid intervals, such a person could make provision for treatments during those intermittent periods when capacity fails. Prior agreement of this sort can be seen as more respectful of patient autonomy than a compulsory treatment order.

While it is acknowledged in common law that a patient cannot *require* a doctor to take specific positive actions, there is arguably scope for an anticipatory statement to authorize medical or other treatment. New ideas take time to permeate society. If society is serious about acknowledging patient rights and choices, including those expressed in advance, people need to become accustomed to anticipatory decision-making as a means of dealing with recurrent or

36   *Death, Dying and the Law*

familiar problems, rather than solely as a method for dealing with the frightening and the unusual.

The Last Resort of the Unheard?

Advance directives have been made in the UK for over 20 years but have only received attention comparatively recently. The way in which they are drafted and the degree to which they are implemented varies, there being no standard format and no statute to enforce them. Many health professionals are confused about the implications of advance directives or erroneously equate them with requests for euthanasia – probably because the earliest guidance and examples of advance directives were drawn up by the Voluntary Euthanasia Societies. In the late 1980s agencies, such as Age Concern,[14] published advice on advance directives, fuelling the assumption that they were likely to be useful only or mainly to the elderly. This is ironic since, both in the UK and the USA, the high-profile legal cases – namely, the US cases of Karen Quinlan and Nancy Cruzan and the UK cases of Tony Bland and 'T' –[15] which discuss the importance of advance directives, but where in fact directives were conspicuous by their absence, involved people under 25 years old.

Recognition of the relevance of advance directives to people of all ages owes much to the *Bland* case and patient advocacy groups. The Terrence Higgins Trust and the Alzheimer's Disease Society have drawn attention to the particular application of directives to the onset of progressive mental impairment. Although these organizations have undoubtedly influenced the public perception of advance directives, the advance directive still retains a residual image as the last resort of marginalized groups.

US surveys[16] showed that advance directives, like organ donor cards, are seen by the public as a 'good thing', but that spontaneous take-up has fallen far short of the number who express theoretical support. A recent UK survey[17] indicated that, while 84 per cent of the 2000 respondents (average age 69.1 years) supported the idea of *everyone* making advance directives, exactly the same percentage said that they did not have one. Only 13 per cent of the respondents had made an advance directive and, in younger age groups, the percentage is likely to be even lower. Another survey demonstrated that the function of an advance directive in relation to incapacity was broadly misunderstood by people who thought that having a legally witnessed document would simply increase their chances of being heard when they (competently) express their views in hospital. Many writers have drawn attention to the fact that advance directives can only really become effective in communities willing to confront their own mortality. One of the perceived advantages of advance directives and other anticipatory statements is that they encourage open discussion of death and mental incapacity. But in practice this only works where individuals are already receptive to the opportunity, and, as stated earlier, death has become marginalized in present day society. Thus, unless they have had specific training or long experience, health professionals are just as likely as other people to distance themselves from potentially disturbing discussions.

Common law recognition of advance directives is recent. If the basic conditions outlined by Lord Donaldson in the 'T' case are fulfilled,[18] the binding force of advance directives at common law in England and Wales seems secure. This means that if a competent, informed and unpressured adult makes a clear anticipatory refusal of treatment and the circumstances envisaged by the patient subsequently arise, health professionals would be bound by that refusal. In Scotland, there has been no case law, although the House of Lords' comments in the *Bland* case about advance directives would be relevant. One of the leading speeches in *Bland* came from a Scottish Law Lord, Lord Keith of Kinkel who stressed that any mentally competent person is at liberty to decline treatment and can also do this in anticipation of later loss of competence. In Lord Keith's view, to administer medical treatment contrary to such a refusal is unlawful and constitutes both a tort and the crime of battery.

The English and Scottish Law Commissions are both working on legislation which will change some aspects of the way decisions are made for people who cannot make decisions for themselves. Advance directives, however, barely gain a mention in the Scottish Law Commission consultation paper of 1991.[19] The Commission reassures us that these directives are used in the USA because of

> ... unnecessary treatment being given to terminally ill patients and expensive private health care which can impoverish patients and deprive their families of their anticipated succession rights. These difficulties do not arise to the same extent in Scotland.[20]

In England, the Law Commission published draft legislation in March 1995,[21] which, if enacted, would legally oblige health professionals to take account of the ascertainable past and present wishes of a mentally incapacitated person in every case. The Commission draws distinction, however, between the legal effect of an advance expression of views or preferences and advance decisions. Its proposed legislation only gives specific statutory recognition to clear decisions to refuse particular forms of treatment. Even if this Bill becomes law, doctors will need to assess the scope of the patient's decision and its applicability to the circumstances. Clause 9(3) of the Bill negates any advance refusal if the patient has not specifically recognized the possibility of death as a result of nontreatment. Effectively, therefore, health professionals will retain a degree of discretion except in cases where the directive unambiguously refuses specific treatment in all circumstances, such as the Jehovah's Witness type of directive.

Eventually, enduring powers of attorney may be extended to cover health care. Both the Scottish and English Law Commissions suggest this as a possible extension of the law and both recommend limits on what such an attorney could agree to or refuse on behalf of an incapacitated person. Feeding, nursing, pain relief or other palliative care could not be refused by the attorney. The Scottish Law Commission has more faith in the medical profession and says that proxy 'power to consent is less important since doctors will generally not propose treatment that is not in the patient's best interests.'[22] The English Law Commission is less sure about this and would not allow attorneys to consent to a range of treatments which doctors might suggest but which require the additional permission of a judicial forum. These would include some sterilizations, donation of non-regenerative tissue or bone marrow and some kinds of medical research.

The House of Lords

In effect, the House of Lords has had two bites at the issue of advance directives. As already mentioned, in the *Bland* case there was agreement that medical treatment could not be given contrary to clear anticipatory instructions refusing it. Lords Browne-Wilkinson and Mustill also stressed that they considered it imperative for Parliament, rather than the courts, to rule on the wider issues raised by the case.

A contradictory view came from the Lords Select Committee on Medical Ethics.[23] After a year of taking evidence on end-of-life issues, the 14 members of Committee astonished some observers by reaching agreement on some contentious issues. They published 21 conclusions, all of which indicate a cautious, conservative handling of the issues and general confirmation of the status quo. Finally, while commending the development of advance directives, they found it unnecessary for Parliament to introduce legislation, although they did recommend that a professional code of practice on advance directives should be developed.

How Important are the Recommendations?

An essential question is: what will become of these recommendations and how much force do they have? The answer is not much, unless other interested bodies choose to take them up. One might expect the Department of Health to act on them but its response[24] to the Lords, published in May 1994, is non-committal on many points and passes the buck on others.

Where Did the Recommendations Come From?

The Lords' recommendations closely reflect the evidence put to them by organizations of health professionals, including the BMA and Royal College of Nursing. In particular, the recommendations on advance directives briefly encapsulate the long flirtation that the BMA has had with the notion of advance directives – except that the BMA changed its traditional view and supported the English Law Commission's proposals for legislation on advance directives during the period in which the House of Lords' Committee was sitting, and this was not mirrored by the Lords' final statement.

Prior to that, the BMA's views had gone through several stages. Initially lukewarm to the notion of advance directives, the BMA saw them as only potentially helpful in a few cases. In the 1990s the relationship developed more spark as the BMA sought opportunities for improved doctor–patient dialogue. Nevertheless, while the Association was happy to live with the concept of advance directives, like a reluctant bridegroom it had cold feet about formalizing the relationship by means of statute. It argued that respect for patient choice could be achieved through improved medical education, clear professional guidance (such as a code of practice) and the changing emphasis on willingness to listen to patients. Statute, the BMA argued, was superfluous - partly (but not only) because long experience had shown that whatever goes into Parliament tends to emerge in quite another form.

Although the BMA no longer objects to statute, its original prediction that legislation would be superfluous now seems closer to becoming reality. Much depends on the reaction to the code of practice published by the BMA in April 1995[25] in response to the House of Lords' report. In time this should set the standard for 'good professional practice' and help ensure consistency in the way advance directives are handled. Although the code of practice has been endorsed by medical and nursing royal colleges, considerable further effort will be required before the guidance is widely known in the mainstream of medical practice.

40　*Death, Dying and the Law*

Do Advance Directives Offer Genuine Advantages?

The House of Lords' report lists advantages and disadvantages which witnesses raised in regard to advance directives. The perceived advantages include giving patients control of their destiny and therefore peace of mind, providing opportunity for dialogue, guiding health professionals in difficult cases and removing responsibility for difficult decisions from relatives.

The primary perceived advantage of advance directives lies in protecting patient autonomy beyond the onset of incapacity but this may arguably be a 'symbolic' rather than a practical expression of autonomy. Many forms of advance directives offer the drafter a choice of specifying personal instructions and/or nominating a proxy to decide. US surveys indicate that people are most likely to select proxy decision-making by their family or their doctor. A US study[26] published in 1992 indicated that, of 104 patients with a life-threatening illness who were offered advance directives, 69 took up the offer and most asked for non-aggressive treatment if 'the burdens of treatment outweigh the expected benefits', although none gave any other personal instructions and all of them designated a proxy. However, other evidence[27] suggests that proxies are more likely than patients themselves to opt for life-prolonging treatment. While choosing to transfer the decision is just as much an expression of autonomy as deciding oneself, it does not require an advance directive to do so.

In any case, people are not entirely autonomous in their decision-making, but are influenced to some degree by the advice and information they receive and how the options are portrayed to them. It is increasingly recognized that the concept of non-directive counselling on complex issues is often no more than a sham.[28] Dialogue with health professionals is an important facet of making an informed advance directive, but health professionals, although exhorted to make their advice non-directive, find this hard to achieve. Nor is it easy to find specialized counselling about the likely future options for patients with specific diseases. Autonomy is only protected if the instructions are available at the right moment and the directive is clear. An ambiguous statement will complicate, rather than simplify, the situation.

Discussions of 'autonomy' sometimes appear to juggle theories but offer little by way of practical guidance. In Dworkin's view, when an individual is conscious but mentally incapacitated, 'two autonomies are in play: the autonomy of the demented patient and the autonomy of the person who became demented. These two autonomies can conflict, and the resulting problems are complex and difficult.[29] Of course, some philosophers resolve this dilemma by attributing no autonomy to the demented person and recognizing the 'residual interests' of the previously competent individual as paramount. A cluster of fascinating psychological and philosophical questions arise here about an individual's ability to make decisions, in advance, on matters of life and death on behalf of the person he or she will be in the future when some part of the individual 'self' – mental faculties, memories and awareness of continuity – has been lost. As Dworkin implies, the competent person who makes the anticipatory decision can be seen as fundamentally different and 'other' to the incapacitated individual who lives out (or does not) the consequences of the decision. While individuals can only make advance directives for 'themselves', a person who becomes severely mentally disordered or brain-damaged is, in some sense, no longer 'herself'.

Much of Western philosophy has been preoccupied with the importance of 'personhood', personal identity and the relationship between mind and body. Harris, for example, sees the individual's capacity to assess and value his life as fundamental[30] to personhood. There is a tradition of trying to resolve problems of identity by citing continuity of mind and mental state as the important criterion. Yet, continuity of the body is irrelevant. If the mind ceases to function as a mind, then that 'person' ceases to exist although the bodily shell may continue. A competent individual therefore is arguably not making advance decisions for him or herself but for the relics of that individual which he or she once was.

Although it is philosophically complex, on a practical level this issue is not necessarily intractable. If we allow 'persons' to make testamentary disposition for their material possessions, why not permit the same for their bodily shell after the cessation of the rational faculties? 'Ownership' of the body was the notion that sparked off the original idea of a living will: Luis Kutner's proposal was that a competent adult should be able to execute a document 'analogous to a revocable or conditional trust, with the patient's body as the *res* (the property or asset), the patient as the beneficiary and grantor, and the doctor and the hospital as trustees'.[31] The concept of property is based on the idea that there is a system of rules governing access to, and control of, some resources, whether material or incorporeal. In this case the property would be very much corporeal, and the owner, when competent, might be assigned legal rights about how it is treated in future. The owner of the body would retain an enduring interest in the body until it decays and would continue to inhabit it or be allowed to vacate it in accordance with his prior direction.

Some modern philosophers, such as Parfit,[32] argue that survival of identity need not be viewed as an 'all or nothing' issue but as a matter of degree, and this has some intuitive plausibility. One of his

42   *Death, Dying and the Law*

arguments is that, in the natural course of life, we experience a series of 'successive selves' and he quotes Proust's notion that:

> ... we are incapable, while we are in love, of acting as fit predecessors of the next persons who, when we are in love no longer, we shall presently have become.[33]

It is trite to observe that people's views change with their circumstances. Parfit imagines the possibility of the diffusion of 'self' along several different potential branches of development. He talks, for example, of 'my most recent self', 'one of my earlier selves' and 'one of my distant selves' – each of these showing a different degree of psychological connectedness with the past self. From a practical perspective, would this mean that a greater weight should be attached to an advance directive made comparatively recently by an individual who is still more or less the same self? If we recognize varying degrees of psychological continuity with former and future selves, it leaves unresolved the same question of whether it is morally correct for subsequent selves to be locked in by the provisions of an advance directive which fails to reflect their current interests. In life, of course, we do recognize that individuals make bad or risky choices in the development of their 'successive selves' but that these should generally be respected.

Theorizing aside, concern for the welfare of people with severe and permanent incapacity or dementia is often used as an argument for imposing limits on the scope of advance directives. The incapacitated individual may show all signs of wanting to be nourished, to receive treatment and to live, oblivious to the views of the former self. Despite such difficulties, it is not my intention to diminish the importance of respect for autonomy, imperfect though the exercise of it may be in practice.

Some disadvantages of advance directives were noted by the House of Lords. They include the difficulties patients experience in making their views known unambiguously, the risks of pressure or other forms of abuse being brought to bear upon the drafter and the danger of misdiagnosis. Unfortunately, however, none of these are restricted to anticipatory decision-making, but may apply to any treatment situation. Admittedly, the matter of ensuring unambiguous expression may be more complex in the case of anticipatory refusals. An example from the *Lancet*[34] drew attention to a dilemma facing doctors treating an elderly woman with advanced cancer of the colon and intestinal obstruction. Her acute pain was unamenable to narcotics but could have been relieved by a colostomy under local anaesthetic. Her advance directive refused any 'heroic' intervention in the case of incurable illness and did not distinguish between life-prolonging and pain-relieving measures. On the brief evidence given, however, such a directive might have been justifiably challenged under the criteria specified by Lord Donaldson in the 'T' case[35], as arguably, the patient had insufficient information when she drafted the directive. It might also be argued that the circumstances which arose were not precisely those envisaged in advance.

A potentially more damaging disadvantage would arise if advance directives were seen as a covert measure for reducing treatment costs or limiting the amount of care given to the elderly and terminally ill. Any encouragement by health professionals for the drafting of directives would then create suspicion and mistrust. A comparison of costs and benefits was offered in the Schneiderman study[36] which, although it admittedly involved relatively small patient numbers, showed that while most patients with advance directives wanted to limit expensive high-technology treatments, in the actual implementation of their directive there was no significant difference in overall provision of terminal care or costs between these patients and others who made no anticipatory choice. This conclusion obviously leads to the question of whether advance directives are likely to work or have any genuine value outside the realm of theoretical debate.

Do Advance Directives Work in the Real World?

The study mentioned above indicated that, in 1992, advance directives made little or no difference to treatment of the seriously ill in the state of California. No significant differences were found between those with and without advance directives in terms of patient satisfaction, general well-being, length of survival and amount of narcotics given. Patients with directives spent more days in hospital than those in the control group without directives, and similar treatment costs were incurred by all patients in the last month of life. The authors identify several reasons for this lack of divergence. They suggest, for example that doctors may simply have ignored the directive or limited 'heroic' treatment in equal measure to those with and without directives or that the document was not applicable to the circumstances. One of the most significant findings is that, contrary to expectation, most of the patients in the study retained decision-making capacity in the terminal stages. For those facing mental incapacity through diseases such as AIDS, 'discussion before death was so extensive it precluded dependence on the advance directive'.[37] Clearly, it is inadvisable to generalize from such limited data, but one inevitable conclusion is that even where advance directives are

44　　*Death, Dying and the Law*

potentially most useful, they are superfluous in practical terms if good opportunities for dialogue already exist.

It is appropriate to ask how meaningful anticipatory decision-making is likely to be in the context of the prevalent social and medical realities in the UK. Not least, it must be questioned whether good opportunities for negotiation and dialogue exist in the context of terminal care. Arguably, if it is difficult to negotiate aspects of terminal care when one is competent to do so then anticipatory attempts stand very little chance. One recently published Scottish study[38] seems to indicate some of the practical problems. The study monitored care given to 50 hospitalized dying patients, of which only two received aggressive interventions before death. More than half the patients retained competence and consciousness until shortly before death, but were unable to obtain basic minimal interventions to maintain their comfort, such as a drink of water on demand. The authors concluded that 'contact between nurses and the dying patients was minimal; distancing and isolation of patients by most medical and nursing staff were evident; this isolation increased as death approached'.[39]

The UK is five years into a managed market of health care. A culture of public expectation about treatment choices has been raised by such measures as the Patient's Charter. But, as yet, the promised patient rights in the market are illusory in practice. Patients do not have control of their health care, and sometimes individual care is fragmented by health authorities changing the hospitals with whom they have block contracts if a better bid is made by another facility. Often, it is not health professionals who make choices but the purchasing authorities. Patient audit, patient satisfaction surveys and new complaints mechanisms have a potential to change the picture. If advance directives are to become commonplace and implemented, this will be achieved from the bottom up by the accelerated 'consumerization' of health care and the need for health facilities increasingly to adapt to client demand within a highly competitive market.

There have been anecdotal reports of a few NHS Trusts saying 'we do not accept advance directives here', in the same way as they decline to offer some loss-making clinical services. But health-care purchasers, including fund-holding GPs, can pick and choose among the hospitals competing for patients. Ultimately those who pay the piper will call the tune on making provisions for advance directives *if* people feel strongly enough about the issue. Sufficient demand from the public could result in purchasers demanding the sort of care that respects advance directives for the proportion of patients who want this. But this brings attention back to the fact that, in the UK, anticipatory decision-making is a minority activity.

Another factor influencing the usefulness of directives concerns the venue where treatment is provided. Community-based services, short-stay hospital or hospice care, community nursing and better liaison between the NHS, social services and voluntary sector can promote patient choice. Even when complicated technical interventions are required, people who die in their own homes supported by carers, specialized nurses or hospice outreach programmes are likely to have greater control over the final stages of life. There are persistent fears, however, that hard-pressed health authority budgets will increasingly be used to purchase acute services rather than provide palliative care for people at home. Funding for hospice and palliative care is no longer ring-fenced as it was in the past. Palliative care services have to win contracts from purchasers who no longer have specific palliative care budgets.

Advance directives refuse life-prolonging measures. Advance statements may also be needed to address issues other than the mere refusal of medical interventions. The current reality is that the NHS is ceasing to fund long-term care of the elderly, and local hospitals are being closed as preference is given to establishing centres of excellence for acute care. There is a danger that the mentally incapacitated and dying will become the object of 'benign neglect' rather than of technological interventions to keep them alive. This might be seen as a practical reflection of the proposal by Erin and Harris[40] of a presumption of non-treatment unless advance effort has been made to rebut that notion.

Fears undoubtedly abound that life-prolonging measures are likely to be increasingly unavailable for patients with poor long-term prognoses, even if they want them. In its position paper to the House of Lords Select Committee, the Alzheimer's Disease Society implies that a concentration on autonomy may distract from broader needs. It suggests that people might be willing to sacrifice the right to consent to treatment if they could use a living will to will themselves appropriate medical care when they need it. The Society goes on to say that the good terminal care for people with dementia is decreasing and 'it is likely that many people in the last stages of Alzheimer's disease will have very little prospect of high quality and appropriate health care in the early part of the next century'.[41] This is not to say that advance directives will become superfluous but rather that they may need to change to allow those who want treatment to register a claim.

In real life the practicalities of combining directives with proxy decision-makers may also raise difficulties. The pattern of population trends is such that the proportion of older people in the UK who may want to appoint proxies will exceed the number of those they know and can be confident will survive them. Women, in particular,

46 *Death, Dying and the Law*

live longer than men, are more likely to experience widowhood and are less likely to remarry. At present half of the women of 65 years and over and a fifth of older men live alone. Dementia occurs in about 5 per cent of the population over 65 and in up to 20 per cent of those over 80. The very old (85 years and over) often live in institutional settings and carry the highest risk of dementia. Will there be trusted proxies available for them in future?

Conclusion

All the signs are that advance directives – at least in their present form – may not be the best or only answer for people with deteriorating mental faculties. Despite the rhetoric, only a small minority of people presently have sufficient confidence to commit themselves about future choices, and they may be aiming wrongly to ward off treatments which are increasingly never even on offer. In a climate of genuine patient choice, advance statements could usefully broaden in scope and offer a way forward to better communication and negotiation. In practice this can only be achieved if opportunities for unhurried or repeated discussion are built into the provision of health care. These are rarely available at present. The attitudes of health professionals are also vital. Hopefully the Code of Practice published by the BMA will establish a baseline and give patients a voice and consistency in the manner they are cared for at the end of life.

Notes

1. *Airedale NHS Trust* v. *Bland* [1993] 1 All ER 821.
2. See, for example, Chapter 16 of Kennedy, I. and Grubb, A. (1994), *Medical Law: Text with materials*, London: Butterworths; or, more briefly, Chapter 15 of Mason, J.K. and McCall Smith, A. (1991), *Law and Medical Ethics*, London: Butterworths.
3. Report of the Select Committee on Medical Ethics, HL Paper 21-1, HMSO 1994, p. 7.
4. *Re C (Adult: Refusal of Medical Treatment)* [1994] 1 WLR 290.
5. Illich, Ivan (1976), *Limits to Medicine: Medical Nemesis: the Expropriation of Health*, New York: Boyars Marion.
6. Law Commission (1991), *Mentally Incapacitated Adults and Decision-Making: An Overview*, Consultation Paper no. 119, London: HMSO, at para. 6.2, p. 137.
7. See, for example, Re J (a minor) (wardship: medical treatment) [1990] 3 All ER 930 where Lord Donaldson stated and reiterated in subsequent cases that 'No one can dictate the treatment to be given', at para. g–h, p. 934.
8. Lush, Denzil (1993), 'The history of living wills', *Eagle Magazine*, August–September.
9. Erin, C.A. and Harris, J. (1994), 'Living Wills: Anticipatory Decisions and Advance Directives', *Reviews in Clinical Gerontology*, **4**, pp. 269–275.

10   Ibid., at p. 270.
11   Ibid.
12   See the discussion by D. Lush in *op. cit.*, note 8 supra.
13   See note 1 above.
14   Age Concern (1988), *The Living Will: Consent to Treatment at the End of Life*, Working Party Report, London: Age Concern Institute of Gerontology and King's College Centre of Medical Law and Ethics.
15   Re Quinlan, 70 NJ, 10, 355, A.2d, 647 (1976); *Cruzan v. Director, Missouri Dept of Health*, 111, L.Ed 2d, 224, 110 S Ct 2841 (1990); *Airedale Trust v Bland, op. cit.* note 1 supra; Re T (adult: refusal of treatment) [1992] 4 All ER 649.
16   Dworkin, for example, mentions an American poll of 1991 in which 87 per cent of interviewees claimed to support withdrawal of treatment in accordance with an advance directive but only 17 per cent of interviewees in another poll had signed one. Dworkin, R. (1993), *Life's Dominion*, London: HarperCollins, p. 180.
17   Survey published in *Yours* magazine, December 1994.
18   *Op. cit.*, note 15 supra.
19   Scottish Law Commission (1991), *Mentally Disabled Adults: Legal Arrangements for Managing their Welfare and Finances*, Discussion Paper no. 94, Edinburgh: HMSO.
20   Ibid., as para. 5.108, p. 312.
21   Law Commission Document 231 (1995), London: HMSO.
22   Ibid. *Op. cit*, at para 5.108, p. 312, note 19 above.
23   *Op. cit.*, note 3 above.
24   Government response to the Report of the Select Committee on Medical Ethics, HMSO, 1994.
25   Advance statements about Medical Treatment (1995), London: BMJ Publishing Group.
26   Schneiderman, L. *et al.* (1992), 'Effects of offering advance directives on medical treatments and costs', *Annals of Internal Medicine*, **117**, pp. 599–606.
27   Seckler, A.B. *et al.* (1991), 'Substituted judgement: how accurate are proxy predictions?', *Annals of Internal Medicine*, **115**, pp. 92–8.
28   See, for example, in the genetic field, Clarke, Angus (1991), 'Is non-directive genetic counselling possible?' *Lancet*, **338**, 19 October, p. 998.
29   Dworkin, R. *op. cit.*, note 16 above, p. 192.
30   Harris, J. (1985), *The Value of Life*, London: Routledge, p. 16.
31   *Indiana Law Journal*, **44**, 1969, pp. 539–554 at p. 552.
32   Parfit, Derek, 'Personal Identity', reprinted in Ted Honderich and Myles Burnyeat (eds) (1979), *Philosophy As It Is*, Harmondsworth: Pelican.
33   Proust, Marcel (1949), *Within a Budding Grove*, London, quoted and translated by Parfit, *op. cit.*, note 32 above, p. 205.
34   Rosner, F. (1994), 'Living Wills', *Lancet*, **343**, 23 April, p. 1041.
35   *Op. cit.*, note 15 above.
36   Schneiderman *et al.*, *op. cit.*, note 26 above.
37   Ibid., p. 605.
38   Mills, M., Davies, H. and Macrae, W. (1994), 'Care of dying patients in hospital', *British Medical Journal*, **309**, pp. 583–6.
39   Ibid., p. 605.
40   *Op. cit.*, note 9 above.
41   Position paper based on written evidence submitted to the House of Lords Committee on Medical Ethics by the Alzheimer's Disease Society, June 1993.

[21]

Euthanasia in the Netherlands: sliding down the slippery slope?

JOHN KEOWN

INTRODUCTION

THERE IS ONLY one country in which euthanasia is officially condoned and widely practised: the Netherlands. Although euthanasia is proscribed by the Dutch Penal Code, the Dutch Supreme Court held in 1984 that a doctor who kills a patient may in certain circumstances successfully invoke the defence of necessity, also contained in the Code, to justify the killing. In the same year, the Royal Dutch Medical Association (KNMG) issued its members with guidelines for euthanasia. Since that time the lives of thousands of Dutch patients have been intentionally shortened by their doctors.

A requirement central to both the legal and medical guidelines has been the free and explicit request of the patient. Defenders of the guidelines have claimed that they permit voluntary euthanasia but not euthanasia without request; that they are sufficiently strict and precise to prevent any slide down a 'slippery slope' to euthanasia without request, and that there has been no evidence of any such slide in the Netherlands.

The question addressed in this chapter can be simply put: Does the Dutch experience of euthanasia lend any support to the claims of supporters of voluntary euthanasia that acceptance of voluntary euthanasia does not lead to acceptance of non-voluntary euthanasia or does it, rather, tend to support the claims of opponents of voluntary euthanasia that voluntary euthanasia leads down a 'slippery slope' to euthanasia without request?

The 'slippery slope' argument is often thought of as one argument but it is more accurately understood as comprising two independent yet related forms: the 'logical' and the 'empirical'. In its logical form, the argument runs that acceptance of voluntary euthanasia leads to acceptance of at least non-voluntary euthanasia (that is, the killing of patients incapable of requesting euthanasia such as newborns or those with advanced senile dementia) because the former rests on the judgment that some lives are not 'worth' living, which judgment can logically be made even if the patient is incapable of requesting euthanasia. Doctors are not automata who simply execute their patient's wishes, however autonomous. They are professionals who form their own judgment about the merits of any request for medical intervention. A responsible doctor would no more euthanatise a patient just because the patient autonomously asked for it any more than the doctor would prescribe anti-depressant drugs for a patient just because the patient autonomously requested them. The doctor, if acting professionally, would decide in each case whether the intervention was truly in the patient's best interests. A responsible doctor would no more kill a patient who had, in the doctor's opinion, a life 'worth' living any more than he would prescribe anti-depressants for a patient who, in the doctor's opinion, was not depressed. Consequently, the alleged justification of voluntary euthanasia rests fundamentally not on the patient's autonomous request *but on the doctor's judgment that the request is justified because the patient no longer has a life 'worth' living.* And, if a doctor can make this judgment in relation to an autonomous patient, he can, logically, make it in relation to an incompetent patient. Moreover, if death is a 'benefit' for competent patients suffering certain conditions, why should it be denied incompetent patients suffering from the same conditions?[1]

In its empirical form, the 'slippery slope' argument runs that even if a line can in principle be drawn between voluntary and non-voluntary euthanasia, a slide will occur in practice because the safeguards to prevent it cannot be made effective. A common illustration of the argument in this form is the story of decriminalised abortion in England, where the law allowing therapeutic abortion has conspicuously failed to prevent widespread abortion for social reasons.

The empirical argument is, of course, dependent on empirical evidence. Invaluable evidence about euthanasia in Holland has of late been provided by a large-scale survey carried out on behalf of a Commission appointed by the Dutch Government to investigate medical decision-making in Holland at the end of life. This chapter makes comprehensive use of this evidence.

The chapter comprises three parts. Part I outlines both the relevant law as laid down by the Dutch Supreme Court and the Guidelines for euthanasia prescribed by the KNMG and considers their alleged precision and strictness.

Part II summarises the evidence, including that contained in the above survey, which indicates widespread breach of those Guidelines, especially the practice of euthanasia without request. The final part examines the slide from voluntary to non-voluntary euthanasia in Dutch practice and the shift in Dutch opinion towards condonation of non-voluntary euthanasia. The chapter concludes in Part III that there is ample evidence from the Dutch experience to substantiate the relevance of the 'slippery slope' argument in both its forms. First, an important word about terminology.

A standard definition of 'euthanasia' is 'The intentional putting to death of a person with an incurable or painful disease'.[2] It is common to refer to euthanasia carried out by an act as 'active' euthanasia and euthanasia by omission as 'passive' euthanasia. A common further sub-division is between 'voluntary', 'non-voluntary' and 'involuntary' euthanasia, which refer respectively to euthanasia at the patient's request, where the patient is incompetent, and where the patient is competent but has made no request.

Dutch definitions of 'euthanasia' are, typically, markedly narrower, such as 'the purposeful acting to terminate life by someone other than the person concerned upon request of the latter'.[3] It will be apparent that this is narrower than the usual definition in two respects: it is limited to cases of *active*[4] killing where there is a *request by the patient*. In short, the Dutch definition corresponds to what is normally called 'active, voluntary euthanasia'.

I. STRICT SAFEGUARDS?

A. The legal and professional guidelines

Taking the life of another person at his request is an offence contrary to Article 293 of the Penal Code (as amended in 1891) and assisting suicide is prohibited by Article 294. In 1984, however, in the *Alkmaar* case, the Dutch Supreme Court allowed a doctor's appeal against conviction for intentionally killing one of his elderly patients at her request. The Court held that the lower courts had wrongly failed to consider whether he had been faced with a 'conflict of duties'[5] (his duty to obey Article 293 on the one hand and his duty to relieve his patient's suffering on the other), whether 'according to responsible medical opinion'[6] measured by the 'prevailing standards of medical ethics'[7] a situation of 'necessity'[8] existed, and whether he had, therefore, been entitled to the defence of necessity, contained in Article 40.[9]

This decision is remarkable for a number of reasons. First, the necessity defence has traditionally been understood as justifying an ostensible breach of the law in order to *save* life (as by pushing someone out of the path of an oncoming car), not to take it. Secondly, the judgment fails to explain *why* the doctor's duty to alleviate suffering overrides his duty not to kill. Finally, the Court appears to abdicate to medical opinion the power to determine the circumstances in which killing attracts the necessity defence.

In a series of decisions straddling this landmark case, lower courts have laid down a number of conditions which have hitherto been understood as being required for a doctor successfully to avail himself of the necessity defence, though there is increasing uncertainty as to which, if any, are required. Subject to this important *caveat*, they were listed in 1989 (by Mrs Borst-Eilers, then Chairman of the Dutch Health Council) as follows:

(1) The request for euthanasia must come only from the patient and must be entirely free and voluntary.
(2) The patient's request must be well-considered, durable and persistent.
(3) The patient must be experiencing intolerable (not necessarily physical) suffering, with no prospect of improvement.
(4) Euthanasia must be a last resort. Other alternatives to alleviate the patient's situation must have been considered and found wanting.
(5) Euthanasia must be performed by a physician.
(6) The physician must consult with an independent physician colleague who has experience in this field.[10]

Moreover, having performed euthanasia, the doctor should *not* certify death by 'natural causes', which would involve the offence of falsifying a death certificate, but should call in the local medical examiner to investigate. The medical examiner should carry out an external inspection of the corpse, interview the doctor and file a report with the local prosecutor, who should decide whether to investigate further or to allow the body to be handed over to the next-of-kin.

Three months before the landmark Supreme Court decision in 1984, the KNMG published a Report setting out its criteria for permissible euthanasia.[11] They are substantially similar to the conditions just listed and require a voluntary request by the patient which is well considered and persistent; unacceptable suffering by the patient, and consultation by the doctor with a colleague working in the same institution and then with an independent doctor.[12] The KNMG subsequently formulated, in collaboration with the National Association of Nurses, certain 'Guidelines for Euthanasia'[13] which embody the above criteria.

B. 'Precisely defined' and 'strict'?

Before considering the evidence which indicates the extent to which the practice of euthanasia conforms to the above requirements, some comment is called for on the nature of those requirements and particularly on the extent to which they are capable of closely regulating the practice of euthanasia.

A leading Dutch defender of euthanasia has claimed (a claim reproduced with uncritical, almost robotic repetition in many newspaper articles on this subject) that the Guidelines are 'strict' and 'precise'.[14] However, even a cursory examination indicates that this is not the case. For one thing, it is not even possible precisely to identify the legal criteria, let alone define them: the Supreme Court omitted to lay down a precise list and lower courts have issued sets of criteria which are far from congruent. For another, as Professor Leenen, a leading Dutch health lawyer (and supporter of legalised euthanasia) has observed, concepts such as 'unbearable pain' (*a fortiori*, one might add, 'suffering') are open to subjective interpretation and are incapable of precise definition.[15] As for the assertion that the Guidelines are 'strict', this too is difficult to sustain, not only because of their imprecision but also because of the absence of any effective independent check on the doctor's decision-making to ensure that they are satisfied.

A hypothetical case may help highlight their inherent vagueness. A leading Dutch practitioner of euthanasia, who is highly respected in Holland, has said that he would be put in a very difficult position if a patient told him that he wanted euthanasia because he felt a nuisance to his relatives who wanted him dead so they could enjoy his estate. Asked whether he would rule out euthanasia in such a case, the doctor replied:

> I . . . think in the end I wouldn't, because that kind of influence – these children wanting the money now – is the same kind of power from the past that . . . shaped us all. The same thing goes for religion . . . education . . . the kind of family he was raised in, all kinds of influences from the past that we can't put aside.[16]

If such a leading practitioner of euthanasia, who had delivered many lectures on the subject inside and outside Holland (including lectures to the Dutch police on how to handle euthanasia cases) can interpret the Guidelines requiring an 'entirely free and voluntary request' and 'unbearable suffering' as possibly extending to such a case, little more need be said about their inherent vagueness and elasticity. In short, the Guidelines are simply incapable, because of their vagueness and the fact that they entrust the decision-making to the individual practitioner, of ensuring that euthanasia is carried out only in accordance with the criteria they specify. The empirical evidence which confirms the inability of the Guidelines effectively to regulate euthanasia is set out in Part II.

II. EUTHANASIA IN PRACTICE: THE EMPIRICAL EVIDENCE

A. The origins of the Remmelink Commission and the van der Maas Survey

The Dutch coalition government which assumed office in 1989 decided to appoint a Commission to report on the 'extent and nature of medical euthanasia practice'.[17] A Commission under the chairmanship of the Attorney-General, Professor Remmelink, was appointed on 17 January 1990 by the Minister of Justice and the State Secretary for Welfare, Health and Culture and asked to report on the practice by physicians of 'performing an act or omission . . . to terminate [the] life of a patient, with or without an explicit and serious request of the patient to this end'.[18]

To assist the discharge of this responsibility, the Commission asked P.J. van der Maas, Professor of Public Health and Social Medicine at the Erasmus University, to carry out a survey which would produce qualitative and quantitative information on the practice of euthanasia. The Commission and van der Maas agreed that the survey should embrace all medical decisions affecting the end of life so that euthanasia could be seen within that broader context. The umbrella term 'Medical Decisions Concerning the End of Life' ('MDELs') includes 'all decisions by physicians concerning courses of action aimed at hastening the end of life of the patient or courses of action for which the physician takes into account the probability that the end of life of the patient is hastened'.[19] MDELs comprise the administration, supply or prescription of a drug; the withdrawal or withholding of a treatment (including resuscitation and tube-feeding), and the refusal of a request for euthanasia or assisted suicide.[20] The Commission's Report[21] and the Survey[22] were published in Dutch in September 1991. One year later, the Survey was published in English.[23]

A previous paper of mine[24] suggested that the Dutch experience lends support to the 'slippery slope' argument in both its 'logical' and 'empirical' forms.[25] Do the Report and Survey require that suggestion to be qualified? The answer, on an uncritical reading of the Report, would be 'Yes'. But a reading of the Report in the light of its Survey yields a contrary answer. Indeed, taken together, the Survey and Report tend forcefully to confirm the application of the argument in both its forms.

B. The findings of the Survey and the conclusions of the Commission

After an outline of the Survey's findings about the incidence of euthanasia, consideration will be given to the light the Survey and the Report throw on the extent to which the criteria laid down by the courts and the KNMG have been observed in practice. Attention will focus on the Survey rather than the Report: the Report contains the Commission's conclusions in the light of the Survey but the Survey is a comprehensive empirical study which stands independently of the Report, and the conclusions drawn in the Report are not infrequently difficult to square with the findings of the Survey.

1. Methodology

Before turning to the Survey's findings, a summary of its methodology is appropriate. The Survey comprised three studies.

(i) The retrospective study.[26] A sample of 406 doctors was drawn from general practitioners, specialists (concerned with MDELs) and nursing home doctors, of whom 91% agreed to participate. The doctors were interviewed on average for two and a half hours and almost always by another doctor.[27] The respondent was asked about relevant types of decision. If he had made a decision of a given type, the last occasion on which he had done so was discussed in greater detail. At most, ten cases were discussed with each.[28]

(ii) The death certificate study.[29] This study examined a stratified sample of 8500 deaths occurring in Holland from July to November 1990 inclusive. The treating doctor was identified from each death certificate and was sent a short questionnaire which could be returned anonymously. The response rate was 73%.[30]

(iii) The prospective study.[31] Each of the doctors interviewed in the retrospective study was asked at interview if he would complete a questionnaire about each of his patients who died in the following six months. This study had several advantages: there would be little memory distortion because the questionnaire would be completed soon after the death; it would provide additional information to strengthen the quantitative basis of the interview study; and the carefully planned selection of respondents meant that the responses were representative of 95% of all deaths. The study ran from mid-November 1990 to the end of May 1991. Eighty per cent of those involved in the first study participated, completing over 2250 questionnaires.[32] In all, each of some 322

doctors supplied information about, on average, seven deaths.[33] The method of collection of data in all three studies was such that anonymity of participants could be guaranteed.[34]

2. The incidence of euthanasia

In 1990, the year covered by the Survey, thee were almost 130 000 deaths in Holland from all causes, of which 49 000 involved a MDEL.[35] Both the Report and the Survey adopted the Dutch definition of euthanasia as 'the intentional action to terminate a person's life, performed by somebody else than the involved person upon the latter's request'.[36] How many cases of 'euthanasia' so defined were there in 1990?

The three studies differed as to the incidence of euthanasia, yielding respective figures of 1.9%, 1.7% and 2.6% of all deaths. The researchers felt that the difference between the second and third estimates was 'probably due to the existence of a boundary area between euthanasia and intensifying of the alleviation of pain and/or symptoms'[37] and to the probability of the third study counting cases of pain alleviation as cases of 'euthanasia', thereby exaggerating its incidence.[38]

Of the three studies it is, however, arguably the third which produces the most accurate estimate of 'euthanasia'. As the authors of the Survey point out, the respondents in the second study had no information other than the questionnaire and an accompanying letter, whereas those in the third had participated in the physician interviews, discussing one or more cases from their practice and the crucial concepts in the questionnaire for over two hours with a trained interviewer. The authors, noting that a 'great number'[39] of interviewees commented that the interview had clarified their thinking about MDELs, suggest the possibility of a learning effect: familiarity with the questionnaire, in which the question about euthanasia followed those relating to other MDELs, may have led the respondents to reply negatively to the earlier questions knowing that the question about euthanasia was to come. The authors conclude that the most important fact was that the respondents in the third study 'changed their approach with respect to their intention when administering morphine due to their recent intensive confrontation with thinking about this complex of problems'.[40] If the thinking of participants in the third study had been clarified by their participation in the first study, their responses are surely more likely to have been reliable than those in the second study, particularly as, the second study being retrospective, there was less risk of memory distortion.

The authors' conclusion, however, is that in the light of all three studies, 'euthanasia' occurred in about 1.8% of all deaths, or about 2300 cases,[41] and that there were almost 400 cases of assisted suicide, some 0.3% of all deaths.[42] More than half the physicians regularly involved with terminal patients indicated that they had performed 'euthanasia' or had assisted suicide and only 12% of doctors said they would never do so.[43]

So much for euthanasia in its narrowest sense: intentional, *active* termination of life *at the patient's request*. But the authors of the Survey themselves go on, rightly, to consider euthanasia in a somewhat wider but still precise and realistic sense. They estimated that in a further 1000 cases (or 0.8% of all deaths) physicians administered a drug 'with the explicit purpose of hastening the end of life without an explicit request of the patient'.[44]

And beyond this, there lies a range of evidence yielded by the Survey, but not adequately considered by the authors in their commentary. For many other MDELs also involved an intent to hasten death. Palliative drugs were administered in 'such high doses . . . that . . . almost certainly would shorten the life of the patient'[45] in 22 500 cases (17.5% of all deaths).[46] In 65% (or 14 625) of these cases the doctor administered the medication merely 'Taking into account the probability that life would be shortened',[47] but in 30% (or 6750 cases) it was administered 'Partly with the purpose of shortening life'[48] and in a further 6% (or 1350 cases) 'With the explicit purpose of shortening life'.[49]

Moreover, doctors withdrew or withheld treatment without request in another 25 000 cases and, by the time of the Survey, some 90% of these patients, or 22 500, had died.[50] In 65% (or 16 250 cases) the treatment was withdrawn or withheld 'Taking into account the probability that life would be shortened',[51] but in 19% (or 4750 cases) 'Partly with the purpose to shorten life'[52] and in a further 16% (or 4000 cases) 'With the explicit purpose to shorten life'.[53]

Further, physicians received some 5800 requests to withdraw or withhold treatment when the patient intended at least in part to hasten death.[54] In 74% of these cases the doctor withdrew or withheld treatment partly with the purpose of shortening life but in 26% 'With the explicit purpose of shortening life'.[55] By the time of the interview, some 82% (or 4756) had died.[56] The above figures are reproduced in Table 1.

Thus, it becomes clear that, while the Commission stated that the figure of 2700 cases of 'euthanasia' and assisted suicide 'does not warrant the assumption that euthanasia in the Netherlands occurs on an excessive scale',[57] the total number of euthanasiast acts and omissions in 1990 was in reality far higher than the Commission claims. To clarify and confirm this conclusion it is necessary to look more closely at the definitions used by the authors of the Survey in classifying their data to produce the figure of 2700.

Table 1. *Medical decisions concerning the end of life in 1990*

Acts or omissions with intent to shorten life[a]

Total deaths (all causes)	129 000	
'Euthanasia'[b]		2 300
Assisted suicide		400
Intentional life-terminating acts without explicit request[c]		1 000 (1 000)
Alleviation of pain/symptoms[d]	22 500	
With the 'explicit purpose' of shortening life		1 350 (450)
'Partly with the purpose' of shortening life		6 750 (5 058)
Withdrawal/withholding of treatment without explicit request[c]	25 000	
With the 'explicit purpose' of shortening life		4 000 (4 000)
'Partly with the purpose' of shortening life		4 750 (4 750)
Withdrawal/withholding of treatment on explicit request[f]	5 800	
With the 'explicit purpose' of shortening life		1 508
'Partly with the purpose' of shortening life		4 292
Sub-total[g]		10 558 (5 450)
Total[h]		26 350 (15 258)

[a]Cases of 'explicit' intent to shorten life are in italics; cases without explicit request in parentheses.
[b]No shortening of life occurred in 1% of these cases. Survey, 49, table 5.13.
[c]No shortening of life occurred in 4% of these cases. Ibid., 66, table 6.10.
[d]No shortening of life occurred in 8% of these cases. Ibid., 73, table 7.3.
[e]Ninety per cent of these patients (22 500) had died by the time of the interview and there had been no shortening of life in 20% of these cases. Ibid., 90, table 8.14.
[f]Eighty-two per cent of these patients (4756) had died by the time of the interview and there had been no shortening of life in 19% of these cases. Ibid., 82, table 8.6.
[g]This sub-total refers to cases where doctors 'explicitly' intended to shorten life by act or omission.
[h]This total refers to cases where doctors intended ('explicitly' or 'partly') to hasten death by act or omission. Both it and the preceding sub-total therefore include (as does the Survey) cases where life may not in fact have been shortened and cases in the two withdrawal/withholding of treatment categories where patients had not died by the time of the Survey.

The definition of euthanasia adopted by the Commission was the *'intentional* action to terminate a person's life, performed by somebody else than the involved person upon the latter's request'.[58] Similarly, the definition adopted in the Survey was 'the *purposeful* acting to terminate life by someone other than the person concerned upon request of the latter'.[59] These definitions echo that embraced by the central committee of the KNMG in its 1984 report on euthanasia as all actions 'aimed at'[60] terminating a patient's life at his explicit request. This report added that a majority of the committee had rejected a sub-division into 'active' and 'passive' as 'morally superfluous'[61] and undesirable: 'All activities or non-activities *with the purpose to terminate a patient's life* are defined as euthanasia'.[62]

The authors of the Survey distinguish the following states of mind:

[acting with] the explicit purpose of hastening the end of life;
[acting] partly with the purpose of hastening the end of life;
[acting while] taking into account the probability that the end of life will be hastened.[63]

They explain that the first category, unlike the third, applied where the patient's death was the intended outcome of the action. The second category was used because sometimes an act was performed with a particular aim (such as pain relief) but the side effect (such as death) was 'not unwelcome'.[64] The authors felt that such an effect should be categorised as intentional because to count as *un*intentional a death 'should not in fact have been desired'.[65] The category related to a situation in which the 'death of the patient was not foremost in the physician's mind but neither was death unwelcome'[66] and was regarded by the author as a 'type' of intention.[67]

As Table 1 reveals, doctors are stated by the Survey to have intended to accelerate death in far more than the 2700 cases classified by the Commission as 'euthanasia' and assisted suicide. This total ignores the 1000 cases of intentional killing without request and, in addition, three further categories where there is said to have been some intention to shorten life: first, the 8100 (1350 + 6750) cases of increasing the dosage of palliative drugs; secondly, the 8750 (4000 + 4750) cases of withholding or withdrawing treatment without request and, finally, the 5800 (1508 + 4292) cases of withholding or withdrawing treatment on request.[68] Adding these 23650 cases to the 2700 produces a total of 26350 cases in which the Survey states that doctors intended, by act or omission, to shorten life. This raises the incidence of euthanasia from around 2% to over 20% of all deaths in Holland.

It could be argued that the 23650 cases are not 'euthanasia' because they are not cases of intentional killing at the patient's request. There are, however, two counter-arguments. First, some of them clearly *are*. In relation, for example, to the 1350 cases in which it was the explicit purpose of the doctor to shorten life by increasing the dosage of palliative drugs, the Survey discloses: 'In all these cases the patient had at some time indicated something about terminating life and an explicit request had been made in two thirds of the cases'.[69] Indeed, the authors comment: 'This situation is therefore rather similar to euthanasia'.[70] It is unclear, therefore, why the Commission does not regard these as cases of 'euthanasia'; they seem to fall squarely within its definition. Interestingly, a member of the Commission (who in fact wrote the

Report) has subsequently agreed with the proposition that those cases where doctors had, with the explicit purpose of shortening the patient's life and at the patient's explicit request, administered palliative drugs, could properly be categorised as euthanasia.[71]

The second counter-argument is that the true scale of euthanasia can only properly be gauged when the Commission's abnormally narrow definition of 'euthanasia' is replaced by a standard definition such as 'when the death of a human being is brought about on purpose as part of the medical care being given to him'.[72] If this more realistic definition is applied, then the Survey's own presentation of the data suggests that there were a further 23 650 deaths by euthanasia.

However, there remains a further question about the proper interpretation of the Survey's definitions, and thus of its figures. Is it appropriate to include the 15 792 cases in which hastening death was only 'partly' the doctor's intention? These cases were distinguished in the Survey from those where the doctor merely foresaw the acceleration of death (where he proceeded 'Taking into account the probability that life would be shortened'[73]). If the doctor's purpose in these cases was, albeit partly, to hasten death, then it seems quite appropriate to regard them as instances of euthanasia. By analogy, if racial discrimination is the intentional (purposeful) treating of one person less favourably than another on racial grounds and, say, an employer takes advantage of a need to make redundancies in order to get rid of his black workers, he may be said to have acted partly with a view to doing just that, even though his primary purpose is to save his company by reducing expenditure on wages.

On the other hand, it is arguable that these are not necessarily cases in which the doctor's purpose was to hasten death. Notwithstanding the researchers' treatment of these as cases of purposeful killing, their explanation of this category and in particular their apparent understanding of the concept of 'purpose' in fact leave the matter unclear. The implication in their explanation that death in these cases was 'desired' does indeed suggest that the doctor intended to shorten life, but the reference to death as a 'not unwelcome' consequence suggests that death, while not regretted, may not, in some of these cases, have been any part of the doctor's purpose or goal.

Although it may well be that the doctor's intention in most if not all of these cases was to shorten life (a conclusion which would be consistent with the finding that no fewer than 88% of Dutch doctors had performed euthanasia or would be willing to do so[74]), the possibility that it was not cannot be ruled out. These cases are, therefore, regarded in this chapter as cases of intentional shortening of life subject to this *caveat*. However, the force of the following critique of Dutch euthanasia in no way depends on their inclusion. For even if they are discounted, the total number of life-shortening acts and omissions where the doctor's *primary* intention (more graphically but less precisely called 'explicit purpose' by the Survey) was to kill, and which are therefore indubitably euthanasiast, is 10 558. That figure is almost 4 times higher than the number of cases categorised as 'euthanasia' and assisted suicide by the Commission and amounts to over 8% of all deaths in Holland. In other words, almost 1 in 12 of all deaths in Holland in 1990 was intentionally accelerated by a doctor.

3. 'Dances with data'?

The authors of the van der Maas Survey recently argued that I (and a number of other commentators on Dutch euthanasia) have misinterpreted their findings.[75] One of their main criticisms (to which I shall limit myself in the interests of conciseness) is that I have inaccurately inflated the number of cases of euthanasia and assisted suicide disclosed by their Survey. I respectfully demur.

It will be recalled that van der Maas *et al.* concluded that there were 2300 cases of euthanasia and 400 cases of assisted suicide[76] and that what largely accounts for the discrepancy between their total of 2700 and mine of 10 558 is their peculiarly narrow definition of 'euthanasia' as '*active, voluntary euthanasia*' as contrasted with my standard definition of euthanasia as the intentional shortening of a patient's life, by act or omission. Their arguments for rejecting my total are quite unpersuasive. Their main argument is that 'intentions cannot carry the full weight of a moral evaluation on their own'[77] because 'intentions are essentially private matters. Ultimately only the agent "decides" what his intentions are, and different agents may describe the same actions in the same situations as performed with different intentions'.[78] And, they add, the agent's purpose may change over time, so what is to count as the 'definitive description'?[79]

This line of argument is remarkable. They agree that euthanasia is to be distinguished from other MDELs in that it involves the intentional ('purposeful') shortening of life; indeed, one of the welcome features of their meticulous Survey is the care they took to ascertain the doctors' state of mind when hastening death. They specifically *asked* whether the doctors shortened life with the 'explicit purpose' of so doing; or 'partly with the purpose' of so doing; or merely 'taking into account the probability' of so doing and the doctors *replied* that in some 10 558 cases it had been their *explicit intention to shorten life*. Why are the doctors' own answers not taken as the 'definitive description' of their intention? If the authors thought it impossible to discern the doctors' intention, why did they bother asking them?

The authors add that no doctor who performs euthanasia does so with the sole intent to kill: 'His or her intention can always be described as trying to relieve the suffering of his or her patient. This is exactly what infuriates Dutch physicians when, after reporting the case they are treated as criminals and murderers'.[80] However, while the doctor's ultimate intention may be to relieve suffering, he intends to do so by shortening the patient's life which is precisely why, in most jurisdictions, the doctor who performs euthanasia is liable for murder. If an heir kills his rich father by slipping a lethal poison into his tea, would they deny that this was murder on the ground that the heir's intention was not to kill and 'can always be described as' trying to accelerate his inheritance?

They continue that it is wrong to rest the moral evaluation entirely on intention: 'For a moral evaluation, more is to be taken into account, such as the presence of a request of the patient, the futility of further medical treatment, the sequelae of the decision to stop treatment (e.g. will this cause heavy distress?), the interests of others involved such as family and so on'.[81] Yet more muddle. The question at issue here is not the *moral evaluation* of cases of euthanasia but their *incidence*, and this is a matter of definition, not evaluation. And standard definitions reckon as euthanasia cases where the doctor, by act or omission, intentionally shortens life.

A further argument they advance is that if the 'context' is taken into account, it can be questioned whether the intentions were euthanasiast. As an example they cite the 6% of cases of alleviation of pain and symptoms in which doctors stated that their explicit intention was to shorten life. The authors seek to distinguish these cases from euthanasia on the ground that they involve a failure of palliative care followed by the use of higher doses which may lead to a point at which 'the physician realises that he or she actually hopes that the patient dies'.[82] His or her intention is 'not necessarily'[83] the same as with euthanasia, where the physician would surely try another lethal drug if the first failed, which would 'never'[84] happen with the administration of opioids.

This argument, too, fails. First, in these 6% of cases doctors stated it was their *explicit*, not partial, intention to shorten life; the authors give no reason to doubt the accuracy of this response. Secondly, the argument appears to rest on the unsubstantiated speculation that, had the higher dose failed to shorten life, the doctor would not have resorted to another method. Even if this were so, the argument is specious, resting on a patent *non sequitur*. If A attempts to kill B by method M1, which fails, his decision not to resort to method M2 in no way establishes he did not intend to kill by method M1.

In sum, the arguments advanced by van der Maas *et al.* against my total of 10 558 backfire, succeeding only in highlighting the inaccurate basis on which they have calculated their own total of 2700.

C. Conformity with the Guidelines?

How many of the 10 558 (or, if partly intended life-shortening is included, 26 350) euthanasiast acts and omissions satisfied the Guidelines laid down by the courts and the KNMG? More specifically, in how many cases was there a 'free and voluntary' request which was 'well-considered, durable and persistent'? In how many was there 'intolerable' suffering for which euthanasia was a 'last resort'? And in how many cases did the doctor consult with a colleague and report the case to the legal authorities, whether prosecutor, police or local medical examiner?[85]

1. An 'entirely free and voluntary' request which was 'well-considered, durable and persistent'

Doctors stated that in the '2700' cases of euthanasia and assisted suicide there was an 'explicit request'[86] in 96%; which was 'wholly made by the patient'[87] in 99% of all cases and 'repeated'[88] in 94%; and that in 100% of cases the patient had a 'good insight'[89] into his disease and its prognosis. Oddly, no specific question was put about the voluntariness of the request and there is no evidence of any mechanism to ensure that the request was voluntary. Moreover, the request was purely oral in 60% of cases[90] and, when made to a general practitioner (GP) in cases where a nurse was caring for the patient, the GP more often than not failed to consult her.[91]

There is no way of gauging the accuracy of the doctors' statements, which are uncorroborated, about the patients' requests. Even if they are true, however, the Survey data show that in the 10 558 cases in which it was the doctor's primary purpose to hasten death, there was in the majority (52%) no explicit request from the patient. Similarly, in a majority (58%) of the 26 350 cases in which it was the doctor's primary or secondary intention to shorten life, the doctor shortened life without the patient's explicit request.

(i) 'Life-terminating acts without the patient's explicit request'. In the light of the three studies, the Survey concludes:

> On an annual basis there are, in the Netherlands, some thousand cases (0.8% of all deaths) for which physicians prescribe, supply or administer a drug with the explicit purpose of hastening the end of life without an explicit request of the patient.[92]

In over half these cases, the decision was discussed with the patient or the patient had previously indicated his wish for the hastening of death, but in 'several hundred cases there was no discussion with the patient and there also was no known wish from the patient for hastening the end of life'.[93] Virtually all cases, state the authors, involved seriously ill and terminal patients who obviously were suffering a great deal and were no longer able to express their wishes, though there was a 'small number'[94] of cases in which the decision could have been discussed with the patient.

The fact that doctors administered a lethal drug without an express request in 1000 cases – almost half as many as they did on request – is striking. So too is the Commission's reaction to this statistic. The Commission observes that the ('few dozen'[95]) cases in which the doctor killed a *competent* patient without request 'must be prevented in future',[96] and that one means would be 'strict compliance with the scrupulous care'[97] required for euthanasia 'including the requirement that all facts of the case are put down in writ[i]ng'.[98] However, the Commission *defends* the other cases of unrequested killing, stating that 'active intervention'[99] by the doctor was usually 'inevitable'[100] because of the patient's 'death agony'.[101] That is why, it explains, it regards these cases as 'care for the dying'.[102] It adds that the ultimate justification for killing in these cases was the patient's 'unbearable suffering'.[103]

The Commission's assertion that most of the 1000 patients were incompetent patients in their 'death agony' should not pass unchallenged. The physician interviews indicate that 14% of the patients were totally competent and a further 11% partly competent;[104] that 21% had a life expectancy of one to four weeks and 7% of one to six months (the Survey classed patients as 'dying' if their life had been shortened only by 'hours or days', not by 'weeks or months'[105]) and that doctors did not list 'agony' as a reason for killing these patients. The reasons given by doctors were the absence of any prospect of improvement (60%); the futility of all medical therapy (39%); avoidance of 'needless prolongation'[106] (33%); the relatives' inability to cope (32%); and 'low quality of life'[107] (31%). Pain or suffering was mentioned by only 30%.[108] And, even in relation to these 30%, if they were essentially cases of increasing pain or symptom treatment to shorten life, why did the doctors not classify them under that heading?[109]

In short, the Commission's defence of these 1000 cases would appear to be based on a shaky factual foundation and its attempted ethical justification amounts to little more than a bare assertion that killing without request, a practice in breach of cardinal criteria for permissible euthanasia, is morally acceptable. On the basis of this assertion, it proceeds to recommend that doctors should report such cases in the same way as they report cases of voluntary euthanasia.[110]

The Government has implemented the Commission's recommendation that euthanasia without request should be reported by incorporating the reporting procedure into the law regulating the disposal of the dead. The procedure makes it clear that it applies whether or not the patient requested euthanasia.[111]

(ii) Other cases of intentional life-shortening without explicit request. In addition to the 1000 cases of active life termination without explicit request there were many more in which the patient made no explicit request that his life be shortened.

In 59% (or 4779) of the 8100 cases in which doctors are said to have intended to hasten death by pain-killing drugs, the patient had 'never indicated anything about terminating life'.[112] and there had been no explicit request in a further 9% (or 729),[113] making 5508 cases in which there had been no explicit request.[114]

Additionally, in 8750 cases treatment is said to have been withheld or withdrawn without explicit request and intentionally to shorten life.[115] The Commission would have it that these were cases of omitting to provide futile treatment. It states:

> After all, a doctor has the right to refrain from (further) treatment, if that treatment would be pointless according to objective medical standards. The commission would define a treatment without any medical use as therapeutical interference that gives no hope whatsoever for any positive effect upon the patient. To the application of this kind of futile medicine, no one is entitled. It is undisputed that the medical decision whether a particular action is useful or not, belongs to normal medical practice.[116]

The Commission appears confused. First, the Survey did not use the concept of futile treatment in relation to withdrawal of treatment as the authors felt its meaning was open to 'variable' interpretation.[117] Secondly, the preamble to the relevant questions suggests that they were not asking about the withdrawal of futile treatment, that is, treatment which was unlikely or incapable of achieving its normal therapeutic purpose, but rather about the withdrawal of treatment which was preserving 'futile' lives, that is, lives which were not thought to be worth preserving:

> In most instances this [decision to withhold or withdraw treatment] concerns situations in which the treating physician does not expect or does not observe sufficient success. However, there are situations in which a considerable life-prolonging effect can be expected from a certain treatment while the decision can nevertheless be made to withhold such treatment or to withdraw it. This implies that under such circumstances considerable prolongation of

life is considered undesirable or even futile. 'Considerable' is taken to mean more than one month.[118]

That the questions were concerned with 'futile' lives rather than ineffectual treatment is further suggested by the authors' explanation of this series of questions:

> Briefly, two types of situations are discussed here. On the one hand therapies are involved which will probably meet with little or no success. Such treatment can be withdrawn or withheld for this reason. On the other hand there are cases in which therapies which can have a considerable (more than one month) life-prolonging effect but in which prolongation of life is undesirable or pointless and treatment is withdrawn or withheld for this reason.[119]

They add that doctors were asked to discuss 'only the second type'[120] of situation.

Thirdly, it seems clear that the question was so understood by at least some of the respondents, 35% of whom replied that their (primary or secondary) intention was to hasten death, not to withdraw a futile treatment.[121]

That the lives of so many patients were shortened without explicit request is striking. Hardly less striking is the fact that by no means all of the patients killed without request were incompetent. It will be recalled that of the 1000 actively killed without request, 14% were (according to the physician interviews) totally competent and a further 11% partly competent. Van der Wal has aptly commented that in these cases the right to self-determination was 'seriously undermined'.[122] Moreover, of the 8100 patients whose deaths are said to have been intentionally accelerated by palliative drugs, 60% (or 2867) of those who had never indicated anything about life termination were competent.[123] Finally, the patient was totally competent in 22%, and partly competent in a further 21%, of all the cases where treatment was withheld or withdrawn without request.[124]

The Commission concludes that the Survey 'disproves the assertion often expressed, that non-voluntary active termination of life occurs more frequently in the Netherlands than voluntary termination'.[125] However, if intentional termination by omission is included, as it should be if an accurate overall picture is to be presented, the Survey indicates that non-voluntary euthanasia is in fact more common than voluntary euthanasia. As Table 1 illustrates, the Survey discloses that in 1990 doctors intentionally sought to shorten more lives without than with the patient's explicit request. It was their primary aim to kill 10 558 patients, 5450 (52%) of whom had not explicitly asked to have their lives shortened. If one includes cases in which the patient's death is referred to as part of what the doctor aimed to achieve, then the total number of intentional killings by doctors may not be far short of 26 350, in 15 258 (58%) of which the patient had not explicitly asked for death to be hastened.

2. 'Intolerable suffering with no prospect of improvement' when euthanasia was a 'last resort'

(i) 'Intolerable suffering'. The Survey throws considerable doubt on whether euthanasia was confined to patients who were 'suffering unbearably' and for whom it was a 'last resort'.[126] For example, doctors were asked in interview which reason(s) patients most often gave for requesting euthanasia. Their replies to this question (and to that about the most important reasons for killing without request[127]) show that in most cases, 57%, it was 'loss of dignity';[128] in 46% 'not dying in a dignified way';[129] in 33% 'dependence'[130] and in 23% 'tiredness of life'.[131] Only 46% mentioned 'pain'.[132]

One recent case concerned a 50-year-old woman who had lost two sons, one to suicide, the other to cancer, and who repeatedly asked her psychiatrist, a Dr Chabot, to help her die. Dr Chabot assisted her to commit suicide and was prosecuted but acquitted. The prosecution's appeal to the Court of Appeal was unsuccessful but an appeal to the Supreme Court resulted in the doctor's conviction on the ground that the doctor should have ensured that one of the doctors he had consulted had personally examined the patient. A novel and disturbing feature of the case is that the woman was not terminally or, indeed, even physically ill. The suffering which was considered sufficient to warrant assisted suicide was purely mental, resulting from a 'depression in a narrower sense without psychotic characteristics in the context of a complicated grieving process'.[133]

In relation to cases of withholding or withdrawal of treatment without explicit request and with intent to hasten death, the basis for the decision appears to have been simply a belief that, in the words of the preamble to the question put, 'considerable prolongation of life'[134] was considered 'undesirable or even futile'.[135]

That Dutch doctors regard 'unbearable suffering' as an essential criterion is, moreover, hardly confirmed by the agreement of two thirds of those interviewed with the proposition that 'Everyone is entitled to decide over their own life and death'.[136]

(ii) A 'last resort'. Nor does it appear that euthanasia was invariably a 'last resort'. Doctors said that treatment alternatives remained in 1 in 5 cases (21%) but that, in almost all of these cases, they were refused.[137] One in three GPs who decided that there were no alternatives had not sought advice from a colleague.[138] When asked to rank the Guidelines in order of importance, only

64% of respondents said absence of treatment alternatives was '(very) important'.[139]

Moreover, even in the 4 out of 5 cases in which the doctors said there were no treatment alternatives, this appears to mean 'alternatives to the current treatment' rather than 'alternatives to euthanasia', an interpretation supported both by the question asked ('Were alternatives available to the treatment given? Here I consider other therapeutic possibilities or possibilities to alleviate pain and/or symptoms'[140]) and by the doctors' response to another question about the aim of the treatment at the time when the decision to carry out euthanasia or assisted suicide was made. Seventy-seven percent replied it was palliative, 10% life prolonging, and 2% curative: only 14% said there was no treatment.[141] In other words, just because there might have been no treatment alternatives to the existing treatment does not mean that the existing treatment was not an alternative to euthanasia.

But even *if* palliative treatment given in 77% of cases was not preventing intolerable suffering and was so ineffectual that euthanasia was thought to be the only alternative, does this (and the fact that in 46% of cases pain was one of the reasons most frequently given by patients as a reason for wanting euthanasia) not raise questions about the quality of the palliative care that the patients were receiving? A report on palliative care published in 1987 by the Dutch Health Council concluded that a majority of cancer patients in pain suffered unnecessarily because of health professionals' lack of expertise.[142] Similarly, more recent research into pain management at the Netherlands Cancer Institute, Amsterdam, contains the 'critical and worrisome overall finding . . . that pain management was judged to be inadequate in slightly more than 50% of evaluated cases'.[143]

Interestingly, 40% of the Dutch doctors interviewed in the van der Maas Survey expressed agreement with the proposition that 'Adequate alleviation of pain and/or symptoms and personal care of the dying patient make euthanasia unnecessary'.[144] Yet the Commission concludes that its total of 2700 cases of 'euthanasia' and assisted suicide shows that 'euthanasia' is not being used as an alternative to good palliative medicine or terminal care.[145] This observation is quite unsupported by the data, which reveal not 2700 but over 10 500 unambiguously euthanasiast acts and omissions. It also sits uneasily with the Commission's later observation about the inadequacy of such care in Holland:

> The research report shows that the medical decision process with regard to the end of life demands more and more expertise in a number of different areas. First of all medical and technical know-how, especially in the field of the

treatment of pain, of prognosis and of alternative options for the treatment of disorders that cause insufferable pain.[146]

It adds:

> Especially doctors, but nurses as well, will have to be trained in terminal care . . . Optimal care for someone who is dying implies that the doctor has knowledge of adequate treatments for pain, of alternatives for the treatment of complaints about unbearable pain and that he is aware of the moment when he must allow the process of dying to run its natural course. Doctors still lack sufficient knowledge of this care . . . In a country that is rated among the best in the world when it comes to birth care, knowledge with regard to care for the dying should not be lacking.[147]

If there is such a lack of knowledge, does this not confirm and help to explain the Survey evidence which indicates that euthanasia is being used as an alternative to appropriate palliative care?[148]

3. Performed by a doctor who has consulted an independent colleague and reported the case to the legal authorities

(i) Consultation. A KMNG-proposed scheme of consultation with two colleagues, one of whom is independent, has never been put into effect. Doctors stated that they had consulted a colleague in 84% of cases of euthanasia and assisted suicide.[149] The Survey does not explain the form, substance or outcome of the consultations. Again, in respect of the 1000 acts of life termination without request – cases where it might be assumed that consultation assumed especial importance – only a minority (48%) of doctors consulted a colleague.[150] Moreover, 40% of GPs stated that they did not think that consultation was very important.[151]

(ii) Reporting. Only a minority of cases of 'euthanasia' were duly reported to the legal authorities. In almost 3 out of 4 cases (72%) doctors (3 out of 4 GPs and 2 out of 3 specialists) certified that death was due to 'natural causes'.[152] By so doing, they not only failed to comply with one of the Guidelines whose importance has been continually stressed by the KNMG, but they also committed the criminal offence of falsifying a death certificate.

Doctors gave as their three most important reasons for falsifying the certificate the 'fuss' of a legal investigation (55%); a desire to protect relatives from a judicial inquiry (52%); and a fear of prosecution (25%).[153]

Similarly, virtually all of the 1000 acts of life termination without request were certified as natural deaths. The most important reasons given by the doctors were the 'fuss' of a legal investigation (47%); the (remarkable) opinion that the death was in fact natural (43%); and the desire to safeguard the relatives from a judicial inquiry (28%).[154]

Interestingly, only 64% of doctors thought that each case of euthanasia should somehow be examined, and the most favoured form of review was by other doctors.[155]

III. THE SLIDE IN PRACTICE AND THE SHIFT IN OPINION

My earlier article suggested that the 'slippery slope' argument in both its logical and practical forms applies to the Dutch experience of euthanasia.[156] The Survey and the Report serve amply to reinforce that contention. The examination of the Guidelines in Part I of this paper concluded that they are vague, loose and incapable of preventing abuse. The Survey bears out this conclusion by indicating that cardinal safeguards – requiring a request which is free and voluntary; well-informed; and durable and persistent – have been widely disregarded. Doctors have killed with impunity. And on a scale previously only guessed at: the Survey discloses that it was the primary purpose of doctors to shorten the lives of over 10 000 patients in 1990, the majority without the patient's explicit request.

How the Remmelink Commission can so confidently conclude, in the light of the evidence unearthed by the Survey, that the 'medical actions and decision process concerning the end of life are of high quality'[157] is puzzling. The Commission's assessment is based solely on the doctors' uncorroborated replies, replies which disclose, surely far more reliably, wholesale breach of the Guidelines. In particular, the scale of intentional life-shortening without explicit request and of illegal certification of death by natural causes must cast grave doubt both on the Commission's conclusion that decision-making is of 'high quality' and on van der Maas's opinion that the Survey shows that doctors are 'prepared to account for their decisions'.[158] As the 1000 cases of unrequested killings vividly illustrate, the existing system cannot realistically hope to detect the doctor who ignores the Guidelines since it essentially relies on him to expose his own wrongdoing.

Moreover, the Remmelink Report's narrow categories of 'euthanasia' and 'intentional killing without request' may suggest to those who have not considered it before a neat way of side-stepping the reporting procedure. A doctor might kill not by a iethal drug, which he would be required to report, but by an overdose of morphine or by withdrawing treatment, which he could claim with at least some show of legitimacy (in the unlikely event of being challenged) to be 'normal medical practice'.

Even though recent statistics indicate a significant increase in the number of cases reported (1424 in 1994[159]) it seems clear that the reporting procedure will continue to provide a wholly inadequate mechanism for regulating euthanasia and that the reports filed will continue to provide no more accurate a picture of the reality of euthanasia than they have hitherto done. Reports of killing without request promise to be particularly unrepresentative: how many doctors are likely to report a practice which has not (yet) been declared lawful by the courts?[160] Further, even if all cases were reported, this would still provide no guarantee of propriety; indeed, were all to be reported, it is doubtful whether prosecutors would have the resources to subject them even to the limited check which reports currently receive.

The Report uses the finding that doctors refused some 4000 serious requests[161] to argue that 'euthanasia' is not used excessively and as an alternative to good palliative care.[162] Leaving aside the evident shortcomings in Dutch terminal care, this is simply illogical, particularly when viewed against the 10 500 occasions on which it was the doctor's primary purpose to shorten life.

That statistic suggests rather the pertinence of the 'slippery slope' argument. The argument's relevance is indeed quite strongly suggested by the fact that doctors had as their primary aim the shortening of the lives of some 5500 patients without their explicit request (and are represented in the Survey as having had as their subordinate aim the shortening of the lives of upwards of a further 10 000 without their explicit request). The relevance is sufficiently striking even if one focuses simply on the 1000 cases involving the administration of a lethal drug without explicit request. Nor were these patients killed by a minority of maverick doctors: a majority of doctors admitted that they either had killed without request or would be prepared to do so.[163]

In any event, it is now apparent that legal and medical authorities in Holland openly condone non-voluntary euthanasia in certain circumstances. The Remmelink Report defends, it will be recalled,[164] the vast majority of the 1000 killings without request as 'care for the dying'.[165] Stating that the absence of a request only serves to make the decision more difficult than when there is a request, it adds:

> The ultimate justification for the intervention is in both cases the patient's unbearable suffering. So medically speaking, there is little difference between these situations and euthanasia, because in both cases patients are involved who suffer terribly. The absence of a special request for the termination of life stems partly from the circumstance that the party in question is not (any longer) able to express his will because he is already in the terminal stage, and partly because the demand for an explicit request is not in order when the

treatment of pain and symptoms is intensified. The degrading condition the patient is in, confronts the doctor with a case of force majeure. According to the commission, the intervention by the doctor can easily be regarded as an action that is justified by necessity, just like euthanasia.[166]

The classification of killing without request as 'care for the dying' could be criticised as tendentious euphemism and is inconsistent even with established Dutch terminology.[167] Moreover, in view of the importance which has long been attached by many Dutch proponents of euthanasia to the need for a request by the patient, it is remarkable that the Commission, rather than setting out a reasoned ethical case to substantiate its opinion that killing without request can be justified, should do scarcely more than simply assert that a request is no longer essential in all cases.

Nevertheless, the Dutch Parliament has implemented the Commission's recommendation that the reporting procedure for euthanasia should clearly allow for such cases. It has amended the Burial Act 1955 to set out the reporting procedure in statutory form, a form which makes it clear that the procedure is to be followed even in cases of euthanasia without request.[168] The amendment, which was passed in 1993 and came into force in June 1994, has not made euthanasia lawful but has enshrined the reporting procedure in statutory form.

Moreover, a committee of the KNMG set up to consider non-voluntary euthanasia has condoned the killing, in certain circumstances, of incompetent patients including babies and patients in persistent coma and has canvassed opinion on the killing of patients with severe dementia.[169] It is surely only a matter of time before such 'responsible' medical opinion receives judicial approval. Indeed, if the criterion for the availability of the defence of necessity is what accords with 'responsible' medical opinion, it is difficult to see how the courts could deny it. The authors of the van der Maas Survey, referring to the 1000 killings without explicit request, state that legally speaking there is no question that these cases should be seen as anything other than murder but that 'the possibility that a court will accept an appeal to force majeure cannot be ruled out'.[170] Similarly, Leenen has recently expressed the opinion (which seems to contradict his earlier opinion,[171] to which he does not refer) that in 'exceptional' cases non-voluntary euthanasia attracts the necessity defence.[172] The approval of the courts may not even be necessary: the Chief Prosecutors have already declined to prosecute in a number of cases of killing without request.

One such case involved a patient in a permanent coma after a heart attack. The local Chief Prosecutor, mindful of the Remmelink Commission's recommendation that such cases should be dealt with in the same way as killing on request, decided against prosecution; after questions had been raised in Parliament, his decision was affirmed at a meeting of all the Chief Prosecutors in February 1992.[173]

Another case concerned a dying, comatose 71-year-old man who had not asked for his life to be shortened. At a meeting in November 1992 the Chief Prosecutors decided against prosecution since 'the action taken . . . amounted to virtually the same as suspending ineffectual medical treatment',[174] even though they regarded the case as 'potentially extending the boundaries of current practice'.[175]

The current and growing condonation of non-voluntary euthanasia contrasts markedly with earlier pronouncements on euthanasia. There was little support for non-voluntary euthanasia in 1984. As has been seen, the very definition of 'euthanasia' adopted by the Dutch incorporated the need for a request. Moreover, the KNMG Report of that year was careful to confine itself to euthanasia on request and three of its five Guidelines were concerned with ensuring not only that there was a request but that it was free, well-considered and persistent. In 1985, a State Commission on Euthanasia concluded that third parties should not be permitted to request euthanasia on behalf of (incompetent) minors and 'other persons incapable of expressing their opinion, such as the mentally handicapped or senile elderly people'.[176] Its Vice-Chairman, Professor Leenen, has since written that the Commission proposed an amendment to the Penal Code to prohibit the intentional termination of an incompetent patient's life on account of serious physical or mental illness and did so in order to 'underline the importance of the request of the patient'.[177] In 1989, Leenen reaffirmed that a request was 'central' to the Dutch definition, adding:

> *Without it the termination of a life is murder.* This means that the family or other relatives, parents for their children, or the doctor cannot decide on behalf of the patient. *People who have become incompetent are no longer eligible for euthanasia,* unless they have made a living will prior to their becoming incompetent, in which they ask for the termination of life.[178]

He added that Article 2 of the European Convention for the Protection of Human Rights and Fundamental Freedoms, which provides that everyone's right to life shall be protected by law, does not (in his view) prohibit the killing of a patient who freely wishes to die but that it *'prohibits the State and others from taking another's life without his request'.*[179] Rejecting the argument that euthanasia would undermine the public's trust in doctors, he stated: 'People's trust in health care will not decrease if they are sure that

euthanasia will not be administered *without their explicit request*.[180] Leenen
was echoed in the same year by Henk Rigter, who wrote in the *Hastings
Center Report*: 'In the absence of a patient request the perpetrator renders
him or herself guilty of manslaughter or murder'.[181] An array of leading
Dutch advocates of voluntary euthanasia wrote endorsing the accuracy of
Rigter's paper, adding that 'problems concerning the termination of life of
incompetent patients, either comatose or newborn, are *not* part of the
euthanasia problem'.[182] One, the Director of the National Hospital Association,
wrote that 'euthanasia' meant killing on request, adding:

> Consequently, it is impossible for people who do not want euthanasia to be
> maneuvred or forced into it. The requirement of voluntariness means no one
> need fear that his or her life is in danger because of age or ill health, and that
> those who cannot express their will, such as psycho-geriatric patients or the
> mentally-handicapped, shall never be in danger as long as they live.[183]

But how much longer will they be allowed to live in view of the common
practice of, and growing support for, non-voluntary euthanasia? The
argument that euthanasia cannot be forced upon competent or incompetent
people, and that such conduct is not part of the euthanasia problem, because
it does not fall within the definition of 'euthanasia', is hardly convincing. If an
advocate of abortion were to define abortion as 'therapeutic' abortion and
dismiss arguments that its legalisation might lead to abortion for social
reasons, or to women being pressured into abortion, on the ground that these
would not be 'abortion' and are not, therefore, 'part of the abortion
problem', he would rightly be given short shrift. The suggestion, by leading
Dutch advocates of euthanasia, that the moral debate about euthanasia can
be resolved by definitional *fiat* serves only to illustrate the intellectual poverty
of the case for euthanasia which has come to prevail in their country.

The widespread readiness to kill without any request contrasts starkly with
the refusal of many serious requests for euthanasia, and serves further to
underline the dispensable role of patient autonomy in the reality, if not the
rhetoric, of the Dutch experience. As ten Have and Welie shrewdly point out,
acceptance of euthanasia is not resulting in greater patient autonomy but in
doctors 'acquiring even more power over the life and death of their patients'.[184]

In 1990 Professor Leenen observed that there is an 'almost total lack of
control on the administration of euthanasia' in Holland.[185] The Report and
the Survey serve only to confirm the accuracy of that observation.[186] The
Commission's Report paints a reassuring picture of the euthanasia landscape
revealed by the Survey, but the scene it depicts is grossly misleading. As Dan
Callahan has pointed out, the reality is quite different: 'The Dutch situation is

a regulatory Potemkin village, a great façade hiding non-enforcement'.[187] The hard evidence of the Survey indicates that, within a remarkably short time, the Dutch have proceeded from voluntary to non-voluntary euthanasia. This is partly because of the inability of the vague and loose Guidelines to ensure that euthanasia is only performed in accordance with the criteria laid down by the courts and the KNMG. It is also because the underlying justification for euthanasia in Holland appears not to be patient self-determination, but rather acceptance of the principle that certain lives are not 'worth' living and that it is right to terminate them. Indeed, the authors of the van der Maas Survey recently lent support to this thesis when they wrote:

> [Is] it not true that once one accepts euthanasia and assisted suicide, the principle of universalizability forces one to accept termination of life without explicit request, at least in some circumstances, as well? In our view the answer to this question must be affirmative.[188]

An objection might be raised that the number of cases has remained static and that the evidence reveals not a slope but a plateau. This objection fails, however, to dent the slippery slope argument in its logical form. Indeed, even the empirical form of the argument is, arguably, not dependent on showing a statistical *in*crease in non-voluntary euthanasia over time. Even if the proportion of non-voluntary euthanasia cases remained stable from the time voluntary euthanasia gained approval, this would hardly disprove either the logical connection or the ineffectiveness of the safeguards; quite the contrary. There would appear, in any event, to be no empirical evidence to support the hypothesis of a plateau. Moreover, the hypothesis seems particularly implausible in the light of the available statistical evidence and the clear shift in opinion since 1984 in favour of the non-voluntary termination of life.

That the evidence from Holland lends support to the 'slippery slope' arguments should come as no surprise. Some twenty years ago a perspicacious warning about the dangers of venturing onto the slope was sounded by Dr John Habgood, now Archbishop of York and a member of the House of Lords Select Committee on Medical Ethics which reported early in 1994:[189]

> Legislation to permit euthanasia would in the long run bring about profound changes in social attitudes towards death, illness, old age and the role of the medical profession. The Abortion Act has shown what happens. Whatever the rights and wrongs concerning the present practice of abortion, there is no doubt about two consequences of the 1967 Act:
> (a) The safeguards and assurances given when the Bill was passed have to a considerable extent been ignored.
> (b) Abortion has now become a live option for *anybody* who is pregnant. This

does not imply that everyone who is facing an unwanted pregnancy automatically attempts to procure an abortion. But because abortion is now on the agenda, the climate of opinion in which such a pregnancy must be faced has radically altered.

One could expect similarly far-reaching and potentially more dangerous consequences from legalized euthanasia.[190]

However, the patent reality of the slide in Holland may not yet be fully appreciated outside (or, indeed, inside) that country. The slide was not *explicitly* identified and criticised by the House of Lords Select Committee on Medical Ethics, even though a delegation from the Committee visited Holland in October 1993. Perhaps the delegation was influenced by the statement made to them by a Ministry of Justice spokesman that 'the government held strongly to the position that euthanasia was not possible for incompetent patients'.[191] This statement was made eight months after the proposed change in the law to provide a mechanism for the reporting of non-voluntary euthanasia had been approved by the Second Chamber of the Dutch Parliament and one month before its approval by the First Chamber. If euthanasia was 'not possible' for incompetent patients, why was the government providing for its reporting?

A welcome recognition of the slide is, however, clearly implicit in the Committee's rejection of the legalisation of euthanasia, in the light of the Dutch experience, on the ground, *inter alia*, 'that it would not be possible to frame adequate safeguards against non-voluntary euthanasia'.[192] Moreover, in the debate on the motion to receive the Report in the Lords, the Committee's Chairman, Lord Walton, observed that those members of the Committee who had visited Holland returned from the visit 'feeling uncomfortable, especially in the light of evidence indicating that non-voluntary euthanasia . . . was commonly performed'.[193] He added that they were 'particularly uncomfortable'[194] about the case of the woman of 50 suffering from mental stress who had been assisted in suicide by her psychiatrist. His Lordship could, of course, have gone much further but took the view (without saying why) that it would not be proper for him to criticize the decisions of the 'medical and legal authorities in another sovereign state'.[195]

Another member of the Committee to comment unfavourably on the Dutch experience, Lord Meston, said:

> it did not seem possible to find any other place beyond the existing law for a firm foothold on an otherwise slippery slope. The evidence of the Dutch experience was not encouraging: in the Netherlands, which apparently lacks much in the way of a hospice movement, there seems to be a gap between the

theory and practice of voluntary euthanasia. One cannot escape the fear that the same could happen here, with pressures on the vulnerable sick and elderly, who may perceive themselves to have become a burden on others, and pressures on the doctors and nurses from relatives and from those who are concerned with resources.[196]

Of course, the reality of the slippery slope may not have been lost on at least some Dutch advocates of voluntary euthanasia, who may have thought it tactically desirable to maintain a discreet silence about it. Professor Alexander Capron, reporting on a euthanasia conference in Holland at which this point was conceded, has written that the Dutch proponents of euthanasia began with a narrow definition of euthanasia 'as a strategy for winning acceptance of the general practice, which would then turn to . . . relief of suffering as its justification in cases in which patients are unable to request euthanasia'.[197] He adds: 'It was an instance, or so it seemed to me, when the candour of our hosts was a little chilling'.[198]

CONCLUSION

The evidence marshalled in this chapter indicates, consistently with that unearthed by others,[199] that the Dutch euthanasia experience lends weighty support to the slippery slope argument in both its forms. Within a decade, the so-called strict safeguards against the slide have proved signally ineffectual; non-voluntary euthanasia is now widely practised and increasingly condoned in the Netherlands. For inhabitants of such a flat country, the Dutch have proved remarkably fast skiers.

As this book goes to press, it is reported that a Dutch court has, as predicted above, held that non-voluntary euthanasia can be lawful. The Alkmaar district court has held (in a case referred to in note 175) that a doctor charged with murder for killing a disabled newborn at the parents' request 'had made a choice which – given the special circumstances of the case – can reasonably be considered justifiable' and enjoyed the defence of necessity.[200] The slide continues apace.

NOTES

1 For an exposition of the argument in its logical form see Luke Gormally's chapter in this book. See also Yale Kamisar, 'Some Non-Religious Views against Proposed "Mercy-Killing" Legislation' (1958) 42 *Minnesota Law Review* 969.

2 *Stedman's Medical Dictionary* (25th ed., 1990) 544. See also n. 72.

3 P.J. van der Maas *et al.*, *Euthanasia and other Medical Decisions Concerning the End of Life* (Amsterdam: Elsevier, 1992) 5. Hereafter 'Survey'. Also published in (1992) 22(1)/(2) *Health Policy*. A summary of the Survey appears in (1991) 338 *Lancet* 669.

4 Though a Report of the KNMG on euthanasia states: 'All activities or non-activities with the purpose to terminate a patient's life are defined as euthanasia'. 'Vision on Euthanasia' (a translation by the KNMG in 1986 of its Report 'Standpunt inzake euthanasie' published in (1984) 39 *Medisch Contact* 990) 15.

5 *Nederlandse Jurisprudentie* ('*N.J.*') (1985) No. 106, 451 452. See also I. J. Keown, 'The Law and Practice of Euthanasia in The Netherlands' (1992) 108 *Law Quarterly Review* 51, 51–57.

6 *N.J.* (1985) No. 106, 453.

7 Ibid.

8 Ibid.

9 Ibid.

10 Keown, op. cit. n.5, 56.

11 Op. cit. n.4.

12 Ibid., 8–11.

13 'Guidelines for Euthanasia' (translated by W. Lagerwey) (1988) 2 *Issues in Law & Medicine* 429. Hereafter 'Guidelines'.

14 Henk Rigter, 'Euthanasia in The Netherlands: Distinguishing Facts from Fiction' (1989) 19(1) *Hastings Center Report* 31.

15 H. J. J. Leenen, 'The Definition of Euthanasia' (1984) 3 *Medicine and Law* 333, 334.

16 Interview by author with Dr Herbert Cohen, 26 July 1989.

17 Survey, 3.

18 Ibid., 4.

19 Ibid., 19–20.

20 Ibid., 20.

21 *Medische beslissingen rond het levenseinde. Rapport van de Commissie onderzoek medische praktijk inzake euthanasie* ('s-Gravenhage: Sdu Uitgeverij, 1991). Hereafter 'Report'.

22 *Medische beslissingen rond het levenseinde. Het onderzoek voor de Commissie Onderzoek Medische Praktijk inzake Euthanasie* ('s-Gravenhage: Sdu Uitgeverij, 1991).

23 Op. cit. n.3. Oddly, the Report has not been translated, though a brief English summary has been produced by the Ministry of Justice: *Outlines [sic] Report Commission Inquiry into Medical Practice with regard to Euthanasia* (nd). Hereafter 'Outline'. Dr Richard Fenigsen's unpublished 'First Reactions to the Report of the Committee on Euthanasia' (1991) contains a translation of key passages of the Report. I am grateful to Dr Fenigsen for permission to rely on his translation. His paper 'The Right of the Dutch Governmental Committee on Euthanasia' is published in (1991) 7 *Issues in Law & Medicine* 3.

24 Op. cit. n.5.

25 Ibid., 61–78.

26 See generally Survey, Part II (chapters 4–10).

27 Ibid., 14–17; 191. The authors considered whether those who refused to participate formed a select group which could lead to serious bias and concluded that, in the light of the total number of refusals (41) and the variety of reasons for refusing (mainly lack of time) this could hardly be so. The 15 who indicated that they disapproved of the Survey, did not wish to comment or opposed euthanasia could only have introduced a 'very modest' bias. Ibid., 228. This reasoning is unpersuasive: does the conclusion excluding bias not depend on answers which are unverified? Is it not possible that some of the 41 who declined to participate frequently performed euthanasia and equally possible that some of these cases fell outside the Guidelines?

28 Ibid., 33.

29 See generally ibid., Part III (chapters 11–13).

30 Ibid., 15; 121–125; 191.

31 See generally ibid., Part IV (chapters 14–15).

32 Ibid., 15; 149–151; 192.

33 Ibid., 160.

34 Ibid., 16.

35 Report, 14.

36 Ibid., 11 (see also Outline, 2); 'the purposeful acting to terminate life by someone other than the person concerned upon request of the latter'. Survey, 5; see also ibid., 23; 193.

37 Survey, 178.

38 Ibid.

39 Ibid., 162.

40 Ibid.
41 Ibid., 178.
42 Ibid., 179.
43 Ibid., 40, table 5.3.
44 Ibid., 182. The third study returned a figure of 1.6%. Ibid., 181.
45 Ibid., 71. The authors were not concerned with cases where palliative drugs were used which had no chance of shortening life. Ibid., 72. Life was shortened by up to one week in 70% of cases and by one to four weeks in 23%. Ibid., 73 table 7.3.
46 Ibid., 183.
47 Ibid., 72, table 7.2.
48 Ibid.
49 Ibid.
50 Ibid., 85; 90, table 8.14.
51 Ibid., 90, table 8.15.
52 Ibid.
53 Ibid.
54 Ibid., 81.
55 Ibid., 84, table 8.7.
56 Ibid., 82, table 8.6.
57 Report, 31; Outline, 2.
58 See n.36. (Emphasis added.)
59 Ibid. (Emphasis added.)
60 Op. cit. n.4, 15.
61 Ibid.
62 Ibid. (Emphasis added.)
63 Survey, 21. They state, confusingly, that death 'may not' have been intended in the third category.
64 Ibid.
65 Ibid.
66 Ibid.
67 Ibid.
68 By no means all of the patients from whom treatment was withdrawn on request were terminal. Life was shortened by one to four weeks in 16%, by one to six months in 43% and even longer in 13%. Ibid., 82, table 8.6. Moreover, three of the four reasons most frequently given by the patient for requesting withdrawal – 'loss of dignity' (31%), 'tiredness of life' (28%) and 'dependence' (24%): ibid., 82, table 8.4 – appear (unlike the remaining reason – 'burden of treatment' (43%)) quite consistent with a suicide intent. However, as the respondent doctors were not given the

opportunity of stating that they withheld or withdrew treatment merely foreseeing that life would be shortened, the figures indicating that doctors intended to shorten life in *all* cases should be treated with some caution, and their categorisation here as cases of euthanasiast omissions is subject to this *caveat*.
69 Ibid., 72.
70 Ibid.
71 Interview by author with Mr A. Kors, Ministry of Justice, The Hague, 29 November 1991.
72 *Euthanasia and Clinical Practice: The Report of a Working Party* (The Linacre Centre, 1982) 2. See also *Dictionary of Medical Ethics* (A. S. Duncan, G. R. Dunstan, R. B. Welbourn eds; 1981) 164 ('. . . "mercy killing", the administration of a drug deliberately and specifically to accelerate death in order to terminate suffering'); and text at n.2.
73 Survey, 73, table 7.2; ibid., 90, table 8.15.
74 Ibid., 40, table 5.3.
75 P.J. van der Maas *et al.*, 'Dances with Data' (1993) 7 *Bioethics* 323.
76 See text at nn.41–42.
77 Op. cit. n.75, 325.
78 Ibid.
79 Ibid.
80 Ibid.
81 Ibid., 325–326.
82 Ibid., 326.
83 Ibid.
84 Ibid.
85 Ninety-eight per cent of doctors stated that they were aware of the 'rules of due care' formulated by the KNMG, the Health Council and the Government. When asked what they were, 89% mentioned consultation but only 66% the need for a seriously considered request; 42% a voluntary request; 37% 'unacceptable' suffering; and 18% a long-standing desire to die. Survey, 95–96, table 9.1. When shown 14 Guidelines, however, and asked to rank them in importance, 98% mentioned voluntariness and only 67% consultation. Ibid., table 9.2.
86 Ibid., 50, table 5.15.
87 Ibid.

88 Ibid.

89 Ibid.

90 Ibid., 43. A smaller, postal survey of euthanasia by nursing home physicians between 1986 and 1990 revealed that in over 1 in 5 cases euthanasia was administered less than a week after the first discussion with the patient (in 7% of cases in less than a day) and in 35% of cases less than a week after the first request. M. T. Muller *et al.*, 'Voluntary Active Euthanasia and Physician-Assisted Suicide in Dutch Nursing Homes: Are the Requirements for Prudent Practice Properly Met?' (1994) 42 *Journal of the American Geriatrics Society* 624, 626, table 2. Hereafter 'Muller'.

91 Survey, 108, table 10.3. (By contrast, 96% of specialists and nursing home doctors consulted nursing staff. Ibid.) Further, two thirds of GPs said they felt it was up to the doctors in certain circumstances to raise the topic of euthanasia. Ibid., 101.

92 Ibid., 182.

93 Ibid.

94 Ibid.

95 Outline, 3.

96 Ibid.

97 Ibid.

98 Ibid.

99 Ibid.

100 Ibid.

101 Ibid.

102 Ibid.

103 Ibid.

104 Seventy-five per cent of the patients were 'totally unable to assess the situation and take a decision adequately'. However, 14% were totally, and 11% partly ('not totally') able to do so. Survey, 61, table 6.4. The authors describe a person 'not totally able' as 'partially able to assess the situation and on this basis adequately take a decision'. Ibid., 23. According to the death certificate study, 36% were competent. Loes Pijnenborg *et al.*, 'Life-terminating Acts without Explicit Request of Patient' (1993) 341 *Lancet* 1196, 1197, table II.

105 Survey, 66, table 6.10. According to the

Survey's (tentative) definition of 'dying' (ibid, 24), therefore, in only 29% of the 2700 cases of euthanasia and assisted suicide was the patient dying. Ibid., 49, table 5.13.

106 Ibid., 64, table 6.7.

107 Ibid.

108 Ibid. Surprisingly, no question was asked about the doctor's intention which, as the authors note, 'complicates the interpretation of the results'. Ibid., 57.

109 Henk Jochemsen, 'Euthanasia in Holland: An Ethical Critique of the New Law' (1994) 20 *Journal of Medical Ethics* 212 at 213.

110 Outline, 6. The Commission excepted from this recommendation cases where 'the vital functions have already and irreversibly begun to fail' on the ground that in such cases a natural death would have ensued anyway. Ibid. The Government has rejected this exception: see Gevers, op. cit. n.111, 140.

111 J. K. M. Gevers, 'Legislation on Euthanasia: recent Developments in the Netherlands' (1992) 18 *Journal of Medical Ethics* 138, 139–40. See text at n.168.

112 Survey, 76, table 7.9.

113 Ibid.

114 In 17% of cases, the patient had indicated something about life termination but the 'request was not strongly explicit'. Ibid. If these cases are included, the number of cases of life shortening without explicit request becomes 6885. In only 15% of cases, therefore, was there a 'strongly explicit' request. Ibid.

115 See text at nn.52–53. In 18% of cases the patient had 'indicated something at some time about terminating life' and in a further 13% there had been some discussion with the patient. Survey, 88, table 8.11.

116 Outline, 3–4.

117 Survey, 24.

118 Ibid., 84–85.

119 Ibid., 85.

120 Ibid.

121 See text at nn.52–53.

122 Gerrit van der Wal, 'Unrequested Termi-

nation of Life: Is It Permissible?' (1993) 7
Bioethics 330, 337.

123 Survey, 77.

124 Ibid., 88. The Survey does not appear to
provide separate figures for those whose
lives were intentionally shortened.

125 Outline, 3; Report, 33.

126 The Commission states that Dutch doctors
regard the 'intolerable suffering of the
patient and/or his natural desire for a
quiet death' as the only grounds on which
to perform euthanasia. Ibid., 32. The
reference to these grounds in the alternative, without disapproval, is revealing: it
confirms that neither all doctors nor the
Commission regard both as essential for
euthanasia to be permissible.

127 See text at nn.106–108.

128 Survey, 45, table 5.8.

129 Ibid.

130 Ibid.

131 Ibid.

132 Similarly, Muller found that the most
common main reason for requesting euthanasia was not 'unbearable suffering'
but 'fear of/avoidance of deterioration of
condition'. Muller, 626, table 3. Nor is
this clearly defined. Muller *et al.* observe
that it means the 'gradual effacement and
loss of personal identity that characterizes
the end of stages [*sic*] of many terminal
illnesses'. Ibid., 628. Further, earlier in
the paper (at 624) they state that requests
arising from fear of pain 'must be refused'.
This makes it even more difficult to
understand why fear of deterioration
should be acceptable.

133 'een depressie in engere zin, zonder psy-
chotische kenmerken, in het kader van
een gecompliceerd rouwproces'. Hoge
Raad, 21 June 1994, Strafkamer, nr. 96.972.
para. 4.5. The Supreme Court rejected the
prosecution's submissions that necessity
required somatic pain and that a psychiatric patient could not make a genuine
request for death. It held, however, that
in cases where the suffering was not
somatic, a proper factual basis for the
necessity defence could be laid only where
the patient had been examined by an

independent doctor who had assessed the
gravity of the suffering and possibilities
for its alleviation. As the Appeal Court
had not made such a finding in this case it
had not been in a position to conclude
that a situation of necessity existed.
Although the doctor's conviction was
restored, he was not punished. For commentaries on the case see T. Schalken,
N.J. (1994) No. 656, 3256–59; J.H.
Hubben, *Nederlands Juristenblad* (1994)
No. 27, 912; H.J.J. Leenen, *Tijdschrift
voor Gezondheidsrecht* (1994) No. 1, 48.

134 Survey, 85.

135 Ibid. For example, the evidence in relation
to the 8750 cases in which doctors stated
that they withheld or withdrew treatment
without request with intent to shorten life
does not indicate that all the patients
were suffering unbearably and that euthanasia was a last resort. For one thing,
58% were incompetent, so how was the
doctor able to assess the extent of the
patients' suffering (if any), particularly as
the patients' conditions varied? Survey,
88, table 8.12.

136 Ibid., 102, table 9.7.

137 Ibid., 45, table 5.7.

138 Ibid., 43. Even in those cases where the
doctors (two thirds of GPs and 80% of
specialists) did consult, there is nothing
to suggest that the colleague consulted
was a specialist in palliative medicine.

139 Ibid., 96, table 9.2.

140 Ibid., 43.

141 Ibid., 45, table 5.6. Why 14% were
receiving no treatment is unexplained.

142 Op. cit. n.5, 65. The British Medical
Association Working Party on Euthanasia
commented that palliative care in Holland
is not as advanced as in Britain. *Euthanasia*
(London: BMA, 1988) 49.

143 Karin L. Dorrepaal *et al.*, 'Pain Experience
and Pain Management among Hospitalized
Cancer Patients' (1989) 63 *Cancer* 593,
598. Referring to this study, Zbigniew
Zylic, Medical Director at Holland's
newest hospice, comments that it does
not warrant a general judgment about
terminal care in Holland but should be

taken as a warning and a stimulus for further studies. He notes that 'cancer pain treatment and symptom control does not receive enough attention and in many places, it is practised at a very poor level. As yet, there is no specific training available in palliative care'. 'The Story Behind the Blank Spot', (July/August 1993) 10 *American Journal of Hospice & Palliative Care* 30, 32. He adds that there are no comprehensive hospices in Holland because the high standard of care in hospitals and nursing-homes and the Government's policy to reduce institutional beds have combined to discourage the hospice system. While hospitals are officially encouraged to provide hospice care, the necessary resources are not provided. Zylic urges the establishment of more hospices. Ibid., 33–34.

144 Survey, 102, table 9.7.

145 Outline, 2; Report, 31.

146 Outline, 7.

147 Ibid.

148 An expert committee of the World Health Organization has concluded: 'now that a practicable alternative to death in pain exists, there should be concentrated efforts to implement programmes of palliative care, rather than a yielding to pressure for legal euthanasia'. *Cancer Pain Relief and Palliative Care* (Geneva: WHO, Technical Report Series No. 804, 1990). Dr Pieter Admiraal, one of Holland's leading practitioners of euthanasia, has written that 'in most cases, pain can be adequately controlled without the normal psychological functions of the patient being adversely affected'. 'Justifiable Euthanasia' (1988) 3 *Issues in Law & Medicine* 361, 362.

149 Survey, 47, table 5.9.

150 Ibid., 64, table 6.8. The reason given for not doing so in 68% of cases was that the doctor felt no need for consultation because the situation was clear. Ibid., 65. Before withholding or withdrawing a treatment without request, doctors consulted a colleague in 54% of cases. Ibid., 89, table 8.13. (When there was a request the figure was 43%. Ibid., 82, table 8.5.) Before

administering palliative drugs in such doses as might shorten life, doctors consulted in 47% of cases. Ibid., 73, table 7.4.

151 Ibid., 96, table 9.2. Muller's survey revealed that, of the doctors consulted, only two thirds talked with the patient, only half studied the medical records and only 17% physically examined the patient. Muller, 627.

152 Survey, 49, table 5.14. Muller found that in 57% of cases doctors certified a natural death. Muller, 628, table 7.

153 Survey, 48. The authors add that 23 doctors actually stated that they had regarded the death as natural.

154 Ibid., 65. Deaths hastened by withholding or withdrawing a treatment without request were almost all certified as natural deaths. Ibid., 89. So too were all deaths hastened by the administration of palliative drugs, in over 90% of cases because the doctor felt the death was natural, but in 9% because he felt that reporting an unnatural death would be 'troublesome'. Ibid., 74.

155 Ibid., 97, table 9.3. See also ibid., 98. It merits mention that in a small number of cases the lethal drug was administered by someone other than the doctor, nurse or patient. See ibid., 140, table 13.10; 143; 193.

156 Op. cit. n.5.

157 Outline, 6. Remarkably, van der Maas also regards them of 'good quality'. Survey, 199. According to the replies to Muller's survey, all the requirements were met in only 41% of cases. Muller, 628. Even this figure, based as it is on self-serving replies, may well be too high.

158 Survey, 205.

159 *See Table at end of these notes.*

160 Op. cit. n.111, 140.

161 Survey, 52.

162 Outline, 2.

163 Survey, 58, table 6.1.

164 See text at nn.99–103.

165 A member of the Commission informed me that these killings came as a 'terrible shock' to its members, who had hoped that they did not exist. Interview by author with Mr A. Kors, 29 November

1991. This makes the Commission's defence of the bulk of these killings all the more puzzling.

166 Outline, 3.

167 See text at nn.178; 181.

168 See *Report of the Select Committee on Medical Ethics* (HL 21-I of 1993–94) appendix 3, 65.

169 Henk Jochemsen, 'Life-prolonging and Life-terminating Treatment of Severely Handicapped Newborn Babies . . .'(1992) 8 *Issues in Law & Medicine* 167; *Doen of laten?* (Utrecht: Nederlandse Vereniging voor Kindergeneeskunde, 1992) 13; 'Dutch Doctors Support Life Termination in Dementia' (1993) 306 BMJ 1364.

170 Johannes J. M. van Delden *et al.*, 'The Remmelink Study: Two Years Later' (1993) 23(6) *Hastings Center Report* 24, 25; cf. Loes Pijnenborg *et al.*, 'Life-terminating Acts without Explicit Request of Patient' (1993) 341 *Lancet* 1196, 1199, where they write that, when all the 'safeguards' are respected and 'only the best interests of the patient are taken into account' such killings are 'certainly not murder'.

171 See text at nn.177–180.

172 H. J. J. Leenen and Chris Ciesielski-Carlucci, '*Force Majeure* (Legal Necessity): Justification for Active Termination of Life in the Case of Severely Handicapped Newborns after Forgoing Treatment' (1993) 2(3) *Cambridge Quarterly of Healthcare Ethics* 271, 274.

173 Personal communication, Staff Office of the Public Prosecutor, The Hague, 12 February 1993.

174 Ibid.

175 Ibid. A third case involved the killing of a 4-year-old handicapped child who was dying. Charges were dropped 'in view of the specific and unusual circumstances of the case, despite the fact that the patient had not expressly requested intervention'. Ibid. It has since been reported that two doctors who allegedly killed gravely ill newborns are to be prosecuted by order of the Minister of Justice in order to ascertain the law relating to non-voluntary

euthanasia. *The Times*, 23 December 1994.

176 H. J. J. Leenen, 'Euthanasia, Assistance to Suicide and the Law: Developments in the Netherlands' (1987) 8 *Health Policy* 197, 204.

177 Ibid.

178 H. J. J. Leenen, 'Dying with Dignity: Developments in the Field of Euthanasia in the Netherlands' (1989) 8 *Medicine and Law* 517, 520. (Emphasis added.)

179 Ibid., 519. (Emphasis added.)

180 Ibid. (Emphasis added.)

181 Op. cit. n.14, 31.

182 Letters (1989) 19(6) *Hastings Center Report* 47–48. (Original emphasis.)

183 Ibid., 48.

184 Henk A. M. J. ten Have and Jos V. M. Welie, 'Euthanasia: Normal Medical Practice?' (1992) 22(2) *Hastings Center Report* 34, 38. See also Jos V. M. Welie, 'The Medical Exception: Physicians, Euthanasia and the Dutch Criminal Law' (1992) 17 *Journal of Medicine and Philosophy* 419, 435.

185 'Legal Aspects of Euthanasia, Assistance to Suicide and Terminating the Medical Treatment of Incompetent Patients' (Unpublished paper delivered at a conference on Euthanasia held at the Institute for Bioethics, Maastricht, 2–4 December 1990) 6.

186 The author of the Remmelink Report agreed that there was no control over cases which had not been reported and that, even in relation to the reported cases, the prosecutor did not know whether the doctor was telling the truth. He maintained that euthanasia occurred even if the law prohibited it, as was the case outside Holland, and that it was preferable to try to control it. Interview by author with Mr A. Kors, 29 November 1991.

187 *The Troubled Dream of Life* (New York: Simon & Schuster, 1993) 115.

188 Op. cit. n.170, 26. (Footnote omitted.)

189 *Report of the Select Committee on Medical Ethics* HL Paper 21-I of 1993–94.

190 Rt Rev. J. S. Habgood, 'Euthanasia – A Christian View' [1974] 3 *Journal of the Royal Society of Health* 124, 126. The

Abortion Act 1967 decriminalised abortion where, in the opinion of two registered medical practitioners, the continuance of the pregnancy involved risk to the life, or to the physical or mental health of the mother, greater than if the pregnancy were terminated, or where there was a substantial risk that if the child were born it would be seriously handicapped.

191 Op. cit. n.189, appendix 3, 68.

192 Ibid., 49.

193 (1993–94) 554 Parl. Deb. H.L. col. 1345, 1346.

194 Ibid. See text at n.133.

195 (1993–94) Parl. Deb. H.L. col. 1346.

196 Ibid., col. 1398. In a recent decision of the Canadian Supreme Court rejecting an alleged right to assisted suicide in Canadian law, Mr Justice Sopinka, delivering the majority judgment, noted the 'worrisome

trend' in Holland toward euthanasia without request, which supported the view that 'a relaxation of the absolute prohibition takes us down the "slippery slope"'. *Rodriguez v. Attorney-General* (1994) 107 D.L.R. (4th) 342 at 403.

197 Alexander Morgan Capron, 'Euthanasia and Assisted Suicide' (1992) 22(2) *Hastings Center Report* 30, 31.

198 Ibid.

199 See e.g., Carlos F. Gomez, *Regulating Death: Euthanasia and the Case of the Netherlands* (New York: Free Press, 1991); the colloquy in (1992) 22(2) *Hastings Center Report*; cf. Margaret Battin 'Voluntary Euthanasia and the Risks of Abuse: Can We Learn Anything from the Netherlands?' (1992) 20 *Law, Medicine & Health Care* 133.

200 *The Independent*, 27 April 1995.

Note 159. *The following table of disposals in euthanasia cases has been translated from the annual report of the public prosecutor for 1994 (Jaaverslaag Openbaar Ministerie 1994, Ministerie van Justitie, Den Haag, 1995).*

Year	Non-prosecution	Prosecution	Non-prosecution after judicial investigation	Prosecution taken further
1984	16	1	0	0
1985	26	4	1	0
1986	81	0	1	2
1987	122	2	1	1
1988	181	2	1	0
1989	336	1	1	0
1990	454	0	0	0
1991	590	1	0	0
1992	1318	4	1	0
1993	1303	15[a]	1	0
1994	1417	7	12	2

[a]The relatively high number of decisions not to prosecute following judicial investigation concerns cases which were reconsidered taking account of the *Chabot* decision (see text at n. 133).

[22]

Assisted Suicide in the Netherlands: The *Chabot* Case

*John Griffiths**

In earlier decisions the Dutch Supreme Court has recognised a defence of 'necessity,'[1] under narrowly-defined circumstances, to a charge of performing euthanasia.[2] Its most recent decision deals with assistance with suicide in the case of a person whose suffering is not of somatic origin. The case is of general interest and has been widely (and not always accurately) invoked in discussions outside the Netherlands. It therefore seems useful to make the Court's decision itself available in English.

The decision of the Supreme Court is presented below. All but some purely formal passages have been translated directly and in full. Direct translation is indicated by quotation marks. All footnotes have been added. The statement of facts is taken from the decision of the Court of Appeals.

The translation is followed by some comments on the decision itself and on some of the reactions to it, ending with a brief reflection on the question: what is slipping from where to where on the notorious 'slippery slope'?

Office of Public Prosecutions v *Chabot*[3]

Supreme Court of the Netherlands, Criminal Chamber, 21 June 1994, nr 96.972. Judges Haak (Vice-President), Mout, Davids, Van Erp Taalman Kip-Nieuwenkamp and Schipper [*Nederlandse Jurisprudentie* 1994, nr 656; *Tijdschrift voor Gezondheidsrecht* 1994/96, nr 47].

1 Procedure

The appeal[4] is from the Court of Appeals, Leeuwarden (30 September 1993), which (like the District Court, Assen, 21 April 1993) found the defendant not

---

*Faculty of Law, University of Groningen.

1 There is a translation difficulty in connection with the legal concept *noodtoestand*. The technically correct translation is '(situation of) necessity,' and the defence of necessity is, in general terms, the same in Dutch law as in the common law. However, in the case of euthanasia the 'necessity' which has been recognised by the Dutch courts is not a general necessity but a specifically *medical* one, measured in terms of the state of medical knowledge and the professional norms of doctors, and it seems clear that no one but a doctor can successfully invoke it. There is, therefore, an argument to be made for translating the term as 'medical necessity.'

2 For current Dutch law on the subject, see Griffiths, 'The Regulation of Euthanasia and Related Medical Procedures that Shorten Life in the Netherlands' (1994) 1 Med Law Int 137–158; Griffiths, 'Recent Developments in the Netherlands Concerning Euthanasia and Other Medical Behavior that Shortens Life' (1994) 1 Med Law Int 347–386, referred to in subsequent notes as Griffiths 1994a and Griffiths 1994b respectively.

3 In the translation of this judgment I have had the invaluable critical assistance of several highly qualified Dutch experts.

4 Technically, request for cassation. The facts as found by the court below are taken as established and, when the prosecution appeals, only those issues specifically presented in the request for cassation are considered by the Supreme Court. In general, if the judgment below is found legally incorrect, the case is assigned to a different Court of Appeals for a new decision.

guilty[5] of the offence charged: 'intentionally assisting another person to commit suicide' as prohibited by Article 294 of the Criminal Code.[6] The Court of Appeals found the defence of necessity well-founded and the question on appeal is whether the Court's interpretation of the scope of the defence was legally correct and whether the facts as found support the decision.

The appeal was brought by the Solicitor General of the Court of Appeals. E.Ph.R. Sutorius represents the accused. The brief of the Advocate General of the Supreme Court, L.C.M. Meijers, recommends rejecting the appeal.

2   Facts

The following facts were established by the Court of Appeals.[7]

The defendant is a psychiatrist who on 28 September 1991 supplied to Mrs B, at her request, lethal drugs which she consumed in the presence of the defendant, a family doctor[8] and her friend Mrs H. She died half an hour later. The defendant reported her death the same day to the local coroner as a suicide which he had assisted. He included what the Court of Appeals characterises as an 'extensive report' of the case, with 'a very detailed account of the discussions with Mrs B (and her sister and brother-in-law), a report of the psychiatric investigation and the defendant's diagnosis, his considerations concerning Mrs B's bereavement process and her refusal of treatment.'

Mrs B was 50 years old. She had married at the age of 22 but the marriage was, from the beginning, not a happy one. She had two sons, Patrick and Rodney. In 1986 her older son, Patrick, committed suicide while in military service in Germany. From that time on her marital problems grew worse and the relationship more violent, and her wish to end her life began to manifest itself. According to her own statements, she only remained alive to care for her other son Rodney. These circumstances led to a brief admission to the psychiatric ward of a local hospital in October 1986,[9] followed by polyclinical psychiatric treatment, neither of which had an effect on her situation: according to the psychiatrist at the time, she was not open to any suggestion of working towards an acceptance of Patrick's death.

In December 1988, shortly after the death of her father, Mrs B left her husband, taking Rodney with her; the divorce followed in February 1990. In November

---

5   Dutch criminal procedure distinguishes between two acquittal verdicts: *vrijspraak* is based on failure of the prosecution to prove the facts charged; if the facts charged are proved, *ontslag van rechtsvervolging* may nevertheless follow, either because the facts charged do not amount to an offence or because the defendant successfully pleads an excuse or a justification. The judgment of the Court of Appeals — as of the District Court — was an acquittal of the last sort.

6   Article 294: 'He who intentionally incites another to commit suicide, assists him to do so, or provides him with the means of doing so, is liable, if the suicide takes place, to a prison term of at most three years.'

7   In Dutch criminal procedure, a Court of Appeals conducts a full trial of the case and makes its own findings of fact. More detail is known about the case than the facts as established by the Court of Appeals (see eg Chabot, *Zelf beschikt* (1993), of which an English translation is being prepared under the title *Chosen Fate*). The following statement is, except where noted, limited to the facts as found by the Court of Appeals, which formed the basis of its judgment and that of the Supreme Court.

8   From the findings of the Court of Appeals, one might assume that this was *her* family doctor. I am informed by Chabot that this was not the case: Mrs B did not want her family doctor to know when the suicide was to take place, because he was also her former husband's doctor and the latter was opposed to her plans. The family doctor present was a friend of Chabot's, asked by him to be present 'to ensure that what I did was proper, in the technical medical sense' (letter BC to JG, 21 August 1994).

9   According to Chabot, the hospital chart shows an admission from Monday 6 (not 3, as stated in the decision of the Court of Appeals) through Monday 20 October, of which two weekends were spent at home, so that a total of 13 days were spent in the hospital (letter BC to JG, 12 October 1994).

1990, Rodney was admitted to hospital in connection with a traffic accident; in the hospital he was found to be suffering from cancer, from which he died on 3 May 1991. That evening, Mrs B attempted suicide with drugs which she had received from her psychiatrist[10] in 1986 but had saved. The attempt was unsuccessful and to her great disappointment she recovered consciousness a day and a half later. She immediately began to save drugs again, with the intention of committing suicide.

Finding a way to die began to dominate her thoughts. She discussed various methods with her sister; she gave an old friend a letter which was to be opened only after her death; she arranged for cemetery plots for herself, her two sons and her former husband, and had her first son reburied so that there was space for her between the graves of her two sons. She attempted to get effective drugs for committing suicide and considered other methods as well, which she discussed with various people. However, she was afraid that a second failure might lead either to an involuntary committal to a mental institution or to continued life with a serious disability. She made it known to others[11] that she wished to die, but in a humane way which would not confront others involuntarily with her suicide.

Mrs B approached the Netherlands Association for Voluntary Euthanasia and in this way came into contact with the defendant, who had indicated his willingness to give psychiatric support[12] to persons who might approach the Association for help. Between 2 August and 7 September 1991, the defendant had four series of discussions with Mrs B, totalling some 24 hours.[13] He also spoke with Mrs B's sister and brother-in-law. Beginning on 11 August, after the second series of discussions with Mrs B, the defendant approached four consultants. He furnished them with an extensive account of his findings and requested suggestions concerning matters which he might have overlooked in the psychiatric investigation of Mrs B or which required further clarification. He also asked whether they were in agreement with his diagnosis. Later, after the third series of discussions, he approached three more consultants.[14]

In considering the question 'whether Mrs B was suffering from any illness,' the Court of Appeals concluded that there was no indication of any somatic condition which might have been the source of Mrs B's wish to die. From the beginning of the defendant's contacts with her, it was clear that she was suffering from psychic traumas which in principle lent themselves to psychiatric treatment so that the defendant was justified in entering into a doctor − patient relationship with her, even though that might ultimately expose him to a conflict of duties.

10 Chabot informs me that the Court of Appeals was mistaken on this point: in fact, Mrs B got the drugs from her family doctor, not from the psychiatrist (letter BC to JG, 7 September 1994).

11 Chabot informs me that these included her family doctor, a psychiatric social worker and a clinical psychologist of the Association for Voluntary Euthanasia, all of whom declined to help or advised her to consult a psychiatrist. She also unsuccessfully sought help from close friends in obtaining lethal medications (letter BC to JG, 21 August 1994).

12 In Dutch: *zich bereid had verklaard tot opvang van mensen*. There is no suggestion in the Dutch word *opvang* (relief, care, support) that the support the defendant was prepared to offer entailed assistance with suicide. Chabot himself states that he had informed the NVVE that he 'was not in principle opposed to assistance with suicide, but that he assumed that in most cases it would be possible to redirect a wish for death into a desire to learn how to live in a different way, on the condition that one can win the confidence of the person concerned and that one takes the wish for death seriously' (letter BC to JG, 21 August 1994).

13 In other accounts of the case, the figure of 30 hours is often mentioned: the difference is due to the distinction between actual hours (24) and billable hours (30). Of the 24 hours, 20 were with Mrs B alone; three in the presence of her sister and brother-in-law; and one in the presence of her friend Mrs H (letter BC to JG, 12 October 1994).

14 The seven consultants included four psychiatrists, a clinical psychologist, a GP and a well-known professor of ethics (of Christian persuasion) (letter BC to JG, 7 September 1994).

The defendant's professional judgment of Mrs B was that there was no question in her case of a psychiatric illness or major depressive episode, but that, according to the classification system of the American Psychiatric Association (DSM-III-R), she was suffering from an adjustment disorder consisting of a depressed mood, without psychotic signs, in the context of a complicated bereavement process.[15] In his opinion, she was experiencing intense, long-term psychic suffering that, for her, was unbearable and without prospect of improvement. Her request for assistance with suicide was well-considered: in letters and discussions with him, she presented the reasons for her decision clearly and consistently, and showed that she understood her situation and the consequences of her decision. In his judgment, her rejection of therapy was also well-considered.

The Court of Appeals found that the defendant was an experienced psychiatrist who made his diagnosis in a very careful way. The experts consulted by him were agreed that Mrs B's decision was well-considered and her suffering long-term and unbearable, and that in the circumstances there was no 'concrete treatment perspective'; the majority agreed without reservation with the way he had handled the case. Several of them observed that it was highly likely that, if not given expert assistance, Mrs B would have continued her efforts to commit suicide, using increasingly violent means. Although her condition was in principle treatable, treatment would probably have been long and the chance of success was small. None of the experts consulted considered that there was in fact any realistic treatment perspective in light of her well-established refusal of treatment. The defendant had repeatedly tried to persuade Mrs B to accept some form of therapy and the Court of Appeals accepted the defendant's testimony to the effect that, if there had been an available treatment with a realistic chance of success within a reasonable period, he would have continued to pressure Mrs B to accept it and, if she continued to refuse, would not have given her the requested assistance.

Although two expert witnesses stated that in their opinion the doctors whom the defendant had consulted ought to have examined Mrs B personally, neither was of the opinion that in this case that would have made any difference, nor that questions were thereby raised concerning the defendant's carefulness. In the opinion of the Court of Appeals, the defendant's conclusions could be adequately checked in this case against the information available from Mrs B's letters, from intimate acquaintances of hers, from her family doctor and from her previous psychiatrist. Furthermore, the defendant's very detailed and extensive reporting of the case was intended by him to make it possible for others to assess what he had done. The doctors consulted by the defendant had been able, on the basis of the defendant's reports, to reach firm conclusions.

The experts consulted in this case, a discussion paper of the Medical Association on the subject,[16] a discussion paper of the Inspectorate for Mental Health[17] and a

---

15   The Court of Appeals observed in this connection that the absence of a somatic basis requires 'great care in establishing that the wish to die is not a direct symptom or consequence of a psychiatric sickness or condition and that — in this connection — the request for assistance with suicide is well-considered and voluntary. Whether the diagnosis which emerges from investigation [of the person concerned] is labelled a psychiatric syndrome, a psychiatric condition or . . . a psychiatric disorder is in the opinion of the Court for these purposes not really relevant.'

16   Commission on the Acceptability of Termination of Life (CAL) of the Royal Dutch Medical Association, discussion papers on termination of life in the case of non-competent patients, Part 4: *Hulp bij zelfdoding bij psychiatrische patiënten* [Assistance with suicide in the case of psychiatric patients] (1993).

17   Geneeskundige Inspectie voor de Geestelijke Volksgezondheid, *De meldingsprocedure euthanasie/ hulp bij zeolfdoding en psychiatrische patiënten* [The reporting procedure for euthanasia/assistance with suicide and psychiatric patients] (1993).

position paper of the Dutch Association for Psychiatry[18] all agree that, from the point of view of medical ethics, there may be circumstances in which assistance with suicide is legitimate in the case of persons whose suffering does not have a somatic origin and who are not in the terminal phase of their disease.

3 Consideration of the issues raised on appeal

On the basis of the above facts, the Court considers the questions presented on appeal.

3.1 General considerations

'Particularly over the past decade there has been a public debate concerning the prohibition of euthanasia and assistance with suicide, which has included the question whether Article 294 of the Criminal Code should be revised. This debate has not, however, led to any revision. Legislative Bills to that end have been rejected or withdrawn. This Court must therefore proceed on the basis that the prohibition has not been modified.

'However, the circumstances of an individual case may be such that rendering assistance with suicide, like performing euthanasia, can be considered justifiable. This is the case when it is proved that the defendant acted in a situation of necessity, that is to say — speaking generally — that, confronted with a choice between mutually conflicting duties, he chose to perform the one of greater weight. In particular, a doctor may be in a situation of necessity if he has to choose between the duty to preserve life and the duty as a doctor to do everything possible to relieve the unbearable suffering, without prospect of improvement,[19] of a patient committed to his care.[20]

'When a doctor who has performed euthanasia or furnished the means for suicide claims that he acted in a situation of necessity, the judge must investigate — this task is *par excellence* that of the trial judge — whether the doctor, especially in the light of scientifically well-founded medical knowledge and according to the norms recognised in medical ethics, made a choice between mutually conflicting duties that, considered objectively and in the context of the specific circumstances of the case, can be considered justifiable. In this connection, it should be observed that the procedure by which the responsible doctor[21] is to report cases of

---

18 Nederlandse Vereniging voor Psychiatrie [NVP], 'Mededelingen bestuur' (1992) *Nieuws en Mededelingen* 86/2, pp 2 – 3.
19 Dutch: *ondraaglijk en uitzichtloos lijden*, one of the established conditions for justifiable euthanasia.
20 The exact formulation of the conflict of duties upon which the justification of necessity rests has taken different forms and the differences may be doctrinally important in connection with the balancing of values on which the defence rests (see Schalken: Note accompanying the decision of the Supreme Court in the *Chabot* case, *Nederlandse Jurisprudentie* (1994) nr 656). In a note to an earlier case, Mulder formulated the conflict as one between 'the legal value of respect for life . . . [and] the legal value of respect for the personal autonomy [*persoonlijkheid*] of the patient' (Note accompanying the decision of the Court of Appeals (The Hague), 10 June and 11 September 1986, *Nederlandse Jurisprudentie* (1987) nr 608).
21 The Dutch term *behandelende arts* refers to a doctor responsible for the care of the patient (at any given time there might be more than one such doctor, responsible for different aspects of the patient's' situation). It is generally assumed that only a *behandelende arts* is authorised to perform euthanasia or to give assistance with suicide. The exact scope of the term has not, however, been fully worked out. The requirement gives rise to problems when the patient's *behandelende arts* (for instance, a family doctor) is not willing to accede to a request for euthanasia/assistance with suicide and also does not refer the patient to a colleague. That Chabot, in the circumstances, acted as Mrs B's *behandelende arts* was not questioned.

euthanasia and assistance with suicide, including thereby information on a number of specified items[22] — a procedure which has been in effect in practice since 1 November 1990[23] and has recently received a legislative foundation[24] ... — contains no substantive criteria which, if met by a doctor who performs euthanasia or renders assistance with suicide, entail that his behaviour is justifiable. The reporting procedure offers a procedural structure within which the responsible doctor can render account of his behaviour and the prosecutorial authorities or the trial judge can assess it.'

3.2 The justifiability of assistance with suicide in the case of non-somatic suffering and a patient who is not in the terminal phase

'The first point on appeal depends on the view that assistance with suicide by a doctor, in the case of a patient like Mrs B whose suffering is not somatic and who is not in the terminal phase,[25] can [as a matter of law] never be justifiable.

'This view cannot be considered correct. The specific nature of the defence of necessity, which, depending upon the trial judge's weighing and evaluation after the fact of the particular circumstances of the case, can lead him to decide that the act was justified, does not allow for any such general limitation. A claim of necessity can therefore not be excluded simply on the ground that the patient's unbearable suffering, without prospect of improvement, does not have a somatic cause and that the patient is not in the terminal phase. The Court of Appeals found, and this is not challenged on appeal, that from the point of view of medical ethics the legitimacy of euthanasia or assistance with suicide in such circumstances is not categorically excluded. In answering the question whether in a particular case a person's suffering must be regarded as so unbearable and lacking in any prospect of improvement that an act which violates Article 294 must be considered justified because performed in a situation of necessity, the suffering must be distinguished from its cause, in the sense that the cause of the suffering does not detract from the extent to which suffering is experienced. But the fact remains that when the suffering of a patient does not demonstrably follow from a somatic illness or condition, consisting simply of the experience of pain and loss of bodily functions, it is more difficult objectively to establish the fact of suffering and in particular its seriousness and lack of prospect of improvement. For this reason, the trial judge must in such cases approach the question whether there was a situation of necessity with exceptional care.'[26]

3.3 The voluntariness of the request in the case of a psychiatric patient

The second ground of appeal challenges the Court of Appeals' holding that it is possible for a psychiatric patient voluntarily to request assistance with suicide; alternatively, it is argued that the judgment of the Court of Appeals that the request

---

22 Dutch: *aandachtspunten* (matters requiring attention).
23 The reporting procedure referred to here was announced by the Ministry of Justice as prosecutorial policy after negotiations with the Royal Dutch Medical Association.
24 Amendment to the Law on Disposal of Corpses (*Staatsblad*, 1993) p 643. This is the recent legislation on euthanasia which was widely reported internationally. See n 33 *infra* on the form prescribed for reporting.
25 Dutch: *die niet in de stervensfase verkeert.*
26 The brief of the Advocate General (paras 11, 12) suggests some additional arguments for the Court's holding on this issue: the distinction between body and mind is artificial; the nature of the conflicting duties which give rise to the situation of necessity (respect for life, respect for the person of the patient) make the cause of suffering irrelevant; the decisions of lower courts and the literature support the view that the terminal phase is not essential.

was voluntary is not based on sufficient evidence. The third ground of appeal challenges the Court of Appeals' holding that the fact that a second psychiatrist had not examined Mrs B is not an obstacle to accepting the defence of necessity. The Supreme Court deals with these various contentions together.

The Court holds that the prosecution's assertion that the request for assistance with suicide of a psychiatric patient cannot be voluntary 'is as a general [legal] proposition incorrect.' The Court of Appeals held 'that the wish to die of a person whose suffering is psychic can be based on an autonomous judgment. That holding is in itself not incorrect.'

The alternative challenge — to the sufficiency of the evidence — is, however, well founded; among other things, in light of the fact that Mrs B had not been examined by a second psychiatrist.

'As stated above, in a case in which the suffering of a patient is not based on a somatic disease or condition, the trial judge must approach the question whether under the circumstances of the case assistance with suicide can be justified as having occurred in a situation of necessity with exceptional care.

'If a doctor who affords his patient assistance with suicide has neglected before acting to check his judgment concerning the situation with which he is confronted against that of an independent colleague, whether or not the latter conducts his own examination of the patient, this need not in general preclude the possibility that the trial judge, based on his own investigation of the circumstances of the case, comes to the conclusion that the doctor acted in a situation of necessity and therefore must be considered not guilty. However, the situation is different in a case like the present one.'

When the case involves 'a patient whose suffering is not based on a somatic disease or condition . . . the trial judge, in considering whether the claim of necessity is well-founded, must — considering the exceptional care with which he is to approach this matter — base his decision among other things on the judgment of an independent medical expert who has at least seen and examined the patient himself. Since the trial judge must decide whether the defence of necessity is compatible with the requirement that the course of conduct chosen be proportional to the harm to be avoided and also the least harmful choice available,[27] the judgment of the independent colleague of the defendant, based partly on his own examination, should deal with the seriousness of the suffering and the lack of prospect for improvement, and in that connection also with other possibilities of providing help.[28] This is because in assessing whether suffering is so unbearable and lacking in any prospect for improvement that assistance with suicide can be deemed a choice justified by a situation of necessity, there can in principle be no question of a lack of prospect for improvement if there is a realistic alternative to relieve the suffering which the patient has in complete freedom rejected. The independent expert must also include in his examination the question whether the patient has made a voluntary and well-considered request, without his competence being influenced by his sickness or condition.

'Absent the judgment of an expert who saw and examined Mrs B, the Court of Appeals could not properly come to the conclusion that the defendant as the responsible psychiatrist was confronted with an unavoidable conflict of duties and

---

27 This requirement is called in Dutch the principle of *proportionaliteit en subsidiariteit*.
28 Dutch: *hulpverlening*; the usual association of the word in everyday Dutch is with more or less institutionalised forms of assistance. It is not clear precisely what the Supreme Court has in mind here: see n 37 *infra*.

in that situation made a justifiable choice. In such a situation, the Court of Appeals should have rejected the defence.'[29]

4   Judgment

The judgment below must be reversed. In general, this would lead to referral of the case to another Court of Appeals. However, in the circumstances of this case, such a referral — considering the absence of the essential report of an independent expert who himself examined Mrs B — could only lead to the conclusion that the defence of necessity must be rejected. In such a case, it is more efficient for the Supreme Court to give final judgment itself.

The defence of necessity is rejected and the defendant, not having made any other defence, is found guilty of the offence as charged.

However, 'the person of the defendant and the circumstances in which the offence was committed . . . have led the Supreme Court to apply Article 9a of the Criminal Code and not to impose any punishment or other measure.'

Comments on the decision

1   The holdings

Holdings on four important questions are given in the Supreme Court's decision in the *Chabot* case:

   (a) Can assistance with suicide be legally justifiable in the case of a patient whose suffering does not have a somatic basis and who is not in the terminal phase? The Court holds that it can be.

   (b) Can the wish to die of a person suffering from a psychiatric sickness or disorder legally be considered the result of an autonomous (competent and voluntary) judgment? The Court holds that it can be.

   (c) Can the suffering of such a person legally be considered 'lacking any prospect for improvement' if he or she has refused a realistic (therapeutic) alternative? The Court holds that in principle it cannot be.

   (d) What are the legal requirements of consultation in such a case, as far as the defence of necessity is concerned? The Court holds that an 'independent colleague' must himself have examined the patient.

I have purposely included the term 'legal' in each case to emphasise something that non-lawyers tend to forget: the decision of the Court concerns a number of legal terms and norms (in particular, those of the criminal law), not psychiatric or other terms or theories.

---

29   The brief of the Advocate General had argued (paras 19—21) that this ground of appeal was unfounded: a categorical requirement of independent examination was in his view inconsistent with the nature of the defence of necessity and not supported in existing case law; the judgment of the Court of Appeals was, he argued, essentially a factual one and adequately supported by its findings.

2 The Supreme Court's reasoning

With all respect to the Court, it is perhaps characteristic of Dutch opinion-writing style that the Court gives rather little argument for its conclusions.[30] Holdings (a) and (b) depend essentially on the Court's position that the defence of necessity cannot be bound by general limitations, as a consequence of which the case is largely decided not on normative, but on factual grounds. Otherwise, the only direct support for holding (a) is the bare assertion (invoking the support of 'medical ethics') that suffering, not the cause of suffering, is determinative. Direct support for holding (b) is limited to the dogmatic observation that the suggestion that the request of a psychiatric patient cannot be voluntary 'is as a general proposition incorrect.'

3 The nature of the defence of necessity

The Court's fundamental point of departure — that there can be no general limitations on the defence of necessity[31] — cannot, it is respectfully submitted, stand up to critical examination. It is, of course, true that the whole point of a general defence of necessity is to deal with unforeseen circumstances in which application of the strict terms of a prohibition would lead to unjust results. In that sense it would defeat the point of the defence to try to specify in advance when it will and will not be available. In effect, the defence allows for future judicial legislation. Once it is invoked in a concrete case, that quasi-legislative process begins: the court has to decide whether the circumstances of the case require — in the name of substantive justice — a qualification on the coverage of the prohibition. A court does so, necessarily, on the basis of general normative considerations. This is precisely what the prosecution invited the Dutch Supreme Court to do. The Court apparently did not agree with the proposed normative considerations but, instead of saying this, it suggested that *any* normative limitations are unacceptable, thereby confusing the situation *before* a concrete set of facts is first presented for adjudication with the situation when the court is considering whether those facts, in light of the relevant normative considerations, amount to a state of necessity. And, of course, *after* a court has made a decision on the scope of the defence, its decision governs future similar cases as well. In fact, having rejected the idea of general limitations on the defence of necessity, the Supreme Court itself imposed one: the special consultation requirement in the case of non-somatic suffering.

---

30 One reason for the absence of extensive argument may have to do with the absence of concurring and dissenting opinions in Dutch judicial practice, with the resultant pressure within a court to arrive at a compromise acceptable to all the members of the court (that the Court found this difficult in the *Chabot* case seems to be indicated by the fact that judgment was twice postponed: see Leenen, Note accompanying the decision of the Supreme Court in the *Chabot* case, *Tijdschrift voor Gezondheidsrecht* (1994/96) nr 47, p 355). On the other hand, the explanation for the Court's oracular style is probably partly historical as well. Dutch cassation practice derives from French practice, in which the court consists both of judges and of an Advocate General, whose brief includes fuller arguments and is to be read together with the rather bare conclusions of the judges (cf Remmelink, 'Plaats en taak van het Openbaar Ministerie bij de Hoge Raad in strafzaken' in *Beginselen: opstellen over strafrecht aangeboden aan G.E. Mulder* (1981) pp 291–308). To the extent that they go further than or are of a different tenor from those of the Court, the arguments of the Advocate General on the various issues in the *Chabot* case have been indicated in footnotes at the appropriate places in the Court's decision.

31 That this position underlies the Court's treatment of the central issues on appeal is more explicit in the brief of the Advocate General than in the Court's opinion.

The history of legal change concerning euthanasia and related medical practices which shorten life has largely taken place in the Netherlands within the scope of the defence of necessity.[32] It has been a history of normative proposals, some of which have been rejected and some accepted by the courts. Once accepted for the purposes of deciding a given case, such norms have governed future cases and in that sense have constituted general limitations on the scope of the defence of necessity. It is on this basis that the lower courts, the prosecutorial authorities and, most recently, the Dutch parliament itself have been able to predict, follow, adjust to and, in the case of the parliament, implicitly ratify what the Supreme Court has done. It would be quite unthinkable for the Supreme Court to announce in a subsequent case, for example, that in that case somatic suffering *is* required. The idea invoked in the Court's decision in the *Chabot* case, that in each case the fate of the defence of necessity has depended on 'the trial judge's weighing and evaluation after the fact of the particular circumstances of the case,' is, it is submitted, impossible as a matter of legal theory and of social practice, and inaccurate as a matter of history.

4 The requirement of consultation

The central holding in the case — the ground on which Chabot's conviction was ultimately based — is that a trial court must have before it the judgment of an independent doctor who himself examined the person concerned. This requirement is based on the Court's view that in a case of non-somatic suffering the trial court must approach the question of necessity with exceptional care. It is respectfully submitted that this part of the Court's decision is unsatisfying for several reasons.

The requirement of consultation is formulated by the Supreme Court as one which governs the fact-finding of the trial court, not as one of the 'rules of careful practice' to which a doctor rendering assistance with suicide must conform. It is true that the Supreme Court is concerned on appeal with the legal correctness of the decision of the Court of Appeals, not (directly) with the defendant. Still, it would have seemed natural to formulate the new condition for the defence of necessity as one resting on the doctor who invokes the defence; the mistake of the Court of Appeals would in that case have been formulated as one concerning what it had supposed the defendant was required to have done in order to be able successfully to invoke the defence.

The Court of Appeals had in fact devoted special care to the question of consultation, concluding that whereas in an ordinary case the special demands resulting from non-somatic suffering might require the judgment of a second doctor who had examined the patient, in the circumstances of this case there was so much information available concerning Mrs B (her letters, information from intimate acquaintances and from her family doctor and psychiatrist), and the

---

32 Contrary to the common assumption that the common law is characterised by flexibility, the civil law by rigid adherence to codes, the Dutch courts have exhibited far more creativity and flexibility than the English courts in dealing with the legal problems posed by euthanasia. Even under the extreme circumstances of the *Cox* case, in which the patient was so close to death that it was not certain that the drug used (potassium chloride) had actually caused death, the House of Lords considered itself not free to find an appropriate substantive solution; the problem of rendering justice to the accused was solved in sentencing: a suspended sentence and a mere 'admonishment' from the disciplinary authorities (see Lord Goff of Chieveley, 'A Matter of Life and Death' (1993) 5 *Juridisk Tidskrift* 1 – 17). However, in Schalken's view (n 20 *supra*, p 14), the Dutch Supreme Court has given such an encompassing interpretation to the idea of necessity that it has 'departed quite far from the classical view in criminal law scholarship,' and he seems to imply that the Court may thereby have gone too far.

consultants approached by Chabot were so sure of their ability to assess the situation on the basis of the extensive report he sent them, that the absence of a second psychiatric investigation of Mrs B was not critical. 'Assuming there were such a requirement,' the Court of Appeals observed, 'in a concrete case the defence of necessity could be honoured even if the requirement had not been fulfilled.' Especially in light of this passage in the decision of the Court of Appeals, an absolute condition of independent examination seems precisely the sort of categorical limitation on the defence of necessity which the Supreme Court earlier in its decision had rejected.

The Court notes in passing that the requirement of consultation is not a condition of the defence in the case of somatic suffering. That is not because the requirement does not obtain (it appears in all the standard formulations of the 'rules of careful practice'), but because it is enforced, if need be, in medical disciplinary proceedings. The Court does not explain why, in a case like *Chabot* in which the facts are not in dispute, failure to conform to the requirement that an independent colleague examine the patient is a condition of the defence of necessity and not a disciplinary offence.

While it seems clear that the examination requirement is desirable, the Court's reasoning, and its application in a criminal case of a new and especially strict consultation requirement (independent examination), gives an unpleasant air of *ex post facto* to the conviction of Chabot. He could easily have complied with such a requirement but had no way of knowing that he needed to persuade at least one consultant to examine Mrs B himself, since no such requirement was to be found in the case law, the guidelines of the Medical Association or the reporting procedure (as it was in 1991).

In the midst of the most detailed discussion in the entire decision, the Court is strangely silent with respect to two especially important aspects of the requirement of consultation: need the second expert be a psychiatrist, and need the second expert agree with the defendant's decision to give assistance with suicide? The Court's decision speaks only of 'an independent colleague/medical expert' and of the topics with which the latter's examination must deal. The report of the Commission on the Acceptability of Termination of Life (CAL) of the Medical Association is far more explicit on the first question. In the case of a psychiatric patient, the second doctor must be a psychiatrist (and if the doctor who is asked to render assistance is not a psychiatrist — being, for example, the patient's GP — then at least two independent psychiatrists must be consulted and there should be 'intensive contact' with the psychiatrist responsible for treatment as well).[33]

On the second question, the CAL seems to assume without specific discussion that the independent consultant(s) must agree with the first doctor on the essential issues. The CAL states that the consultant need not necessarily examine the patient, but 'a conclusion of the psychiatrist consulted which agrees [with the proposal to carry out assistance with suicide] must . . . always be based on an examination of the patient,'[34] a formulation which would be peculiar if the CAL contemplated the possibility that a decision to render assistance could follow on a

---

33 n 16 *supra*, pp 36–37. The form prescribed for reporting a case of euthanasia or assistance with suicide contemplates, in a case of non-somatic suffering, consultation with two independent colleagues (of whom one is a psychiatrist), both of whom have examined the person concerned (Ministerial Decree of 17 December 1993, *Staatsblad* (1993) nr 688). The exact status of the items on which the form requires information is not clear, and in any case the courts will not necessarily regard these items as defining the contours of a successful defence of necessity.

34 *ibid.*

negative consultation. Without pretending that it is clear what the ultimate solution to this problem should or will be, two difficulties with the CAL's apparent position should be noted. In the first place, the CAL assumes one of two quite different views concerning the function of consultation: that this is one of collectivising the decision-making, taking it out of the hands of the first doctor (alone), not one of supporting the first doctor's decision-making and ensuring that the facts of the case can be attested to by an independent expert witness.[35] Given the insistence of the medical profession throughout the entire euthanasia discussion on the final responsibility of the individual doctor for his or her decisions, it seems peculiar that that position should be abandoned here without further discussion. A second difficulty with the CAL's position is that, if the doctor consulted must agree with the decision, there will have to be subsidiary rules governing 'consultant-shopping' and the situation (as in the *Chabot* case) that more than one or two consultants are involved.

In short, the whole matter of consultation is rather more complex than the Supreme Court's decision seems to suppose. Whatever the ultimate rule may be, it will have to undergo quite a lot of fine-tuning to deal with a large variety of possible situations. It may therefore, with all respect, not have been wise to impose consultation as a condition of the defence of necessity, a vehicle which does not lend itself very well to detailed rule making.

5 The existence of alternatives

The Court's observation in passing (in connection with the report of an independent colleague) that 'there can in principle be no question of lack of prospect for improvement if there is a realistic alternative to relieve the suffering which the patient has in complete freedom rejected' appears, with respect, to be *obiter dictum*, since the issue had not explicitly been raised on appeal and there is no suggestion that the stricture applied to the case of Mrs B (precisely this question having been extensively examined by the Court of Appeals). The Supreme Court does not use the reasonably well-defined term 'concrete treatment perspective' which the Court of Appeals had adopted from the Medical Association's discussion paper on the subject[36]; but it is not clear whether there is a reason behind the Court's use of a different and seemingly vague expression 'realistic alternative.'[37] Nor is it clear what the idea of a rejection of treatment 'in complete freedom' implies. The Court also does not explain why rejection of treatment stands in the way of necessity in the case of non-somatic suffering, whereas it is pretty well established that this does not apply to somatic suffering.[38] In short, the Court's observation in this regard exhibits the difficulties characteristic of *obiter dicta*.

---

35 That Chabot's conception of the requirement of consultation was of the second variety is plain, among other things, from the fact that his consultations took place *before* he had himself come to a decision.

36 See n 16 *supra*. The discussion paper identifies three aspects of the concept: (1) whether there is a real prospect of improvement; (2) whether this will take place within a reasonable time; and (3) whether the results are proportionate to the burden for the patient.

37 The Court of Appeals had not considered whether there were non-medical alternatives available. Perhaps this is what the Supreme Court had in mind by using the term 'other possibilities of providing help' (cf the brief of the Advocate General, para 25, to such an effect). If so, the term used by the Court is unfortunately ambiguous (see n 28 *supra*).

38 Seen Leenen, n 30 *supra*. In one earlier case, for example, the defence of necessity was allowed (in a situation of somatic suffering), despite the patient's refusal of treatment with psychofarmaca (Supreme Court, 27 November 1984, *Nederlandse Jurisprudentie* (1985) nr 106; Court of Appeals, The Hague, 10 June and 11 September 1986, *Nederlandse Jurisprudentie* (1987) nr 608).

Nevertheless, since everyone (Chabot, Medical Association, Psychiatric Association, Court of Appeals, Supreme Court) seems to be agreed that there should be some such requirement, it seems likely that there will be. Its precise contours will have to be worked out in the future.[39]

6 The limits of psychiatric practice

In considering the situation of a psychiatrist who assists a patient to commit suicide, the Court pays relatively little attention to those aspects of the situation which have particularly troubled some members of the psychiatric community. There are, of course, psychiatrists who, as a matter of professional ideology, deny the very possibility of a 'voluntary' or 'balanced' request for suicide. As far as the criminal law is concerned, the Court rejects this categorical approach. This holding, however, does not address the more specifically professional concern for the delicate and dangerous nature of the psychiatrist—patient relationship, with its problems of transference and counter-transference (misplaced anger, need for control), of blackmail (if you don't agree to help me, I will do it in a horrible way), etc.[40] The requirement of an examination by a second, independent psychiatist — however it be enforced — does go some way towards coming to terms with such concerns. Nevertheless, there are those who argue that the very nature of the relationship excludes the possibility of a psychiatrist acceding to a request for assistance with suicide, and this is certainly a respectable position. What seems to be involved here is not a legal issue — at least, not an issue of criminal liability — but competing professional views among psychiatrists. The medical and psychiatric professions in the Netherlands[41] have on the whole taken a less restrictive view of the limitations of the relationship between psychiatrist and patient than some psychiatrists (especially outside the Netherlands) consider appropriate.

7 Euthanasia versus assistance with suicide

Although strictly speaking only assistance with suicide, not euthanasia (killing on request),[42] was at issue in the *Chabot* case, the Court treats the two sorts of behaviour as one, at least for the purposes of the defence of necessity. The discussion within the medical profession seems to assume, without explicit argument, that only assistance with suicide is appropriate in the case of suffering of non-somatic origin.[43] The possibility that the requirements for the justification of necessity in the two cases may be different has received no attention in the Dutch literature. There are, of course, things to be said in favour of assistance with suicide (final guarantee of voluntariness; less moral buck-passing from patient to

---

39 A recent case presents the question squarely (District Court, Haarlem, 4 July 1994, *Tijdschrift voor Gezondheidsrecht* (1994/96) nr 48): the court concluded on the basis of expert testimony that there were realistic possibilities for dealing with the patient's suffering (the result of paralysis due to several strokes) and held that the doctor had too readily accepted the patient's refusal of any alternative to assistance with suicide.

40 Needless to say, the risk of transference and other psychological threats to the medical rationality of the psychiatrist's decision making is equally present when the decision is to *refuse* assistance with suicide.

41 See the report of the CAL, n 16 *supra*; NVP, n 18 *supra*.

42 Article 293 of the Criminal Code: 'He who kills another person at the latter's express and serious request is punishable with a prison term of up to 12 years.'

43 CAL, n 16 *supra*; see also Griffiths (1994b), n 2 *supra*.

doctor), but it is not at all clear that these parallel the somatic/non-somatic line (many persons dying of an incurable somatic disease being capable of performing suicide with the assistance of a doctor).

It would probably be a mistake, however, to exaggerate the brightness of the line between the two sorts of behaviour or to put too much weight on it as the indicator for substantially different sorts of legal treatment. Assistance with suicide varies from behaviour scarcely distinguishable from euthanasia (in the presence of the doctor, the patient opens the valve on a lethal intravenous drip), through the situation involved in the *Chabot* case, to the situation in which the doctor makes pills available to a patient who may or may not use them at some future time. It is doubtful that this whole range can be dealt with as one regulatory category, distinct from euthanasia.

8 Suffering of somatic and non-somatic origin

What, ultimately, is the relevance of the somatic/non-somatic distinction? Euthanasia or assistance with suicide in a case of suffering of non-somatic origin generally involve a more substantial loss of life than the hours, days or weeks characteristic of cases of somatically-based suffering.[44] The Court presumably had this in mind in referring specifically to the requirement of 'proportionality' in the case of a patient whose suffering is non-somatic and who has refused a realistic alternative to assistance with suicide: the burden for the patient of treatment less easily outweighs the benefits when the amount of life to be won is significant. Is this, then, a reason to distinguish cases of somatic and of non-somatic suffering so far as the defence of necessity is concerned?

Not all cases of non-somatic suffering involve a substantial remaining life expectancy.[45] It is not clear that this was true in the *Chabot* case. The various experts Chabot consulted were agreed that Mrs B was likely to attempt suicide again within a month if not given assistance, it being well known that 'persistently suicidal patients' generally go on trying until they succeed.[46] The argument that a patient's life expectancy should be considered in isolation from his or her suicidality was rejected by one of them as irrelevant, since in that case the patient would be a different person.[47] So the distinction somatic/non-somatic is not congruent with the problem of proportionality.

The idea that in cases of non-somatic suffering there is more reason to doubt whether the patient's request is voluntary and well considered does not, on further inspection, support the distinction[48]: a patient suffering from somatic causes may also suffer from diminished competence, and the competence of patients whose suffering is non-somatic need not necessarily be in question at all. In short, the distinction is not congruent with the problem of competency.

Euthanasia or assistance with suicide in the case of non-somatically-based suffering may entail serious problems of establishing after the fact that the patient

---

44 See, for relevant data, Van der Maas *et al*, *Medische beslissingen rond het levenseinde* [report of the research for the Remmelink Commission]; English translation: *Euthanasia and other Medical Decisions Concerning the End of Life* (1992); also published as a special supplement of *Health Policy* (1992) 22/1+2.
45 Nor, of course, do all cases of somatically-based suffering necessarily entail a limited life expectancy (eg some AIDS patients).
46 Letter BC to JG, 12 October 1994.
47 Compare CAL, n 16 *supra*.
48 Compare Griffiths (1994b), n 2 *supra*.

was suffering unbearably, was competent and wanted to die. This seems an obvious reason for wanting to impose special procedural requirements in cases of non-somatic suffering. Until recently, cancer was the main occasion for euthanasia in the Netherlands, and cancer leaves a substantial trail of corroborating evidence behind. Where X-rays, laboratory reports and autopsy evidence are lacking, the reports and the testimony of other doctors who examined the patient can be particularly important. However, as the *Chabot* case illustrates, the distinction somatic/non-somatic is not congruent with the need for such corroborating evidence: there was in fact a wealth of corroboration concerning the situation of Mrs B.

Finally, whatever the merits or demerits of the distinction between somatic and non-somatic suffering, it seems highly questionable whether it can be made to stick in practice. Suffering itself is always psychic, and 'pain' is not the only sort of suffering that leads patients to request euthanasia.[49] Increasingly, forms of suffering which used to be considered non-somatic in origin are being found to derive from a somatic condition; it is known, for instance, that this is true of many cases of depression. Instead of the sharp lines which the criminal law requires for a categorical treatment of the defence of necessity, there seems to be a considerable grey area that is gradually gobbling up larger and larger chunks of the supposedly distinct categories on either side of it. With respect, it seems unlikely that the distinction somatic/non-somatic can be made to do the major work which the decision of the Supreme Court expects of it.

9   Assistance with suicide for the non-'sick'?

Assistance with suicide in the case of non-somatic suffering is only in a residual sense 'medical.' The fundamental basis for Dutch euthanasia law therefore seems, with the decision in the *Chabot* case, to have taken a decisive step away from the doctor-centred approach which has dominated legal development up to now (euthanasia and assistance with suicide being justified as a special empowerment of doctors, subject to the request of the patient) toward patient self-determination.[50] It will be interesting to see whether the Dutch courts will hold assistance with suicide justifiable in several categories of cases in which the person concerned is not 'sick' at all (eg the case of very elderly persons who are incapacitated in various ways and simply 'tired of life'). From there it is only a small additional step to the case in which the person concerned is not suffering at all at the time the request is made but, in anticipation of coming deterioration, wants to be in a position to choose the time of death in advance of becoming incapacitated and dependent.[51]

---

49   See Van der Maas *et al*, n 44 *supra*.
50   Compare Schalken, n 20 *supra*.
51   The place of these various sorts of 'rational suicide' in the context of recent Dutch legal developments is discussed briefly in Griffiths (1994b), n 2 *supra*.

Reactions to the decision and the problem of the 'slippery slope'

In general, the Dutch response to the decision in the *Chabot* case — in legal, medical and political circles — has been positive.[52] The new government promptly announced a revision of its prosecutorial guidelines to reflect the holdings of the court, and 11 of the 15 pending prosecutions (involving non-somatic suffering or patients not in the 'terminal phase') were dropped.[53]

Hendin characterises the Dutch experience as 'an increasing tendency to free the physician from legal control' and asserts that legalisation of euthanasia has 'encourage[d] involuntary euthanasia [*sic*]' in the Netherlands.[54] In thus invoking the hoary spectre of a 'slippery slope' in apparent criticism not only of the Supreme Court's decision in the *Chabot* case, but of the entire preceding legal development in the Netherlands, Hendin and others like him appear to overlook some fundamental facts. The Dutch data on medical practices which shorten life, in the cases of non-competent or of competent but not-consulted patients, are indeed a matter of concern.[55] However, some differentiation is in order. Almost all of the behaviour concerned involves abstaining from or terminating life-prolonging treatment, or administration of heavy doses of painkillers, in circumstances in which remaining life expectancy was (very) short and the doctor's behaviour may, as far as we know, have been entirely appropriate. There is really not a shred of evidence that the frequency of this sort of behaviour is higher in the Netherlands than, for example, in the United States; the only thing that is clear is that more is known about it in the Netherlands. In short, there is no reason to assume, as Hendin does, a causal relationship between limited legalisation of euthanasia and 'lack of control' over other sorts of medical behaviour.

Looking more specifically at psychiatric patients, where is the feared 'slippery slope'? Anecdotal evidence suggests that psychiatrists have long engaged in practices which amount to assistance with suicide and there is no apparent reason to suppose they do so more often in the Netherlands than in the United States. Psychiatrists turn a blind eye to the fact that their patients are storing up medicines for a suicide attempt; they allow release of suicidal patients from institutions to enable them to commit suicide; they refer patients to organisations such as the Hemlock Society or call their attention to do-it-yourself books on suicide. How

---

52 Critical commentary has been addressed not so much to the Supreme Court's decision as to what Chabot did. The most important criticisms are those of Hendin ('Seduced by Death: Doctors, Patients and the Dutch Cure' (1994) 10 *Issues in Law and Medicine* 123–168) and Koerselman ('Balanussuïcide als mythe' (1994) 49 *Maandblad Geestelijke Volksgezondheid* 515–527), an American and a Dutch psychiatrist, respectively. Each of them takes Chabot to task for supposed oversights in his diagnostic examination of Mrs B and for his conclusion that her request was well considered. Unfortunately, both Hendin and Koerselman base their criticisms on numerous and serious errors of fact in their accounts of Mrs B and of Chabot's interaction with her; neither of them made use of the extensive psychiatric report of the case, which Chabot furnished to the various consultants and which was later relied upon by the courts. Their position seems to be that a request for assistance with suicide *cannot* be well considered and Chabot therefore *cannot* have done his work well. Their treatment of the facts is systematically manipulated to conform to this ideological preconception and their conclusion — quite different from that of all the professionals involved in the case itself — that Chabot's behaviour was unprofessional is really only a logical, not a factual one.

53 See *Staatscourant* nr 179 (19 September 1994) p 1.

54 Hendin, n 52 *supra*, pp 163, 165.

55 cf Griffiths (1994a), n 2 *supra*.

247

much of this goes on, we cannot say. The only thing we can safely say is that, so long as it is underground, it is quite beyond any form of legal or other control.

Hendin and others who invoke the metaphor to criticise Dutch legal developments seem quite confused about the direction in which the 'slippery slope' is tilting. While many Americans and other foreign observers invoke taboos as if these describe actual practice in their own countries, the Dutch are busy trying to bring a number of socially dangerous medical practices which exist everywhere under a regime of effective societal control. They began with euthanasia (in the technical Dutch sense of killing on request) and have moved on to medical practices which shorten life in the case of seriously defective newborn babies, coma patients, seriously demented patients and now psychiatric patients.[56] They still have a long way to go. But triumphantly pointing out the shortcomings of Dutch control, as if these were a sufficient argument against the whole tendency of Dutch legal development, is to confuse a cure with a disease. The appropriate Dutch response to this sort of criticism is to concede the imperfections, but to point out that working step-by-step towards effective control is surely better than denial.[57]

---

56 Recent developments in the Netherlands concerning all of these categories are discussed in Griffiths (1995), n 2 *supra*.
57 Compare Miller, 'Regulating Physician-Assisted Death' (1994) 331 New Eng J Med 119−123. The courts in the United States and in the United Kingdom are in fact presently engaged in an effort comparable to that of the Dutch courts to subject medical practices which shorten life to legal control, beginning with the situation of patients in a coma or 'persistent vegetative state.' See eg Lord Goff of Chieveley, n 32 *supra*; Weinberg, 'Demystifying the Right to Die: The New Jersey Experience' (1988) 7 *Medicine and Law* 323−345.

Assisted Suicide in the Netherlands: Postscript to *Chabot*

*John Griffiths**

The decision of the Dutch Supreme Court in the *Chabot* case — involving the criminal prosecution of a psychiatrist who had acceded to the request of a psychically traumatised but not otherwise 'sick' woman (Mrs B) for assistance with suicide — was reported in an earlier issue of MLR (58:2, March 1995, pp 232–248). The Court held that the defence of necessity, upon which the legalisation of euthanasia and assistance with suicide in the Netherlands has been based, could in principle be invoked in such a case but was not available to Chabot because of his failure to meet an essential procedural requirement (personal examination by a second doctor).

The prosecution had requested the responsible Medical Inspector, who was contemplating a medical disciplinary proceeding, not to go ahead with it while the criminal case was pending. When, with the decision of the Supreme Court on 21 June 1994, the criminal case was over, the disciplinary proceedings against Chabot got underway. The regional Medical Disciplinary Tribunal rendered a decision on 6 February 1995.[1] It concluded that what Chabot had done 'undermined confidence in the medical profession' (the basic disciplinary norm).[2] Chabot received a relatively severe sanction: 'reprimand.' On 19 April 1995, Chabot announced that he had had enough of legal proceedings and would not appeal this decision, which means that the case is now finally closed.

The purpose of this brief postscript to the earlier report of the Supreme Court's decision in the criminal case is to provide some basic information about and comments on the subsequent decision of the Medical Disciplinary Tribunal. The facts in the case are set forth in the report of the Supreme Court's decision.[3]

Chabot wanted vindication on the merits from a tribunal of his peers (of the five members of a medical disciplinary tribunal, all but the president — a lawyer — are doctors), so he instructed his lawyer not to raise the difficult issue of double jeopardy. The Tribunal was therefore not forced to confront the question whether, in the circumstances of this case in which no issue was involved in the second proceeding that was not, or could not have been, raised in the first proceeding, it is not fundamentally unfair that the state should have two opportunities to make its case. Nor did the Tribunal address itself to the relationship between the substantive and procedural norms for euthanasia and assistance with suicide as worked out by

*Faculty of Law, University of Groningen.

1 *Gerritsen v Chabot*, Medisch Tuchtcollege Amsterdam, nr 93/185; *Medisch Contact* nr 21 (1995) pp 668–674. A companion complaint by the Inspector against the general practitioner present at the suicide at Chabot's request resulted in the holding that under the circumstances (in which he was only present as a witness to the proceedings and it was not 'plainly apparent' that what Chabot proposed to do was inconsistent with the medical disciplinary norm) he was not responsible for what Chabot did: *Gerrisen v Beukman*, Medisch Tuchtcollege Amsterdam, nr 93/186; *Medisch Contact* nr 21 (1995) pp 675–676.

2 For a discussion of Dutch medical disciplinary law, see Verkruisen, *Dissatisfied Patients: Their Experiences, Interpretations and Actions* (Groningen, 1993).

3 The statement of facts in the judgment of the Medical Disciplinary Tribunal is particularly careful and complete, and sheds additional light on some aspects of the case.

the courts in criminal cases on the one hand, and medical disciplinary norms on the other. The Tribunal seems to have accepted the contours of the defence of necessity to a criminal charge as delimiting acceptable professional conduct. This is not surprising since, although there is neither a doctrinal requirement nor an institutional guarantee of congruence between criminal and medical disciplinary law, the courts have in fact largely based their decisions on the scope of the defence of necessity in euthanasia cases on expert testimony concerning the norms of the medical profession. It would have been embarrassing if the Medical Disciplinary Tribunal had taken quite a different view of the matter from that of the Supreme Court.

The Medical Disciplinary Tribunal held, as had the Supreme Court, that assistance with suicide can be legitimate in the case of a person whose suffering is of non-somatic origin and who is not terminally ill. The request must be the result of an 'autonomous decision' and not relate to a treatable disorder. The consulted doctors must have personally examined the person concerned (the Tribunal is not entirely clear whether more than one doctor must be consulted, nor whether this must be a psychiatrist).

The Tribunal also found that in the specific circumstances of the case Chabot had not adequately preserved his professional distance, particularly in light of the frequency and length of his sessions with Mrs B and the fact that these took place at Chabot's house in the countryside (where Mrs B, together with a couple who accompanied her, resided in a guest cottage on Chabot's property).

Finally, the Tribunal adopted a significantly more restrictive view than the Supreme Court on one crucial aspect of the case: the extent to which a doctor must insist on treatment as an alternative to assistance with suicide.[4] The Supreme Court explicitly recognised that there may be no realistic possibility of treatment if the patient rejects it. But the Tribunal took the position that Chabot could not properly conclude that Mrs B's disorder was untreatable until after treatment had in fact been tried: 'The patient's refusal of treatment should have been a reason for [Chabot] to refuse the requested assistance with suicide, at least for the time being.'

This difference between the two decisions seems explainable in terms of a fundamental difference of opinion between the experts whom Chabot had consulted and who testified in the criminal case, and one expert called by the Tribunal in the disciplinary proceeding. The Tribunal adopted the latter's view that there was a realistic possibility of treatment in the circumstances of the case and that the patient's refusal ought not to have been honoured. With respect, there is something profoundly unsatisfying about this aspect of the Tribunal's decision. First, it seems unacceptable that the result on such an important matter should be so dependent upon the particular expert(s) who happen to testify. There is, more generally, an element of arbitrariness involved in the role of expert witnesses in these cases, a matter which the courts and tribunals involved have so far not adequately addressed. Secondly, if anything was indisputable after all the evidence in the two proceedings had been heard, it was that the psychiatric profession is

---

4   In the Supreme Court's decision, the existence of a possibility of treatment is important in connection with the requirement that the patient's suffering lacks any prospect of improvement; in the Tribunal's decision, the importance of a treatment alternative is emphasised in connection with the question whether the request is an 'autonomous' one. It is, by the way, fairly clear that in a case of somatically-based suffering the patient's refusal of treatment is no bar to euthanasia.

deeply divided on the question whether in the circumstances of Mrs B — including her well-considered refusal of treatment — there was any realistic treatment perspective. It is hard to understand how the fact that Chabot acted on one of two apparently equally respectable medical opinions could be considered a breach of the medical disciplinary norm.[5]

---

5   Dutch periodicals were at the time full of statements of the opposing professional views. After the decision of the Medical Disciplinary Tribunal, four expert witnesses involved in the two proceedings protested publicly that the Tribunal had simply, without argument, rejected their professional opinion and preferred that of another expert witness (*Trouw*, 29 April 1995).

[23]

Jonathan Glover

Not Striving to Keep Alive

Thou shalt have one God only; who
Would be at the expense of two?
No graven images may be
Worshipped, except the currency

Thou shalt not kill, but need'st not strive
Officiously to keep alive . . .

A.H. Clough: *The Latest Decalogue*

You are eating a hearty meal, while somewhere a baby is
starving. As the charitable appeals point out, you might have
saved it. But pleading guilty to the charge does not give you
license to strangle a neighbour's infant with your bare hands, as
though to say 'What's the difference? Both babies are dead,
aren't they?'

Mary McCarthy: *Medina*

But each one of us is guilty in so far as he remained inactive.
The guilt of passivity is different. Impotence excuses; no moral
law demands a spectacular death . . . But passivity knows itself
morally guilty of every failure, every neglect to act whenever
possible, to shield the imperilled, to relieve wrong, to countervail.

Karl Jaspers: *The Question of German Guilt*

Is it worse to kill someone than not to save his life? What we
may call the 'acts and omissions doctrine' says that, in certain contexts, failure to perform an act, with certain foreseen bad consequences of that failure, is morally less bad than to perform a
different act which has the identical foreseen bad consequences.

92

NOT STRIVING TO KEEP ALIVE

It is worse to kill someone than to allow them to die. Philippa Foot has discussed a case which illustrates this view.[1] She says, 'most of us allow people to die of starvation in India and Africa, and there is surely something wrong with us that we do; it would be nonsense, however, to pretend that it is only in law that we make a distinction between allowing people in the underdeveloped countries to die of starvation and sending them poisoned food'.

Another case where our intuitive response to killing differs from our response to not striving to keep alive concerns old-age pensioners. Until the introduction of automatic regular increases, the Chancellor of the Exchequer in his annual budget normally either failed to increase the old-age pension or else put it up by an inadequate amount. In either case, it was predictable that a certain number of old-age pensioners would not be able to afford enough heating in winter, and so would die of cold. We think that the decision of such a Chancellor was not a good one, but we do not think it nearly as bad as if he had decided to take a machine-gun to an old people's home and to kill at once the same number of people.

Apart from this support the acts and omissions doctrine derives from our intuitive responses to such cases, it might be argued that to abandon it would place an intolerable burden on people. For, we may think that, without it, we would have morally to carry the whole world on our shoulders. It is arguable that we would have to give money to fight starvation up to the point where we needed it more than those we were helping: perhaps to the point where we would die without it. For not to do so would be to allow more people to die, and this would be like murder. And, apart from this huge reduction in our standard of living, we should also have to give up our spare time, either to raising money or else to persuading the government to give more money. For, if a few pounds saves a life, not to raise that money would again be like murder.

Finally, it could be said that for us the acts and omissions

1. Philippa Foot: The Problem of Abortion and the Doctrine of the Double Effect, *The Oxford Review*, 1967.

MORAL THEORY

doctrine is a 'natural' one: that it is presupposed by the way in which we use moral language. There is in our vocabulary a distinction between duties and those good acts that go beyond the call of duty. A doctor has no duty to risk his life by going from England to a plague-infested town in an Asian country at war in order to save lives there, and we do not blame him if he does not do so. If he does go, we think of him as a hero. But, if we abandoned the acts and omissions doctrine, we might have to abandon our present distinction between acts of moral duty and supererogation.

1 The Sources of Strength of the Acts and Omissions Doctrine

It will be argued here that we ought to reject the acts and omissions doctrine. I have no formal argument to show that it is self-contradictory or in any way incoherent. I cannot show that it is a doctrine which any rational person must reject. The argument to be used is less conclusive than that. I shall present a diagnosis of why people hold the doctrine, a cluster of reasons which seem more impressive before they are separated out than after critical examination.

The acts and omissions doctrine draws its strength from the following sources:

(*a*) Confusions between different kinds of omission.

(*b*) The fact that the doctrine is itself confused with negative utilitarianism.

(*c*) Other factors only contingently associated with the act-omission distinction.

(*d*) Other moral priorities that are themselves questionable.

(*e*) A failure to separate the standpoint of the agent from the standpoint of the moral critic or judge.

94

2 Varieties of Omission

Sometimes when I do not do something, it would be entirely unreasonable to blame me for this. If someone I have never heard of killed himself last week in Brazil, without my knowing or doing anything about it, I cannot be blamed for it. Even if we took the view denied by the acts and omissions doctrine (that I ought to do everything in my power to further the good and frustrate the bad) I still cannot be blamed. For my ignorance of the whole episode meant I had no opportunity to intervene, and this ignorance was not itself the result of negligence: I had in advance no reason to suppose that good would come or harm be avoided if I took the trouble to find out anything about that man.

But some omissions are at the other extreme of blameworthiness. A man who will inherit a fortune when his father dies, and, with this in mind, omits to give him medicine necessary for keeping him alive, is very culpable. His culpability is such that many people would want to say that this is not a mere omission, but a positive act of withholding the medicine. Supporters of the acts and omissions doctrine who also take this view are faced with the problem of explaining where they draw the line between acts and omissions. Is consciously failing to send money to Oxfam also a positive act of withholding? Presumably supporters of the doctrine do not want to make it an empty analytic truth, by insisting that anything we consider culpable must be counted as an act rather than an omission.

Between these extremes are other kinds of omission. Some are the result of ignorance that is negligent, where the agent could and should have avoided being ignorant. Other omissions are conscious, but are the result of some such factor as laziness, rather than some discreditable motive. It seems possible that some of the force of the acts and omissions doctrine derives from tacitly thinking of omissions in terms of examples drawn from the non-culpable end of the spectrum. The doctrine certainly seems less plausible where the omission is deliberate and results from a bad motive. But such a simple lack of discrimination is

95

clearly by no means the whole explanation of the popularity of the doctrine.

3 Acts, Omissions and Negative Utilitarianism

In some of the cases to which the doctrine is applied, it seems to derive part of its strength from the fact that often the forbidden act would harm someone, while the permitted omission is merely a failure to benefit someone. Stealing five pounds from you is a forbidden act that harms you, while failing to make you a present of five pounds is a permitted failure to benefit you. Because of such cases, those who are attracted to negative utilitarianism, which tells us not to promote happiness, but rather to eliminate misery, often also feel attracted to the acts and omissions doctrine.

Doubt has often been cast on the attractiveness of negative utilitarianism, at least without severe restriction or modification, as the basis of a morality. (The only certain way of eliminating all misery would be the painless extermination of all conscious life.) And the distinction it depends upon is not very clear: the size of a man's income is likely to be relevant to whether stealing five pounds from him is a matter of making him unhappy or merely of reducing his happiness. And the same holds for the failure to give him five pounds.

But it can be seen, in cases where the line between positive and negative utilitarianism is intuitively relatively clear, that negative utilitarianism does not support the acts and omissions doctrine. For sending money to help the starving could reasonably be held to reduce misery, as could raising the old-age pension, and yet the failure to do either of these can shelter behind the acts and omissions doctrine. Even if we were to accept both that there was a clear distinction between eliminating unhappiness and promoting happiness, and that this was of great moral importance, we would be wrong to suppose this relevant to the defence of a view that an act and an omission *with identical consequences* can vary in moral value.

96

Philippa Foot has proposed a variant on the acts and omissions doctrine which at the same time has considerable appeal
and seems to bring the doctrine closer to negative utilitarianism.
For her, it is the distinction between what we do and what we
allow that is crucial. On the basis of this distinction, she proposes a doctrine of positive and negative duties. Positive duties
are to help people, and are taken to include acts of charity,
which might normally not count as 'duties' at all. Negative
duties are to refrain from injuring or harming people. Negative
duties are seen as more important than positive ones. Mrs Foot
says, 'It is interesting that, even where the strictest duty of positive aid exists, this still does not weigh as if a negative duty were
involved. It is not, for instance, permissible to commit a murder
to bring one's starving children food.'

For Mrs Foot, the distinction between negative and positive
duties is not reducible to the distinction between acts and omissions. She says that 'An actor who fails to turn up for a performance will generally spoil it rather than allow it to be
spoiled. I mention the distinction between omission and commission only to set it aside.' Yet, despite this disclaimer, it is not
clear that the two kinds of duty can be distinguished except on
the basis of the act-omission distinction. For, if I do not bring
my starving children food, they will die. The harm to them may
be at least as great as to someone I murder. So, if it is not
permissible to commit a murder to bring one's starving children food, this prohibition cannot be based on the view that
the murder would do more harm. It is hard to see how the
overriding negative duty can be distinguished here from the
mere positive duty to the children except by using the act-omission distinction. It is not clear that there is any acceptable half-
way house between straightforward negative utilitarianism and
the acts and omissions doctrine.

4 Probability of Outcome

Many acts can reasonably be said to be worse than their apparently corresponding omissions, because their bad consequences are either less avoidable or else worse. The difference in our responses to some of the cases already mentioned could be largely explained in these terms.

When the Chancellor of the Exchequer failed to raise old-age pensions, there was still some possibility of saving the lives of those who would otherwise die of cold next winter. There was still the possibility that relations, friends or private charities would step in with sufficient money, fuel, food or clothes to save those at risk. But, if someone goes to an old people's home and machine-guns the inhabitants, the deaths of most of them are inevitable. In thinking of the old-age pensioners, it would have been self-deception to suppose that adequate private rescue operations were likely, for in no year was enough done privately. And we may prefer that adequate pensions should be given to everyone as of right than that old people should have to accept private charity. But, despite these points, it remains true that probable death is preferable to certain death, and so we have at least one reason here for thinking the act worse than the omission.

But this difference is insufficient to save the acts and omissions doctrine in general, since some omissions create just as strong a probability of death as their corresponding acts. If someone is being kept alive on a respirator and I switch it off, this makes death no more certain than if, when attaching the patient to the machine, I fail to switch it on. In either case there is a chance that someone passing by will see it is off and switch it on. But the probability of this is not increased by the fact that it was on before.

98

5 Side-Effects

There are also differences of side-effects between the massacre
and the failure to raise the old-age pension. In part they stem
from the fact that people resent hostile acts more than equally
hostile omissions. The Chancellor of the Exchequer allowed
pensioners to die, but, if he massacred some of them, this would
indicate that he actually wanted them to die. The resentment
felt against the man who does not care enough to do what is
necessary to keep people alive is nothing to the resentment felt
against the man who wants people to die.

Another factor is that a massacre is a scene of horror. The
man responsible for it may find it hard to forget and is likely to
have feelings of guilt. But those who do not raise the pension
(and those of us who do not campaign for higher pensions) do
not have sleepless nights. This claim about differential guilt, like
that about differential resentment, depends on the fact that
people's responses are in line with the acts and omissions doctrine. Our present tendency to feel less guilty about allowing
someone to die than about killing him might be eradicated if we
renounced the acts and omissions doctrine. But, to the extent to
which these psychological responses are outside our control,
'irrational' differences in strength of guilt feelings might persist
after such a decision. And, even if we ourselves change our
attitudes, the resentment of others who have not changed theirs
will remain a factor to take into account.

Other harmful side-effects are independent of resentment or
guilt. A massacre undermines our sense of security. We all feel
more comfortable because we know that almost everyone in the
country observes an absolute taboo on killing his fellow citizens. Our sense of security is not undermined to the same extent
when we hear of old people dying quietly of cold in their rooms.
This may be irrational, for we will all be old one day, and our
society is still arranged so that most people have the prospect
of being poor when old. But, even so, many of us are irrational
in this way, and, while we stay so, there remains this differ-

99

MORAL THEORY

ence between the side-effects of the act and of the omission.

These side-effects do not always seem great enough to justify the different moral value often placed on acts and omissions. The man responsible for a massacre has caused deaths that are more certain than those caused by the failure to raise the pension. He has also terrified his victims, aroused resentment and insecurity among other people, perhaps made himself feel guilty, and set a bad example. (The bad example carries no weight in favour of the acts and omissions doctrine, for the man who does not raise old-age pensions also sets a bad example to his successors.) The side-effects other than the bad example, harmful as they are, are not *clearly* so great as to outweigh factors on the other side. For example, although being shot in a massacre must be a terrifying experience, it may be far worse to die slowly of cold. And the extra suffering involved could possibly outweigh the extra bad effects of the act of shooting.

But even if the differences of side-effects between acts and omissions are sometimes exaggerated, it must often still be true that killing has worse total consequences than letting someone die has. Yet this is no help to the acts and omissions doctrine as it stands. That doctrine cannot explicitly be argued for on the basis of side-effects, for it claims that there is a moral difference between acts and omissions with the same total consequences. If the appeal of the acts and omissions doctrine lies in these differences of side-effects, its supporters are simply confused. For the plausible claim that many acts have worse total consequences than the omissions that apparently correspond to them supports the claim only that *these* acts are more to be avoided than *these* omissions. It provides no support for the view that, morally speaking, harmful acts are intrinsically worse than equally harmful omissions.

6 Who is Wronged?

One argument sometimes used in favour of the acts and omissions doctrine is that an act, say, of killing is always an act of

100

killing someone in particular. But many cases of letting die do
not involve knowing who it is that dies. The murderer chooses
his victim, or at least knows under some description whom he is
killing. But when we let people die of starvation in India or let
pensioners die of cold, we are not able to say in advance which
people will lose their lives. And, even after they have died, there
is often no clear way of saying which people my own money
could have saved. If, over the years, millions die of starvation, I
could not have saved them all. Even my best efforts could only
have saved some of them. And any decision that these deaths
rather than those ones would have been saved by my action is
bound to be fairly arbitrary. The suggestion is that killing some
particular person is worse than allowing some unidentified
person to die.

But it is hard to see just how this is to be taken. Is the crucial
factor the lack of knowledge in advance who it is will die? If so,
it is hard to see why this should be thought of any moral importance. Suppose a technician in hospital maliciously sab-
otages a kidney machine so that the next person to use it will
not have his life saved. Why should this act be more wrong if he
happens to have looked at a list and seen that the next patient
to use the machine will be Mr Hedley-Smythe, proprietor of a
hotel in Basingstoke? The plea 'My act was not as bad as it
might have been, for only later did I discover the identity of the
person whose death I caused' seems to have no mitigating force
at all.

The claim may not rest on whether we know in advance
whose life is at stake. If this can be found out afterwards, as in
the kidney machine case, it is clear that there is a particular
person whose death has been caused. But there are other cases,
as when many more people die of starvation than I could have
saved, where even afterwards we cannot say which lives have
been lost through my inaction. But, as long as it is clear that my
omission added to the number of deaths, why is it a mitigating
factor that I cannot tell *which* deaths were caused by me? This
certainly seems totally irrelevant to the wrongness of my failure
to act. If five gunmen each fire once into a crowd, each killing

101

MORAL THEORY

one person, it may be unclear which person was killed by which gunman. Whatever the legal position, the uncertainty as to who killed whom does not reduce the moral wrong of the gunmen's acts. If it turned out that their bullets had each been numbered, their acts would not then be regarded as worse. Why should the case be any different with omissions?

7 Not Playing God

A case in which there was a choice between saving the lives of two different lots of people occurred during the Second World War.[2] A German 'spy ring' in Britain consisted of a double agent on the British side and a string of fictitious people. It was on this supposed network of agents that the German government relied for information about where the V1 and V2 rockets were falling. The aiming was broadly accurate, hitting the target of London. It was proposed that the double agent should send back reports indicating that most of them had fallen well north of London, so that the rocket ranges would correct their aim a number of miles to the south. The result of this would have been to make most of the rockets fall in Kent, Surrey or Sussex, killing far fewer people than they did in London. This proposal is said to have been resisted successfully by Herbert Morrison, on the grounds that the British government was not justified in choosing to sacrifice one lot of citizens in order to save another lot.

I do not know the details of the argument actually used, but it may have been a reluctance to play a God-like role, deciding who is to live and who is to die, that made members of the government resist the proposal. Such reluctance is very understandable.

For most of us, situations where we have to choose between saving one life or another are a nightmare we are glad not to experience. Some people, especially those concerned with the allocation of scarce medical resources, do have to face such

2. Sefton Delmer: *The Counterfeit Spy*, London, 1971, Ch. 12.

decisions, and most other people prefer not to be consulted. But the feeling that we ought not to play God in such matters can stem from something more admirable than the desire to avoid a painful choice. This is a desire not to place ourselves above other people. Choosing which of two others should live and which should die, it is natural that one may feel conscious of being presumptuous. If I regard other people as my equals, what right have I to decide between their lives? It may seem less objectionable to decide randomly than to try to judge between them.

The question of whether a choice of which person of two to save ought to be made randomly will be discussed later on. But Morrison's view about the V1 and V2 targets can be criticized independently. For here the choice was not between equal numbers of people. It was between allowing the rockets to continue to fall where they killed a larger number of people, and diverting them so that they killed a different (smaller) lot of people. Mr Morrison's view seems to depend either on the belief that numbers of deaths need be of no moral importance, or else on the belief that positive intervention is more presumptuously God-like than letting things take their course.

Objections will be made in a later chapter to the view that numbers of deaths can be morally irrelevant. But there are also problems for Morrison's other possible line of argument: that acts are more God-like than omissions. For this claim depends on holding that I am less responsible for someone's death where it is the result of my deliberate non-intervention than where it is the result of my act. This is plausible only when we make the mistake of overlooking the different varieties of omission and their corresponding degrees of culpability, or when we hold the acts and omissions doctrine which is the subject of this chapter. The belief that acts are more objectionably God-like than omissions cannot be used as an argument in support of the acts and omissions doctrine which it presupposes.

MORAL THEORY

8 The View of Father Zossima's Brother, and the Impossibility of Doing All Good Things

In *The Brothers Karamazov*, there is a passage where Father Zossima narrates a conversation between his younger brother and his mother.

'And let me tell you this, too, Mother: everyone of us is responsible for everyone else in every way, and I most of all.' Mother could not help smiling at that. She wept and smiled at the same time. 'How are you,' she said, 'most of all responsible for everyone? There are murderers and robbers in the world, and what terrible sin have you committed that you should accuse yourself before everyone else?' 'Mother, my dearest heart,' he said (he had begun using such caressing, such unexpected words just then), 'my dearest heart, my joy, you must realize that everyone is really responsible for everyone and everything.'

This view of Father Zossima's brother bears an obvious resemblance to what has been argued in this chapter, but seems to have nightmare implications. There is so much misery in the world that, however hard one person tries, he cannot remove more than a fraction. Does rejection of the acts and omissions doctrine commit us to being responsible for all that is left? This seems so unreasonable that people may be attracted by the acts and omissions doctrine as an alternative. It is clearly absurd that a man who devotes his whole life to a campaign against poverty should reproach himself for, say, not having done any useful research into the causes of muscular dystrophy.

This brings out one difference between acts and omissions that is of some moral importance. Actions take time, while omissions do not. There is no end to the list of a person's omissions, while the actions he has time for during his life are limited. However heroic he is, he cannot do all the good things which, ignoring pressure of time, would be in his power. Harmful omissions are unavoidable, while most harmful acts can be avoided.

104

In allocating our time between actions, we have to work out priorities. The moral approach advocated here does not commit us, absurdly, to remedying all the evil in the world. It does not even commit us to spending our whole time trying to save lives. What we should do is work out what things are most important and then try to see where we ourselves have a contribution to make. We should then be able to justify the pattern of our lives. This is still a very demanding morality, which hardly anyone succeeds in living up to, but it is not the totally impossible demand made by Father Zossima's brother.

If this is not emphasized, the views argued for here are rightly open to criticism on grounds of an objectionable puritanism. This puritanism would take the form of suggesting that the only acceptable pattern of life would be one of continuous activity to save lives. But there is more to life than saving lives. Many other activities enrich people's lives, and only a view that recognized no trade-off between saving lives and other values would disallow these other activities. What is argued here does not *entail* the view that an actor rehearsing for a play, a civil servant drawing up laws to regulate pollution, or parents playing with their children, ought to be trying to raise money for Oxfam instead. (But it does make us ask the disturbing question: would we kill people if it were necessary for our pursuit of these activities?)

As well as recognizing the variety of ways in which people can contribute to the world, it is also necessary to accept the desirability of people protecting things that are worth-while in their own lives as well. This is partly because Yeats was right that too long a sacrifice makes a stone of the heart. People who make too many altruistic demands on themselves may after a time lose the inclination to go on doing good works, with the result that over the course of their lives they do less good than they would have done by starting at a sustainable rate. But it is also partly because someone's own worth-while life is a good thing in itself, not merely an instrument for creating benefits for others.

The distinction between acts and omissions can legitimately

105

MORAL THEORY

be used at some points in drawing up rules of thumb by which to guide one's life. Consider a man who buys his children some chocolate and wonders whether to throw away the paper in the street. He disapproves of litter, but sees that other people have dropped their wrappers. If he does not accept the acts and omissions doctrine, he might think that throwing down one more bit of rubbish would be no worse than failing to clear up someone else's bit of rubbish, so he might either throw it down or else spend some time clearing up the street. But these alternatives are clearly unsatisfactory. We sometimes want to follow a middle course between contributing to an evil or spending our time setting it right. Either to protect our own free time or because we could make a more useful contribution to society by doing something else, we are entitled to make a rule of thumb saying that, in general, we will make the easy negative contribution of not dropping rubbish ourselves, without feeling committed to picking up any rubbish we see. Father Zossima's brother might feel responsible for all the litter in the world, but the rest of us need not share his feelings of guilt.

But it remains true that rules of thumb allowing omissions have to be justified, and there may be circumstances in which even a justifiable rule should be broken. It is hard to believe that many of us would be able to justify the degree to which we protect what we like in our own lives at the cost of starvation and death to others. (There is always the disturbing question, for those of us who reject the acts and omissions doctrine, of the extent to which we would think it legitimate to kill people, either in order to bring about things that make life interesting for the rest of us, or to protect our own lives from intolerable pressures. This Dostoyevskian question, when taken seriously, is likely to force us to reconsider *both* how justifiable it is for us to spend time playing with our children rather than helping fight starvation *and* the matter of whether positive acts of killing are quite as hard to justify as we usually suppose. The concessions made to conventional morality in the last few paragraphs are far less substantial than may first appear.) It is also hard to believe that the medical policy of refraining from killing in

106

cases where 'not striving to keep alive' is thought morally right
is a justifiable rule of thumb when the importance of what is at
stake is fully appreciated.

9 Laws and Conventional Moral Rules

Macaulay, commenting on *A Penal Code Prepared by the
Indian Law Commissioners*, points out the absurdity of having
legislation which treats *all* deliberate omissions as on a par with
acts having the same foreseen consequences:

> It will hardly be maintained that a man should be punished as a
> murderer because he omitted to relieve a beggar, even though there
> might be the clearest proof that the death of the beggar was the
> effect of this omission, and that the man who omitted to give the
> alms knew that the death of the beggar was likely to be the effect of
> the omission. It will hardly be maintained that a surgeon ought to be
> treated as a murderer for refusing to go from Calcutta to Meerut to
> perform an operation, although it should be absolutely certain that
> this surgeon was the only person in India who could perform it, and
> that if it were not performed the person who required it would die.[3]

There are obvious reasons for agreeing with Macaulay. The
standard set would be so high that almost all of us could be
found guilty of murder. And it would be quite unclear which
omissions people should be prosecuted for: if yesterday I read a
novel, am I to be prosecuted for not saving lives by working
for Oxfam, or for not doing so by holding a road-safety class at
the local school?

But, from the point that the law should not punish certain
harmful omissions, it does not follow that they are morally
acceptable. If I see a child for whom I have no special responsibility drowning in a river and deliberately do nothing
when I could save him, the law does not punish me, largely
because of the difficulties of drawing clear-cut and sensible

3. Quoted in Charles Fried: *Medical Experimentation, Personal Integrity
and Social Policy*, 1974.

107

MORAL THEORY

boundaries around any proposed offence. But few of us would feel entitled to conclude that my omission is immune from criticism.

Legality does not establish that something is morally justified, but legality and illegality can make a moral difference. Doctors who think it justifiable to allow someone to die rather than prolong a painful terminal illness are no doubt right to count the risk of a murder charge as a possible reason for not administering a lethal dose of a drug. It is debatable what the law should forbid here, and debatable how strong a reason illegality is against killing in such circumstance. But some weight should be given both to the general undesirability of breaking the law and to the bad consequences of being caught.

A similar point can be made about the preservation of beneficial conventional moral rules. On the whole, the rules of conventional morality are stronger in prohibiting actions than in enjoining them. Not rescuing the drowning child is less frowned on than pushing him in to start with. Even if the conventional rules are not the best ones imaginable, there may still be a case for preserving them rather than setting a precedent which may undermine them. This is an additional reason for not killing someone which may not always apply to taking positive steps to save people.

But these reasons, which have to do with the law and with conventional practices and attitudes, may not always be decisive against killing: the question is whether killing averts a great enough evil to be justified, bearing in mind both the direct objections to killing and the side-effects, including any weakening either of the law or of a desirable common attitude. And, while the conventional revulsion against killing is an additional reason against it, this line of reasoning may not work the other way. The conventional casualness about letting people die from hunger or lack of medical care is something we should be better off without.

108

10 Agents and Moral Critics

Some of the plausibility of the acts and omissions doctrine may depend on confusing two different moral standpoints. There is the standpoint of the person deciding how he himself ought to act, and the standpoint of someone else wondering whether the act or omission of the first person is blameworthy. (The standpoints of the agent and of the moral judge or critic.) Because it seems reasonable to adopt a more lenient attitude in making moral judgements in many cases of harmful omission than in many cases of comparably harmful action, it is easy to assume that we are entitled to see harmful omissions as less bad when we ourselves are in the position of the agent deciding what to do. But this is doubtful, as we see when we think why it may be reasonable to judge others more leniently for omissions.

The straightforward utilitarian doctrine, according to which omissions and acts with identical consequences are equally bad, should not be interpreted crudely. That is, we should be sure that an act and an apparently corresponding omission really do have the same consequences. We have seen that there are often importantly different side-effects between what at first sight seem a corresponding pair. The utilitarian does not deny that killing someone may have worse total consequences than letting someone die has. But he does claim that, in arguing which is morally worse, we should go directly to the different consequences rather than base our view on a general principle about acts and omissions.

It is clear that, even taking side-effects into account, this utilitarian morality is a very demanding one. Although there are substantial differences of side-effects, deliberately failing to send money to Oxfam, without being able to justify our alternative spending as more important, is in the same league as murder. If this is so, a lot of us are living far below the moral standards we believe in. To deny the acts and omissions doctrine is to propose a radical and very demanding morality. I should spend my time on good works right up to the point

MORAL THEORY

where I can justify the claim that the disadvantage to me out-weighs the benefit to others.

Living up to this demanding morality is to many of us a very unattractive prospect: it is the prospect of a huge reduction in income and the loss of a lot of our spare time. The alternatives also are not very comfortable. One is to invent some ration-alization to save the acts and omissions doctrine, fitting our beliefs to our conduct rather than our conduct to our beliefs. The other approach, which I adopt, is to accept the utilitarian view, but to allow a huge discrepancy between professed beliefs and actual conduct. This is not very admirable, either.

In our present world, most of us who think about the matter fall into one of the last two categories, while only a few saints live up to the utilitarian view. Because this view sets standards so much higher than those prevailing in our present world, we are reluctant to blame the ordinary person who does not live up to them. For blame is normally apportioned at least partly in ac-cordance with the standards of the time. We do not think that those who executed men for heresy in the sixteenth century were wicked men, although we now think that what they did was wrong. The reason why we do not think they were wicked is that we make allowances for the moral standards of the day and judge them by comparison with others in that context. The same may be said of the ordinary man who in our day fails to do enough about the evils of the world. We are reluctant to say that he is wicked, because he is not worse than other men in our historical period. But this reluctance to blame others for not living up to the utilitarian morality does not justify us in ignor-ing it when we are in the position of the agent.

11 The Effects of Blame for Omissions

It might be suggested that to undermine the general belief in the acts and omissions doctrine would have very bad consequences. Our greater willingness to blame people for harmful acts than for equally harmful omissions may be thought to serve a useful

110

social purpose. What would happen if people came to view not giving to Oxfam as not very different from murder? It could be argued that this would make them, not more willing to give to Oxfam, but less reluctant to murder.

It might also be said that harmful acts often manifest different character traits from equally harmful omissions, and that it is more important to blame people for those different character traits. The man who massacres the old people exhibits some hostile motive or an unrestrained violence. The Chancellor who fails to put up the pension merely exhibits lack of imagination or concern. The suggestion is that it is more important to discourage hostility or violence than to discourage unconcern or lack of imagination, and so blame in accordance with the acts and omissions doctrine has good consequences.

None of this, even if accepted, would amount to an argument that to reject the acts and omissions doctrine would be mistaken. At best it would show that widespread rejection of it would be harmful. Arguments of this kind invite the reply made in a different context by Hume: 'There is no method of reasoning more common, and yet none more blameable, than in philosophical debates to endeavour to refute any hypothesis by a pretext of its dangerous consequences to religion and morality. When any opinion leads us into absurdities, 'tis certainly false; but 'tis not certain an opinion is false, because 'tis of dangerous consequence.' Although moral beliefs are not in any straightforward way true or false, there is something both objectionable and absurd about trying to argue for a moral view by saying how harmful its widespread rejection would be.

It may be thought that this misses the point. The suggestion may not be that the acts and omissions doctrine is defensible, but that it is a beneficial irrationality that ought not to be publicly criticized. Some people would object to this advocacy of one morality for us and another to be fostered in other people on grounds of the dishonesty and apparent condescension it involves. But it is in any case not clear that it would be harmful to undermine public belief in the acts and omissions doctrine. If we came to think of not giving to Oxfam as being very similar

111

MORAL THEORY

to a positive act of killing, this might not undermine the taboo on murder. It would obviously be a long time before most of us lived up to the high standards the belief demands, but it seems just as likely that we should move a bit in that direction as that we should relax our views on murder.

And the other claim, that it is more important to discourage positive acts of hostility than to encourage people to care more about what happens to each other, is not obviously true either. It is arguable that indifference plays as large a part in causing the world's misery as positive hostility. The existence of wars, poverty and many of the other things that destroy or stunt people's lives may be as dependent on widespread unconcern as on any positively bad motives. It may well be because of tacit acceptance of the acts and omissions doctrine that we acquiesce in the worst evils in the world.

Some Conclusions

Since much of the argument so far has been opposing some influential alternative approaches to the morality of killing, the positive conclusions can be stated briefly.

It has been argued that the reasons why it is wrong to kill are not the intrinsic value of life or consciousness, nor that people have a right to life. The reasons that have been given are of two kinds. Some make killing directly wrong, while others relate to the harmful side-effects on other people.

1 The Direct Wrongness of Killing

A. It is wrong to reduce the length of a worth-while life.

B. Except in the most extreme circumstances, it is wrong to kill someone who wants to go on living, even if there is reason to think this desire not in his own interests.

c. It is wrong to kill someone where the process of being killed is frightening or painful. (This is mentioned for the sake of completeness. It is less central than the other two reasons: painless killing is not *much* less bad than other kinds.)

Reason B will normally rule out involuntary euthanasia: someone's autonomy should almost always in practice be given priority over reasons for killing him that appeal to his own interests. Do similar arguments make it wrong to kill someone in order to benefit other people? This brings up the whole question of side-effects.

113

MORAL THEORY

2 Side-Effects and the Wrongness of Killing

Most of the side-effects which often count strongly against kill-ing someone have been mentioned. It is obvious that no exhaustive list of all possible relevant side-effects can be given. The sight of someone being murdered may so upset another man that he does not compose what would have been a great piece of music. There is no end to the possible reverberations of a single act. But some objections that will often be serious can be listed.

(i) There are the effects on the family and friends of the person killed. These can include their grief at his death, lone-liness, poverty and possible other psychological damage.

(ii) The person's contribution to the community is lost. This can be an economic contribution, if he does useful work, but can also be more intangible. The community is enriched, not only by the goods and services, inventions and works of art which someone produces, but also by the contribution that his personality and his relationship with other people make to the whole social atmosphere. (I thought this did not need saying until I read some of the economics literature on the value of human life.)

(iii) The act of killing may arouse hatred and resentment. This may be especially so where there is a tradition of family vendetta, or where a community is divided into hostile camps, as in Northern Ireland.

(iv) Killing someone may undermine the sense of security that other people have. Perhaps, if the general murder rate goes up, many will feel more scared when alone or in places they think dangerous. This danger of insecurity is particularly relevant to euthanasia, for it is very important that people going into hos-pital are not made to fear the doctor as a potential killer.

(v) Killing a person may encourage others to take killing more lightly and may also undermine one's own reluctance to kill again. Most people have a revulsion, possibly 'instinctive', against killing. (This applies at least to killing humans at close

114

range. Many mind less about animals, and dropping bombs or firing missiles and long-range guns seem to be easier to do than killing with a bayonet.) There is often an immense resistance to killing, which armies in war often have to overcome by rigid discipline, the encouragement of patriotic or ideological fervour and by attempts to make the enemy seem less than human.

Even if our revulsion against killing is a basic human instinct, it does not follow that killing is always wrong. Instincts sometimes ought to be controlled. But the existence of this revulsion may be a restraint upon our actions that is of immense value to the human race. If so, the argument that a particular act of killing will weaken this revulsion should be taken very seriously.

3 The Possibility of Beneficial Side-Effects

The direct objections to killing, although very strong, are not being presented here as ones that cannot ever be overridden. It is possible that Hitler had a life which, from his own point of view, was worth living. He probably did not want to die. Yet it is still open to someone who holds the principles outlined here to think that, all things considered, it would have been right to assassinate him. It has not been argued that side-effects must always have less weight than the direct objections to killing.

The Hitler case is both trite and extreme. But other cases where the side-effects of killing may on the whole be beneficial are more disputable and far more morally disturbing. Some senile old people and some children born with gross abnormalities may be such an emotional burden on their families that, thinking purely of side-effects, it would arguably be better if they were dead. These situations are some of the hardest to think about, but one way not to solve the problems they raise is by supposing they do not arise.

115

MORAL THEORY

4 Saving Lives

To kill is to shorten a life, while to save a life is merely to extend it. The conscious failure to save a life is in some circumstances conventionally regarded either as killing or as morally equivalent to it, but in other circumstances the conventional view is that they are neither identical nor morally on a par. The argument here has suggested that this conventional difference of moral evaluation is defensible to the extent that it reflects differences of side-effects. But in so far as it results from thinking that an act and deliberate omission with *identical* consequences can vary in moral value, the conventional view should be rejected. This suggests that, except for differences of side-effects, the arguments against killing are equally good arguments in favour of saving lives.

116

BIBLIOGRAPHY

Graham Hughes: 'Criminal Omissions', *Yale Law Journal*, 1958.

J. O. Urmson: 'Saints and Heroes', in A. I. Melden: *Essays in Moral Philosophy*, Washington, 1958.

Joel Feinberg: 'Supererogation and Rules', *Ethics*, 1961, reprinted in Joel Feinberg: *Doing and Deserving*, Princeton, 1970.

Eric D'Arcy: *Human Acts*, Oxford, 1963, Ch. 1.

Jonathan Bennett: 'Whatever the Consequences', *Analysis*, 1966.

P. J. FitzGerald: 'Acting and Refraining', *Analysis*, 1967.

Philippa Foot: 'The Problem of Abortion and the Doctrine of the Double Effect', *The Oxford Review*, 1967.

Daniel Dinello: 'On Killing and Letting Die', *Analysis*, 1971.

John Casey: 'Actions and Consequences', in John Casey (ed.): *Morality and Conduct*, London, 1971.

Myles Brand: 'The Language of Not Doing', *American Philosophical Quarterly*, 1971.

Peter Singer: 'Famine, Affluence and Morality', *Philosophy and Public Affairs*, 1972.

Michael Tooley: 'Abortion and Infanticide', *Philosophy and Public Affairs*, 1972.

J. M. Freeman: 'Is There a Right to Die – Quickly?' *Journal of Paediatrics*, 1972.

Michael Walzer: 'Political Action: The Problem of Dirty Hands', *Philosophy and Public Affairs*, 1973.

Bernard Williams: 'A Critique of Utilitarianism' (Sections 3, 4 and 5), in J. J. C. Smart and Bernard Williams: *Utilitarianism, For and Against*, Cambridge, 1973.

John Harris: 'The Marxist Conception of Violence', *Philosophy and Public Affairs*, 1974.

BIBLIOGRAPHY

John Harris: 'Williams on Negative Responsibility', *Philosophical Quarterly*, 1974.

Charles Fried: *Medical Experimentation: Personal Integrity and Social Policy*, Oxford, 1974, Ch. 3.

John Harris: 'The Survival Lottery', *Philosophy*, 1975.

Gerard Hughes: 'Killing and Letting Die', *The Month*, 1975.

Richard L. Trammell: 'Saving Life and Taking Life', *Journal of Philosophy*, 1975.

James Rachels: 'Active and Passive Euthanasia', *New England Journal of Medicine*, January 1975.

Name Index